T0319340

Nan Jing

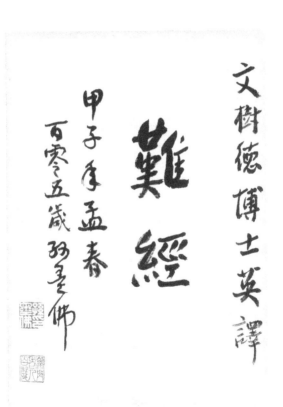

文樹德博士英譯

難經

甲子年孟春
百零五歲孫兀佛

The Chinese Medical Classics

Nan Jing

The Classic of Difficult Issues

With commentaries by Chinese and Japanese authors
from the Third through the Twentieth century

The Complete Chinese Text with
an Annotated Translation

by Paul U. Unschuld

University of California Press

University of California Press, one of the most distinguished university presses in the United States, enriches lives around the world by advancing scholarship in the humanities, social sciences, and natural sciences. Its activities are supported by the UC Press Foundation and by philanthropic contributions from individuals and institutions. For more information, visit www.ucpress.edu.

University of California Press
Oakland, California

Library of Congress Control Number: 2016939466

25 24 23 22 21 20 19 18 17 16
10 9 8 7 6 5 4 3 2 1

CONTENTS

Part I.
Prolegomena / 1

Introductory Remarks / 1

Historical Significance of the *Nan jing* / 6

The Contents of the *Nan jing* / 10

The Origin of the *Nan jing* / 21

The Reception of the *Nan jing* in Later Centuries / 27

Part II
Text, Translation, Commentaries, and Notes / 47

Preliminary Note / 47

Chapter One
The Movement in the Vessels and Its Diagnostic Significance / 49

The First Difficult Issue / 49

The Second Difficult Issue / 63

The Third Difficult Issue / 71

The Fourth Difficult Issue / 80

The Fifth Difficult Issue / 91

The Sixth Difficult Issue / 96

The Seventh Difficult Issue / 100

The Eighth Difficult Issue / 107

The Ninth Difficult Issue / 115

The Tenth Difficult Issue / 121

The Eleventh Difficult Issue / 130

The Twelfth Difficult Issue / 135

The Thirteenth Difficult Issue / 141

The Fourteenth Difficult Issue / 151

The Fifteenth Difficult Issue / 168

The Sixteenth Difficult Issue / 184

The Seventeenth Difficult Issue / 200

The Eighteenth Difficult Issue / 205

The Nineteenth Difficult Issue / 218

The Twentieth Difficult Issue / 226

The Twenty-First Difficult Issue / 230

The Twenty-Second Difficult Issue / 235

Chapter Two
The Conduits and the Network vessels / 240

The Twenty-Third Difficult Issue / 240

The Twenty-Fourth Difficult Issue / 253

The Twenty-Fifth Difficult Issue / 262

The Twenty-Sixth Difficult Issue / 268

The Twenty-Seventh Difficult Issue / 272

The Twenty-Eighth Difficult Issue / 276

The Twenty-Ninth Difficult Issue / 281

Chapter Three
The Long-Term Depots and the Short-Term Repositories / 286

The Thirtieth Difficult Issue / 286

The Thirty-First Difficult Issue / 291

The Thirty-Second Difficult Issue / 300

The Thirty-Third Difficult Issue / 302

The Thirty-Fourth Difficult Issue / 307

The Thirty-Fifth Difficult Issue / 313

The Thirty-Sixth Difficult Issue / 320

The Thirty-Seventh Difficult Issue / 324

The Thirty-Eighth Difficult Issue / 331

The Thirty-Ninth Difficult Issue / 335

The Fortieth Difficult Issue / 339

The Forty-First Difficult Issue / 345

The Forty-Second Difficult Issue / 349

The Forty-Third Difficult Issue / 357

The Forty-Fourth Difficult Issue / 359

The Forty-Fifth Difficult Issue / 363

The Forty-Sixth Difficult Issue / 370

The Forty-Seventh Difficult Issue / 374

Chapter Four
On Diseases / 377

The Forty-Eighth Difficult Issue / 377

The Forty-Ninth Difficult Issue / 383

The Fiftieth Difficult Issue / 398

The Fifty-First Difficult Issue / 403

The Fifty-Second Difficult Issue / 406

The Fifty-Third Difficult Issue / 408

The Fifty-Fourth Difficult Issue / 414

The Fifty-Fifth Difficult Issue / 417

The Fifty-Sixth Difficult Issue / 420

The Fifty-Seventh Difficult Issue / 429

The Fifty-Eighth Difficult Issue / 433

The Fifty-Ninth Difficult Issue / 444

The Sixtieth Difficult Issue / 448

The Sixty-First Difficult Issue / 454

Chapter Five
Transportation Holes / 459

The Sixty-Second Difficult Issue / 459

The Sixty-Third Difficult Issue / 464

The Sixty-Fourth Difficult Issue / 467

The Sixty-Fifth Difficult Issue / 471

The Sixty-Sixth Difficult Issue / 473

The Sixty-Seventh Difficult Issue / 482

The Sixty-Eighth Difficult Issue / 487

Chapter Six
Needling Patterns / 492

The Sixty-Ninth Difficult Issue / 492

The Seventieth Difficult Issue / 497

The Seventy-First Difficult Issue / 502

The Seventy-Second Difficult Issue / 505

The Seventy-Third Difficult Issue / 510

The Seventy-Fourth Difficult Issue / 514

The Seventy-Fifth Difficult Issue / 521

The Seventy-Sixth Difficult Issue / 529

The Seventy-Seventh Difficult Issue / 532

The Seventy-Eighth Difficult Issue / 536

The Seventy-Ninth Difficult Issue / 541

The Eightieth Difficult Issue / 545

The Eighty-First Difficult Issue / 547

Appendices / 551

Appendix A
Survey of Commentated *Nan jing* Editions by Chinese Authors from the Third
through Twentieth Century / 553

Appendix B
Chinese Twentieth-Century Essays on the Nan jing / 563

Appendix C
Commentated *Nan jing* Editions by Japanese Authors in the Takeda and Fujikawa
Libraries, as well as Lost Titles of Past Centuries / 567

Appendix D
Zhang Zhixian's Graphs Depicting the Eighty-One Difficult Issues (1510) / 573

Glossary of Technical Terms in the *Nan Jing* / 595

Index to Prolegomena, Commentaries, and Notes / 619

Comparative Studies of Health Systems and Medical Care / 639

PART I.
PROLEGOMENA

Introductory Remarks

The *Nan jing* 難經 is an ancient Chinese medical classic; it was compiled, probably, at some time during the first or second century CE. For the past eight or nine centuries, the *Nan jing* has been overshadowed by the reputation and authority of the "original" classic, the *Huang Di nei jing* 黃帝內經 ("The Yellow Thearch's Inner Classic") with its two largely different segments, the *Huang Di nei jing Su wen* (or *Su wen* 素問) and the *Huang Di nei jing Ling shu* (or *Ling shu* 靈樞). The present edition of the *Nan jing* combines a translation of its *textus receptus* and of selected commentaries by twenty Chinese and Japanese authors of the past seventeen centuries with an interpretation by this author. One of its goals is to demonstrate that the *Nan jing* should once again (as was the case until early the second millennium) be regarded as a significant and innovative work that marks the apex, and also the conclusion, of the developmental phase of the conceptual system known as the medicine of systematic correspondence.

The contents of the *Nei jing* texts, in contrast, should be appreciated as a collection of extremely valuable transitory stages in this developmental phase—valuable because they reflect various historical steps as well as a wide range of diverging (and even contradictory) theoretical arguments.[1] These arguments characterize the genesis of a system of therapeutic ideas and practices which has a formative period that can be traced from its first extant documented sources (the so-called Ma wang dui texts of about the late third century BCE) to the heterogeneous contents of the

---

[1] For further details on the heterogeneous nature of the *Huang Di nei jing* texts, and a preliminary analysis of historical developments reflected in these texts, see Paul U. Unschuld, *Huang Di Nei Jing Su Wen: Nature, Knowledge, Imagery in an Ancient Chinese Medical Text*. Berkeley: University of California Press, 2006 (second printing).

Nei jing texts, and, finally, to the homogeneous and highly systematized message of the *Nan jing*.

Among the *Su wen*, the *Ling shu* and the *Nan jing*, the *Su wen* is the most difficult one to read. Apparently, at the time of Wang Bing in the ninth century, and according to his introductory remarks to the edition he had prepared, only fragments of the original text were available. The *Ling shu*, in contrast, is much more homogeneous. Presumably, it, too, is a compilation including the thoughts and writings of different ancient authors, arranged by an editor unknown to us, and at a time undefinable today. But the *Ling shu* is much more systematic than the *Su wen*, and it has a clear focus: needle therapy, both in the sense of modern acupuncture and in terms of bloodletting. The origin and contents of the *Nan jing* justify an identification of this work as one of the three classics of the medicine of systematic correspondence in general.

Whether this was intended by its original (unknown) author or whether it is the result of editorial work by later scholars, the *Nan jing* covers—in an unusually systematic fashion—all aspects of theoretical and practical health care perceivable within the confines of the yin-yang and Five Phases doctrines, as defined by the original medicine of systematic correspondence. I speak here of the "original" medicine of systematic correspondence because later admixtures to this conceptual system—such as the utilization of drugs (far reaching attempts to create a pharmacology of systematic correspondence were not undertaken before the twelfth century CE)[2]—do not appear in the *Nan jing*. Such persistent elements of traditional Chinese health care as demonological medicine and religious healing were not taken into consideration either (apparently irreconcilable with the classic concepts of systematic correspondence, a demonology of systematic correspondence was developed only as late as the early Qing dynasty).[3]

The *Nan jing* is comprehensive: it addresses questions concerning the location, size, and normal functions of the basic units that constitute the organism; it dis-

---

2   For a detailed account of efforts undertaken from the twelfth through the fourteenth century to combine the use of pharmaceutical drugs with the concepts of systematic correspondence, see Paul U. Unschuld, *Medicine in China: A History of Pharmaceutics*, section C.II. Berkeley: University of California Press, 1986. On the developments during the Song era more recently: Asaf Goldschmidt, *The Evolution of Chinese Medicine: Song Dynasty, 960–1200*. London: Routledge, 2008.

3   From the seventeenth through the early nineteenth century, eminent Chinese physicians discussed the nature and the reality of demonic apparitions. In this context attempts were made to explain such phenomena on the basis of the concepts of systematic correspondence. For a detailed account see Paul U. Unschuld, *Medicine in China: A History of Ideas*, section 8.2.3. Berkeley: University of California Press, 1985.

cusses the origins and the nature of diseases; it outlines a system of therapeutic needling; and it develops—in great detail—an innovative approach to diagnosis.

Chinese medicine differs from European science in that it appears to be based on what one might call patterned knowledge. Various patterns of knowledge—sometimes overlapping, sometimes antagonistic and mutually exclusive—exist side by side in the literature and probably, in the minds of the people. There have been Chinese authors who, for reasons about which we can only speculate, have rejected some and accepted only a limited number of other very specific patterns. This is true both on the level of macro-patterns (in that some intellectuals objected to demonological knowledge while acknowledging the paradigm of systematic correspondence) and on the level of micro-patterns (in that some proponents of the paradigm of systematic correspondence rejected the Five Phases concepts, which represent one pattern of knowledge within the paradigm of systematic correspondence, while relying solely on the yin-yang doctrine which represents another pattern within that paradigm).

In general, however, a notion seems to have prevailed in China that lent some justification to all patterns of human knowledge. A specific pattern might be useful for handling a certain issue or situation successfully, and it might be contradicted logically by another pattern of knowledge that had also proven to be useful for handling the same (or another) issue. Both patterns—and this seems to have been the dominant attitude in Chinese history—were therefore legitimized. The "either/or" approach that springs to a mind trained in the Western tradition appears to have been posed with much less persistence in Chinese medicine.

Hence authors did not find it difficult to propose, in one and the same book, therapeutic guidelines derived from, as a Western reader might conclude, logically mutually exclusive paradigms or patterns of knowledge. Such "pragmatic" tendencies have been observed in the behavior of patients and practitioners all over the world: wherever two or more conceptual systems of health care coexist, the population is known to oscillate between these systems and utilize them eclectically or syncretically according to its perceived needs. What appears particularly characteristic of China is the fact that this conciliatory attitude toward differing patterns of knowledge is so enormously pervasive. True, heated polemics were exchanged between the proponents of contradictory paradigms, but once a new pattern had existed long enough, its antagonistic relation with older paradigms tended to decrease in importance until it was accepted into the heterogeneous pool of patterns from which a patient or practitioner could select the one most suitable for coping successfully with the specific problem at hand.

In its outline of diagnosis, the *Nan jing* itself provides ample evidence of a harmonious coexistence of micro-patterns within the paradigm of systematic correspondence—micro-patterns that have a common theoretical basis but that are, nevertheless, difficult to reconcile with one another. Within his accepted conceptual framework, the author of the *Nan jing* linked differing patterns of diagnosis without posing the either/or question that is implicit in all Western secondary literature on traditional Chinese medicine. Western authors seem to be continually forced to decide which single pattern of knowledge (whether on the macro- or on the micro-level) they should present to their readers. Almost unanimously, they have not accepted Chinese demonological and religious therapies as facets of traditional or contemporary Chinese medicine, despite the fact that these patterns of knowledge have exerted a tremendous impact on health care in China from remote antiquity up to the most recent times. On a smaller scale, to give another example, the either/or approach demands an answer to whether terms like *xin* 心 ("heart"), *gan* 肝 ("liver"), and *pi* 脾 ("spleen") must be understood solely as references to abstract functional systems that do not necessarily correspond to tangible anatomical structures (as some passages in ancient Chinese literature suggest) or as designations of concrete structures within the organism (as other passages suggest). Clearly, both notions have coexisted in traditional Chinese medical literature, so it should be a moot point as to which interpretation of the Chinese terms is correct.

As a consequence of decisions in favor of one or another notion or pattern of knowledge, Western authors writing on traditional Chinese medicine tend to be selective and to omit all patterns of knowledge that fail to correspond to the demands of conceptual coherency or stringency (perhaps this attitude is motivated by an underlying fear that Chinese medicine otherwise might appear "unscientific" to a contemporary audience). In the short run, such a streamlined Chinese medicine may indeed generate the attraction intended by its advocates, especially if it appears clad in Greco-Latin terminology and based on the Western concept of energy. In the long run, however, this does a disservice not only to those who wish to learn about the real nature of Chinese medicine but also to the traditional conciliatory worldview underlying the patterned knowledge of traditional Chinese health care —and to whatever beneficial effects that worldview may still promise to humanity in general.

The present edition of the *Nan jing* shall point to a different direction. Because it includes not only the entire text itself but also selected commentaries from twenty authors of the third through the twentieth century, the reader will become familiar both with the contents and general history of the reception of this text through the centuries and with differences in opinion voiced by medical authors over time. Consequently, a vivid portrait of an ongoing discussion should emerge which reflects some (and only some) of the dynamics inherent in historical Chinese medicine and which documents some of the strengths and weaknesses of the concepts that underlie the medicine of systematic correspondence.

However, this annotated translation of the *Nan jing* should serve primarily as a research tool. When its first edition appeared in 1986, I expressed in this preface a hope that the publication of this book might stimulate others to embark on the difficult task of philological analysis of further writings from the history of Chinese medicine, and to develop ever-improving methodologies for conveying the concepts they contain to a Western readership. It is only with the understanding resulting from such analysis that historians, anthropologists, sociologists, and others concerned with the exploration of science and knowledge will have the tools that permit them to pose comparative and other questions. And it is only with this kind of access to the primary sources that those interested in the practice of Chinese medicine as an alternative to Western medicine will be in a position to determine whether the concepts of historical Chinese medicine are indeed applicable to a contemporary Western clientele in any meaningful way.

In concluding the 1986 preface, I pointed out, with sincere gratitude, the unconditional support I received from the China Research Institute for the History of Medicine and Medical Literature at the Academy of Traditional Chinese Medicine in Beijing, where I enjoyed ideal working conditions during two study periods in 1982 and 1983. My special thanks went to Professors Ma Jixing and Ma Kanwen, who found the time to discuss with me a number of problematic passages, and who enabled me to gain access to rare sources unavailable in the United States or Europe. I am happy to know that thirty years later both are still among us. Similar thanks went to the Research Institute for Humanistic Studies of Kyoto University, and especially to Dr. Akira Akahori, who sadly has passed away in the meantime, for his valuable suggestions and for his part in compiling the list of commentated *Nan jing* editions published by Japanese authors. Financial assistance for conducting this study and traveling to East Asia was provided by a Heisenberg grant and by travel subsidies awarded by the German Research Association (DFG), to whose officers and consultants I am most grateful for the understanding my project received. Finally, my thanks go to the academic editorial board of the *Münchener Medizinische Wochenschrift* for a grant that assisted in the production of this volume. With the current revised edition I wish to add Dr. Horst Görtz to this list of benefactors. The Horst-Görtz-Institute for the Theory, History, and Ethics of Chinese Life Sciences endowed by him offered me a unique opportunity to continue my philological and historical studies of ancient Chinese medical texts and to complete both a new translation of the *Nan jing* adapted to my changing understanding of the terminology of ancient Chinese medicine, and a first-time annotated philological translation of the *Ling shu*. With the availability on an identical level of the *Su wen*, the *Ling shu*, and the *Nan jing* to non-Chinese readers, a foundation is laid to compare these texts not only with their contemporary equivalents, such as the ancient Greek Corpus Hippocraticum, but also with the writings of more recent time as vestiges of an ancient knowledge that was most revolutionary from its beginning.

Historical Significance of the *Nan jing*

The prehistory of the *Nan jing* as a work marking the apex of the application of the concepts of yin-yang and of the Five Phases to medicine in Chinese antiquity may have begun at some time in the third century BCE with the emergence of the medicine of systematic correspondence. As far as we can judge from the evidence available today, before the third century BCE, health care in China was based on a recognition of an ancestral responsibility in matters of disease and health (a doctrine that seems to have dominated during the Shang and early Zhou), and on an awareness of the activities of malevolent demons as causative agents of human disease.[4] In addition, although less well documented, it must be assumed that pharmaceutical drugs played an important role in health care (without necessarily being linked to either demonological or ancestral concepts). Historical sources, such as the *Zuo zhuan* 左傳, contain many references to nonmetaphysical concepts of etiology that allegedly date back as far as the sixth century BCE. Yet whether, for instance, the remarks made by the physician He (when he reproached the Marquis of Jin for his excessive intercourse with women) to the effect that "the six heavenly qi 氣 [i.e., yin, yang, wind, rain, obscurity, and brightness]—when they are in excess—produce the six diseases" do indeed reflect a mode of thinking existing at that time, or whether they constitute a retrospective political metaphor phrased from the perspective of half a millennium later, can hardly be decided as long as no evidence from the era in question has come to light.[5]

The earliest extant Chinese medical texts are the texts discovered at Ma wang dui 馬王堆. Together with the data in historical and philosophical sources of the last centuries BCE, these texts suggest that, concurrently with the first unification of the Chinese empire between the third and the first centuries BCE, ancestral and

---

4   Ibid., chapters 1 and 2.

5   See *Chun qiu Zuo zhuan* 春秋左傳, Book X, Duke Chao, First Year.

demonological concepts of health care were supplemented by a conceptual system employing nonmetaphysical notions of natural law.[6] This new medicine appears to have been developed as a consequence of the emergence of at least two philosophical schools (with origins traceable to the fifth century BCE) that introduced paradigms of systematic correspondence to China. The doctrines they expounded were based on the yin-yang and Five Phases paradigms. The representatives of the two doctrines opposed each other vehemently in the beginning, and yet—in a manner typical of subsequent developments—neither was the contradiction between the two doctrines solved in a true synthesis, nor did one paradigm win over the other. Rather, the two were linked (although this proved by no means an easy task). Thereafter, the rise, transformation, and disappearance of any phenomenon in the real world or in the world of concepts could be interpreted by referring to its correspondence to the interactive dynamics of the yin-yang categories of all existence, to the interactive dynamics of the Five Phases of all existence, or to both—whichever appeared to be most conclusive.

Throughout its history of two thousand years, the medicine of systematic correspondence has been transformed and expanded. It has even been linked to originally rival paradigms—when the *Zeitgeist* allowed for such bridges. The medicine of systematic correspondence has always been the subject of probing debates among intellectuals and practitioners of historical Chinese medicine; over the centuries, there have been countless attempts at reconciling its basic tenets with thoughts and experience gained by physicians in actual clinical therapy. Yet the formative period of the medicine of systematic correspondence appears to have been marked by extraordinary dynamics within a relatively short span of time—dynamics that were unsurpassed even by the developments between the twelfth and fifteenth century.

The medicine of systematic correspondence may be traced from a collection of individual writings of the late third or early second century BCE (unearthed from the tombs at Ma wang dui in the early 1970s), which recommend health care and therapy based on demonology, concepts of magic and systematic correspondence, as well as surgical and pharmaceutical knowledge that may have been derived in part from experience and observation (without theoretical underpinnings).[7] From here, it may be traced to the *Huang Di nei jing Su wen* and *Ling shu* anthologies of

---

6   See Unschuld, *Medicine in China: A History of Ideas,* chapter 3.

7   For a survey of all fourteen medical manuscripts unearthed from the Ma wang dui tombs, see Donald Harper, *Early Chinese Medical Literature. The Mawangdui Medical Manuscripts.* New York: Routledge, 1997. These manuscripts demonstrate the coexistence of demonological, magic, empirico-pharmaceutical, petty surgical, and further therapeutic concepts and practices in Chinese medicine around 200 BCE.

systematic correspondence of the second or first century BCE, in which only a few allusions to demonology and drug lore remain, and thence to its conclusion—that is, to the compilation of the *Nan jing* around the first century CE.

This early phase of development included the struggle between the yin-yang and Five Phases doctrines and their convergence in the field of medicine; the transition of the concept of "wind" from a spirit entity to a non-metaphysical natural phenomenon responsible for disease; and the partial replacement—of the concept of "wind" by a concept of "vapors" (*qi* 氣) that underlie all physiological and pathological change. This phase also included an innovative understanding of the functional structure of the organism and the introduction of a therapeutic technique hitherto unknown (or at least undocumented) in China—namely, needling or acupuncture.

The significance of the *Nan jing* in this historical context is twofold. First, its unknown author contributed to the formative period of the medicine of systematic correspondence by creating a conceptual system of medical theory and practice that for the first time consistently accounted for the "discovery" of a circulatory movement in the organism (documented earlier in the *Huang Di nei jing* texts).[8] Second, the *Nan jing* marks the end of this formative epoch because it discarded all the irrelevant ballast of the past and concentrated—in a most coherent manner—on nothing but the most advanced concepts of systematic correspondence. No similar work has since been written.

In devising his conceptual system, the author of the *Nan jing* adopted, with no change, a number of concepts from the *Huang Di nei jing* texts. In addition, he borrowed some older terms but adapted them to his own ideas by presenting them with a modified meaning. Finally, he introduced a series of innovative terms and concepts to complete the doctrine he intended to teach.

The core idea around which the entire *Nan jing* appears to be centered is a modification of diagnosis and therapy in accordance with the "discovery" of a circulatory movement of qi (and blood) in the organism—a discovery that may have occurred some time during the second century BCE.[9] Two of the Mawangdui manuscripts

---

8   See, for instance, *Su wen* treatise 39, "Ju tong lun" 舉痛論.

9   Lu and Needham *(Celestial Lancets,* Cambridge, 1980, 23) have suggested an even earlier emergence of a concept of physiological circulation in China. As evidence they quoted a passage from the *Guanzi* 管子 (identified by Lu and Needham as a text from the fourth century BCE): *shui zhe di zhi xue qi ru jin mai zhi tong liu zhe ye* 水者地之血氣如筋脈 之通流者也. In Lu's and Needham's translation this passage reads: "[One can say that] water is the blood and the *chhi* of the earth, because it flows and penetrates everywhere [just in the same manner] as the circulation [of the *chhi* and the blood] in the *ching-chin* [nerve, muscle and tendon] and the *ching-mo* [tract and channel, including blood vessel] systems." Rendered literally, this passage reads: "Water is the blood and the *qi* of the earth; it flows and penetrates everywhere just as the sinews and the vessels." One might

of around 200 BCE (i.e., the *Shi yi mai jiu jing* 十一脈灸經 texts) refer to eleven vessels that permeate—separately and without mutual interconnection—the human body. Six of these vessels extend upward from the feet into abdomen and chest (some of them reaching the head); five are described as extending from the hands into the chest or head. These vessels are filled with qi vapors; they may suffer from depletion or repletion, or from unusual movements of their contents.

Each of these vessels has its own diseases that produce characteristic symptoms. The sole treatment recommended for manipulating the contents of the eleven vessels is heat, applied by burning a particular herbal substance on the courses the afflicted vessels are believed to take. No specific points at which to conduct such treatment are identified.

By the time those sections of the *Huang Di nei jing* texts that are concerned with physiology and needling were compiled, significant changes had taken place. Twelve vessels were named, which take different courses in comparison to the eleven vessels of the Mawangdui scripts, and which form an interconnected system of "streams" or "conduits" (*jing* 經) that extends throughout the body. The circuit of these conduits represented the central structure of a fine net of passageways formed—in addition to the main conduits—by so-called network vessels (*luo mai* 絡脈) and "tertiary vessels" (*sun mai* 孫脈).

Through these conduits, an endless flow of qi was believed to pass, partially taken in from the outside environment and partially generated by the organism itself. Each of the vessels was known to correspond to one of the basic functional units in the body, and to signal—through changes occurring in the movement inside it—diseases affecting the corresponding unit. The movement in the vessels caused the vessels themselves to pulsate in a particular way. Points were defined all over the body where the individual conduit vessels could be palpated to assess, through the condition of their movement, the condition of the functional units with which they were associated.

For treatment, the *Huang Di nei jing* recommended primarily the insertion of needles at specific locations on all twelve conduit vessels. Since needling was first mentioned in China in the *Shi ji* 史記 of 90 BCE, and since it obviously was not known to the authors of the manuscripts unearthed from the Ma wang dui tombs

go a little further and accept the following interpretation: "Water is the blood and the *qi* of the earth; it flows and penetrates everywhere just as [the blood and the *qi* in] the sinews and vessels [of the human body]." *Guanzi* appears to refer here to a physiological concept reflecting the image of waterways and their contents (above and below the surface of the earth) permeating the entire country. The Chinese wording suggests neither a physiological concept of circulation nor a "meteorological water cycle." For further details on the origin of the circulation concept in Chinese medicine, see Unschuld, *Medicine in China: A History of Ideas,* chapter 3.3.2.

(who recorded every other possible mode of treatment), we may assume that the acupuncture sections of the *Nei jing* were conceptualized and compiled not earlier than during the late second or first century BCE.[10]

The author of the *Nan jing* may have recognized a contradiction between the notion of an ongoing circulatory movement in the vessels and the idea that each vessel has to be diagnosed and treated as if it constituted an individual entity. If the qi pass through an endless circle of conduits again and again, as the text repeatedly states, "like in a ring without end", it is difficult to imagine that the quality of their movement changes when they leave one section of the circuit to enter the next. Hence it is almost irrelevant where the movement is examined: one point on the circuit should reveal all the information needed.

Consequently, the author of the *Nan jing* discarded all locations on the body hitherto used for palpating the vessels, with the exception of one (or, under certain circumstances, two). A problem arose from this concentration—that is, how could one gain from a single point the same information on the condition of the individual functional units of the organism that had been gathered previously from locations spread all over the body?

The information needed to assess a patient's health and to devise and conduct a proper treatment on the basis of the concepts of systematic correspondence was quite complex. It is one of the merits of the author of the *Nan jing* that he developed adequately sophisticated diagnostic patterns by linking some forty-seven perceivable types of movement in the conduit vessels (palpable in various surface or vertical sections at the wrist of one or both hands) to all the normal and abnormal states known to affect the functional units of the organism in the course of the annual seasons. All these patterns were, of course, grounded in the concepts of systematic correspondence.

In devising his system of therapy, the author of the *Nan jing* may have started from conclusions similar to those upon which he based his diagnostic system. Why pierce the individual sections of the circuit through holes scattered all over that circuit if the qi passing through the sections are one and the same? Hence it should be no surprise that the *Nan jing* does not mention conventional circuit-needling at all, but recommends, first, the needling of "accumulation holes" on the back and front of a patient where certain undesired qi gather and can be removed. Second, the *Nan jing* outlines what we may call "limbs needling," a scheme previously documented in the *Ling shu*. In this scheme, twelve streams (running from hands or feet to elbows or knees, respectively) are conceptualized, with five (or six) holes on each. These

---

10 For a more detailed discussion of the earliest references to needling therapy in Chinese literary sources, see Unschuld, *Medicine in China: A History of Ideas*, chapter 3.3.4.

streams (*jing* 經) are associated with the basic functional units of the organism, but they are not seen as part of a circuit. Through inserting needles into the holes (bearing such telling names as "well," "creek," "rapids/transportation," "stream," and "confluence"), it is possible, according to the *Nan jing*, to influence the organism's basic functional units in any way desired.

The Contents of the *Nan jing*

An innovative diagnostic approach and a coherent concept of needling therapy are, on first glance, the two central messages conveyed by the *Nan jing*; they represent, however, only two ingredients of a virtually complete conceptual system of medical care that also includes a detailed discussion of physiology, etiology, and pathology.

As is the case with the editions of the *Su wen* and the *Ling shu* that are extant, the *textus receptus* of the *Nan jing* consists of eighty-one sections. In the *Su wen*, all eighty-one sections are designated by a specific topic to which is added consistently the term *lun* 論 ("discussion" or simply "on ..."); in the *Ling shu*, only a fraction of the eighty-one section titles carries the adjunct *lun*, while the majority have only the topic discussed as their title. In the *Nan jing*, in contrast, all eighty-one sections are merely called *nan* 難, and they are numbered consecutively with no topics appearing as titles. The term *nan* has been interpreted by Eastern and Western authors in various ways. Xu Dachun 徐大椿, an eminent eighteenth century author of conservative medical writings and a commentator on the *Nan jing*, read *nan* as "question-and-answer dialogue" or "examination." He concluded: "The aim [of the *Nan jing*] is to explain difficult issues in the text of the classic. Hence it poses questions concerning these difficult issues (*wen nan* 問難) and, then, clarifies them. Therefore it is called *Nan jing*."[11] Okanishi Tameto 岡西為人, the late Japanese historian of Chinese medical literature, followed Xu Dachun here when he identified *nan* as *wennan*,[12] and so, most recently, did Gu Weicheng 賈維誠, the editor of *San bai zhong yi ji lu* 三百种醫籍錄.[13]

Rather than emphasizing the question-and-answer structure of the *Nan jing*, other authors have understood *nan* as referring to the "difficult" nature of the issues discussed. Li Jiong 李駉, a thirteenth century author of a commentated *Nan jing*

---

11 Xu Dachun, "Nan jing lun" 難經論, *Yi xue yuan liu lun* 醫學源流論, in *Xu Lingtai yi shu quan ji* 徐霛胎醫書全集. Taipei. 1969, 113.

12 Okanishi Tameto , 岡西爲人 *Chugoku Isho Honzo-ko* 中國醫書本草考 Osaka, 1974. 14–15.

13 Gu Weicheng 賈維誠, *San bai zhong yi ji lu* 三百种醫籍錄 Harbin, 1982. 25.

edition, wrote in his preface that the *Nan jing* "was structured as a fictitious dialogue in order to elucidate doubtful and difficult meanings. In all, it consists of eighty-one sections. Hence it is called the 'Classic of Eighty-One Difficult Issues'."[14]

A third noteworthy explanation of the title was offered by Itō Kaoru 伊籐馨, author of a thoughtful etymological *Nan jing* commentary (which was never published; his original manuscript is in the Fujikawa Library of Kyoto University). Itō may have had in mind the title of section twelve of *Han fei zi* 韓非子 ("Shuo nan" 說難) when he stated: "The meaning of the character *nan* is that of *shuo* 說 [here 'to instruct', 'to persuade'] as in *shuo nan* ['the difficulties of persuasion'].[15] It was used in antiquity to express the meaning of 'instruction'. It is, therefore, quite appropriate to consider [the wording] *ba shi yi nan* 八十一難 as carrying the meaning *ba shi yi shuo* 八十一說 ['eighty-one instructions']."[16]

Over the centuries, various schemes have been introduced to group the eighty-one difficult issues. Allegedly dating back to the Tang commentator Yang Xuancao 楊玄操 (eighth century) is a system of thirteen chapters that was repeated by the *Nan jing ji zhu* 難經集註 edition of the early sixteenth century.[17] Other editions followed a classification initiated by Wu Cheng 吳澄 (1247-1331), a *literatus* who grouped the eighty-one difficult issues into only six chapters.[18] These two approaches to dividing the eighty-one sections of the *Nan jing* into meaningful groups or related subjects adopted an identical order of the individual difficult issues. Yet a few commentators, especially those of more recent times, have felt the need to re-arrange—and even cut apart—a number of difficult issues to recombine segments

---

14 Taki Mototane 多紀元胤, *Zhong guo yi ji kao* 中國醫籍考 Peking, 1956. 45.

15 See *Shi ji* 史記, ch. 63.

16 Ito Kaoru, *Nan jing wenzi kao*, n.d., n.p. (see appendix C).

17 See Yang's preface reprinted in Okanishi Tameto, *Song yi qian yi ji kao* 宋以前醫籍考 (Taipei, 1969), 107. The thirteen chapters adopted by the *Nan jing ji zhu* edition are: 1. Diagnosing the [movement in the] conduit vessels (sections 1–24); 2. Enumeration of [main] conduits and network [vessels] (sections 25 and 26); 3. The eight single-conduit vessels (sections 27–29); 4. camp and guard [qi] and the Triple Burner (sections 30 and 31); 5. The long-term depots and the short-term repositories and their correspondences (sections 32–37); 6. Enumeration and measurements of the long-term depots and short-term repositories (sections 38–47); 7. Depletion, repletion, evil [qi], and proper [qi] (sections 48–52); 8. Transmission of diseases through long-term depots and short-term repositories (sections 53 and 54); 9. Accumulation and collection [illnesses] in the long-term depots and short-term repositories (sections 55 and 56); 10. The five diarrheas and harm caused by cold (sections 57–60); 11. Spirits, sages, artisans, and workmen (section 61); 12. Wells [and other] transportation holes [associated with the] long-term depots and short-term repositories (sections 62–68); 13. Supplementing and draining with needles (sections, 69–81).

18 Okanishi Tameto 1974, 15.

of the text they interpreted as originally belonging together.[19] And concurrent with contemporary attempts to filter out of the entirety of traditional Chinese medicine those elements that some authors consider worth preserving and utilizing in practice, a few editions have been published recently which—in contrast to all former editions (which included even those sections of the *Nan jing* considered to be wrong or absurd)—present not the complete text but only selected passages.[20] In the present edition of the complete text, the eighty-one difficult issues are presented in the traditional order adopted by all the pre-eighteenth-century editions I have seen. Since the original division of the text into "chapters" prior to Yang Xuancao—if there was one—is no longer known, I have adopted the six-chapter scheme introduced by Wu Cheng for its conciseness and clarity.

The following is a survey of the contents of each of the eighty-one difficult issues grouped in six chapters.

Chapter One: The Movement in the Vessels and its Diagnostic Significance

The first difficult issue
Explanation of the significance of the inch opening for diagnosing diseases through investigating the movement in the vessels.

The second difficult issue
Introduction of the first subdivision of the inch opening into an "inch section" and a "foot section," divided by a line called "gate."

The third difficult issue
Discussion of the terms "great excess," "insufficiency," "mutual takeover by yin and yang," "turnover," "overflow," "closure," and "barrier" as diagnostic parameters indicated by specific movements in the vessels.

The fourth difficult issue
Explanation of yin and yang patterns of movement in the vessels, and introduction of the concept of three longitudinal levels in the movement in the vessels.

The fifth difficult issue
Introduction of the concept of five longitudinal levels in the movement in the vessels, and of a method to distinguish these levels.

The sixth difficult issue

---

19 For instance, Katō Bankei in his *Nan jing gu yi* of 1784 (see appendix B) and Huang Weisan in his *Nan jing zhi yao* of 1967 (see appendix A). See also He Aihua, "Guan yu *Nan jing* de bian ci wen ti," *Ha er bin zhong yi* 8 (1965): 41–43 (see appendix B).

20 For instance, Yan Hongchen and Gao Guangzhen in their *Nei Nan jing xuan shi* of 1979 (see appendix A).

Discussion of the terms "yin abundance, yang depletion" and "yang abundance, yin depletion" as diagnostic parameters indicated by specific movements in the vessels.

The seventh difficult issue
Explanation of the significance of the appearance of any of the three yin and three yang kinds of movement in the vessels as they are related to the six periods within one year.

The eighth difficult issue
Explanation of the significance of the "moving qi" (also called "vital qi") in the organism, as appearing at the inch opening.

The ninth difficult issue
How to distinguish diseases in the long-term depots and short-term repositories by the speed of the movement in the vessels.

The tenth difficult issue
Introduction of the concept of "ten variations" in the movement in the vessels, as can be felt in the different sections at the wrist that are associated with specific long-term depots.

The eleventh difficult issue
Explanation of the concept that one long-term depot is void of qi if the movement in the vessels stops once in less than fifty arrivals.

The twelfth difficult issue
Introduction of the concept that the internal or external parts of the organism may be cut off from the movement in the vessels.

The thirteenth difficult issue
Introduction of the concept of a correspondence between a person's complexion, the movement in the vessels as felt at the inch opening, and the condition of the skin in the foot section of the lower arm.

The fourteenth difficult issue
Introduction of the concepts of "injured" (i.e., slower than usual) and "arriving" (i.e., faster than usual) movements in the vessels; also, discussion of the significance of the presence of a movement in the vessels at the inch section when no movement can be perceived at the foot section, and vice versa.

The fifteenth difficult issue
Elucidation of the changes in the movements in the vessels in accordance with the passing of the four seasons.

The sixteenth difficult issue
Discussion of various methods to diagnose diseases by taking internal and external evidence into account.

The seventeenth difficult issue
How to predict a patient's impending death or survival by comparing the movement in his vessels with other manifestations of his disease.

The eighteenth difficult issue
Systematized presentation of the correspondences of the yin and yang conduits with the inch, gate, and foot sections near the wrist where the movement in the vessels can be felt, on the basis of the mutual generation order of the Five Phases. Also, discussion of methods for recognizing internal accumulations and chronic diseases through the movement in the vessels.

The nineteenth difficult issue
Introduction of the concept of differences in the movement in the vessels in males and females.

The twentieth difficult issue
Introduction of the concepts of hidden and concealed movements in the vessels, of doubled qi, and of lost qi.

The twenty-first difficult issue
On the prognostic significance of situations where a patient's bodily appearance shows signs of disease while the movement in his vessels does not, and vice versa.

The twenty-second difficult issue
Elaboration of the concepts of diseases in the vessels that are "excited" and of those that are "generated."

Chapter Two: The Conduits and the Network Vessels

The twenty-third difficult issue
Systematized presentation of the lengths and courses of the conduit vessels as sections of a large circulatory system. Also, reference to the significance of feeling the movement in the vessels at the wrists of both hands, and explanation of the concepts of "end" and "beginning."

The twenty-fourth difficult issue
Systematized presentation and prognostic evaluation of external symptoms indicating that a specific conduit vessel has been cut off from the movement in the vessels.

The twenty-fifth difficult issue

Explanation of the concept of "twelve conduits" in the presence of five long-term depots and six short-term repositories through the introduction of the concepts of "heart enclosing network" and "Triple Burner" as carrying a name (i.e., fulfilling a function) without having a form (i.e., an anatomical substratum).

The twenty-sixth difficult issue

Remarks on the fifteen network vessels.

The twenty-seventh difficult issue

Introduction of the term "eight single-conduit vessels," and of the concept that they function as "ditches and reservoirs" absorbing surplus contents of the main conduits.

The twenty-eighth difficult issue

Description of the courses of the eight single-conduit vessels in the organism.

The twenty-ninth difficult issue

List of signs and symptoms caused by diseases in the eight single-conduit vessels.

Chapter Three: The Long-Term Depots and the Short-Term Repositories

The thirtieth difficult issue

Elucidation of the concepts of camp qi and guard qi, and introduction of the idea that the long-term depots and short-term repositories are supplied with qi by the stomach directly.

The thirty-first difficult issue

Innovative reinterpretation of the concept of the Triple Burner as a functional description of the upper, central, and lower groups of organs in the body.

The thirty-second difficult issue

Explanation of why the heart and the lung are the only long-term depots located above the diaphragm.

The thirty-third difficult issue

Discussion of apparent contradictions resulting from the association of the liver and kidneys with the phases wood and metal, respectively.

The thirty-fourth difficult issue

Pattern of the five long-term depots and their corresponding sounds, complexions, odors, liquids, and flavors. Association of the five long-term depots with the seven spirits.

The thirty-fifth difficult issue
Discussion of theoretical issues concerning the functions and locations of the six short-term repositories, especially as they are related to the five long-term depots.

The thirty-sixth difficult issue
Introduction of the concept that the organism has two kidneys, one of them constituting the "gate of life."

The thirty-seventh difficult issue
Elucidation of the concept that the qi of the five long-term depots pass through specific orifices, thus maintaining the functions of these orifices. Also, further discussion of the concepts of closure and barrier, and reference to the concepts of turnover and overflow.

The thirty-eighth difficult issue
Further elucidation of the nature and function of the Triple Burner as an answer to the question of why there are six short-term repositories but only five long-term depots in the body.

The thirty-ninth difficult issue
Further elucidation of the nature and function of the gate of life and of the Triple Burner in reference to the existence of six short-term repositories but only five long-term depots.

The fortieth difficult issue
Discussion of apparent contradictions resulting from the association of the nose with the lung (which is responsible for the sounds, while the nose is responsible for distinguishing the odors) and from the association of the ears with the kidneys (which are responsible for the liquids, while the ears are responsible for distinguishing the sounds).

The forty-first difficult issue
Explanation of why the liver is the only long-term depot that has two lobes.

The forty-second difficult issue
Description of all long-term depots and short-term repositories in terms of length, diameter, weight, and capacity.

The forty-third difficult issue
Explanation of the phenomenon that someone who does not eat or drink will die after seven days.

The forty-fourth difficult issue
List of the names and locations of the seven through-gates.

The forty-fifth difficult issue
Introduction of the concept of the eight gathering points.

The forty-sixth difficult issue
On different sleeping patterns in old and young people.

The forty-seventh difficult issue
Why the face can stand cold.

Chapter Four: On diseases

The forty-eighth difficult issue
Introduction of various diagnostic patterns allowing one to distinguish whether a person suffers from a depletion or from a repletion.

The forty-ninth difficult issue
Introduction of the concepts of primary affection by the five evil qi from outside the organism, and of secondary affection by evil qi transmitted within the organism.

The fiftieth difficult issue
Introduction of the concepts of "depletion evil," "repletion evil," "robber evil," "weakness evil," and "regular evil," denoting the five possibilities of internal secondary affliction.

The fifty-first difficult issue
Explanation of different preferences and aversions on the side of the patient permitting one to distinguish whether a disease is located in the long-term depots or short-term repositories.

The fifty-second difficult issue
On the static nature of diseases in the long-term depots and on the mobile nature of diseases in the short-term repositories.

The fifty-third difficult issue
Introduction of the concepts of "transmission of a disease through seven long-term depots" and of "transmission skipping a depot."

The fifty-fourth difficult issue
Diseases in the long-term depots are difficult to cure; diseases in the short-term repositories are easy to cure.

The fifty-fifth difficult issue
Reinterpretation of the concepts of "accumulation" and "collection" diseases.

The fifty-sixth difficult issue
Reinterpretation of terms and concepts related to accumulation diseases, and introduction of a systematic theory of the generation of the five accumulation diseases.

The fifty-seventh difficult issue
Introduction of a fivefold classification of different diarrheas.

The fifty-eighth difficult issue
Introduction of a fivefold classification of "harm caused by cold" diseases and of the different movements in the vessels resulting from these diseases. Also, a list of signs and symptoms allowing for a diagnosis of diseases caused by heat and cold.

The fifty-ninth difficult issue
How to distinguish peak-illness from madness.

The sixtieth difficult issue
Discussion of the concepts of "stagnant pain" and "true pain" in head and heart.

The sixty-first difficult issue
Introduction of a categorization of healers as "spirits," "sages," "artisans," and "workmen," based on their respective approaches to diagnosing a disease.

Chapter Five: Transportation Holes

The sixty-second difficult issue
Explanation of why the conduits associated with the short-term repositories have six transportation holes, while those associated with the long-term depots have only five.

The sixty-third difficult issue
Explanation of why each conduit has a "spring" as its first transportation hole.

The sixty-fourth difficult issue
Introduction of a systematic categorization of the transportation holes according to yin and yang and the Five Phases.

The sixty-fifth difficult issue
Remarks concerning the "spring" and "confluence" transportation holes.

The sixty-sixth difficult issue
Discussion of the "origin" transportation holes as outlets of the "original qi" of the six long-term depots and six short-term repositories.

The sixty-seventh difficult issue
Explanation of the location of "levy holes" on the front and of "transportation holes" on the back of one's body.

The sixty-eighth difficult issue
Introduction of a list of diseases that can be cured by needling the respective transportation holes associated with them.

Chapter Six: Needling Patterns

The sixty-ninth difficult issue
General advice on how to supplement a depletion and drain a repletion, and when to remove a disease from an affected conduit itself.

The seventieth difficult issue
Introduction of a pattern of two different needling techniques to be applied during the spring-summer and autumn-winter seasons, respectively.

The seventy-first difficult issue
Advice for needling the camp qi and the guard qi.

The seventy-second difficult issue
Reinterpretation of the terms "moving against" and "following" as concepts referring to the direction of the movement in the vessels.

The seventy-third difficult issue
Advice to needle a "creek" transportation hole if theory requires needling a "well" hole.

The seventy-fourth difficult issue
Introduction of a pattern of needling different holes in the course of the five seasons.

The seventy-fifth difficult issue
Elucidation of the theoretical basis underlying the therapeutic approach of supplementing a so-called depletion and of draining a so-called repletion.

The seventy-sixth difficult issue
Discussion of the concepts of "supplementing" and "draining."

The seventy-seventh difficult issue
Introduction of a classification of healers as "superior" or "mediocre" practitioners according to their understanding of the transmission of diseases within the organism.

The seventy-eighth difficult issue
Reinterpretation of the techniques of supplementing and draining by means of needling.

The seventy-ninth difficult issue
Further elucidation of the theoretical basis underlying the treatment of states of depletion and repletion.

The eightieth difficult issue
Comments on the techniques of inserting and withdrawing a needle.

The eighty-first difficult issue
Warning against "replenishing a repletion" and "depleting a depletion."

The Origin of the *Nan jing*

The compilation date of the *Nan jing* remains a matter of controversy. Decades ago, Fan Xingzhun suggested that the *Nan jing* was written at some time during the era of the Six Dynasties, probably during the fifth or sixth century CE.[21] In an essay elucidating his arguments, Fan Xingzhun 范行准 (1906-1998) quoted Liao Ping 廖平 (1851-1914?), who was the first to propose such a late compilation date. Among other arguments, Liao Ping pointed out that a new attitude toward women, beginning at the time of the Qi and Liang dynasties, had forced physicians to modify their diagnostic techniques: "Since the times of Qi and Liang it was no longer a matter of course to touch the throat or feet of women for diagnosis. Hence this method [of pulse diagnosis at the wrist] was established so that [physicians could continue] to earn their livelihood."[22]

Taki Mototane (Tamba Genkan) 多紀元胤 (1789-1827), author of a comprehensive medical bibliography (*Zhong guo yi ji kao* 中國醫籍考), had reached different conclusions when he suggested a compilation date during the Eastern Han dynasty (that is, during the first or second century CE). He pointed out that the concept of *yuan qi* 元氣 ("original qi"), although introduced by Dong Zhongshu 董仲舒 of the second century BCE, found entrance into common usage only during the Eastern Han. Similarly, the concepts of "males are born at *yin* 寅; females are born at *shen*

---

21 Fan Xingzhun, "*Huang di zhong nan jing zhu yu hui zhen jing zuo zhe Lü Guang de nian dai wen ti,*" *Shang hai yi xue za zhi* 10 (1957): 32–35 (see appendix B).

22 Ibid., 34.

申,"[23] "this is why wood sinks into the depth, while metal floats at the surface,"[24] and "metal is generated at *ji* 己, water is generated at *shen* 申; drain the fire of the South, supplement the water of the North"[25]—none of which had been included in either the *Su wen* or the *Ling shu*—should also be regarded as facets of Eastern Han thought.[26]

A later compilation date had already been excluded by Taki Mototane's father, Taki Motohiro 多紀元閏 (1755-1810), who had interpreted a line in the preface to the *Shang han lun* 傷寒論 of Zhang Ji 張機 (142-220?) as referring to the *Nan jing*.[27] This line is worded *xuan yong Su wen Jiu juan Ba shi yi nan Yin yang da lun tai lu yao lu* 選用素問九卷八十一難陰陽大論胎臚藥錄. It had been read by Zhang Zhicong 張志聰 (1610-1674) as "in compiling [the *Shang han lun*] I made use of the *Su wen* with its eighty-one difficult issues discussed in nine chapters." Zhang failed to realize that *Jiu juan* 九卷 referred to a separate book—quoted, for instance, by the *Mai jing* 脈經 and in the *Ishinpo* 醫心方 as *Jiu juan yun* 九卷云 ("The Nine Chapters state ..."), possibly for lack of a proper title.[28] Also, in the eleventh century edition of the *Shang han lun* (preserved in Japan), the line quoted appears as a commentary added to Zhang Ji's 張繼 text by a later editor. Still later editors may have included these remarks in the main text. Hence, as Fan Xingzhun concluded, there is no evidence that Zhang Ji knew of the *Nan jing*, and the first ten characters of the line in question should be read as "in compiling [the *Shang han lun* 傷寒論] I made use of the *Su wen* and of the *Jiu juan*, both having eighty-one sections."[29]

Soon after Fan Xingzhun had voiced his views, He Aihua—in two essays published in 1958 and 1960—rejected these arguments and suggested a compilation date at some time during the Western Han dynasty (that is, during the second or first century BCE). He pointed out that in analysing the line in the preface to the *Shang han lun*, one should take into account not only its first ten characters but also the entire sentence, because two more book titles were mentioned in it, and he saw no reason not to interpret *Jiu juan* and *Ba shi yi nan* as book titles too. He Aihua suggested reading the line in question as follows: "in compiling [the *Shang han lun*] I made use of the *Su wen*, the *Jiu juan*, the *Ba shi yi nan*, the *Yin yang da lun*, and the

---

23 See "difficult issue" 19.

24 See "difficult issue" 33.

25 See "difficult issue" 75.

26 Taki Mototane 1956, 79.

27 Ibid.

28 Fan Xingzhun 1957, 35.

29 Ibid.

Tai lu yao lu."[30] He took it for granted that this phrase had been written by Zhang Ji himself (he did not discuss the "commentary" interpretation), and he quoted another sentence from Zhang Ji's preface to prove that the *Nan jing* had been written earlier. The *Nan jing*, He argued, had introduced pulse diagnosis at the wrists, an innovation that had led to the disregarding of the *Nei jing* methods of vessel diagnosis—that is, of pulse feeling at the side of the larynx and at the feet, in addition to palpation of the wrists. Ho stated that this development must have taken place before Zhang Ji's time because in his preface, Chang complained:

> Today's physicians do not take great pains to seek instructions from the classics in order to expand their knowledge; they rely only on abilities transmitted in their families. From beginning to end they follow their old precepts. When they are confronted with a disease, they approach the patient with smart speeches. Disregarding what would be essential in such [a situation], they simply prescribe decoctions and feel [the vessels at] the inch[-section]—but not even at the foot [section]. They rely on [an examination of the vessels at] the hands and disregard the feet; they do not care about an investigation of all three diagnostic sections [of the body, which would include an examination] at the *ren ying* [points at the throat] and at the ankles, in order to assess the frequency [of the movement in the vessels] and of [the patient's] breathing .... They act like someone who gazes through a narrow tube in order to observe heaven![31]

He Aihua saw further evidence for Zhang Ji's awareness of the teaching of the *Nan jing* in numerous references, in the *Shang han lun* itself, to wrist diagnosis at the inch, gate, and foot sections, arguing that Zhang Ji was most probably quoting from the *Nan jing* (since these concepts had been introduced by the *Nan jing*). Similarly, He Aihua regarded Wang Shuhe's 王叔和 (210-285) *Jia yi jing* 甲乙經 and Huangfu Mi's 皇甫謐 (214-282) *Mai jing* 脈經 as influenced, beyond any doubt, by various *Nan jing* innovations in vessel diagnosis.[32]

A significant number of the questions raised in the eighty-one sections of the *Nan jing* are introduced by the phrase *jing yun* 經云 ("the scripture states" or "the classic states"). An exact title of that scripture or classic is not mentioned. Also, while some of the issues referred to as statements quoted from that scripture may

---

30 He Aihua, "Wo dui *Nan jing* zhu zuo nian dai wen ti de shang que," *Shang hai zhong yi za zhi* 4 (1958): 42; and He Aihua, "Guan yu *Nan jing* de ji ge wen ti," *Ren min bao jian* 2 (1960): 169 (see appendix B).

31 See Zhang Ji 張繼 *Shang han lun* 傷寒論, (Shanghai, 1983), preface, 4.

32 He Aihua 1958, 42.

indeed be found—in identical or somewhat altered wording—in the *Su wen* or the *Ling shu*, other statements introduced by *jing yun* 經云 do not appear in the *textus receptus* of these ancient classics. He Aihua did not consider the possibility, voiced by other authors, that these statements may have been part of *Su wen* or *Ling shu* passages that have been lost in the meantime, or that they may be fictitious quotations designed merely to raise and discuss a specific issue. He wrote:

> When the text of the *Nan jing* quotes the text of the *Nei jing*, it does not distinguish between *Su wen* and *Ling shu* but says in all instances merely "the classic states." This is sufficient evidence not only to fully disclose the erroneous and commonly held view that the *Su wen* appeared first while the *Ling shu* is of later origin, but also to prove that the *Nan jing* must have been written before the *Nei jing* was split into *Su wen* and *Ling shu*.[33]

He Aihua, in contrast to Taki Mototane, considered the diagnostic scheme outlined in the *Nan jing* to be identical with the scheme followed by the physician Chunyu Yi 淳于意, whose approach to diagnosis is referred to (if in less detail than is needed to substantiate He's conclusion) in the *Shi ji*. Thus He concluded that the *Nan jing* was written either by Chunyu Yi himself or by some other author of Chunyu Yi's school.[34] Traditionally, though, most commentators have attributed the *Nan jing* to semi-legendary or legendary personalities, who are assumed to have lived and spread their wisdom many centuries before Chunyu Yi. Bian Que 扁鵲, a shadowy physician of about the fifth or sixth century BCE whose biography appears in the *Shi ji*, seems to have been linked to the *Nan jing* since the Sui-Tang era. The name Bian Que has been associated with itinerant shaman-healers from Shandong province who clad themselves in feathers, suggesting an ability to rise into the skies;[35] it may also have been a designation conferred upon or adopted by various healers during the time of the Zhou (this is suggested by records hinting at the

---

33 He Aihua 1960, 169.

34 Ibid.

35 Kanō Yoshimitsu 加納喜光, "Isho ni miero kiron" 醫書見氣論, in Onozawa Seiichi 小野 et al. (eds.), *Ki no shisō* (Tokyo, 1980), 284–285. Liu Dunyuan 劉敦, the discoverer of the Han reliefs depicting Bian Que as a human-headed bird, suggested that the latter might have been influenced by the Indian *gandharva* myth of human-headed birds acting as skilled physicians. Cf. Liu Dunyuan, "Han hua xiang shi shang de zhen jiu tu" 漢畫像上的鍼灸圖, *Wen wu can kao zi liao* 文物參考資料 6 (1972): 47 f. Bian Que and his innovative art had already been linked to Indian qi by Wei Juxian in his essay "Bian Que de yi shu lai zi yin du," *Xin zhong yi kan* (October 1939). For a refutation of Wei's arguments, see Lu Jue-fei, "Bian Qu yi shu lai zi yin du zhi yi," *Hua xi yi yao za zhi* (November 1947); see also appendix B.

existence of a Bian Que in different centuries).[36] In his *Shi ji* of 90 BC, Sima Qian identified Bian Que as a man called Qin Yueren, but he did not give any details concerning Bian's actual dates. According to Sima Qian, Qin Yueren "made himself a name especially with vessel diagnosis," and "to this time, whoever discusses vessel [diagnosis] bases [his arguments] on Bian Que."[37] Yet no reference appears in this biography to a specific book written by Bian Que. (According to the biography, Bian Que promised to his mysterious teacher Changsang jun not to transmit his knowledge to anyone else before the latter transferred his abilities to Bian Que.) At the time of the Han, at least two texts existed which had allegedly been compiled by Bian Que himself. The official history of the Han dynasty lists a *Bian Que nei jing* 扁鵲内經 and a *Bian Que wai jing* 扁鵲外景 (in addition to a *Huang Di nei jing* 黃帝内經, a *Huang Di wai jing* 黃帝外經, and other *nei jing* and *wai jing* titles), but we have no clues suggesting any relationship between these Bian Que titles and the *Nan jing* that is extant. In fact, Taki Mototane discovered what is currently regarded as the earliest known reference to Bian Que as the author of the *Nan jing*. Wang Dao 王燾, in his *Wai tai mi yao* 外臺秘要 (ca. 725 CE), quoted from the *Shan fan fang* 刪繁方, a prescription work compiled around 600 CE by Xie Shitai 謝士泰 who, in turn, quoted a Bian Que as making statements that appear in today's *Nan jing*.[38] Not much later, Yang Xuancao 楊玄操 (seventh or eighth century) began the preface to his *Nan jing* commentary with the unambiguous statement: "The *Huang Di ba shi yi nan jing* was compiled by Qin Yueren 秦越人 from Bo hai 渤海," i.e., by the Bian Que of the *Shi ji*.[39]

The appearance of a reference to the Yellow Thearch in the title named by Yang Xuancao may indicate a separate—and possibly earlier—tradition crediting the legendary Huang Di (the Yellow Thearch) with the authorship. In what may be the earliest known reference to the *Nan jing* and its origin (if we disregard the controversial line in the *Shang han lun* for a moment), the Yellow Thearch appears as the originator of the *Nan jing* because the text resulted from a discussion between Huang Di and two of his consultants. Huangfu Mi 皇甫謐 (214-282) wrote in his *Di wang shi ji* 帝王世紀: "Huang Di ordered Lei gong and Qi Bo to discuss [with

---

36 Wei Juxian suggested that all the different "Bian Ques" mentioned in the *Han fei zi* 韓非子, the *Zhan guo ce* 戰國策, the *Shi ji* 史記 and other sources of that time refer to healers practicing "Western medicine" (i.e., Indian medicine). See Chen Bangxian 陳邦賢, *Zhong guo yi xue shi* 中國醫學史 Taipei, 1969. 24.

37 See *Shi ji*, ch. 105.

38 Taki Mototane 1956, 79–80.

39 See Okanishi Tameto 1969, 106.

him] the courses of the conduit vessels. He questioned them about eighty-one issues and created the *Nan jing*."⁴⁰

Wang Bo 王勃 (648-676), an exceptionally gifted scholar of the Tang era, may have attempted a compromise between the Yellow Thearch tradition and the Bian Que tradition when he wrote:

> The *Huang Di ba shi yi nan jing* is a secretly recorded medical classic. In ancient times [this text] was handed over by Qi Bo to [the Yellow Thearch] Huang Di. From Huang Di it was handed over, through nine [generations of] instructors, to Yi Yin. Yi Yin handed it over to Tang, and from Tang it was handed over, through six [generations of] instructors, to Tai gong. Tai gong handed it over to Wen wang. From Wen wang it was handed over, through nine [generations of] instructors, to the physician He. From the physician He it was handed over, through six [generations of] instructors, to Qin Yueren. Qin Yueren was the first to put [this text] down in writing.⁴¹

It was only in the late nineteenth century that Liao Ping, the conservative author of the *Nan jing jing shi bu zheng* (see the following section of this Introduction and appendix A), found it difficult to link a work that he considered to be in many respects far from the truth conveyed by the "classic" *Huang Di nei jing* with an author who had lived in classical antiquity. To make his point, Liao did not shrink from manipulating the preface of his conservative but far less rigid predecessor Xu Dachun, whose *Nan jing* commentary entitled *Nan jing jing shi* Liao had selected as a basis for his own comments. While Xu had attributed the *Nan jing* to a pre-Han origin, Liao changed the line in his edition of Xu's work so that Xu appeared to have suggested a Western Jin (265-317) origin of the *Nan jing*. In his own commentary to this line, Liao then refuted this as too early and suggested an even later compilation date during the era of the Six Dynasties (i.e., during the fifth or sixth century).⁴²

Earlier in these prolegomena, I have referred to the *Nan jing* as a work of the first or early second century CE; it may even have been written a few decades before the first century CE. I concur with the opinion that the *Shang han lun* was influenced by the *Nan jing*, and I agree with those commentators who saw a significant gap between the language and the concepts used by the *Nan jing* and those found in

---

40 See *Tai ping yu lan* 太平御覽, ch. 721.

41 Quoted in *Wen yuan ying hua* 文苑英華, ch. 735, "Xu" 序 37, "Za xu" 雜序 1: *Huang di ba shi yi nan.*

42 See Xu Dachun's preface to his *Nan jing jing shi* in Liao Ping's *Nan jing jing shi bu zheng*; where the last sentence reads *ran shi xi Jin yi hou shu yun* 然實西晉以後書云. Compare with Xu Dachun 1969, preface, 2; Taki Mototane 1956, 94–95; and Okanishi Tameto 1969, 99, where this line reads *ran shi liang Han yi qian shu yun* 然實兩漢以前書云.

the *Nei jing*—a gap that signals development as well as difference. I am convinced (as shall be elucidated further in my notes to the individual difficult issues) that the *Nan jing* was compiled to overcome the heterogeneity and unsystematic nature of the *Huang Di nei jing* anthology of medical schools and concepts—and especially to draw the conceptual and clinical consequences from the "discovery" of the circulation of qi in the organism. In my opinion, the *Nei jing* texts on needling and diagnosis reveal a stage of development that is not only later than that indicated by the texts unearthed from the Ma wang dui tombs (168 BCE) but also later than that indicated in the biography of Chunyu Yi (216-150?) in the *Shi ji* (compiled in 90 BCE). Thus the *Nei jing* texts cannot have been compiled before the late second or first century CE. (although some parts of the *Nei jing*—for instance, those on wind divination—appear to be older, and some are much younger).[43] The *Nan jing*, then, could have been written after the appearance of the *Nei jing* texts on needling and vessel diagnosis, and before the appearance of the *Shang han lun* in the second century and of Huangfu Mi's *Di wang shi ji* in the third century CE.

The Reception of the *Nan jing* in Later Centuries

The message offered by the *Nan jing* must have been quite convincing in at least one respect. Vessel diagnosis concentrating on the wrists was adopted not only by many physicians (who were criticized by Zhang Ji—or by a later commentator to his preface—for an all too simplistic practice both of diagnosis in general and of wrist diagnosis as well) but also by the leading pre-Song authors of medical works with sections on diagnosis that have been transmitted to us from pre-Song times. This applies—in addition to the *Shang han lun*—to the *Jia yi jing* 甲乙經 and the *Mai jing* 脈經 (both of the third century CE), as well as to Sun Simiao's 孫思邈 *Qian jin yi fang* 千金翼方 of the early seventh century.

The impact of and interest in the *Nan jing* must have been considerable in subsequent centuries: the *Nan jing* provoked an endless series of commentaries attempting to plumb the depths of its message. The bibliographical section of the Sui History (compiled during the seventh century) mentions a *Huang Di ba shi yi nan jing* and adds the remark: "The *Liang (Qilu)* refers to a *Huang Di zhong nan jing*,1 *juan*., with a commentary by Lü Bowang 呂博望. [The work is] lost." If the usual interpretation that this remark in the Sui History was indeed based on Ruan Xiaoxu's 阮孝緒 (479-536) *Qi lu* 七錄 is correct, one should assume that the first commentary on the *Nan jing* was published before the year 500, but did not

---

43 For details, see Unschuld, *Medicine in China: A History of Ideas*, section 3.3.

survive (at least as an independent work) until the early Tang era. Yang Xuancao, the second *Nan jing* commentator, referred to his predecessor as "Wu tai yi ling Lü Guang" 吳太醫令呂廣. As Japanese scholars have pointed out, several persons are known whose personal name Guang 廣 was changed into Bo 博 following a taboo placed on the former after the ascension to the throne of the Sui emperor Yang di in 605.[44] And Fan Xingzhun observed that it was quite common, during the era of the Six Dynasties, to drop the central or final character of a person's name in literary references. Hence the original name of the man who is generally considered to have written the first *Nan jing* commentary may have been Lü Guangwang 呂廣望.[45]

The dating of Lü's lifetime, though, is more problematic than the identification of his personal name. The usual reading of *Wu tai yi ling* would be "Head of the Imperial Physicians during the Wu dynasty." This interpretation appears to be substantiated by a statement found in section *Yi si* 醫四 of chapter 724 of the Song encyclopedia *Tai ping yu lan* 太平御覽 of 983, where the preface to a "Needle Scripture from the Jade Chest" (*Yu kui zhen jing* 玉匱鍼經) is quoted with the following information:

> Lü Bo was still young when he made himself a name with his medical practice. He was an expert in the differentiation of diseases on the basis of vessel diagnosis. He wrote a lot about this. In the second year of *chi wu* 赤烏 of the [dynasty] Wu he became Head of the Imperial Physicians *(tai yi ling)*. He compiled the *Yu kui zhen jing* and wrote a commentary on the *Ba shi yi nan jing*. [His works] became very popular.

Accordingly, Lü Bo—alias Lü Guang(wang)—was a man of the Eastern Wu dynasty; the second year of *zhi wu* corresponds to 239 CE.

This dating of Lü's lifetime was contested in 1957 by Fan Xingzhun, who had at least one earlier witness for a different opinion. In a book by the Song author Dang Yongnian 黨永年 entitled *Shen mi ming yi lu* 神秘名醫錄, one Fan Shumi 范樞密 wrote that the *Nan jing* "was transmitted until the time of the Sui when Lü Guang from Wu wrote a commentary on it."[46] (Lü Fu's remarks from the Yuan era—also quoted by Fan Xingzhun—that "during the times of the Sui a commentary version by Lü Bowang existed, but is no longer transmitted" cannot be taken as hinting at Sui dates for Lü himself.) Fan Xingzhun went a long way to prove his point that "Wu" 吳 refers to a place name, and that "second year of *chi wu*" and "Head of the

---

44 Fan Xingzhun 1957, 32.

45 Ibid.

46 Ibid., quoted from *Tai ping yu lan*, ch. 724.

Imperial Physicians" are data that were made up by unknown authors of the sixth, seventh, or early eighth century.

Fan Xingzhun construed two arguments. First, Fan interpreted the wording of the title of a third book associated with Lü—the "Golden Sheath and Jade Mirror" (*Jin tao yu jian* 金韜玉鑑)—as well as a reference to "obscure teachings" (*xuan zong* 玄宗) in Yang Xuancao's characterization of Lü's commentary, as evidence that Lü had been an adherent of the doctrines of Daoism. Fan concluded that because the Eastern Wu under Emperor Song Quan were known to have been opposed to Daoism, no follower of Daoism could have risen to a dominant position in the medical offices of the court.[47] Yet even if Lü had been a Daoist and Song Quan an anti-Daoist, one could point out examples of emperors disregarding such ideological discrepancies when they called in a physician who had demonstrated superior clinical abilities.

Secondly, Fan Xingzhun argued that Lü's *Yu kui zhen jing* must have been written later than the fourth century for the following reason. The bibliographical section of the Sui History mentions a *Chi wu shen zhen jing* 赤烏神鍼經 (but without naming an author). The two Tang Histories attributed this book to a man named Zhang Zicun 張子存 (without providing details on his lifetime). The *Da Tang liu dian* 大唐六典, compiled in the early eighth century, referred to this book as a teaching manual on needling for professors and students of the imperial medical office. And the Ming author Yao Zhenzong 姚振宗, stated, "The *Chi wu shen zhen jing* seems to have been written on the basis of Lü Guang's *Yu kui zhen jing*. Hence the title of the reigning period [during which Lü Guang served as *tai yi ling*] was added [to the title *Shen zhen jing*]."[48] Fan Xingzhun identified Zhang Zicun—the otherwise unknown author of the *Chi wu shen zhen jing*—as Zhang Cun, the author of a treatise on needling who may have lived during the fourth century. Fan concluded that if the *Chi wu shen zhen jing* and the *Yu kui zhen jing* did indeed show similarities (both texts have been lost for centuries), then the former was written first (during the fourth century by Zhang Cun) and the latter was written afterwards (but prior to the Sui dynasty). Fan explained the *Chi wu* in the title as a reference to an ancient place name, used centuries before Zhang Cun's lifetime for an area where Zhang may have lived (he also provided further examples where place names associated with an author had been adopted to precede the title of a book). Later, *Chi wu* was misinterpreted by authors, Fan wrote, as a reference to the *chi wu* reigning period of the Eastern Wu dynasty; similarly, because Lü's work was so similar in contents to the *Chi wu shen zhen jing*, Lü's own native town of Wu was misinterpreted as anoth-

47 Ibid., 34.
48 Ibid., 32.

er reference to the Eastern Wu dynasty. Finally, Fan suggested, someone invented the "second year" and the official title *tai yi ling*, thus laying the foundations for the "erroneous" statements by Yang Xuancao and the authors of the *Tai ping yu lan*.

Perhaps the facts are as complicated as Fan Xingzhun saw them. We should, however, keep in mind that it must have been rather difficult for him to reconcile Liao Ping's and his own idea of a fifth or sixth century origin of the *Nan jing* with a third century appearance of the first *Nan jing* commentary. If we assume an Eastern Han compilation date for the *Nan jing*, there is little reason to doubt Yang Xuancao of the eighth century and the *Tai ping yu lan* of the tenth century, and to follow instead a hint by the obscure Fan Shumi of the eleventh century. Until further evidence to the contrary has come to light, I shall consider Lü Guang(wang) as a third century author.

Yang Xuancao 楊玄操, the author of the second *Nan jing* commentary, has been surrounded by much less controversy than his predecessor. Inthe closing words of the preface to his commentary, he identified himself as a district military official. He is commonly assumed to have lived during the first century of the Tang era (seventh and early eighth century) because a first reference to his work appeared in Zhang Shoujie's 張守節 *Shi ji zheng yi* 史記正義, which was written during the first half of the eighth century.[49]

Although the remark, in the Sui History, on Lü Guang(wang's) *Nan jing* commentary classified Lü's work as "lost," at least fragments of it must have come to the attention of Yang Xuancao. Yang's reference, in his preface, to his predecessor's work leaves it open as to whether Lü himself had commented on only a fraction of the *Nan jing* or whether the "missing half" had been lost in the meantime:

> [Lü's] explanations do not even comprise half of the entire [text of the *Nan jing*], the rest is missing .... I have commented on those parts [of the text] now that had not been elucidated by Mr Lü; where Mr. Lü's comments remained insufficient, I have expanded them.[50]

In addition to this commentary, Yang wrote a second treatise on the *Nan jing*, the *Ba shi yi nan yin yi* 八十一難音義, in which he analyzed, as we learn from the title of the long-lost book, "the pronunciation and meaning" of individual characters appearing in the *Nan jing*.

Yang Xuancao may have been a virtuous Confucian because his career as an official did not prevent him from continuing a profound interest in medicine. "I am very much interested in therapeutics," he wrote, "and I have always sought instruc-

---

49 Taki Mototane 1956, 81.

50 Ibid.

tion in its principles. In particular, I have been taught the contents of this classic, and I have been absorbed in its analysis for the past ten years without interruption. Although I still have not penetrated its deepest levels of meaning, I think I have been able to grasp its general message."[51]

Yang Xuancao accepted the message of the *Nan jing* without reservation. His and Lü's commentary (as well as some early Song commentaries) mark the first phase in the reception of the *Nan jing* in Chinese medical history—a phase characterized by an unquestioned faith in the *Nan jing* as the authoritative exegesis of the fundamental principles of the medicine of systematic correspondence:

> The *Huang Di Ba shi yi nan jing* was compiled by Qin Yueren from Bo hai. Yueren had been instructed by [Chang] Sang jun in his secret arts and, as a result, he understood the principles of medicine. He was quite capable of penetrating [the body with his eyes], of recognizing the long-term depots and the short-term repositories, and of opening the intestines and exposing the heart. Because he stood on one level with the Bian Que of the times of Xian Yuan, he was given the honorary name Bian Que. His home was the state of Lu. Hence he was called the "physician from Lu." Some people believe that the [physician from] Lu and Bian [Que] were two different persons. That is a mistake, though. The *Huang Di nei jing* consists of two volumes with nine chapters each. Its meaning is quite obscure, and it is extremely difficult to analyze it in its entirety. Hence Yueren selected only the most essential elements [of the *Nei jing*], and he combined its two sections in [this *Nan*]jing, with its total of eighty-one sections. [Qin Yueren] wrote scroll after scroll in order to widen access to the [principles of medicine]; he inquired about the obscure and traced out hidden meanings in order to transmit them to posterity. He called [his work] "Eighty-One Difficult Issues" because the principles [dealt with in this book] are very profound and comprehensive, and not easily understandable. [The book] contains the all-encompassing doctrine of a sage. Hence the name of Huang Di precedes [the title. The book] represents the heart and the marrow of medical literature, it is the pivot in one's rescue from disease! As one says, its author has made use of the elephant's teeth and of the unicorn's horn; he has gathered the feathers of the kingfisher male, and the down of the kingfisher female.[52]

---

51 Ibid.
52 Ibid., 80-81.

We cannot yet be totally sure, but it is quite possible that the *Nan jing* superseded the *Nei jing* as "the pivot in one's rescue from disease"—that is, as a standard work for the concepts of the medicine of systematic correspondence—and that its doctrine acquired an authoritative dominance that may have continued, in some very limited circles, well into the second millennium. It was only then, though, that the *Nan jing* received extraordinary attention among medical authors: during the Song era alone at least twenty commentaries were written, while almost no one took the pains to lay open the secrets of the more voluminous *Nei jing*. The *Su wen*, despite significant editing of the remnants available by Wang Bing 王冰 during the Tang era, appears to have been too complex and corrupt to attract the interest of practitioners. The *Ling shu*, for reasons one can only speculate about, received hardly any attention following the Tang era, if it was not lost entirely in China.

The *Nan jing* may already have reached Japan, together with the *Nei jing*, in the sixth century; Japanese authors published at least fifty commentated *Nan jing* editions in subsequent centuries.[53] A first reference to the *Nan jing* from Korea dates from the year 1058.[54] When the Mongols decided, after their invasion of China, to translate representative works from various realms of Chinese knowledge into their own language, they did not choose the *Nei jing Su wen* or *Ling shu* but selected the *Nan jing* as the sole medical classic to be rendered into Mongolian.[55] At the same time, a Persian version of the *Nan jing* appeared.[56]

Despite all this interest in the *Nan jing*, its impact obviously remained restricted to theoretical discussions and to the practice of diagnosis. Actual therapeutic practice in traditional Chinese medicine hardly followed the conceptual stringency advocated by the author of the *Nan jing*, and the conclusions drawn from the "discovery" of circulation achieved only partial recognition. To this day, physicians practicing the medicine of systematic correspondence rely almost exclusively on wrist palpation as a means for assessing the movement in the vessels. In contrast,

---

53 See appendix C.

54 Okanishi Tameto 1974, 18.

55 Walter Fuchs, "Analecta zur mongolischen Übersetzungsliteratur der Yuan Zeit," *Monumenta Serica* 11 (1946): 42. See also Herbert Franke, "Chinese Historiography under Mongol Rule," *Mongolian Studies. Journal of the Mongolian Society* 1 (1974): 23.

56 Karl Jahn, "Wissenschaftliche Kontakte zwischen Iran und China in der Mongolenzeit," *Anzeiger der phil.-hist.Kl. der Österreichischen Akademie der Wissenschaften* 106 (1969):202. It should be noted that, in addition to the *Nan jing*, the *Mai jue* 脈訣 existed in Persian translation, a work attributed to Wang Shuhe (it may have been written under Wang's name many centuries later) that has been published in China together with the *Nan jing* in numerous editions. See also Jutta Rall, "Zur persischen Übersetzng eines Mo-jue," *Oriens Extremus* 7 (1960): 152–157. I am grateful to Professor H. Franke for bringing these references to the Mongolian and Persian translations of the *Nan jing* to my attention.

actual needling therapy continues to apply "pre-circulation" concepts, in that the conduits are still pierced as if they, together with their contents, constitute twelve separate units. Could it be that the strict and consistent application of the theories of systematic correspondence advocated by the *Nan jing* failed to correspond to clinical experience? One might argue that the needling of specific points spread all over the body produces certain physiological effects that were observed and reaffirmed by Chinese clinicians and that were theorized, first, in terms of an understanding of eleven separate vessels distributed in the body (see the Mawangdui manuscripts) and, later, in terms of a belief in twelve (and more) conduits penetrating the organism. (And it may well be that these two stages were preceded by a demonological interpretation of the need for and effects of penetrating the skin with "celestial lancets".)[57] The third stage in this development (or fourth, if one includes a demonological phase)—namely, the integration of the concept of a circulation of the contents of these twelve main conduits—may have overtaxed the paradigm of systematic correspondence; it remained a theoretical achievement that was only partially accepted by practitioners (i.e., in diagnosis). Therapeutic practice—that is, circuit-needling—continued along the lines dictated by experience, not by theory. The basic contradiction in traditional Chinese medicine that resulted from this partial rejection and partial acceptance of the *Nan jing*'s level of theory and practice should be a matter of further consideration.

The fate of attempts during the Song Jin Yuan era to reconcile pharmaceutical experience and practice with the doctrines of systematic correspondence,[58] and the insignificance of the yin-yang and Five Phases theories compared to the persisting dominance of concepts not related to the paradigms of systematic correspondence in the combat of tangible disease entities (in contrast to functional disorders)—all this might be interpreted as further evidence suggesting certain limits in these theories' ability to reflect processes occurring in the real world and, hence, limits in their actual therapeutic applicability.

Such thoughts, however, may have plagued only a minority of those medical intellectuals during the Song era who took a closer look at the *Nan jing*, although some of them did find it difficult to reconcile the apparent discrepancies and contradictions between the *Nei jing* and the *Nan jing*. In this second phase in the reception of the *Nan jing* in later centuries, we witness a growing emphasis on such differences—an emphasis, though, that was combined with efforts to understand these differences as two possible expressions of one and the same issue (if not sim-

---

57 For details on a possible demonological context of early needling, see Unschuld, *Medicine in China: A History of Ideas*, section 3.3.4.

58 Ibid., section 7.2.3.

ply as errors in writing committed by later copyists). Hence the authors of this period sought to explain why the *Nei jing* and the *Nan jing* differed (in contrast to the third phase, when a tendency emerged simply to blame the author of the *Nan jing* for misunderstanding the *Nei jing* wherever the former differed from the latter).

The fourth year of the reigning period *tian sheng* 天聖 of the Northern Song (1026 CE) marks the first firm date in the history of *Nan jing* editions. According to Wang Yinglin's 王應麟 *Yu hai* 玉海, Zhao Zongjue 晁宗愨 and Wang Quanzheng 王拳正, two officials occupied with the edition of classic texts, were ordered by Emperor Ren zong to prepare a revised edition not only of the *Su wen* and the *Zhu bing yuan hou lun* 諸病源候論 but also of the *Nan jing*. In their efforts to edit the latter, they may have been joined by Wang Weiyi 王惟一, the renowned author of the *Tong ren shu xue zhen jiu tu jing* 銅人腧穴鍼灸圖經 ("Illustrated Scripture on the Transportation Holes of the Bronze Man for Needling and Cauterization") and an official of the Hanlin academy—although we lack final proof for his participation. The resulting Tiansheng edition of the *Nan jing* was published five years later, in 1031 CE, by the Imperial Academy. It has been lost in the meantime. However, a man named Li Yuanli 李元立 of the Southern Song dynasty (1127-1280) appears to have collected materials from all commentated and uncommentated *Nan jing* editions known to him (separate manuscripts with Lü's and Yang Xuancao's commentaries seem to have existed in private libraries until Yuan times),[59] and to have published them in a combined edition. This work was lost in China but was rediscovered in Japanese libraries and reprinted in Japan during the Edō period (1764-1849); it was then brought back to China.[60] The front page of the Japanese Edō edition lists the following persons and their contributions:

Qin Yueren 秦越人	author
Lü Guang 呂廣	commentated
Ding Deyong 丁德用	wrote a supplementary commentary
Yang Xuancao 楊玄操	elucidated
Yu Shu 虞庶	elucidated again
Yang Kanghou 楊康侯	continued to elucidate
Wang Jiusi 王九思	revised
Wang Zhixiang 王哲象	revised again
Shi Youliang 石友諒	pronunciation and explanation
Wang Weiyi 王惟一	revised once again

59 According to Ma Jixing's 馬繼興 *Zhong yi wen xian xue* 中医文献学, the famous Ming bibliophile, printer, and scholar Mao Jin 毛晉 (1599-1659) was still able to localize such manuscripts.

60 Okanishi Tameto 1974, 17–18.

Chinese bibliographical works, like Ruan Yuan's 阮元 *Si ku wei shou shu mu ti yao* 四庫未收書目提要, the *Si bu cong kan shu lu* 四部叢刊書錄, and Lin Heng's 林衡 *Yi cun cong shu* 依存叢書, have identified Wang Jiusi as the Wang Jiusi of the Ming History, and they have listed him, as the latest of the persons just named, as the editor responsible for this edition (the 1955 Commercial Press edition of the *Nan jing ji zhu* repeated this information). However, as Taki Mototane[61] and Ma Jixing have demonstrated,[62] the Wang Jiusi who appears as the first *Nan jing* "reviser" cannot have been the man of the same name listed in the Ming History: the birthplaces associated with the two are different; Wang Jiusi appears before Wang Weiyi in the listing quoted above; and Li Jiong 李駉, the thirteenth century Southern Song *Nan jing* commentator, spoke of "ten commentators" before him, possibly referring to the same persons listed in the *Nan jing ji zhu* edition of Li Yuanli. Still, the list of ten includes both Qin Yueren, the presumed author of the *Nan jing* (Li Jiong may have thought of him as a commentator to the *Nei jing),* and Wang Weiyi, who is not referred to anywhere else as a *Nan jing* editor or commentator. The full title of the Li Yuanli edition is *Wang Han lin ji zhu Huang Di Ba shi yi nan jing* 王翰林集注黃帝八十一難經, and it is quite possible that Wang Weiyi, the famous "Hanlin scholar Wang," was added to the list only to give this particular edition the attractive name that Li Yuanli himself did not have.

The *Nan jing ji zhu,* we may assume, combines six Song and pre-Song commentators in addition to Shi Yuliang's notes on individual characters. Unfortunately, Yang Xuancao and Yang Kanghou are both designated simply as "Yang" and—except for two instances in which the latter obviously mentions the former—their commentaries can hardly be distinguished; the contributions of Wang Jiusi and Wang Dingxiang 王鼎象 (referred to in the list as Wang Zhixiang) are not clearly differentiated, either.

Ding Deyong 丁德用 (fl. 1056-1063) is known for two medical works, including his *Nan jing* commentary and a collection of prescriptions against diseases caused by cold. He may have been the first to use graphic tables to illustrate the meaning of individual difficult issues. The preface to his *Nan jing* commentary has been preserved and should be noted for an early acknowledgment of what he terms "defects and omissions":

> Throughout the centuries, the *Nan jing* was handed on by single persons only until Hua Tuo 華佗 of the Wei [dynasty] burned the text while he was in prison. Still, the writings of [Zhang] Zhongjing 張仲景 and [Wang]

61 Taki Mototane 1956, 84.

62 Ma Jixing, *Zhong yi wen xian xue* 中医文献学, unpublished ms.

Shuhe 王叔和—who lived between the Jin and Song [dynasties]—quote this text and amply use its teachings. The Head of the Imperial Physicians of Wu, Lü Guang, has rearranged this classic; he changed its original meaning considerably. That is to say, given the fact that the remnants of the text of the *Nan jing* were rearranged in many instances under the hands of Lü Guang, it is obvious that it must be marked by defects and omissions.[63]

Yu Shu 虞庶 (fl. 1064-1067), also named in Li Yuanli's list, was a scholar who left his Confucian civil service career to study medicine; nothing is known about the background or person of Shi Youliang 石友諒.

Growing doubts developed during the Song era concerning the value of the classics in general and the classical nature of the *Nan jing* in particular; these may have prompted a number of authors to stress the authority of the *Nan jing* as a classic and to defend its views as totally in line with the wisdom of antiquity. Su Dongpo 蘇東坡, the famous poet of the eleventh century who is also known to have had a profound interest in medicine, wrote:

> The Classic of Difficult Issues in medicine is supplemented with reason in each of its sentences, and expresses laws in each of its words .... If someone puts forth new ideas and discards the old learning because—in his eyes—it is of no use, this person is either stupid or crazy! Vulgar physicians, for example, do not discuss [diseases] on the basis of the classics. They issue drug prescriptions to heal diseases, and they do indeed achieve some successes with this approach. But when it comes to diseases where one must act on the spot, and where one must arrive at a decision whether [the patient] is bound to die or will survive, in such cases they are not worth speaking about on the same day together with those who know the classics and study the old! Today's people vainly expect [the vulgar physicians] to achieve success after success, or to win out against the people in antiquity. Hence they say that one can get along without studying the *Nan jing*. This is definitely a mistake![64]

About two hundred years later, Li Jiong reiterated this emphasis on the orthodox nature of the teachings conveyed by the *Nan jing* when he stated in a preface to his own commentated *Nan jing* edition:

> The first medical classic dates back to the Yellow Thearch. The [*Nan jing*] was associated [through the wording of its title] with the Yellow Thearch

---

63 Taki Mototane 1956, 74.

64 Ibid.

in order to clarify its purpose [of elucidating difficult issues in the Yellow Thearch's classic]. From beginning to end this book is grounded on [principles] handed down [from antiquity]; it contains no personal views or strange doctrines.[65]

Concurrent with the general rejection of the "personal views and strange doctrines" associated with the so-called Song teaching, and following a renewed emphasis on the "original" Han (and pre-Han) sources of Confucianism, the many discrepancies between the *Nei jing* and the *Nan jing* began to be seen in a different light. During the first millennium, the innovations presented by the *Nan jing* appear to have been accepted as such, but the search for the "true" classics during Ming and Qing times seems to have lacked any understanding of the concept of "progress" beyond these authoritative origins of wisdom and knowledge. The *Nei jing* is the classic, it was pointed out, and what need could there be to improve on it? The extreme conservatism of the Chinese renaissance stood in fundamental contrast to the European renaissance (although occurring almost simultaneously). The latter took classic learning as a starting point for advances into ever-changing, ever-expanding realms of knowledge, while Chinese renaissance placed a final moratorium on the change and expansion of ancient theories and paradigms—a moratorium that was not observed ubiquitously but appears to have been effective enough to reverse the former Chinese lead in knowledge and technology.

Lü Fu 呂復, a Ming commentator of the *Nan jing* whose exact lifetime is unknown, signaled the transition to this third phase of the reception of the *Nan jing* in Chinese medical history. He defended the *Nan jing* as a classic and at the same time acknowledged that it was not grounded in the *Nei jing* in its entirety. The possibility that the author of the *Nan jing* may have contributed some ideas of his own in order to overcome certain deficiencies of the *Nei jing* was not an acceptable solution to the problem:

> In the thirteen chapters of the *Nan jing,* Qin Yueren has meticulously related the classic of the Yellow Thearch as if the latter had been his ancestor. He used questions and answers in order to elucidate [the classic's meaning] to its students. Of the [statements introduced by] "the scripture states" many do not correspond to the original text of the *Ling* [*shu*]or *Su* [*wen*]. Hence there must have been such a book in antiquity that was lost in the meantime.[66]

---

65 Ibid., 75.
66 Ibid., 77.

Other commentators followed Ding Deyong and blamed the discrepancies simply on errors committed by copyists of later times, on partial losses of the manuscript resulting from various catastrophes, and on faulty reconstruction attempts by later editors.

It was Xu Dachun 徐大椿, the eminent physician and author of the early eighteenth century and an outstanding representative of Han teaching in medicine, who for the first time openly denied the *Nan jing* the status of a classic. He began two essays on the *Nan jing* (both worthy of being quoted in full) with a very unambiguous statement to this effect:

> The *Nan jing* is not a classic. Its aim is to explain difficult issues in the text of the classic. Hence it poses questions concerning these difficult issues and, then, clarifies them. Therefore it is called *Nan jing*. That is to say, it provides an explanation of difficult issues (*nan*) in the text of the classic (*jing*). The purpose of this book, therefore, is to investigate the meaning of the original classic, to elucidate its final principles, to dissolve doubtful aspects, and to provide guidance for students of later times. It is, indeed, of great help for anybody who reads the *Nei jing*. However, some parts of it lack final perfection. In the dialogues, sometimes text passages from the classic are quoted for explanation where the text of the classic was quite clear originally. [In the *Nan jing*,] however, the decisive points are either omitted, or the wording of the classic is even obscured [by the commentary]. In other cases nothing is explained at all, or [the *Nan jing*] contradicts the two [books of the *Nei*] *jing*, or [the *Nan jing*] misinterprets [the *Nei jing*]. These are its shortcomings. [The *Nan jing*] contains several passages, and elucidates [a number of] subtle principles that did not appear in the *Nei jing* but that are, in fact, suitable for clarifying some obscure meanings of the *Nei jing* and for supplementing what had not been sufficiently developed in the *Nei jing*. Hence [the *Nan jing*] can be considered as an additional instruction that is well worth being handed down together with the *Nei jing* into eternity. I am not sure whether [the *Nan jing*] was compiled by Yueren. Maybe Yueren was introduced [as the author] simply to demonstrate that this book existed in antiquity. From Sui-Tang times on, [the *Nan jing*] received great attention; very many people highly appreciated it, and there was nobody to approach it critically. As a consequence, practicing physicians read the *Nan jing* and [believed it to] comprehend all the meaning of medicine. They considered [this book] to be the main stream. How could they have [known that one] penetrates even deeper [into medicine] by investigating the *Nei jing*, by searching for differences

and agreements [between the *Nan jing* and the *Nei jing*], and by seeking to discover what was a gain and what was a loss [in the compilation of the *Nan jing*]? All writings handed down through the ages have deficiencies and errors; if no one dares to criticize [these errors], they will be repeated forever. Why should the *Nan jing* be an exception?! Further details can be found in my "Explanation of the *Nan jing* on the Basis of the Classic."[67]

The *Nan jing* is not a classic; it [is a work] that takes up, in the form of questions and answers, all those subtle statements and unclear thoughts of the *Ling* [*shu*] and the *Su* [*wen*] which had underlying principles that had not been elaborated completely. In this way, [the *Nan jing*] elucidated the meaning [of the *Ling shu* and of the *Su wen*]. When the people in ancient times devised the meaning of the title of some book or treatise, they never did this without great care. When they used the term *nan*, they meant "discussion" (*bian lun* 辨論). How, on earth, could a classic be titled a "discussion"? Hence one knows that the *Nan jing* is not a classic. Since antiquity, all those who speak about medicine base their arguments on the *Nei jing*. It was only during Han times that the *Nei jing* teaching was divided [into several currents]. That is, Cang gong specialized in diagnosis, Mr. [Zhang] Zhongjing specialized in prescriptions, and Mr. Hua Tuo specialized in various methods of needling and [moxa] cauterization. None of them departed from the *Nei jing*, but each of them followed separate instructions. Beginning with the Jin and Tang era, the number of different traditions increased steadily. But [the followers of these traditions] argued merely about the techniques of medicine, not about the basic principles of medicine. Hence they departed from the sages [who wrote the *Ling shu* and the *Su wen*] more and more. The *Nan jing* remained the only work that was based entirely on the words of the *Nei jing* in order to expound the latter's meaning. Here and nowhere else did the transmission of the teaching of the sages begin.

Still, I have some doubts concerning this [work]. In some of its statements, [the *Nan jing*] provides explanations along the lines of the text in the [*Nei*] *jing*. Elsewhere, its explanations contradict the text of the classic. And, occasionally, its explanations turn the text of the classic upside down, as if [the *Nan jing*] had followed here instructions from a very different book. Someone has established here his own teachings, and it is impossible to check the origin or history [of these ideas]. They were meant to contradict the teachings of the sages entirely, but there is no basis to be used as evi-

---

67 Xu Dachun 1969, 113.

dence that they are right or wrong. If, of course, one draws on the text of the *Nei jing* itself to explain the *Nei jing*, then everything is based on the *Nei jing*. If one proves the classic with the classic, it will be obvious what is right and wrong.

The present book already has a history of more than two thousand years. Tens of authors have written commentaries on it, but none of them has ever dared to attest to its heterodox meanings. And even though, among [the statements in the *Nan jing*], there are some that are extremely dubious, the [commentators] have twisted themselves to explain them [as being rooted in the *Nei jing*]. On the contrary, they have criticized parts of this book that are correct. It is beyond my apprehension how all the people of earlier times could be so ignorant!

One reason may be that the critical study of the classics has begun only recently. All that is known so far is how to trace the history [of the classics] in order to find out their origins; if the origins cannot be discovered, [the people conducting such studies] stop in the middle of the way. So far, no one has started from the sources to trace the history. Now, if one looks at the *Nan jing* from the perspective of the *Nan jing*, there is nothing that could be criticized. If, however, one looks at the *Nan jing* from the perspective of the meaning conveyed by the *Nei jing*, then the *Nan jing* has many flaws, indeed!

In the beginning, I greatly revered this [book]. After studying it for a long time I gradually developed some doubts as to whether it might be wrong in some aspects. When I studied it even longer, I lost my faith even in [some statements] which until then I had believed must be correct. What I believe [now] is that the *Nan jing* cannot [have been written to] disobey the *Nei jing*. Hence, because it was written to elucidate difficult issues [of the *Nei jing*], I have, first of all, pointed out the basic concepts of the *Nei jing*, and I have investigated its logic structure. By adding my comments and explanations alongside the text [of the *Nan jing*], I have demonstrated where it differs from and where it agrees with [the *Nei jing*], and I have distinguished what is right and wrong [in the *Nan jing*]. Some sections [of the *Nan jing*] contain unusual patterns and strange ideas that are not based on the *Nei jing*; they serve, however, to clarify [certain statements of] the *Nei jing*. These must have come from a separate school of instructions. In some cases I had to discuss whether or not these [unusual patterns and strange ideas] can be accepted without being able to refer to [any specific statements in] the *Nei jing*. I have pointed out those sections [of the *Nan jing*] where a commentary based on the *Nei jing* would have led to contradictions and have added the necessary evidence. The *Nan jing* cannot serve as a basis for criticizing the classic. All I intend is to elucidate the [nature of the] *Nan jing* to the world and to later generations. I wish them to know that the *Nan jing* is a commentary to the *Nei jing*, with origins which reach back that far. Hence I have called [my work] *jing shi* 經釋 ("explanation on the basis of the classic"). The *Nan jing* was compiled to explain the classic; I now, in turn, use the classic to explain the *Nan* [*jing*]. If one uses the *Nan*[*jing*] to explain the classic, the [meaning of the] classic will become clear; if one uses the classic to explain the *Nan* [*jing*], the *Nan*[*jing*] will become clear. All this concerns the principles of medicine which I mentioned [in the beginning], not the techniques [of medicine].[68]

If Xu Dachun was insightful enough to acknowledge the fact that some of the *Nan jing's* "passages and principles not appearing in the *Nei jing* are suitable for clarifying some obscure meanings in the *Nei jing* and for supplementing what had not been sufficiently developed in the *Nei jing*," Liao Ping 廖平 (1851-1914?), a prolific author and medical conservative, did not indulge in such attempts to appreciate the value of the *Nan jing*. In his commentated edition of Xu Dachun's *Nan jing jing shi*, the *Nan jing jing shi bu zheng* 難經經釋補証, he blasted the *Nan jing* for its "absurdities," for its "murderous qualities," and for the "crimes" of its author which, Liao assumed, must have led to the killing of countless people by physicians who accepted the teaching of the *Nan jing* as their clinical guideline. Liao—who was the first to assign a fifth or sixth century compilation date to the *Nan jing*—also called "apocryphal" all those medical texts of the first millennium that had been influenced by the teachings of the *Nan jing*. I have included Liao Ping's views among the commentaries quoted in the present edition because they mark both an extreme opinion and the conclusion of the discussion of the merits and shortcomings of the *Nan jing* in traditional, imperial China.

Quite a few commentaries on the *Nan jing* have been published since the founding of the Republic, but they reflect a different era—an era marked by the need to defend traditional Chinese medicine against Western medicine (and to play down the internal contradictions), and by the need to reinterpret the concepts of traditional medicine in the light of Marxist ideology (thus demonstrating their value in a socialist society).

Three views, quoted in full from recent publications in the People's Republic of China, provide some insight into the current state of an ongoing discussion:

68 Ibid., preface, 1–2.

Yan Hongchen 阎洪臣 and Gao Guangzhen 高光振
on the *Nan Jing* (1978)

The original title of the *Nan jing* was *Huang Di Ba shi yi nan jing*. According to tradition it has been compiled by the famous physician Bian Que from the era of the
Warring States. The book is written as a commentary, using a question-and-answer
style. Starting from diagnosis, the long-term depots and the short-term repositories, as well as the conduits and the methods to supplement or drain, it elucidates
the central meaning of the *Nei jing*. It exerted a great influence on the medical
people of later times.

The *Nei jing* and the *Nan jing* are the most valuable items contained in the great
treasure-house of Chinese medicine and pharmacy. The rich theoretical knowledge
and the practical experience contained in these [two works] have guided all sections of Chinese medicine for the past two thousand years without interruption,
and have contributed positively not only to the development of the medicine of
mankind in its entirety but also, in particular, to the development of the medicine of
the East. As time progresses, Chinese medicine must undergo further development
too. The future development of Chinese medicine must be sought in a combination
of Chinese and Western medicine, in the generation of a new, integrated medicine
and pharmacy for China. That is the great mission bestowed on us by history. In
the course of the combination of Chinese and Western medicine, medical depart-
ments from all over the country have already undertaken great efforts, and they
have been rewarded with tremendous success. The facts prove beyond all doubt
that these recent successes have been achieved only because the foundations of the
fundamental theories of Chinese medicine expounded in the *Nei jing* and in the
Nan jing have been analyzed and combined with the positive aspects of modern
medicine. Research and analysis of the *Nei jing* and of the *Nan jing*—that is to
say, the adoption and further development of the heritage in the treasure-house of
Chinese medicine—are of extraordinarily realistic and far-reaching historical significance. Still, the compilation of the *Nei jing* and of the *Nan jing* occurred in the
distant past. Their literary style is old and creates considerable difficulties for anyone
venturing to study them. Most of all, they were influenced by the limitations of the
historical conditions in those times, and it was, therefore, unavoidable that both of
them contain a certain amount of garbage. Here a clear line of separation must be
drawn: the valuable has to be adopted; any garbage has to be eliminated. This way
it can be achieved that both [works] will exert an even stronger guiding influence.[69]

---

69 Yan Hongchen and Gao Guangzhen, Nei Nan jing xuan shi, Ji lin, 1979. 1–2 (see appen-
    dix A).

Gu Dedao 贾得道 on the *Nan Jing* (1979)

Long ago, the authorship of the *Nan jing* was ascribed to Qin Yueren (Bian Que); however, this has been doubted by many in the past because this book is mentioned neither in the Bian Que biography of the *Shi ji,* nor in the [bibliographical] section "Yi wen zhi" of the official history of the Han dynasty. The fact that the *Nan jing* was not compiled before the Western Han era can be seen most of all from its content; it was influenced, quite obviously, by the "divination" doctrines which exerted a mystifying influence on the yin-yang and Five Phases [theories]. There are some people who believe that the [*Nan jing*] was compiled during the era of the Six Dynasties; such a date, though, must be too late. First of all, a *Ba shi yi nan* was already mentioned in the author's preface to the *Shang han za bing lun* and second, the bibliographical section of the Sui History refers to a commentary of [the *Nan jing*] that was compiled by Lü Guang of the era of the Three Kingdoms. That would imply that [the *Nan jing*] cannot have been written later than during the Eastern Han. When, in more recent times, some authors have stated that this book was compiled by a person living during the time of the Eastern Han, this appears quite believable.

The *Nan jing* is a theoretical work that was compiled in an ask-about-difficult-issues style to explain an ancient medical classic; altogether the book discusses eighty-one problems. Hence its title is "Eighty-One Difficult Issues." Most of the problems discussed were taken from the *Nei jing*; they include pulse diagnosis, the conduits, the long-term depots and the short-term repositories, the transportation holes, needling, and a section on diseases. In the section on pulse diagnosis, the *san bu jiu hou* 三部九候 of the *Nei jing* are interpreted as the three sections (*san bu* 三部)—inch, gate, and foot—of the inch opening, each of which has three indicator [levels] (*san hou* 九候) called "near the surface," "center," and "in the depth." That reflects a concentration of pulse diagnosis on the one location of the inch opening. Inthe section on the conduits, the doctrine of the "eight single-conduit vessels" appears for the first time. Also, [this section] contains a relatively systematic explanation [of the system of conduits], thus eliminating a weakness of the *Nei jing,* where [this particular subject was treated] in a rather disorderly fashion. In the section on the long-term depots and short-term repositories, [the *Nan jing*] introduced the doctrine "the left kidney is the kidney, the right kidney is the gate of life," and it emphasized the function of the so-called moving qi between the kidneys. In this way, it laid the foundation for the "gate of life" theories of later centuries. In addition, [the *Nan jing*] introduced the doctrine "the Triple Burner has a name but no physical appearance," thus initiating a senseless and unproductive struggle that continued for more than a thousand years. In the section on diseases, [the *Nan jing*] differentiated [the disease] "harm caused by cold" into five kinds—namely, "to be struck by wind," "to be harmed by cold," "[to be harmed by] moisture and warmth," "heat diseases," and "warmth diseases." Also, with respect to accumulation diseases, it distinguished between those occurring in the long-term depots and those occurring in the short-term repositories, maintaining that the long-term depots are subject to *ji*-accumulations while the short-term repositories may be subject to *zhu*-accumulations. Furthermore, [this section] contains references to names and symptoms of accumulations in the five long-term depots. With regard to needling, [the *Nan jing*] introduced the principle "in the case of a depletion, supplement its mother; in the case of a repletion, drain its child." All of these [doctrines] exerted a significant influence on the development of Chinese medicine.

And yet, because this book itself had been influenced by "divinatory" doctrines, it has spread quite a lot of mystical and obscure poison by making absurd statements such as "male infants are born in *yin* 寅[periods], and belong to the yang; female infants are born in *shen* 申 [periods], and belong to the yin"; "when the vessels lose the yang, one sees demons"; "metal is generated in *ji* 己 [periods], wood is generated in *shen* 申 [periods], drain the fire in the South, replenish the water in the North"; and also when it discusses the question of why the liver—which is associated with the [phase of] wood—is located in the lower [section of the body] and why the lung—which is associated with the [phase of] metal—is located in the upper [section of the body], although wood floats on water while metal sinks down, and so on. All such [statements] exerted a horrible influence on the healthy development of the theories of Chinese medicine.

In conclusion one may say that, by and large, the *Nan jing* serves to explain the *Nei jing;* it does not contain anything really new. Those elements that were introduced by this book are, as indicated above, partly useful, partly harmful; they contain minor positive and major negative aspects. Hence it would be quite inappropriate to assign too great a value to this book or to rank it together with the *Nei jing* and call it a "classic."[70]

The Teaching and Research Staff For Ancient Literature
at the Shanghai College of Chinese Medicine on the *Nan Jing* (1980)

Another name for the *Nan jing* is *Huang Di Ba shi yi nan jing.* The entire book was written in a question-and-answer style; it discusses eighty-one medical issues from the areas of physiology, pathology, diagnosis, and therapy. It is concerned mainly with an explanation of the most important contents of the *Nei jing.* The content [of the *Nan jing*] is rich; its wording is concise. It contains comprehensive theoretical treatises, and it offers innovative concepts when it introduces, for instance, the

---

70 Gu Dedao 贾得道, *Zhong guo yi xue shi lüe* 中国医学史略, Taiyuan 1979. 87–88.

technique of "using only the inch opening" for diagnosing the [movement in the] vessels, or when it states "the yang network [vessel] is the network [vessel] of the yang walker; the yin network [vessel] is the network [vessel] of the yin walker." The *Nan jing* enjoyed great appreciation by the physicians at all times; together with the *Nei jing* it is called the classic of medicine. It is an important medical book of our country's ancient times.[71]

---

71 Anonymous collective (the teaching and research staff for ancient literature at the Shanghai College of Chinese Medicine), *Gu dai yi xue wen xuan* 古代医学文献, Shanghai, 1980. 24.

PART II
TEXT, TRANSLATION, COMMENTARIES, AND NOTES

Preliminary Note

The oldest version of the *Nan jing* documented today is probably Li Jiong's edition of 1269; it is preserved in the *zheng tong* 正统 edition of the *Dao zang* 道藏 of the mid-fifteenth century. If not marked otherwise, I have made use of the *Dao zang* version as the basis of the present edition. The textual differences among the *Dao zang* version and other early editions available today (such as the 1590 printing of Hua Shou's *Nan jing ben yi* or the 1472 Japanese printing of Xiong Zongli's *Wu ting zi su jie Ba shi yi nan jing*) are almost negligible (references to those differences will be found in the Notes). It is difficult to state whether all the editions extant date back to one common source compiled later than the original *Nan jing*, or to the original *Nan jing* itself.

To present a translation as true to the original Chinese text as possible, I have put in brackets all additions necessitated in English by the succinctness of the original Chinese wording. Hence, by reading between the brackets the reader will gain an idea of the original style of the *Nan jing*.

Altogether, twenty commentators are quoted. The numbers to the left of their names in the Commentaries section of each difficult issue refer to the sentences or groups of sentences marked with corresponding numbers in the Chinese and English versions of the *Nan jing* text. Wherever several authors are quoted on one and the same sentence or group of sentences in the *Nan jing*, their comments are listed in chronological order. The names of the commentators quoted, the dates of their original writings, and the editions of their works used here are as follows (for details and Chinese characters, see appendix A):

Commentator	Date of Writing	Editions used
Lü Guang(wang)	3d c.	1. *Nan jing ji zhu.*
Yang Xuancao	7/8th c.	*Si bu bei yao* 四部备要, Taibei 1973
Ding Deyong	1062	2. *Nan jing ji zhu.*
Yu Shu	1067	Ed. Qian Xizuo 錢熙祚
Yang Kanghou	1098	*(19th c.), Shanghai 1955*

(Yang Xuancao and Yang Kanghou were quoted as Yang in the *Nan jing ji zhu;* except for a few passages it is impossible to identify which of the two Yangs is the author of a specific comment.)

Commentator	Date	Editions used
Li Jiong	1269	*Huang Di ba shi yi nan jing zuan tu ju jie Zheng tong dao zang* 正統道藏, Taibei 1977
Hua Shou (with quotations from commentaries by Ji Tianxi, Chen Siming [i.e., Chen Ruisun], and Xie [Jinsun?])	1361	1. *Nan jing ben yi Yi tong zheng mai quan shu* 醫統正脈全書, Taibei 1975 2. *Bian Que Nan jing Gu jin tu shu ji cheng* 古今圖書集成, Taibei 1958
Zhang Shixian	1510	*Jiao zheng tu zhu ba shi yi nan jing* n.p. (Hong bao zhai shu ju 鴻寶齋書局) 1912
Xu Dachun	1727	*Nan jing jing shi Xu Lingtai yi shu quan ji* 徐霛胎醫書全集, Taibei 1969
Ding Jin	1736	*Gu ben nan jing chan zhu* *Zhen ben yi shu ji cheng*
Katō Bankei	1784	*Nan jing gu yi* Taibei 1971
Ye Lin	1895	*Nan jing zheng yi* 珍本醫書集成
Tamba Genkan (alias Taki Mototane)	1819	*Nan jing shu cheng*, Gao xiong 1961
Liao Ping	1913	*Nan jing jing shi bu zheng Liu yi guan cong shu* 六譯舘叢書, n.p. 1913
Wang Yiren	1936	*Nan jing du ben*, Taibei 1973
Nan jing	1962	*Nan jing yi shi*, Nan jing 1962
Huang Weisan	1969	*Nan jing zhi yao*, Taibei 1969

Chapter One
The Movement in the Vessels and Its Diagnostic Significance

THE FIRST DIFFICULT ISSUE

一難曰：（一）動脈，（二）獨取寸口，以決五藏六府死生吉凶之法，何謂也？
（三）然：寸口者，脈之大會，手太陰之脈動也。（四）人一呼脈行三寸，一
吸脈行三寸，呼吸定息，脈行六寸。（五）人一日一夜，凡一萬三千五百
息，脈行五十度，周於身。漏水下百刻，榮衛行陽二十五度，行陰亦二十
五度，為一周也，故五十度復會於手太陰。寸口者，五藏六府之所終始，
故法取於寸口也。

The first difficult issue: (1) All the twelve conduits have [sections where the] move-ment [in these] vessels¹ [can be felt]. (2) Still, one selects only the inch opening in order to determine whether the [body's] five long-term depots and six short-term repositories [harbor a] pattern² of death or life, of good or evil auspices. What does that mean?

(3) It is like this. The inch opening constitutes the great meeting point of the [con-tents passing through] the vessels; it is the [section of the] hand major yin [conduit where the] movement [in that] vessel [can be felt]. (4) When a [normal] person ex-hales once, [the contents of] the vessels proceed three inches; when [a normal per-son] inhales once, [the contents of] the vessels proceed three inches [too]. Exhaling and inhaling [constitute one] breathing [period]. During this period, [the contents of] the vessels proceed six inches. (5) A person, in the course of one day and one

---

1   The term *dong mai* 動脈 may have originated at a time when the *mai* 脈 in the body were still considered to be thread-like entities, displaying a throbbing movement. Here, in the *Nan jing* and its commentaries, *mai* is generally used in the sense of hollow ves-sels through which specific contents move. The movement in these vessels also causes a movement of the vessels themselves which can be felt at specific locations. Thus, *dong mai* refers here to sections of the body's vessels where the movement in the vessels can be felt as a movement of these vessels themselves. The first difficult issue focuses on the question of which *dong mai* should be selected for diagnostic purposes. See also note 3.

2   *Fa* 法 ("pattern") could also be rendered as "method": "The [diagnostic] method of only selecting the inch opening in order to determine whether the five long-term depots and six short-term repositories [harbor] death or life, good or evil auspices; what does that mean?"

night, breathes altogether 13,500 times. [During that time, the contents of] the vessels proceed through 50 passages. [That is,] they circulate through the body [in the
period needed by] the [clepsydra's] dripping water to move down by 100 markings.
The camp and the guard [qi] proceed through 25 passages [during a] yang [period],
and they proceed through 25 passages [during a] yin [period]. This constitutes one
cycle. Because [the contents of the vessels] meet again, after 50 passages, with the
inch opening, [this section] is the beginning and the end of [the movement of the
contents of the vessels through the body's] five long-term depots and six short-term
repositories. Hence, the pattern [of death or life, of good or evil auspices harbored
by the body's five long-term depots and six short-term repositories] is obtained
from the inch opening.³

---

3   This difficult issue raises several questions which were discussed by commentators in
    subsequent centuries. They include: (1) The restrictive advice of taking one's diagnostic
    information from examining the movement in the vessels only at the wrist. We witness
    here the controversy around the emergence of pulse diagnosis as it is commonly applied
    by practitioners of Chinese medicine today. The conceptual issue to be solved was diffi-
    cult. Originally (as documented by the Ma wang dui texts), eleven or twelve independent
    vessels were recognized as permeating the body; they were not seen as part of a circulato-
    ry system, and their contents moved up and down or suffered from repletion or depletion
    individually. All of these independent vessels had their respective diseases and symptoms,
    and to examine their respective condition, each had to be examined individually. Then,
    at some time during the second century BCE, all conduit vessels were realized to be
    linked by network vessels, allowing for a continuous circulation of their contents through
    the entire system. This conceptual innovation appears to have stimulated the idea that
    it was sufficient to examine the flow in these vessels at but one location. Various discus-
    sions between the Yellow Thearch and his advisers documented in the *Nei jing* reflect the
    initial uncertainty about whether this was indeed the case. A problem resulting from a
    concentration on but one location was the necessity of finding a method for determining
    the individual conditions of the twelve functional units constituting the organism, all of
    which were now known to be passed by the contents of the vessels. The first 22 chap-
    ters of the *Nan jing* are devoted to this issue; they reflect an increasing sophistication,
    achieved by inductive logic, (a) in the differentiation of various longitudinal sections and
    different levels of the one location selected for diagnosis, (b) in distinguishing differences
    in the kinds of movement to be felt, and (c) in associating all of these parameters with
    categories of the yinyang and Five Phases paradigms. (2) The meaning of the term *hui*
    會 ("meeting-point"). It is not clear from the wording of the *Nan jing* (a) whether its
    author(s) believed, in fact, that all conduit vessels "meet" at the inch opening in the wrist,
    (b) whether they conceptualized different streams of qi, associated with the different
    functional units, as passing on different levels within one vessel, or (c) whether they saw
    one stream of qi within one vessel but alternating its speed and location (for instance,
    "in the depth" or "near the surface"), thus reflecting specific conditions of the organism.
    Commentators debating this issue appear to have represented all three of these under-
    standings, which seem to be transitional consequences related to the conceptual move
    from the individual conduits to a circulatory system. Most authors agreed, however, in
    their interpretation of the term *hui* in the sense of "returning to an origin," thus excluding
    the first of the three understandings just listed. (3) The meaning of the phrase *xing yang*

(1) *Lü Guang*: These are the twelve vessels of the conduits in the hands and feet. The movement of the foot major yang [conduit can be felt] in the bend [of the knee]. The movement of the foot minor yang [conduit can be felt] in front of the ear.

Yang: This is the *xia guan* 下關 hole. [This conduit's] movement can also [be felt] at the *xian zhong* 縣鍾 [hole].

Lü Guang: The movement of the foot yang brilliance [conduit can be felt] above the instep.

Yang: This is the *chong yang* 衝陽 hole which is located above the instep, hence its name. [This conduit's] movement can also [be felt] in the neck at the *ren ying* 人迎 [hole] and also at the *da ying* 大迎 [hole].

Lü Guang: The movement of the hand major yang [conduit can be felt] at the outer corner of the eye.

Yang: This is the *tong zi jiao* 瞳子窌 hole.

Lü Guang: The movement of the hand minor yin [conduit can be felt] at the *ke zhu ren* 客主人 [hole].

Yang: [This conduit's] movement can also [be felt] at the *ting hui* 聽會 [hole].

Lü Guang: The movement of the hand yang brilliance [conduit can be felt] at the corner of the mouth.

Yang: This is the *di cang* 地倉 hole.

Lü Guang: [This conduit's] movement can also [be felt] at the *yang xi* 陽谿 [hole]. The movement of the foot ceasing yin [conduit can be felt] at the *ren ying* 人迎 [hole].

Yang: The *ren ying* [hole] is located on the foot yang brilliance vessel, not on the foot ceasing yin [vessel]. When Lü states that the ceasing yin [vessel's] movement [can be felt] at the *ren ying* [hole], that is a mistake. At the *ren ying* [hole] one may examine the qi of all the five long-term depots; the movement there is not caused by the ceasing yin [vessel] only. The ceasing yin vessel's movement [can be felt] at the *hui gu* 回骨 [hole].

Lü Guang: The movement [of the] foot minor yin [conduit can be felt] below the inner ankle.

---

er shi wu du xing yin er shi wu du 行陽二十五度行陰二十五度 created a debate in that commentators could not agree on the meaning of yang and yin here. Among the explanations offered were yang and yin sections of the body, "day" and "night," and yang and yin sections of a year. For source materials related to the first difficult issue, cf. the *Nei jing* treatises *Ling shu* 10, "Jing mai" 經脈; 15, "Wu shi ying" 五十營; 18, "Ying wei sheng hui" 營衛生會; 62, "Yun shu" 運輸; 76, "Wei qi xing" 衛氣行; and *Su wen*, "Yin yang bie lun" 陰陽別論; 17, "Mai yao jing wei lun" 脈要精微論; 19, "Yu ji zhen zang lun" 玉機真藏論; 21, "Jing mai bie lun" 經脈別論.

Yang: This is the *tai xi* 太谿 hole. The movement [that can be felt] here is not [caused by] the minor yin vessel. The movement [of the] throughway vessel [can be] felt here. The throughway vessel and the minor yin [vessel] run parallel here. Hence, [Lü] states that the minor yin vessel's movement [can be felt] here. In fact, this is not so. This is yet another of the errors committed by Mr. Lü, the movement of the minor yin vessel [can be felt] within five inches above the inner ankle.

Lü Guang: The movement of the foot major yin [conduit can be felt] above the thigh.

Yang: This is the *ji men* 箕門 hole.

Lü Guang: The movement of the hand minor yin [conduit can be felt] below the armpit.

Yang: This is the *ji quan* 極泉 hole. [This conduit's] movement can also [be felt] at the *ling dao* 靈道 [hole] and at the *shao hai* 少海 [hole].

Lü Guang: The movement of the hand heart ruler [conduit can be felt] at the *lao gong* 勞宮 [hole]. The movement of the hand major yin [conduit can be felt] at the *da yuan* 大淵 [hole].

Yang: [This conduit's] movement can also [be felt] at the *chi ze* 尺澤 [hole], at the *xia bai* 俠白 [hole], and at the *tian fu* 天府 [hole].

Ding Deyong: [The statement] "all the twelve conduits have [sections where the] movement [in these] vessels [can be felt]" refers to the three yin and three yang conduits in each of the two hands and feet. Each of them contains, in correspondence to heaven and earth, the three yin and three yang qi. When it is said [elsewhere] that the three yin and three yang [qi] of heaven and earth all have a specific time [of the year] during which they rule, [this is as follows]. The ninety days from after spring equinox to before summer solstice are ruled by the three yang [qi] of heaven. The ninety days from after summer solstice to before autumn equinox are ruled by the three yin [qi] of heaven. The ninety days from after autumn equinox to before winter solstice are ruled by the three yin [qi] of the earth. The ninety days from after winter solstice to before spring equinox are ruled by the yang [qi] of the earth. Everywhere to the left or right, above or below, do these three yin and three yang qi exist; they add up to twelve qi. Hence, man also has twelve conduits. [The qi passing through these conduits] rule [his body's] left and right, upper and lower sections. The section above man's diaphragm is ruled by the three yin and three yang [conduits] of the hands; they are penetrated by the qi of heaven. The section below the diaphragm is ruled by the three yin and three yang [conduits] of the feet; they are penetrated by the qi of the earth. The passage of the qi of heaven [through the body] accounts for the generation of qi and for [their movement through] the vessels; the passage of the qi of the earth [through the body] is responsible for the transformation of [substances carrying] flavor into form. Hence, the twelve conduits pass yin and yang [qi]; they move the qi and the blood. Furthermore, *jing* 經 ("conduit") stands for *jing* 徑 ("direct way"). The [conduits] transmit [their contents] by pouring them into each other, and there is no place [in the body] which is not penetrated by them. This is why the Yellow Thearch has stated: The twelve conduits house all diseases. It is essential to know them in order [to be able] to judge [whether a person's disease will end in] death or survival. When [the *Nan jing*] states that all the twelve conduits have [sections where the] movement [in these] vessels [can be felt], that refers to the three sections at both hands where vessels are located whose movement can [be felt]. The inch section at the left hand[4] is where the movement of the vessels of the heart and of the small intestine appear. The vessel of the heart is called hand minor yin [conduit]; the vessel of the small intestine is called hand major yang [conduit]. Both of them correspond to the ruler fire of the South-East; they are included in the [diagram] *sun* 巽. The gate-section at the left hand is where the movement of the vessels of liver and gall bladder appears. The vessel of the liver is called foot ceasing yin [conduit]; the vessel of the gall bladder is called foot minor yang [conduit]. Both of them correspond to the wood of the East; they are included in the [diagram] *zhen* 震. The foot section at the left hand is where the movement of the vessels of the kidneys and of the urinary bladder appears. The vessel of the kidneys is called foot minor yin [conduit]; the vessel of the urinary bladder is called foot major yang [conduit]. Both of them correspond to the water of the North; they are included in the diagram *kan* 坎. The inch section at the right hand is where the movement of the lung and of the large intestine appears. The vessel of the lung is called hand major yin [conduit]; the vessel of the large intestine is called hand yang brilliance [conduit]. Both of them correspond to the metal of the West; they are included in the [diagram] *dui* 兌. The gate-section at the right hand is where the movement of the vessels of the spleen and of the stomach appears. The vessel of the spleen is called foot major yin [conduit]; the vessel of the stomach is called foot yang brilliance [conduit]. Both of them correspond to the soil of the center; they are included in the [diagram] *kun* 坤. The foot section at the right hand is where the movement of the vessels of the heart enclosing network and of the Triple Burner appears. The [vessel of the] heart enclosing network is called hand ceasing yin[conduit]; the vessel of the Triple Burner is

---

4 For a discussion of the inch, gate, and foot sections at the wrist, see difficult issue 2 and its commentaries.

called hand minor yang [conduit]. Both of them correspond to the minister fire
of the South; they are included in the [diagram] *li* 離. Because the movement of
the vessels appears at these three sections [of both hands], the [*Nan*] *jing* states:
"All [the twelve conduits] have [sections where the] movement [in these] vessels
[can be felt]."

Yu Shu: In their comments, Lü and Yang have in all instances picked holes from
which the flow of the respective conduit vessels proceeds. When they call these
[holes sections where the] movement of the vessels [can be felt], this does not
correspond to the meaning further down in the text of the [*Nan*] *jing* itself,
namely to solely rely on the inch opening. Thus, [I] shall take up this issue now.
The scripture states: The vessels meet at the *da yuan* 大淵 [hole]. The *da yuan*
[hole] is located in between behind the palm and the fish-line[5] of both hands.
Now, this is where the movement of the hand major yin vessel [appears]. The
[long-term depot associated with the hand] major yin [conduit] is responsible
for the qi. Thus one knows that the twelve conduit vessels meet at the *da yuan*
[hole]. Hence, the sages have defined this important meeting point of the vessels as being located in between the palm and the fish-line of both hands. [This
area] is divided into three sections, named inch, foot, and gate. In these three
sections one examines the movement of the vessels in order to know about [a
person's] pathological conditions of depletion and repletion, of cold and heat, as
they may have affected his five long-term depots and six short-term repositories.
That is to say, one single conduit has an interior and an exterior [section]; those
[qi] that come are yang; those that go are yin. Together, both hands have six
sections. In these six sections are united, altogether, twelve conduits. The principle behind this has become obvious now. Through checking the yang [qi] one
knows the place where a disease is located; through checking the yin [qi] one
knows the schedule of death and life. Hence, [the text] states: "All the twelve
conduits have [sections where the] movement [in these] vessels [can be felt]."

Li Jiong: *Jing* 經 ("conduit") stands for *jing* 徑 ("direct way"), and for *chang* 常
("regular"); it refers to "direct roads which are passed regularly." These are the
three yin and three yang [conduits] of the hands and the three yin and three
yang [conduits] of the feet – [namely,] the hand minor yin conduit of the heart,
the hand major yang conduit of the small intestine, the foot ceasing yin conduit
of the liver, the foot minor yang conduit of the gall bladder, the foot minor yin
conduit of the kidneys, the foot major yang conduit of the urinary bladder, the
hand major yin conduit of the lung, the hand yang brilliance conduit of the
large intestine, the foot major yin conduit of the spleen, the foot yang brilliance

_____
5   The "fish-line" is the borderline between palm and lower arm.

conduit of the stomach, the hand ceasing yin conduit of the heart enclosing network, and the hand minor yang conduit of the Triple Burner. All the twelve conduits just listed have a breathing in these vessels which takes the shape of a movement.

Hua Shou: "The twelve conduits" refers to the three yin and three yang [conduits] of the hands and feet, which add up to twelve conduits ... [here follows an outline of the twelve conduits similar to that provided by Ding Deyong and Li Jiong]. "They all have [sections where the] movement [in the] vessels [can be felt]" means the following]. The movement of the hand major yin vessel [appears] in the *zhong fu* 中府, *yun men* 雲門, *tian fu* 天府, and *xia bai* 俠白 [holes]. The movement of the hand yang brilliance vessel [appears] in the *he gu* 合谷 and *yang xi* 陽谿 [holes]. The movement of the hand minor yin vessel [appears] at the *ji quan* 極泉 [hole]. The movement of the hand major yang vessel [appears] at the *tian chuang* 天窗 [hole]. The movement of the hand ceasing yin vessel [appears] at the *lao gong* 勞宮 [hole]. The movement of the hand minor yang vessel [appears] at the *he jiao* 禾窌 [hole]. The movement of the foot major yin vessel [appears] at the *ji men* 箕門 and at the *chong men* 衝門 [holes]. The movement of the foot yang brilliance vessel [appears] at the *chong yang* 衝陽, *da ying* 大迎, *ren ying* 人迎, and *qi chong* 氣衝 [holes]. The movement of the foot minor yin vessel [appears] at the *tai xi* 太谿 and *yin gu* 陰谷 [holes]. The movement of the foot major yang vessel [appears] at the *wei zhong* 委中 [hole]. The movement of the foot ceasing yin vessel [appears] at the *tai chong* 太衝, *wu li* 五里, and *yin lian* 陰廉 [holes]. The movement of the foot minor yang vessel [appears] at the *xia guan* 下關 and *ting hui* 聽會 [holes] .... The meaning conveyed by Yueren's [question] is that all the twelve conduits have [sections where the] movement [in these] vessels [appears at the surface and can be felt] as are listed above. Now, however, [these sections are not] used any longer and one has selected only the inch opening in order to determine auspicious or inauspicious signs in the short-term repositories and long-term depots indicating death or survival. Why is that so?

Xu Dachun: This first difficult issue does not correspond to [the contents of] the *Ling* [*shu*] and of the *Su* [*wen*]. In the [treatise] "San bu jiu hou lun" 三部九候論 of the *Su wen*, it is made clear that all the vessels [the] movement [of which can be felt] at the head and in the face constitute the upper three sections, that the vessels [the] movement [of which can be felt] at both hands constitute the central three sections, and that the vessels [the] movements [of which can be felt] at the thighs and feet constitute the lower three sections. Also, the [movement in the] vessel at the *ren ying* 人迎 [hole] at the side of the larynx is often considered to be as important as [that felt at] the inch opening. The two scriptures do not agree in their discussions of this [issue]. To take advantage of only the inch opening is a doctrine of Yueren. From his time on the diagnostic methods have been subtle,[6] yet they have never been put in order .... A further comment on the *dong mai* 動脈 ("locations where the movement in a vessel can be felt") of the twelve conduits. Books like the *Ming tang zhen jiu tu* 明堂鍼灸 圖 and the *Jia yi jing* 甲乙經 refer to more than twenty holes as *dong mai*. However, the movement [at these locations] differs slightly from that [which can be felt] at the inch opening. In the treatise "Yun shu" 運輸 of the *Ling shu*, the Thearch asked why among the twelve conduit vessels only the hand major yin, the foot minor yin, and the [foot] yang brilliance [conduits display] a ceaseless movement. In his subsequent reply Qi Bo pointed out that only three holes can be called *dong mai* and may, therefore, be used for diagnostic purposes; these include the *jing qu* 經渠 [hole] of the major yin [conduit], the *tai xi* 太谿 [hole] of the minor yin [conduit], and the *ren ying* 人迎 [hole] of the yang brilliance [conduit]. The remaining [holes display a] movement that is so weak that it can be used for nothing but to test whether [a specific location] is indeed a true hole [that can be used for therapeutic piercing] or not. They do not deserve the name *dong mai*.

(2) *Ding Deyong*: The examination method of taking [one's information] solely from the inch opening is based on lowering the index finger [at that specific location. The various kinds of movement in the vessels that can be felt there] include the following: high, low, left, right,[7] long, short, near the surface, in the depth, smooth, rough, slow, and frequent. [These movements allow one] to recognize whether a disease has good or evil auspices. This method constitutes the essential meaning of the Yellow Thearch's "subtle discussions of the important aspects of [examining] the vessels."[8] Yueren has chosen this treatise to be the first among all the others [of his book]. In ancient times the Yellow Thearch asked: "What are the laws of diagnosis?" Qi Bo responded: "The laws of diagnosis [are as follows]. As a rule, it is at dawn, before the yin qi has begun its movement,[9]

---

6   Liao Ping suggested that *jing* 精 ("subtle") should be replaced by *luan* 亂 ("chaotic").

7   "Left, right" is unclear here. The terms could refer to movements that can be felt in the left or right half of a vessel.

8   Title of *Su wen* treatise 17, "Mai yao jing wei lun" 脈要精微論, from which the following dialogue between the Yellow Thearch and Qi Bo is quoted.

9   "Yin qi" may refer to the qi of the earth; they dominate at night and move back into the earth at dawn. Wang Bing, in his commentary to *Su wen* treatise 17, explained *dong* 動 ("to move") as "a descending movement" (*dong er jiang bei* 動而降卑).

before the yang qi is dispersed,[10] before beverages and food have been consumed, before the conduit vessels are filled to abundance, when the [contents of the] network vessels are balanced, before the qi and the blood move in disorder, that, hence, one can diagnose an abnormal [movement in the] vessels. Squeeze the vessels [to determine whether their movement] is excited or quiet, and observe the essence brilliance. Investigate the five complexions. Observe whether the five depots have a surplus or an insufficiency, whether the six short-term repositories are strong or weak, and whether the physical appearance is marked by abundance or decays. All this is brought together to reach a conclusion [concerning] a differentiation between [the patient's] death and survival." Here, only the method [to check] the inch opening has been taken [into consideration].

Li Jiong: The distance of one inch from the fish-line bone [toward the elbow] is called inch opening. Liver, heart, spleen, lung, and kidneys are the five long-term depots; gall bladder, stomach, large intestine, small intestine, urinary bladder, and Triple Burner are the six short-term repositories.

Hua Shou: *Cun kou* 寸口 ("inch opening") stands for *qi kou* 氣口 ("qi opening"). It is located in the distance of one inch from the fish-line on the hand minor yin [conduit]. The [sections] below the qi opening are called "gate" and "foot." They all represent locations touched by the hand major yin [conduit], and this hand major yin [conduit] itself constitutes the beginning of the convergence of the flow in the hundred vessels.

(3) *Lü Guang*: The major yin [conduit] is the vessel of the lung. The lung is the cover above all the long-term depots; it is responsible for the penetration of yin and yang [qi through the body]. Hence, all the twelve conduits meet at the inch opening of the hand major yin [conduit]. One uses [the inch opening] to determine good or evil auspices because if any of the twelve conduits has a disease, one observes the inch opening and may know which conduit's movement [prevails]. It may be at the surface or in the depth, smooth or rough; it may be contrary to or in accordance with the seasons, and [from all this] one knows whether [the patient] will die or survive.

Yu Shu: [Food items carrying] the five flavors enter the stomach. There they are transformed to generate the five qi. The five flavors are sweet, salty, bitter, sour, and acrid; the five qi are rank, frowzy, aromatic, burned, and foul.[11] These are the

---

10 "Yang qi" may refer to the qi of heaven; they dominate during the daytime. Wang Bing, ibid., explained *san* ("to disperse") as "dispersing and emerging" (*san bu er chu* 散布而出).

11 *Su wen* treatise 9, "Liu jie zang xiang lun" 六節藏象論, states: "Heaven feeds man with the five qi; earth feeds man with the five flavors." Wang Bing commented: "Fetid qi accumulate in the liver; burned qi accumulate in the heart; aromatic qi accumulate in the spleen; frowzy qi accumulate in the lung; foul qi accumulate in the kidneys .... Sour flavor

qi and flavors [associated with] the Five Phases. After the flavors have been transformed into qi, [the latter] are transmitted [from the stomach] upward into the hand major yin [conduit]. The major yin [conduit] is responsible for the qi. It receives the five qi in order to pour them into the five long-term depots. If the stomach loses its harmony, it cannot transform [flavor into] qi. As a consequence, there is nothing for the hand major yin [conduit] to receive. Hence, from [examining at] the inch opening [whether the movement in the vessels is] at the surface or in the depth, whether it is extensive or short, smooth or rough, one can know in which long-term depot a disease has developed. This is why the scripture states: "The inch opening constitutes the great meeting point of [all] the vessels."

Li Jiong: This inch opening is the inch opening of the hand major yin vessel of the right hand [below] the index finger.

Liao Ping: The vessels do not meet at the inch opening. The "great meeting" referred to in the [treatise] "Ying wei yun xing"[12] 營衛運行 refers to nothing but the [convergence of the] camp and guard [qi at midnight]. All the vessels follow their respective courses; at no time do they meet [anywhere].

(4) *Lü Guang*: The twenty-seven qi in the twelve conduits and fifteen network [vessels] all show up at the inch opening. According to exhalation and inhalation they move up and down. During exhalation, the [contents of the] vessels move three inches upward; during inhalation, the [contents of the] vessels move three inches downward. Exhalation and inhalation are defined as breathing [period; during this time the contents of] the vessels move six inches. All the twenty-seven qi move upward and downward accordingly. As long as one is awake, they proceed through the body; when one is asleep, they proceed through the long-term depots. At no time does [this movement] stop.

(5) *Lü Guang*: When a [normal] person breathes once, the [contents of his] vessels move six inches. During ten breathing [periods the contents of] his vessels move six feet. During 100 breathing [periods, the contents of] his vessels move six *zhang* 丈. During 1,000 breathing [periods the contents of] his vessels move 60 *zhang*. During 10,000 breathing [periods the contents of] his vessels move 600 *zhang*. During 13,500 breathing [periods the contents of his vessels move] altogether 810 *zhang*. This constitutes one cycle. The yang vessels face toward outside and [the contents] proceed through them twenty-five times. The yin

---

enters the liver; bitter flavor enters the heart; sweet flavor enters the spleen; acrid flavor enters the lung; salty flavor enters the kidneys." For a further discussion of the role of odors in the organism, see difficult issue 34.

12   Liao Ping appears to refer here to *Ling shu* treatise 18, "Ying wei sheng hui."

vessels face toward inside and the [contents] proceed through them twenty-five times, too. Together this adds up to 50 passages. With exhalation and inhalation, yin and yang [qi] repeat their circulation [through the body] until the [standard] number of passages has been completed. After the [contents of the] vessels have completed their circulation through the body, the clepsydra's dripping water has completed 100 markings, too. That is to say, in the course of one day and one night, the dripping water has completed its markings. The brilliant sun of heaven emerges from the East; the [contents of the] vessels return to the inch opening, from which they begin [their course] anew. Hence, [the text] states: "The inch opening is the beginning and the end of [the movement of the contents of the vessels through the body's] five long-term depots and six short-term repositories."

Ding Deyong: According to older comments on the [*Nan*] *jing*, the breathings [of one day cause the contents of] the vessels [to move] 810 *zhang*. While the [clepsydra's] water moves down by two markings, [the contents of the vessels] achieve one passage circulating through the body. When [the water has moved down by] 100 markings, the circulation [of the contents of the vessels] through the body has completed 50 passages. If this were so, [the contents of the vessels] would proceed 50 times through the yang and 50 times through the yin [sections of the body]. This, however, differs greatly from the meaning of the scripture. In the scripture it is stated: "They proceed 25 times in the yang and they proceed 25 times in the yin. This amounts to 50 passages after which they meet again." This so-called passing through the yang and passing through the yin refers to the yin and yang [sections] of one year. [The year] begins [its course] with "spring begins." It passes through the seasons consecutively until, finally, it meets with "spring begins" again. Hence, [the contents of the vessels] pass through a total of 50 passages. Light and darkness of the day, as well as man's being awake or asleep, all of this [starts] at dawn. A day proceeds through 24 hours and then it meets with this [time of the morning] again. Man's qi start [their course] at the Central Burner, from which they flow into the hand major yin [conduit]. Then they proceed through a total of 24 [main] conduits and network [vessels] before they, too, meet once again with the hand major yin [conduit]. At the right [hand] in the "inch-interior" [section] is the hole *tai yuan* 太淵. This is the great meeting point of the vessels; it represents the beginning and end [of the movement of the contents of the vessels]. Hence, [yin and yang] are allotted 25 passages each, and one speaks of the inch opening as the beginning and end of [the movement in] the vessels.

Li Jiong: The camp [qi] are the blood; they belong to the yin. The camp [qi] proceed inside the vessels. The guard [qi] are the qi; they belong to the yang. The
guard [qi] proceed outside of the vessels. The qi and the blood proceed through
the body while one is awake; they proceed through the long-term depots while
one is asleep. They never stop, neither at day nor at night. During 270 breathing
[periods], the [contents of the] vessels proceed 16 *zhang* and two feet. This corresponds to two markings of the clepsydra. Within 13,500 breathing [periods, the
qi in the] vessels proceed 810 *zhang*, corresponding to 100 markings of the clepsydra. They proceed through 25 passages during the yang [section] and through
25 passages during the yin [section of one day]. This amounts to one completion
of the clepsydra's dripping. Hence, the [contents of the vessels] need one day
and one night to circulate everywhere through the entire body. The yang vessels
face toward outside and [the qi] proceed through them 25 times. The yin vessels
face toward inside and [the qi] proceed through them 25 times, too.[13] Together
this adds up to 50 passages. The camp and the guard [qi] start from the Central
Burner and flow into the hand major yin and [hand] yang brilliance [conduits.
From the hand] yang brilliance [conduit] they flow into the foot yang brilliance
and [foot] major yin [conduits. From the foot] major yin [conduit] they flow
into the hand minor yin and [hand] major yang [conduits. From the [hand]
major yang [conduit] they flow into the foot major yang and [foot] minor yin
[conduits. From the foot] minor yin [conduit] they flow into the hand heart ruler and [hand] minor yang [conduits. From the hand]minor yang [conduit] they
flow into the foot minor yang and [foot] ceasing yin [conduits. From the foot]
ceasing yin conduit they flow back into the hand major yin [conduit].
The inch opening: [The movement of the qi in the vessels] starts from the lung
conduit at the right hand. From the lung and large intestine it reaches stomach
and spleen. From the spleen it reaches heart and small intestine. From the small
intestine it reaches urinary bladder and kidneys. From the kidneys it reaches
heart enclosing network and Triple Burner. From the Triple Burner it reaches
gall bladder and liver, and that is the end. When [the qi have reached] the end,
they start again from the lung. Consequently, if one examines the pattern [of the
movement of the qi through the] vessels, one must take [his information] from
the inch opening [in order to be able] to judge [whether a patient must] die or
will survive – that is, whether there are good or evil auspices [for his fate].

Xu Dachun: The text of the scripture states clearly: "One cycle in the body amounts
to sixteen *zhang* and two feet. This constitutes one passage." That is extremely

---

13 The meaning of these two sentences here, repeated from Lü Guang's commentary (see
above), is not clear.

clear. Here [in the *Nan jing*] this one sentence is omitted. But on what basis shall the fifty passages be calculated now? The *Nan jing* was written to clarify the [unclear portions in the] scripture. Here now, the text of the scripture is nothing but copied and its important points are even omitted! Thus, contrary [to what was intended, the meaning of] the scripture is further obscured.

Ding Jin: The circulation in man's blood vessels reaches everywhere in his body and it never stops. When it is stated [in the *Nan jing*] that the [qi in the] vessels move six inches during one breathing [period], this refers to the hand major yin vessel of the lung as start and returning point [of that movement]. One may compare [the movement in the vessels] with the counting of the [rosary] pearls while reciting Buddhist [prayers. The pearls, too,] have a first one and a last one, and they are moved around one by one in a way that all the pearls revolve. To proceed from start to end, one considers the first pearl to be the leader and then determines the number [of rosaries] to be counted. Similarly, the lung vessel is the [place where the] first movement over six inches takes place, but the same movement of six inches takes place in all vessels throughout the body [at the same time]. Now, because each of the twelve conduits passes [its contents] along its path, the camp [qi] and the guard [qi] proceed relatively fast. During one day and one night they circulate through the body fifty times and, of course, they also return to the inch opening fifty times.

Liao Ping: The ancient scriptures issued severe prohibitions against a diagnosis solely [relying on] the inch opening. In the [treatise] "Zheng si shi lun" 徵四失 論 of the *Su wen* it is stated: "If someone hastily grasps the inch opening, which disease could he hit? To issue absurd statements and to make up [disease] names, these are activities pursued by uneducated practitioners to exhaustion." [The same treatise] states further: "If someone at random feels the inch opening, in his diagnosis [he] fails to [correctly] identify the five [movements in the] vessels, and where the one hundred diseases emerge." Thus, if we talk [about diagnosis] in accordance with the ancient methods, it is essential to examine the [locations where] the movement [in the] vessels of all the twelve conduits [can be felt]. A diagnostic method which [takes its information] solely from the [vessels at the] hands is extremely simple. Those in ancient times who resorted to such an abridged [technique] did so because they feared that a thorough examination of all [the locations] was too troublesome [for the patient]. Or they checked only the inch opening when they made up a prescription in the course of a treatment. At that time they would use but one finger to examine just one [of the patient's] hands. That is different from this book, which arranges the twelve conduit vessels at the inch [locations] of both [hands] so that one must distinguish between left [hand] and right [hand], and between the three sections [inch, gate, and foot at each of them]. In transmitting their methods, the ancient scriptures issued severe prohibitions against a diagnosis based specifically on [information taken from] the two inch [openings]. This book, however, strictly prohibits a comprehensive diagnosis and emphasizes specifically the inch opening. Every reader must develop some doubts here. Still, many [commentators] have assumed that this [book] was written by Yueren, and nobody has dared to take issue [with this opinion]. I have had books on diagnostic methods in my hands that were compiled by Bian Que, and none of them contained the doctrine of diagnosing at the inch, gate, and foot [sections] of both hands. Thus, one does not have to say much more to prove that this book is counterfeit.

二難曰：（一）脈有尺寸，何謂也？

（二）然：尺寸者，脈之大要會也。（三）從關至尺是尺內，陰之所治也；從關至魚際是寸內，陽之所治也。（四）故分寸為尺，分尺為寸。（五）故陰得尺內一寸，陽得寸內九分，（六）尺寸終始一寸九分，故曰尺寸也。

The second difficult issue: (1) The vessels have a [section called] "foot and inch." What does that mean?

(2) It is like this. The foot and inch [section] is the great important meeting point of the [movements in the] vessels. (3) [The distance] from the "gate" to the "foot[-marsh" hole in the elbow] represents the "foot-interior" [section]; it is ruled by the yin [qi of the organism. The distance] from the gate to the fish-line represents the inch-interior [section]; it is ruled by the yang [qi of the organism]. (4) Hence, [one] inch is separated [from the entire distance between the gate and the elbow] to represent the foot [long section; one] foot is divided to become an inch. (5) Hence, [the condition of] the yin [qi can be] comprehended from a one inch [section] of the foot-interior [section; the condition of] the yang [qi can be] comprehended from a nine *fen* [section] of the inch-interior [section]. (6) The total length of the foot and inch [section thus] extends over one inch and nine *fen*. Hence, one speaks of a "foot and inch" [section].[1]

---

[1] The wording of this difficult issue suggests that its author distinguished two subsections of the location at the wrist where the movement in the vessels was to be examined for diagnostic purposes. These two subsections were separated by the so-called *guan*. The term *guan* 關, rendered here as "gate," implies a meaning of "frontier pass" or "frontier gate." While this gate itself seems to have been understood, in the second difficult issue, as an imaginary line not occupying any space itself, the section above it (seen from the perspective of a raised arm) was considered to be nine *fen* long and was called "inch-interior." In contrast, the section below the gate was considered to be one inch (i.e., ten *fen*) long, and it was called "foot-interior."

(1) *Liao Ping*: [Zhang] Zhongjing 張仲景[2] and the *Mai jing* 脈經[3] [refer to] three
sections on the head and at the feet [as locations to carry out diagnostic] examinations. Anybody who reads just a little in medical books knows about these
[techniques]. Because it is inconvenient to examine head and feet of females,
the [diagnosis of the] neck was transferred to the inch [section at the wrist, and
the diagnosis of] the feet was confined to the foot [section of the lower arm].
At first [this altered diagnostic technique] was used only with female [patients];

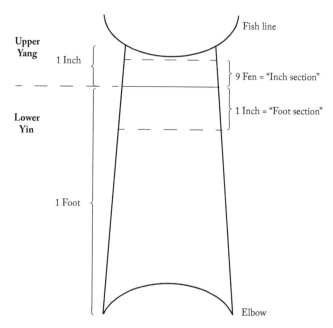

Obviously, no corresponding concept exists in the *Nei jing* scriptures, and the discussion
of this difficult issue among commentators of subsequent centuries focused partly on
this discrepancy between the contents of the ancient classics. It is quite obvious from the
arguments offered that the very existence of such discrepancies was incomprehensible
for a number of authors. However, the fact that diverging doctrines were offered by the
Nei jing, by the *Nan jing*, and in later works demonstrates that individuals emerged from
time to time who introduced new ideas and innovative techniques. A second controversy
related to this difficult issue centers around the nature of the gate. Some later authors
could not perceive the idea of an imaginary line, as proposed here; they preferred a concept which distinguished between three subsections of the *dong mai* section at the wrist.
Such a concept was not alien to the *Nan jing*; it appears in difficult issue 18.

2   This is Zhang Ji (142-220?), the author of the prescription works *Shang han lun* 傷寒論
     and *Jin kui yao lue* 金匱要略,

3   The *Mai jing* 脈經 was written by Wang Xi (210-285).

after a while it was applied generally. The terms "foot" and "inch" have their origins in the terms "foot-marsh"⁴ and "inch opening."

(2) *Lü Guang*: Whenever there is a disease in any of the three sections or on any of the nine indicator [levels]⁵ of the twelve conduit vessels, it will become apparent in the foot and inch [section]. Therefore it is called "the great important meeting point of the [movements in the] vessels."

Li Jiong: The inch [section] is a yang section; it is the important meeting point of the yang [qi]. The foot [section] is a yin [section]; it is the important meeting point of the yin [qi]. Thus, the great important meeting point of the [movement in the] vessels is at the foot and inch section.

(3) *Lü Guang*: "To the foot" means from the foot[-marsh hole in the elbow] to the gate. The [movement in the] vessel appears here for a length of one inch. [The entire section between the foot-marsh hole and the gate] is called "foot" because it represents the basis. The inch opening is one inch long; here the [movement in the] vessel appears for a length of nine *fen*. Yang numbers are odd; yin numbers are even.

Li Jiong: The gate section is the guard station at the borderline between the yin and yang [sections]. In front of the gate is the yang [section]; behind the gate is the yin [section. The distance] from the gate to the foot-marsh hole should be one foot long. This is the "foot section interior," which is ruled by yin [qi. The movement in] the vessel appears in the foot section for one inch; [this short distance] is called "foot," though, because it is based [in the foot section. The distance] from the gate to the fish-line bone is the "inch opening interior," which is ruled by yang [qi]. The inch opening is one inch long and the [movement in the] vessel appears here for nine *fen*.

Hua Shou: The "gate" is the dividing line formed by the elevated bone behind the palms. It lies behind the "inch" and in front of the "foot" as a borderline between the two areas of yin and yang.

Xu Dachun: The *Nei jing* refers to "inch opening," "vessel opening," and "foot and inch," but the term "gate" does not appear. [The section] below the inch opening is always called "foot opening." If we talk about the *ren ying* 人迎,⁶ this is the foot and inch [section]; it is generally called inch opening or "vessel opening."

---

4 The "foot-marsh" (*chi ze* 尺澤) hole is located in the elbow.

5 See difficult issue 18, sentences 6 ff., for an explanation of the concept of *san bu jiu hou* 三部九候 ("three longitudinal sections and nine indicator levels").

6 The term *ren ying* 人迎 denotes two locations to the left and right of the throat where the movement in the vessels can be felt (cf. *Ling shu* treatise 21, "Han re bing" 寒熱病). Here, though – and in the *Mai jing* 脈經 – this term is used to denote the inch opening of the

Katō Bankei: The first difficult issue has recommended [the examination of] one
section – that is, the inch opening – in order to determine death or survival [on
the basis of the conditions] of the long-term depots and short-term repositories,
because it assumed that the [qi moving through the] hundred vessels converge
in the lung. It did not imply that [the inch opening] is linked to the remaining eleven conduits. Thus it utilized the image of the original unity[7] before its
differentiation [into the categories of yin and yang]. In this paragraph now the
doctrine of a differentiation between inch and foot is introduced, based on the
principle that yin and yang [qi] appear and recede in the vessels. Hence, within
the [section of the] vessel [used for diagnosis, this second difficult issue] distinguishes [the subsections] "in front of the gate" and "behind the gate" in order to
establish foot and inch locations [associated with] yin and yang. Here the image
of the differentiation of the original unity into two [aspects] is reflected. Hence,
"nine" refers to the inch [section and to] yang; "ten" refers to the foot [section
and to] yin. The gate is established as a borderline between the inch and foot
sections. The entire length [of both subsections] amounts to one inch and nine
fen. This is the location where one applies pressure with the three fingers. Sun
Simiao 孫思邈 assumed that the three sections – inch, gate, and foot – were a
doctrine of Qi Bo 岐伯.[8] But nothing like this appears in the *Nei jing*. When
the terms "foot" and "inch" were used there, "foot" referred to the skin of the foot
[section], while "inch" referred to the vessel in the one section of the inch opening. The differentiation between three (sub)sections within the inch opening
and foot-interior [sections] is an innovation introduced by the *Nan jing*.

Tamba Genkan: The first difficult issue discusses the method of [just] utilizing the
inch opening to obtain diagnostic information. This paragraph here penetrates
further into this issue. It distinguishes between a foot and an inch location,
but this is different from a differentiation of "three sections" in the eighteenth
difficult issue. The student should not read only one ruling. Yang's comments[9]
do not investigate the reasons of these [differences]. He randomly drew on the

left hand, while the inch opening of the right hand was called the "qi-opening." It is not
clear whether Xu Dachun's comment here reflects his original wording.

7   The Chinese is *tai ji* 太極. According to ancient Chinese cosmological doctrines, the
     tai ji represents the first phase in the ordering of the phenomena. The term translates
     literally as "supreme ridgepole." The *tai ji* phase was preceded by the absence of any such
     ordering structure (*wu ji* 無極), and it was followed by the differentiation of the yin and
     yang and, later, of more complex categories of phenomena.

8   One of the legendary advisers – mentioned in the *Nei jing* – with whom the Yellow
     Thearch discussed medical issues.

9   Tamba appears to refer here to the commentary of Yang [Xuancao] quoted below.

instructions of various authors concerning [a diagnosis of the movement in] the vessels in order to teach them to others, and he took up the theory of correspondences between the long-term depots and short-term repositories on the one hand and the locations [of the sections at the lower arm] on the other hand, as a rule for diagnostic examinations. But there is not enough evidence to prove that this [was meant in the ancient scripture]. His ideas were based on Sun Simiao, who had stated: "[The distance] from the elbow joint to the 'fish-line' is one foot. If one divides it by ten one gets ten inches. Take the one inch of the ninth division, that is the location of the foot [section] of the vessel." This, however, was even more at variance with the message of the scripture. It, too, cannot be followed. In the treatise "Yin yang ying xiang da lun" 陰陽應象大論 of the *Su wen* it is stated: "The 'foot and inch' is the [section] where one examines depth and surface, smoothness and roughness, in order to know where a disease has emerged." Furthermore, in the treatise "Mai yao jing wei lun" 脈要精微論 it is stated: "The inside of the foot-long section, on both sides, this is [the region of] the free ribs." Then follows a comment [by Wang Bing 王冰: "'Foot-interior' means 'inside the foot-marsh [hole]'." The treatise "Xie qi zang fu bing xing" 邪氣藏府病形 of the *Ling shu* states: "when the [movement in the] vessels is tight, the skin of the 'foot-long-section' is also tight. When the [movement in the] vessels is relaxed, the skin of the 'foot-long section' is also relaxed." These statements are all in accordance with the diagnostic method of pressing the skin of the foot [section]. The *Nei jing* does not talk about separating a foot location from the inch opening. Students cannot take advantage of anybody else's explanations of this. Ji Tianxi 紀天錫[10] has also discussed the nonsense of associating the long-term depots and short-term repositories with [specific] locations [at the lower arm]; his arguments are quite subtle and appropriate.

(4) *Ding Deyong*: "[One] inch is separated to represent the foot" [means the following]: In man, the distance between the gate and the foot-marsh hole is one foot long. From within this foot[-long section] one inch[-long section] is separated to represent the pattern of the [entire] foot[-long section). Thus, "[one] inch is separated [from the entire distance between the gate and the elbow] to represent the foot[-long section; one] foot is divided to become an inch."

(5) *Ding Deyong*: Yin numbers are even; yang numbers are odd.

(6) *Yang*: Most authors who have written about the three locations of inch, gate, and foot have disagreed. Let me therefore put this in order and discuss [their arguments] so that the correct meaning will become apparent. Now, Mr. Huangfu,

---

10 The twelfth-century author of a now lost *Nan jing* commentary entitled *Ji zhu Nan jing* 集註難經.

in his instructions on [diagnosing] the vessels, considered a three-finger [broad section] behind the palm as the "three sections." Each finger covers six *fen*; the three sections thus add up to a total of one inch and eight *fen*. Hua Tuo 華佗[11] in his instructions on the vessels, has stated: "Both the "inch" and the "foot" locations are eight *fen* [long]. The "gate" location is three *fen* [long]. Together this amounts to one inch and nine *fen*." Wang Shuhe 王叔和[12] in his instructions on the vessels, has stated: "The locations of the three sections extend over one inch each. This adds up to three inches." All writings differ like this, causing severe doubts and utter confusion in later students. But it is not like this: The diagnosis of the patterns displayed in the vessels originated from the Yellow Thearch. The *Nan jing* originated from Bian Que. Both [persons and their] works represent ancestors, while all [later] authors and their discourses are but branches and leaves. Indeed, one must regard the sources as fundamental, and one may forget about the rest! Let us rely on the important principles that are clear! According to the true scripture of the Yellow Thearch, the three inches behind the palm constitute the three sections. These are the inch, as well as the gate and the foot.[13] Each covers one inch in order to provide [sections for the manifestation of] the three powers. This pattern is set for eternity; nothing can ever be changed about it. One may say that Wang Shuhe understood this. Whenever one diagnoses the [movement in the] vessels, one must first know the principal locations of the three sections and of the nine indicator[levels[14] of these sections, respectively, because this is] where the [conditions of] the five long-term depots and six short-term repositories become apparent. Then one may investigate the latters' good or bad condition by distinguishing between [the movements near the] surface and in the depth. As long as one is unsure about the principal locations [of the three sections and nine indicator levels], one has no way of differentiating the origins of the diseases. And if one intends to heal a disease, this will be difficult, too. The three [longitudinal] sections are the inch, the gate, and the foot. The nine indicator [levels] are "heaven," "earth," and "man." Each section has

---

11 Famous physician and author of various works (all lost now) who lived 110 to 207.

12 *Zi* name of Wang Xi. See note 3.

13 This statement by Yang [Xuancao?] does not correspond to the facts; it may have been formulated to provide historical legitimacy for a concept which, in reality, deviated considerably from the meaning of the term *san bu* 三部 as used in the *Nei jing*. See Xu Dachun's commentary on sentences 6 ff. of difficult issue 18.

14 Despite these words, Yang [Xuancao?] does not take into account the concept of the nine indicator-levels (later in the same comment) when he outlines the significance of the movements in the vessels as they can be perceived near the wrist. Rather than distinguishing three indicator-levels for each longitudinal section – as the concept of *jiu hou* 九候 would imply – he only distinguishes two: one in the depth and one near the surface.

heaven, earth, and man levels – that is, the three sections [together] have nine indicator [levels] where one may examine the qi of the five long-term depots. As far as the appearance of [the conditions of] the five long-term depots and six short-term repositories [at these locations] is concerned, the inch opening of the left hand is where the [movement in the] vessels [associated with] the heart and the small intestine appears. On top of the gate is where the [movement in the] vessels [associated with] the liver and the gall bladder appears. In the center of the foot is where the [movement in the] vessels [associated with] the kidneys and the urinary bladder appears. One *fen* in front of the gate is the location of the *ren ying* 人迎; one *fen* behind the gate is the location of the "spirit gate."[15] The inch opening of the right hand is where the [movement in the] vessels [associated with] the lung and the large intestine appears. On top of the gate is where the [movement in the] vessels [associated with] the spleen and the stomach appears. In the center of the foot is where the [movement in the] vessels [associated with] the gate of life and the Triple Burner appears. One *fen* in front of the gate is the location of the qi opening; one *fen* behind the gate is the location of the spirit gate. All the vessels of the five long-term depots belong to the yin [category]; all yin vessels are in the depth. All the vessels of the six short-term repositories belong to the yang [category]; all yang vessels are near the surface. If, for example, a vessel [is located] near the surface at the inch opening of the left hand, that is the vessel of the small intestine. The one in the depth is the vessel of the heart. All the others are like this. Such are the rules of the positions of the vessels; such are the methods of examining the indicator [levels].

Ding Deyong: An older comment concerning the pattern of the foot and inch [section] in the [*Nan*] *jing* stated that all previous authors who have written about it are in disagreement.[16] That comment pointed out that each of the three sections [i.e., foot, gate, and inch] extends over one inch, amounting to a total of three inches, and it did not see the reason for [a measurement of only] one inch and nine *fen* [as suggested here by the *Nan jing*]. The pattern [displayed] at the one inch and nine *fen* [section] is as follows. Each of the foot and inch locations is associated with the start and end of [the flow of] the yin and yang [qi]. The yang qi emerge at the foot and move at the inch. The yin qi emerge at the inch and move at the foot. Thus, in order to [diagnose the] pattern of the

---

15 "Spirit gate" (*shen men* 神門) is the designation for two holes that belong to a set of 36 gate holes (*san shi liu men* 三十六門) distributed all over the body and recommended for the treatment of diseases caused by wind-evil. The two spirit gate holes are located at the wrist of the left and right hand, respectively, and are considered to be situated on the hand minor yin conduit, which is associated with the heart.

16 This may be a reference to the preceding commentary by Yang [Xuancao?].

yang qi, [the following has to be considered]. They first emerge at "spring begins" and they rise until the "grain-in-ear" [solar term of the year]. The number [of solar terms passed] is nine.[17] The three yang [qi] rule in the front [section of the lower arm – that is,] their pattern is [manifest] near the surface in the nine *fen* [section] within the inch. At "summer solstice" these qi descend; their [course] ends at "winter begins." The number [of solar terms passed] is ten. The three yin [qi] rule in the back [section, that is,] their pattern is [manifest] in the depth of the one inch [section] within the foot. Thus one knows that both the foot and the inch are associated with the beginning and end [of the course of the yin and yang qi]. Yueren alludes here to the existence of yin and yang [subcategories] as well as of beginning and end in the yang. As far as yin and yang [subcategories] as well as beginning and end in the yin are concerned, the yin qi reemerge at "autumn begins." They descend until "winter solstice." The number [of solar terms passed] is ten. After winter solstice they follow the minor yang and rise until "summer begins." The number [of solar terms passed] is nine. These are the beginning and end of [the rise and descent of] the yin and yang [qi of] heaven and earth. Hence, this pattern [is reflected in the fact that the flow of] both yin and yang [qi] through the foot and inch [section] also has beginning and end. The important gates for the convergence of [the qi of] heaven and earth are the beginnings of the four [seasons]. They are named "celestial gate," "earth gate," "human gate," and "demons' gate." Man's qi opening and *ren ying*, as well as the [two] spirit gates at the left and at the right [hand, reflect] the same pattern.

(1)–(6)Liao Ping: When the author of this book established – at his time – terms to signify an upper, a central, and a lower [section], he did not provide other people with a handle [to grasp what he meant]. Nobody can understand why he called an inch a foot. Those who have discussed this for two thousand years now have been ingenious in setting up theories and they have undertaken the greatest efforts in their attempts to understand [the meaning of these sentences]. But they never could agree because the basis of their [discussions itself] was not firmly established.

---

17   The entire year is divided into twenty-four solar terms, each two weeks apart.

三難曰：（一）脈有大過，有不及，有陰陽相乘，有覆有溢，有關有格，何謂也？

（二）然：關之前者，陽之動，（三）脈當見九分而浮。（四）過者，法曰大過；（五）減者，法曰不及。（六）遂上魚為溢，（七）為外關內格，（八）此陰乘之脈也。（九）關以後者，陰之動也，（十）脈當見一寸而沉。（十一）過者，法曰大過；（十二）減者，法曰不及。（十三）遂入尺為覆，（十四）為內關外格，（十五）此陽乘之脈也。（十六）故曰覆溢，（十七）是其真藏之脈，人不病而死也。

The third difficult issue: (1) The [movement in the] vessels may [display the following conditions]: "great excess" and "insufficiency," "mutual takeover by yin and yang," "turnover" and "overflow," "closure" and "barrier." What does that mean?

(2) It is like this. [The section] in front of the gate is where the yang [qi] move. (3) The [perceptible movement in the] vessels should extend [here] over nine *fen* and be near the surface. (4) [If this movement] exceeds [the nine *fen* section], that is a pattern indicating great excess. (5) [If the movement] falls short [of covering the entire nine *fen* section], that is a pattern indicating insufficiency. (6) [If the movement] extends upward to the fish[-line], that constitutes an overflow. (7) It signals external closure and internal barrier. (8) [In this case] the yin [qi] have seized [that section of] the vessel [where normally only yang qi should be]. (9) [The section] behind the gate is where the yin [qi] move. (10) The [perceptible movement in the] vessel should extend [here] over one inch and be in the depth. (11) [If this movement] exceeds [the one inch section], that is a pattern indicating great excess. (12) [If the movement] falls short [of covering the entire one inch section], that is a pattern indicating insufficiency. (13) [If the movement] extends downward into the foot [long section towards the elbow], that constitutes a turnover. (14) It signals internal closure and external barrier. (15) [In this case] the yang [qi] have seized [that section of] the vessel [where normally only yin qi should be]. (16) Hence, one speaks of "turnover" and "overflow." (17) This [reflects the movement in] the vessels of the true[1] long-term depots [themselves]. The [afflicted] person has no disease and yet he will die.[2]

1 Yang Shangshan 楊上善, *Huang Di nei jing Tai su* 黃帝內經太素, (Beijing 1981, 249) in commenting on the treatise "Zhen zang mai xing" 真藏脈形 of the *Tai su*, noted that the term *zhen* 真 ("true") may have been introduced during the Qin dynasty to replace the term *zheng* 正 ("proper"), since the latter became taboo because it was part of the name of the first Emperor.

2 This third difficult issue contains a straightforward explanation of symptoms and terms related to imbalances of yin and yang qi in the body. It elucidates how such imbalances

(1) *Liao Ping*: None of the authors [of previous centuries] has, in his commentaries, responded to the errors of [this] difficult issue. On the contrary, if one looks at older comments it seems as if they had succeeded in increasingly giving some shape to its mistakes and absurdities!

(2)–(16) *Hua Shou*: "Great excess" and "insufficiency" refer to vessel [movements] in the state of disease; "closure," "barrier," "turnover," and "overflow" refer to vessels in the state of [impending] death. As for closure and barrier, the treatise "Liu jie zang xiang lun" 六節藏象論 of the *Su wen* as well as the ninth and for-

---

can be recognized through examining the movements of the qi as they appear in the two sections "in front of the gate" (that is, the "external" section – i.e., the yang section which extends over nine *fen* from the gate toward the palm) and "behind the gate" (that is, the "internal" section – i.e., the yin section which extends over ten fen, or one inch, from the gate toward the elbow).

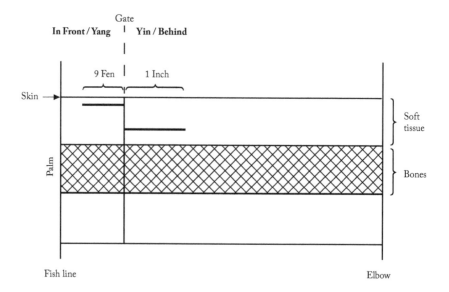

The author of this *Nan jing* paragraph then used terms that had already been employed in the *Nei jing* – but with partially different meanings – to explain the mechanics causing the symptoms displayed at the two wrist sections. The ensuing problem of terminological ambiguity is reflected in the commentaries of later writers. Some of these commentators acknowledged the innovative concepts of the *Nan jing*; others expressed their dislike of what they considered to be an erroneous usage of concepts the true meanings of which were to be found only in the *Nei jing*. A third category of authors simply appears to have been utterly confused; their attempts to reconcile the contents of the *Nan jing* with those of the *Nei jing* reflect their inability to comprehend the real issue at hand.

ty-ninth treatises of the *Ling shu* all focus on the qi opening and on the *ren ying* 人迎 [locations. Information on the movement in the] yang conduits is taken, [according to the *Su wen* and the *Ling shu*,] from the *ren ying*; [information on the movement in the] yin conduits is taken from the qi opening.³ Now, Yueren speaks of "in front of the gate" and "behind the gate," considering the inch [section] as yang and the foot [section] as yin.

Zhang Shixian: "Great excess" and "insufficiency" [refer to movements in] the vessels at their original location; "mutual takeover by yin and yang" [refers to movements] leaving their original location. The nine *fen* [section] is the location of the yang [movement in the vessels]; the one inch [section] is the location of the yin [movement in the vessels]. Near the surface is the yang [movement in the] vessels; in the depth is the yin [movement in the] vessels. *Fa* ("pattern") means here "diagnostic pattern" (*zhen zhi fa* 診之法); *sui* ("to extend") stands for *jing xing* 徑行 ("to proceed directly"). The yang [movement in the] vessels should be perceptible in front of the gate for a distance of nine *fen*; it should be at the surface. The yin [movement in the] vessels should be perceptible behind the gate for a distance of one inch; it should be in the depth. In the case of great excess or insufficiency, either the yin or the yang [qi] prevail unilaterally. In extreme cases turnover and overflow, closure and barrier [conditions may] appear. *Fu* 覆 ("turnover") is a movement from above downward; *yi* 溢 ("overflow") is a movement from below upward. *Guan* 関 ("closure") means there is no source from which to move out; *ge* 格 ("barrier") means there is no way to move in. In the treatise "Mai du" 脈度 of the *Ling shu* it is stated: "When the yin qi abound excessively, then the yang qi are unable to circulate.⁴ Hence that is called 'closure'. When the yang qi abound excessively, then the yin qi are unable to circulate. Hence that is called 'barrier'." If the yang qi cannot circulate through the yin [sections], the yin [qi] will ascend, leaving [their original location], and flow over the fish-line. That constitutes external closure and internal barrier. In

---

3   Hua Shou referred here to the categorization of the left as yang and of the right as yin. Accordingly, the *Nei jing* statements cited consider the *ren ying* 人迎 location near the wrist of the left hand as a place where the condition of the yang conduits (and their respective long-term depots) may be examined, and they regard the "qi opening" (*qi kou* 氣口) near the wrist of the right hand as a suitable place to examine the condition of the yin conduits and their respective long-term depots. In contrast, the author(s) of this difficult issue appear(s) to have distinguished a yin and a yang section on one lower arm only by referring to the categorization of "above," "outside," and "in front" (of the gate) as yang, and of "below," "inside," and "behind" (the gate) as yin.

4   ZJY: „The classic uses the two characters 榮 *ying* and 營 *ying* interchangeably. ‚Unable to circulate' is to say: when the yin and the yang [qi] are in disorder, they are unable to circulate because a closure blocks their passage."

the case of external closure and internal barrier, the [qi from the] yin vessels have availed themselves of the yang [location]. The yang [qi suffer from] external closure and cannot move downward as the yin [qi] come out from inside and meet them with a barrier. The resulting disease is external heat and ceaseless sweating together with internal cold, a sensation of fullness in the chest, and vomiting of food. When the yin qi cannot circulate through the yang [sections], the yang [qi] will move down directly and return into the foot section. That constitutes internal closure and external barrier. In the case of internal closure and external barrier, the [qi from the] yang vessels have availed themselves of the yin [location]. The yin [qi suffer from] internal closure and cannot move upward as the yang [qi] enter from outside and meet them with barrier. The resulting disease is internal heat and constipation of both urine and stool, together with external cold and a cooling of hands and feet.

(2) *Li Jiong*: The yang qi emerge in the foot [section] and [display their] movement in the inch [section. The section] in front of the gate is called the inch opening; that is the location where the yang qi move.

Liao Ping: To have divided the inch opening into three sections is the number one crime of this book. In their attempts to associate [these sections with the categories of yin and yang and with the functional units of the organism], people of later times have developed about ten different doctrines.

(3) *Li Jiong*: Yang numbers are odd; the [yang] amount is nine. Yang [movements in the] vessels are near the surface. Consequently, the [perceptible movement in the] vessels at the inch opening extends over nine *fen* and is near the surface.

(4) *Lü Guang*: "Excess" means that the [movement in the] vessel exceeds the nine *fen* [section] or leaves the one inch [section]. That is called "great excess."

Ding Deyong: "Great excess" means that the vessel in the inch [section] is originally near the surface. When [its movement] increases, when it is replete and strong, that is called "great excess of yang [qi]." When its movement extends upward toward the fish[-line], that would be a "yang overflow." When [the movement remains] at the surface but is diminished and weak, that is an "insufficiency of yang [qi]." When the yang [qi] are insufficient, the yin [qi] will move out to take over their [location]. Another name for this [condition] is "yin overflow"; it is [caused by] an external closure and by internal barrier. [Furthermore,] "great excess" means that the [movement in the] vessels in the foot [section] is originally in the depth. When [this movement] increases, when it is replete and strong, that is called "great excess of yin [qi]." When [the movement remains] in the depth and is diminished and weak, that is indicated by the term "insufficiency." When the yin [qi] are insufficient, the yang [qi] will enter [their location] to take it over. That is called "yang turnover," or internal "closure" and external "barrier."

Li Jiong: "Exceeds" means that the [movement in the] vessel exceeds the nine *fen* [section] or leaves the one inch[section], or that a [movement in a] vessel which is originally located near the surface is increased, replete and strong. That would be an "excessive [movement in the] vessels."

(5) *Lü Guang*: "To fall short" means that [the movement in] the vessel does not reach through the entire nine *fen* but extends only over eight *fen*, seven *fen*, or six *fen*. That is an "insufficient [movement in the] vessels."

Li Jiong: "Falls short" means that [the movement in] the vessel does not reach through the [entire] nine *fen* but extends only over eight *fen*, seven *fen*, or six *fen*. Also, yang [movements in the] vessels are originally near the surface; they are felt by light hand pressure. If [this movement is] diminished and weak, that indicates insufficiency.

(6) *Lü Guang*: "If [the movement] extends upwards to the fish[-line" means that] it leaves the one inch[section] and reaches the fish-line. Another name [for this condition] is "overflow [movement in the] vessels." Another name [for this condition] is "external closure [movement in the] vessels." Another name [for this condition] is "internal barrier [movement in the] vessels." Another name [for this condition] is "yin takeover [movement in the] vessels." Thus, one single vessel [movement] has four different names.

Tamba Genkan: In Lü Guang's commentary it is said: "One single vessel [movement] has four different names." That is wrong.

Li Jiong: An extension upward to the fish-line bone indicates that the vessel is supplemented to overflow. If [the movement is] near the surface, replete and strong, extending upward to the fish[-line], that indicates a yang overflow. If it is near the surface, diminished and weak, that is an insufficiency of yang [qi]. If the yang [qi] are insufficient, the yin [qi] will enter [their location] to take it over, indicating a yin overflow.

(7) *Li Jiong*: "External closure" means that [the qi of] the vessel inside [of the gate – i.e., the qi of the foot section] - cannot leave [into the inch section]. One therefore speaks of an "insufficiency" or of "vessels taken over by yin [qi]." An "inner barrier" is present when the [qi of the] vessel outside [of the gate – i.e., those in the inch section] - cannot return toward inside [of the gate]. One therefore speaks of "great excess" or of "vessels overflowing."

(9) *Li Jiong*: The yin [qi] emerge in the inch [section] and [display their] movement in the foot [section. The section] behind the gate is the foot section; that is the place where the yin qi move.

(10) *Li Jiong*: Yin numbers are even; the [yin] amount is ten. A yin [movement in the] vessels is in the depth. Consequently, the [movement in the] vessel of the foot [section] should extend over one inch [i.e., ten *fen*] and be in the depth.

(11) *Lü Guang*: "Exceeds" means that the [movement in the] vessel exceeds the one inch [section], exceeding it by one *fen*, two *fen*, three *fen* or four *fen*. That is a "great excess" [movement in the] vessels.

  Li Jiong: "Exceeds" means that the [movement in the] vessel exceeds the one inch [section], extending over one inch and two *fen*, three *fen*, four *fen* or five *fen*. The [movement in the] vessel of the foot [section] is originally in the depth. It is felt by heavy hand pressure. If [this movement] is increased, replete, and strong, that indicates a great excess of yin [qi].

(12) *Lü Guang*: "Falls short" means that the [movement in the] vessel does not cover the entire one inch [section] but is perceptible only over eight *fen* or seven *fen* or even only over six *fen* or five *fen*. That is an insufficient [movement in the] vessels.

  Li Jiong: "Falls short" means that the [movement in the] vessel does not supplement the entire one inch [section] but is perceptible only over eight *fen*, seven *fen*, or six *fen*. Also, yin [movements in the] vessels are originally in the depth and soft. They are felt by heavy hand pressure. If [this movement] is diminished and weak, that indicates a "yin insufficiency."

(13) *Lü Guang*: As for [the statement: "If the movement] extends downward into the foot [long section towards the elbow], that constitutes a turnover," a turnover [movement in the] vessel exists when the [movement in the] vessel is perceptible from the gate to the foot-marsh [hole in the elbow]. That is a [movement in the] vessels which "comes again and again." Therefore one speaks of "overturn." The [movement in the] vessel that extends from the gate to the foot-marsh [hole] is [normally] perceptible for one inch [only]. For the remaining portion it proceeds hidden and cannot be perceived. When it becomes perceptible now from the gate [all the way] to the foot-marsh [hole], one consequently speaks of "coming again and again" – in other words, that is a "turnover" [movement in the] vessel; it is also named internal "closure" or external "barrier."

(14) *Li Jiong*: "Internal closure" means that the [qi in the] vessel outside [of the gate] cannot enter [the section inside the gate, i.e., the foot section], indicating a yin insufficiency. As a result, the yang [qi] enter [the inch section] for takeover. "External barrier" means that [the qi in] the vessels inside [of the gate] cannot leave, indicating a yin excess and a yang turnover.

  Liao Ping: The terms "closure" and "barrier" are used here to denote [specific movements in the] vessels. That corresponds to [their usage in] the *Nei jing*.

However, in the thirty-seventh difficult issue, [these terms are employed to] denote a disease, contradicting this [paragraph here].

(15) *Li Jiong*: This means that the yin [section of the] vessel has been seized by the [qi of the] vessel of the yang section.

(16) *Lü Guang*: The [different kinds of] arrivals of the [qi in the] vessels [as described] here refer in each case to [conditions] where a disease results from the mutual taking over or overpowering [of the qi of the yin and yang sections]. An intrusion of an outside evil, [such as] to be struck by wind or to be harmed by cold, are not implied here. [The problem] is perceptible [through the movement] in the vessels already. The respective person may not yet have a disease,[5] but he suffers from a fatal affliction which cannot be cured.

Li Jiong: Whenever there are not enough yin [qi, a condition which allows for] an intrusion and takeover [of their location] by yang [qi], that is a turnover. Whenever there are not enough yang [qi, a condition allowing for] an intrusion and takeover [of their location] by yin [qi], that is an overflow.

Hua Shou: Fu 覆 ("turnover") is used here like "some item is falling down"; something falls downward from above. Yi 溢 ("overflow") is used here like "overflow of water"; [water flows] from inside toward outside.

Katō Bankei: [The terms] *fu* 覆 ("turnover") and *yi* 溢 ("overflow") as used in this paragraph correspond to what is called *guan* 関 ("closure") and *ge* 格 ("barrier") in the *Nei jing*. The so-called *guan* and *ge* in this difficult issue refer to a disease where yin and yang [qi have] mutually availed themselves of each other's [location]. The terms are the same but their meaning is different. Now, someone might ask: "How can the literal meaning of *guan* and *ge* in this paragraph be outlined?" The answer would be: "Look at the [movement in the] vessels [called] 'overflow'. It indicates 'external closure' *(guan)* and 'internal barrier' *(ge)*. Similarly, a [movement in the] vessels [called] 'turnover' indicates 'internal closure' and 'external barrier'. Thus, it becomes obvious that turnover and overflow are nothing but fatal [movements in the] vessels of the true [qi of the] long-term depots. If these vessel [movements] appear externally, there must be corresponding changes of closure and barrier among the long-term depots and short-term repositories internally." The *Su wen* states: "When the yin and the yang [qi] do not correspond to each other, that disease is called 'closure and barrier'." Obviously, *guan* and *ge* are not simply terms denoting [a particular movement in the] vessels. Hence, Mr. Chen 陳 from Siming 四明 has stated: "In the case of 'closure', [the passage of] urine and stool is blocked. In the case of 'barrier', [the body] objects to food and beverages and does not permit them to move down."

---

5   That is to say, the respective person may not yet feel ill.

That is correct. When the disease of "closure and barrier" was mentioned in the prescription literature of later centuries, "turnover" and "overflow" were obviously terms used to denote [movements in the] vessels of only yin or just yang [qi], while "closure" and "barrier" signified conditions where the yin or the yang [qi] have lost their location. Thus, the use of the term "closure and barrier" as a name of a disease originated from this paragraph.

(17) *Xu Dachun*: "[The movement in] the vessels of the true long-term depots [themselves]" means that the [flow of the] qi of the long-term depots has already been cut off; the true shape [of the long-term depots] is manifest only externally [in the movement of the vessels. The patient] does not necessarily suffer from a disease but one may determine already that he will have to die.[6] According to the [treatise] "Yu ji zhen zang lun" 玉機真藏論 of the *Su wen*, each of the five long-term depots is associated with [a movement in] the vessels [that is called] "true [qi of the] long-term depots [movement]" (*zhen zang* 真藏). [By discovering these movements one may] find out details about the shape of the [long-term depots]. Now, if the stomach qi cannot pass together with the long-term depot qi through the hand major yin [conduit], only the [qi from the] vessels of the long-term depots themselves appear.[7] There is no reference [in this context], however, to any closure or barrier. From a close look at the treatise "Zhong shi" 終始 of the *Ling shu* and at the [treatise] "Liu jie zang xiang lun" 六節藏象論 of the *Su wen*, [where one finds] the terms closure and barrier mentioned, [one may learn] that [these terms] have nothing to do with the true [qi of the] long-term depots [movement]. How could it happen that it was all mixed up?! The theory of distinguishing between closure and barrier is dealt with in detail in the thirty-seventh difficult issue.

Ding Jin: In the case of a [movement in the] vessels of only the true [qi of the] long-term depots, no stomach qi are present to achieve their harmonization. "The [afflicted] person has no disease and yet he will die" means that he will not suffer from a disease for long; death comes suddenly.

Liao Ping: The doctrine of the "true [qi of the] long-term depots" in the [*Nei*] *jing* was originally associated with symptoms of [impending] death. One searched

6   *Xing* 形 ("shape") is to be read here metaphorically, as in "to be in shape."

7   The meaning of the *Nei jing* passage referred to here by Xu Dachun is that in case of no illness, or in the presence of only a minor illness, the person examining the movement in the vessels should perceive both a movement of qi associated with the particular long-term depot dominating at the time of the examination, and of qi from the stomach. If the latter are absent, the patient must be fatally ill because the "foundation of the long-term depots" (i.e., the stomach, which supplies the long-term depots with qi) has ceased to function. Yet the meaning implied in sentence 17 of the third difficult issue appears unrelated to the usage of the term *zhen zang* 真藏 In the *Nei jing*.

especially for the true [qi of the] long-term depots in order to determine the date [of death]. It was not used as a method to diagnose the [movement in the] vessels. Also, there is no reference to an "absence of disease" in this regard.

四難曰：（一）脈有陰陽之法，何謂也？

（二）然：呼出心與肺，吸入腎與肝，呼吸之間，脾受穀味也，其脈在中。（三）浮者陽也，沉者陰也，故曰陰陽也。

（四）心肺俱浮，何以別之？

（五）然：浮而大散者，心也；浮而短濇者，肺也。

（六）腎、肝俱沉，何以別之？

（七）然：牢而長者，肝也；（八）按之濡，舉指來實者，腎也。（九）脾者中州，故其脈在中，（十）是陰陽之法也。

（十一）脈有一陰一陽，一陰二陽，一陰三陽；有一陽一陰，一陽二陰，一陽三陰。如此之言，寸口有六脈俱動耶？

（十二）然：此言者，非有六脈俱動也，（十三）謂浮、沉、長、短、滑、濇也。（十四）浮者陽也，滑者陽也，長者陽也；沉者陰也，短者陰也，濇者陰也。（十五）所謂一陰一陽者，謂脈來沉而滑也；（十六）一陰二陽者，謂脈來沉滑而長也；（十七）一陰三陽者，謂脈來沉滑而長，時一沉也。（十八）所言一陽一陰者，謂脈來浮而濇也；（十九）一陽二陰者，謂脈來長而沉濇也；（二十）一陽三陰者，謂脈來沉濇而短，時一浮也。（二十一）各以其經所在，名病逆順也。

The fourth difficult issue: (1) The [movement in the] vessels may display patterns of yin and yang. What does that mean?

(2) It is like this. [That which is] exhaled originates from the heart and from the lung; [that which is] inhaled enters the kidneys and the liver. Between exhalation and inhalation the spleen receives the flavor [qi] of the grains; its [movement in the] vessels is located in the center. (3) Those [movements in the vessels that can be felt] at the surface are yang [movements; those that can be felt] in the depth are yin [movements]. Hence, one speaks of yin and yang [patterns].

(4) Heart and lung [movements] are both located near the surface; how can they be distinguished?

(5) It is like this. A strong but dispersed [movement] at the surface is [associated with] the heart. A rough [movement] of short periods at the surface is [associated with] the lung.

(6) [The movements associated with] the liver and with the kidneys are both located in the depth; how can they be distinguished?

(7) It is like this. A firm and extensive [movement in the depth is associated with] the liver. (8) A [movement in the depth that is] soft and appears replete when the

finger is [pressed down to the bone first and then] lifted is [associated with] the kidneys. (9) The spleen is [associated with] the central region, therefore its [movement in the] vessels is located in the center. (10) These are the patterns of yin and yang.

(11) The [movement in the] vessels may display, it is said, "one yin one yang," "one yin two yang," [or] "one yin three yang," [or] it may display "one yang one yin," "one yang two yin," [or] "one yang three yin." Does [that mean that] there are six vessels at the inch opening, all displaying a movement at the same time?

(12) It is like this. These terms do not imply that there are six vessels all moving at the same time. (13) What is meant is [that there are movements that can be felt] at the surface or in the depth which are extensive or short, smooth or rough. (14) [A movement] at the surface is a yang [movement]. A smooth [movement] is a yang [movement]. An extensive [movement] is a yang [movement. A movement] in the depth is a yin [movement]. A short [movement] is a yin [movement]. A rough [movement] is a yin [movement]. (15)"One yin one yang" means that the [movement in the] vessels comes in the depth and is smooth. (16) "One yin two yang" means that the [movement in the] vessels comes in the depth and is smooth and extensive, (17) "One yin three yang" means that the [movement in the] vessels comes at the surface, is rough and extensive, and appears, once in a while, in the depth. (18) "One yang one yin" means that the [movement in the] vessels comes at the surface and is rough. (19) "One yang two yin" means that the [movement in the] vessels comes in long strides, is situated in the depth, and is rough. (20) "One yang three yin" means that the [movement in the] vessels comes in the depth, is rough and short, and appears, once in a while, at the surface. (21) In each case, one determines on the basis of the location of the [movement in the] conduits whether [the qi] – in the case of a disease – proceed contrary to or in accordance with their proper course.[1]

---

1 The first difficult issue introduced one single location (i.e., the inch opening at the wrist) as sufficient to examine the movement in the vessels. The second and third difficult issues introduced a differentiation among three cross-sections (foot, gate, and inch) within the inch opening. By outlining the yin and yang correspondences of the foot and inch sections, the second and the third difficult issues indicated a first possibility of how to examine the status of yin and yang functional units in the organism by simply checking the vessel movements at these sections. Here, in the fourth difficult issue, two further diagnostic patterns are introduced, allowing for an even more sophisticated differential examination of the condition of the various long-term depots and short-term repositories on the basis of their yin or yang categorization. The first of these new patterns was developed through a differentiation among three longitudinal levels of the inch opening – namely, upper (i.e., "at the surface"), central, and lower (i.e., "in the depth"); these three levels correspond to yang, neither yin nor yang, and yin, respectively. See figure 3:

(1)*Liao Ping*: In Yang [Shangshan's 楊上善] commentary on the *Tai su*, the *ren ying* 人迎 [location at the wrist of the left hand] is [categorized as] yang, while the inch opening [at the wrist of the right hand] is [categorized as] yin. There is no differentiation between yin and yang [subsections] of the inch section.

(2) *Lü Guang*: Heart and lung are located above the diaphragm; they constitute the yang [aspect] among the long-term depots. Thus, during exhalation their qi move out. Kidneys and liver are located below the diaphragm; they constitute the yin [aspect] among the long-term depots. Thus, during inhalation their qi move in. The spleen is [associated with] the central district; it nourishes the [remaining] four long-term depots. Hence, [the text] states: "It receives the qi of the grains between exhalation and inhalation."[2]

Ding Deyong: When the [*Nan*] *jing* states, "[that which is] exhaled originates from," this is not to say that the [breathing] qi leave from the heart or lung. It means [the following]. Kidneys and liver are located below the diaphragm. They rule the interior. Consequently, exhalation [means that the qi] move [from the interior, i.e., lower sections of the organism] outward toward heart and lung. Thus, [one should read:] "Upon exhalation, [the qi of the kidneys and of the

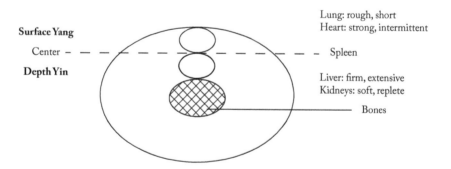

Surface Yang		Lung: rough, short
		Heart: strong, intermittent
Center – — —		Spleen
Depth Yin		Liver: firm, extensive
		Kidneys: soft, replete
		Bones

The second new diagnostic pattern resulted from an identification – on the basis of the sixfold subcategorization of yin and yang – of three characteristic yin and yang movements in the vessels, associated, again, with the individual functional units of the organism. In difficult issue 18, the concept of these three longitudinal levels is applied to all three cross-sections, with the latter still being called *bu* 部 ("section") but the former having their names changed from *bu* to *hou* 候 ("indicator").

2   The character 以 here may be a mistake for *jian* 間 ("between").

liver] move out toward heart and lung." Furthermore, heart and lung are located above the diaphragm. They rule the exterior. Consequently, inhalation [means that the qi] follow the yin and move inward toward kidneys and liver. Hence, the [*Nan*] *jing* states: "[The qi a person] exhales leave [the organism] through yang [long-term depots. The qi a person] inhales enter [the organism] through yin long-term depots."[3]

Xu Dachun: The three words *shou gu wei* 受穀味 ("receives the flavor qi of the grains") are meaningless here. "In the center" means: it is situated between yin and yang.

Liao Ping: *Shen* 腎 ("kidneys") should be read as *dan* 膽 ("gall bladder"). Liver and gall bladder are located together in the lower [section of the organism] .... This forced explanation, namely to associate exhalation and inhalation with the images of the long-term depots, is another invention of this book. If it were so [as it is written here], the upper [section of the organism, i.e., heart and lung] would be entirely responsible for exhalation, while the lower [section of the organism, i.e., kidneys and liver] would be entirely responsible for inhalation. Is there such a principle? Each inhalation must necessarily be tied to an exhalation, and each exhalation must necessarily be tied to an inhalation. One simply cannot separate [inhalation and exhalation] and cut them into two distinct [processes]. Still, the people cling to such queer talk and praise it; they do not care whether it is based on any reason.

(3) *Ding Deyong*: ["At the surface"] means that the [movement in the] vessels proceeds between skin and blood vessels, above the flesh. That is called "at the surface." ["In the depth"] means that the [movement in the] vessels is near the joints and close to the bones. That is called "in the depth."

Yang: [The qi appear to be] not enough when [the vessels are] pressed, and they appear to have a surplus when [the fingers are] lifted. Hence, one speaks of "at the surface." [The qi appear to have a] surplus when [the vessels are] pressed, and [they appear to be] not enough when [the figures are] lifted. Hence, one speaks of "in the depth."

Yu Shu: Yang is represented by fire; flames move upward. Hence, [the text] speaks of "at the surface." Yin is represented by water, which softens what is below. Hence, [the text] speaks of "in the depth."

(4) *Liao Ping*: Only five long-term depots [are mentioned here]; the [heart] enclosing network *(bao luo* 包絡) and the gate of life *(ming men* 命門) are not referred to.

(5) *Ding Deyong*: The heart is [associated with] the Southern regions and with fire. Hence, its [movement in the] vessels arrives near the surface and is strong and

---

3   This is a reference to difficult issue 11, sentence 2.

intermittent. The strong [aspect of it derives from] the long-term depot; the
intermittent [aspect of it derives from] the short-term repository.⁴ The lung is
[associated with] the Western regions and with metal. Metal controls dryness.
Its [movement in the] vessels is near the surface, rough, and short.

Yang: When [the movement of the qi is] fine and slow, when the coming and
going [of the qi seems to be plagued by] difficulties and is intermittent, or when
it even comes to a halt once in a while, that is called a "rough" [movement].

Yu Shu: The heart represents the fire; [fire] illuminates the exterior. Hence, [the
movement of its qi is] near the surface, strong and intermittent. The lung belongs to the metal. Its location is high. Hence, [the movement of its qi is] near
the surface, short, and rough.

Liao Ping: The two terms ["strong" and "intermittent"] do not appear below as
one of the six [possible movements in the] vessels [listed there].

(7) *Ding Deyong:* The liver is [associated with] the Eastern regions and with wood.
[The movement of] its [qi in the] vessels is firm and extended. The firm [aspect
of it derives from] the long-term depot; the extended [aspect of it derives from]
the short-term repository.⁵

Yang: Upon pressing [the vessel], one perceives but an extremely robust [move-
ment]. Hence, it is called "firm."

Yu Shu: The liver belongs to the wood, the roots of which emerge from the earth.
That makes the meaning of "firm" understandable. Branches and leaves extend
toward heaven. The reason for the "extended" [nature of a movement associated
with the liver] originates from this [correspondence].

(8) *Ding Deyong:* The kidneys are [associated with] the Northern regions and with
water, [both of which] control the cold. It is the nature [of water] to be soft and
to be in the depth, [and the same applies to the movement of the qi associated
with the kidneys in the vessels]. The soft [aspect of it derives from] the long-
term depot; the deep [aspect of it derives from] the short-term repository.⁶

Yang: Upon pressing [the vessel, the qi appear to be] not enough; when the [fin-
ger] is lifted they appear to have a surplus. That is called "soft." When [the
movement is] strong and extended, and slightly vigorous, and when it responds
to the finger pressure as if it were oppressed, that is called "replete."

Yu Shu: The nature of fire is an external softness. It is soft when pressed. The nature of water is an internal hardness. When the finger is lifted it comes replete.
That is what was meant here.

---

4 The small intestine is the short-term repository associated with the heart.
5 The gall bladder is the short-term repository associated with the liver.
6 The urinary bladder is the short-term repository associated with the kidneys.

Liao Ping: The term ["replete"] does not appear below as one of the six [possible movements in the] vessels.

(9) *Yu Shu*: It is said above that "between exhalation and inhalation, the spleen receives the flavor [qi] of the grains." Here now it is said that "the spleen is [associated with] the central district; its [movement in the] vessels is located in the center." *Gu* 穀 ("grains") stands for *gu* 谷 ("hollow"), and *gu* ("hollow") implies *kong* 空 ("voidness"). That is to say, the qi of man's exhalation and inhalation are obtained from the grains. The spleen is [associated with] the soil and belongs to the soil. Its location is in the center. The soil is the origin and the end of all things in the five cardinal directions.[7] Hence, it receives the flavor [qi] of the grains, and, hence, it is located in the central region. Hence, [the text] states: "Its [movement in the] vessels is located in the center."

(11) *Ding Deyong*: Earlier, the [*Nan*] *jing has* referred to the [movements in the] vessels as they are associated with the five long-term depots, linking them to the Five Phases. Here now, [the *Nan jing*] refers to the three yin and three yang [movements in the] vessels, linking them to the six [possible movements of the] qi. Those [movements] that are at the surface, smooth, and extended are the three yang [movements]; those [movements that are] in the depth, short, and rough are the three yin [movements]. One feels the three sections[8] [near the wrist] in order to investigate these [six different kinds of movement in the] vessels. This enables one to perceive the hidden patterns of yin and yang. Thus, the area below the skin is the upper[9] [level of the] vessels, constituting the yang section. If [any of] the three yin [kinds of movement in the] vessels appears here, this [implies that] the yin [qi] have moved upward to avail themselves of the yang [level]. Also, the area below the flesh is the lower [level] of the vessels, constituting the yin section. If [any of] the three yang [kinds of movement in the] vessels appears here, this [implies that] the yang [qi] have moved downward to take over the yin [level]. That is [how] to examine the pattern of yin and yang in the upper and lower [levels of the vessels].

Li Jiong: The heart is a yang long-term depot. It is located in the [region of the] Upper Burner. Because a yang [long-term depot] is located here in a yang [region, the heart is subcategorized as] yang-in-yang. The lung is a yin long-term depot.[10] It is located in the [region of the] Upper Burner. Because a yin [long-

---

7   These include East, North, West, South, and Center.

8   The term *bu* 部 ("section") refers here to the three longitudinal levels of the inch opening.

9   The text has *xia* 下 ("lower"). That may be a mistake.

10 In this difficult issue, the *Nan jing* classifies the lung as a yang long-term depot because it is located in the upper section of the organism. Li Jiong, in classifying it as a yin depot,

term depot] is located here in a yang [region, the lung is subcategorized as] yin-in-yang. The kidneys are a yin long-term depot. They are located in the [region of the] Lower Burner. Because a yin [long-term depot] is located here in a yin [region, the kidneys are subcategorized as] yin-in-yin. The liver is a yang long-term depot.[11] It is located in the [region of the] Central Burner. Because a yang [long-term depot] is located here in a yin [region, the liver is subcategorized as] yang-in-yin. The spleen is a yin long-term depot. It is located in the [region of the] Central Burner. Because a long-term depot [categorized as] major yin is located here in a yin [region, the spleen is subcategorized as] extreme yin-in-yin.

(13) *Li Jiong*: This [statement] refers to the three yin and three yang [movements in the] vessels which correspond to the six qi.[12] At the surface, smooth, and extended are the three yang [movements in the] vessels; in the depth, short, and rough are the three yin [movements in the] vessels.

Hua Shou: This question-and-answer [dialogue] is designed to explain the appearance of the yin and yang vessel [movements] in the three sections,[13] and [also to elucidate the phenomenon that] they do not appear individually. They do not appear individually because they appear in combinations. [A movement] at the surface can be perceived with light [pressure of the] hand; an extended [movement] exceeds the measures of its original location; a smooth [movement] comes and goes, flowing easily. All these are yang [movements in the] vessels. [A movement] in the depth can be perceived with heavy [pressure of the] hand; a short [movement] does not reach over its [entire] original location; a rough [movement] comes congealed and restrained. All these are yin [movements in the] vessels.

(14) *Li Jiong*: "At the surface" is a minor yang [movement in the] vessels. "Smooth" is a yang brilliance [movement in the] vessels. "Extended" is a major yang [movement in the] vessels. "In the depth" is a minor yin [movement in the]

---

may refer here to the *Su wen* treatise "Liu jie zang xiang lun" 六節藏象論, in which the lung is defined as belonging to the major yin subcategory of yang.

11 In this difficult issue, the liver is classified as a yin long-term depot because it is located in the lower section of the organism. Li Jiong classified it as a yang depot, again possibly in accordance with the *Su wen* treatise "Liu jie zang xiang lun" 六節藏象論," in which the liver is defined as belonging to the minor yang subcategory of yang.

12 Li Jiong may refer here to a correspondence between the six possible movements in the vessels and the six climatic qi dominating during different periods of the year. The latter include fire, cold, and dryness as yang qi, and heat, humidity, and wind as yin qi.

13 Cf. note 8.

vessels. "Short" is a ceasing yin [movement in the] vessels. "Rough" is a major yin [movement in the] vessels.¹⁴

Liao Ping: The appearances of the [movement in the] vessels are associated here with the five long-term depots. Yang [movements] represent the upper long-term depots; yin [movements] represent the lower long-term depots. Really, that is strange talk! The [*Nei*] *jing* states: "[The movement that can be felt at] the *ren* [*ying*] may be twice, three times, or four times as strong as that [which can be felt] at the inch [opening]," and "[the movement that can be felt at] the inch [opening] can be twice, three times, or four times as strong as that at the *ren* [*ying*]." These are correct statements.

(15) *Ding Deyong*: When this kind of vessel [movement] appears in the foot section of the left hand, it indicates that [the qi in] kidneys and bladder, [i.e.,] in long-term depot and short-term repository – the one representing the exterior and the other representing the interior [aspect] – follow their proper course. When [this kind of movement appears] in the inch opening of the left hand, one suffers from a disease, in that [qi move] contrary to their proper course.

Li Jiong: "One yin" refers to a vessel [movement] in the depth. "One yang" refers to a smooth [movement in the] vessels.

(16) *Ding Deyong*: When this kind of vessel [movement] appears in the yin section, that indicates that the yang [qi] have moved downward to take over the yin section.

Li Jiong:"One yin" refers to a vessel [movement] in the depth. "Two yang" refers to a [movement in the] vessels that is smooth and extended.

(17) *Ding Deyong*: This [condition indicates that] yang [qi] lie hidden in the yin [section].

Li Jiong: "One yin" refers to a vessel [movement] in the depth. "Three yang" refers to a [movement in the] vessels that is at the surface, smooth, and extended. If such a vessel [movement] appears in the foot section at the surface and is smooth and extended, but occasionally also in the depth, it indicates yin [qi] which lie hidden in the yang [section].

(18) *Ding Deyong*: A vessel [movement] that is at the surface and rough is a [movement in the] vessels [that is associated with] the lung. It should appear in the inch opening of the right hand. [If so, this indicates that] the yin and yang [qi] of that specific section follow their proper course. If [such a movement] appears

---

14 Li Jiong, in his comments on sentence 11, applied the fourfold subcategorization of yin and yang (including yin-in-yin, yang-in-yin, yang-in-yang, and yin-in-yang) to classify the long-term depots. Here, he drew on the sixfold subcategorization of yin and yang to classify the vessel movements.

in the gate of the left hand, [this indicates that the person] suffers from a disease, in that [qi move] contrary to their proper course.

Li Jiong: "One yang" refers to a vessel [movement] at the surface. One yin refers to a rough [movement in the] vessels.

(19) *Ding Deyong*: In this case blood and qi are deficient. [The movement of] both of them is rough.

Li Jiong: "One yang" refers to an extended[15] [movement in the] vessels. "Two yin" refers to a [movement in the] vessels that is in the depth and rough. [This kind of a movement in] the vessels is situated in the yang section. If now, in contrast, a yin vessel [movement] appears here, that indicates that both the blood and the qi are depleted, and that yin [qi] have taken over the yang [section].

(20) *Ding Deyong*: If such [a condition] appears in the yang section, it indicates that yin [qi] lie hidden in the yang section.

Li Jiong: "One yang" refers to a vessel [movement] at the surface. "Three yin" refers to a [movement in the] vessels that is in the depth, rough, and short. If the [movement] in the inch section appears in the depth and is rough and short, but occasionally also near the surface, it [indicates] yang [qi] which lie hidden in the yin [section].

Xu Dachun: These [sentences refer to] the parallel appearance of several [movements in the] vessels. Here only this one example is provided but other combinations are possible as well. It must not necessarily be as it is stated here. However, one should also know that [movements] near the surface and in the depth can occur simultaneously, while a smooth [movement] cannot appear together with a rough [movement], and an extended [movement] cannot appear together with a short [movement].

(21) *Yang*: One must examine the changes of the six [kinds of movement in the] vessels as they are related to spring, summer, autumn, and winter. Then it will be obvious whether [the qi] – in the case of a disease – proceed contrary to or in accordance with their proper course.

Xu Dachun: The text above [this last sentence] talks about the appearances of the [movement in the] vessels but does not yet touch on the auspicious or inauspicious [nature of a particular movement]. Here now [the text] refers to how to arrive at a decision [concerning the seriousness of a disease]. The "conduits" are the three yin and three yang [conduits] of hands and feet. "Proceed contrary to or in accordance with their proper course" means, for instance, the following. A [movement in the] vessels [associated with] the heart should be near the surface; a [movement in the] vessels [associated with] the kidneys should be in the

_____

15 "Extended" may be a mistake here for "at the surface."

depth. These would be [movements] "in accordance with their proper course." However, if a vessel [movement associated with] the heart appears in the depth; or if a vessel [movement associated with the] kidneys appears near the surface, these are [movements] "contrary to their proper course." This makes it obvious once again that the [movement in the] vessels does not have a fixed structure. The method for determining – on the basis of the [location of the movement in the] conduits – whether the qi proceed contrary to or in accordance with their proper course is discussed satisfactorily in both scriptures [i.e., in the *Nei jing* and in the *Nan jing*].

(1)–(21) *Nan jing*: Historically, there are two perspectives on how to examine the [movements in the] vessels for differentiating [the conditions of the] yin and yang [aspects of the organism]. The first is based on a differentiation of [the three sections] inch, gate, and foot. Here the inch [section] is yang; it is ruled by heart and lung. The gate is located in the middle; it is ruled by spleen and stomach. The foot [section] is yin; it is ruled by the kidneys and by the liver. The second [perspective] is based on a differentiation of surface, center, and depth. Here the "surface" is yang; it is ruled by heart and lung. The "depth" is yin; it is ruled by the kidneys and by the liver. What is neither at the surface nor in the depth is called "center"; it is ruled by the spleen. If we follow the spirit of the [*Nan jing*] text itself, yin and yang are discussed in this difficult issue mainly according to [the differentiation of] surface and depth. After determining that what is "near the surface" is ruled by heart and lung, while "the depth" is ruled by the kidneys and by the liver, [the discourse] moves a step further in its analysis, [pointing out the following classifications]. The heart is the yang-in-yang; thus, its [movement in the] vessels is at the surface, intermittent, and strong. The lung is yin-in-yang; thus, its [movement in the] vessels is at the surface, short, and rough. The liver is yang-in-yin; thus, its [movement in the] vessels is in the depth, replete, and extended. The kidneys are yin-in-yin; their [movement in the] vessels is soft when pressed, and it comes to fill itself when the finger is lifted. It is soft externally and hard internally. The spleen is located below the heart and lung, and above the liver and the kidneys. Therefore it is called "central district." Ye Lin has stated: "The spleen belongs to the soil and is located in the center. It reigns in all four seasons, and it nourishes the four [remaining] long-term depots. Its [movement in] the vessels comes easily and is relaxed; it is neither in the depth nor at the surface. Hence, [the text] states: 'Its [movement in the] vessels is in the center'." This, then, is the differentiation of yin and yang by taking into account surface and depth. According to an even finer analysis, there are, in addition, the three yin and the three yang [movements in the] vessels.

Surface, smooth, and extended – these three [movements] belong to the yang; depth, rough, and short – these three belong to the yin. One searches at the surface and in the depth for the six [kinds of] vessel [movement]. If, for instance, in the surface section three yin vessel [movements] are apparent, this indicates that the yin [qi] have moved upward to take over the yang [section]. If in the depth section three yang vessel [movements] are apparent, that indicates that the yang [qi] have moved down to take over the yin [section]. As for "one yin one yang; one yin two yang," and so on, these are complex vessel images appearing together at the same time. They too reflect a one-sided flourishing or weakness of yin or yang [aspects of the organism], or a takeover of a yang [section] by yin [qi], and vice versa. On the basis of all of this we may understand the appearance of the three yin and three yang vessel [movements] at the foot and inch sections, near the surface and in the depth. If they do not correspond to their respective [theoretical] locations, that indicates a takeover of yin [locations] by yang [qi], or vice versa.

五難曰：(一)脈有輕重，何謂也？

(二)然：初持脈，如三菽1之重，與皮毛相得者，肺部也。(三)如六菽
之重，與血脈相得者，心部也。(四)如九菽之重，與肌肉相得者，脾部
也。(五)如十二菽之重，與筋平者，肝部也。(六)按之至骨，舉指來疾
者，腎也。(七)故曰輕重也。

The fifth difficult issue. (1) The [movement in the] vessels may be light or heavy.
What does that mean?

(2) It is like this. First one touches the vessel [at the inch opening by exerting a pres-
sure] as heavy as three beans and he will reach the lung section on the [level of the]
skin [and its] hair. (3) If [one exerts a pressure] as heavy as six beans, he will reach
the heart section on the [level of the] blood vessels. (4) If [one exerts a pressure] as
heavy as nine beans, he will reach the spleen section on the level of the flesh. (5) If
[one exerts a pressure] as heavy as twelve beans, he will reach the liver section on the
level of the muscles.[1] (6) If one presses down to the bones and then lifts the fingers
until a swift [movement of qi] arrives, [the level reached] is the kidneys [section].[2]
(7) Hence, one speaks of "light" and "heavy."[3]

---

1 The term *jin* 筋 is not as specific in a modern anatomical sense as its rendering here with
   "muscles" might imply; it includes sinews as well.

2 Except for the *Nan jing ji zhu,* virtually all other editions consulted have added the term
   bu 部 here.

3 This difficult issue introduces a fivefold differentiation of the longitudinal levels on which
   the qi associated with the five long-term depots move. No other difficult issue returns to
   this idea. It may be illustrated as follows:

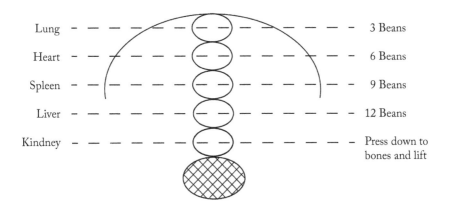

(1) *Li Jiong*: In examining the [movement in the] vessels [one may exert] light or heavy [pressure] in order to investigate the yin and yang [qi on levels that are] high or low.

Liao Ping: The [concepts of] "at the surface" and "in the depth" of the [*Nei*] *jing* are quite intelligible.[4] Here now, the bean method is established and that gives it a confusing turn. One can call [the movement in the vessels] "at the surface" or "in the depth," but one cannot call it "light" or "heavy." The [*Nei*] *jing* has no such doctrine.

(2) *Lü Guang*: *Shu* ("pulse") stands for *dou* 豆 ("bean"). [This difficult issue] discusses the light and heavy [pressure to be exerted in examining the movements] of the vessels. If [the pressure exerted by one's fingers is] as heavy as three beans, one reaches the area of the skin [and of its] hair. The skin [and its] hair are where the qi of the lung proceed. [This level] is called the "lung section."

Li Jiong: Whenever one examines the lung [movement in the] vessels, he should exert only light pressure with his hand.

Hua Shou: The lung is located highest [in the body]. It rules the indicator [level] of the skin [and of its] hair. Hence, its vessel [movement can be located by a pressure] as heavy as three beans.

(3) *Lü Guang*: The heart rules the [movement in the] blood vessels. It comes next to the lung. [Its qi can be felt with a pressure] as heavy as six beans.

Li Jiong: Whenever one examines the [movement in the] vessels [associated with] the heart, he should exert a pressure with his hand that is slightly heavier [than that used to examine the lung movement].

(4) *Lü Guang*: The spleen occupies the center [of the body]; it rules the flesh. Hence, it comes next to the heart. [Its qi can be felt with a pressure] as heavy as nine beans.

Li Jiong: Whenever one examines the [movement in the] vessels [associated with] the spleen, he should exert a pressure with his hand that is neither light nor heavy.

Liao Ping: How can one distinguish in what depth [below the skin] flesh and blood vessels are situated?

(5) *Lü Guang*: The liver rules the muscles; it is located below the spleen. Hence, [the level where its qi can be felt] comes next.

---

4 The concepts of *fu* 浮 ("at the surface") and s*hen* 沈 ("in the depth") appear as diagnostic tools in *Su wen* treatise 17, "Mai yao jing wei lun" 脈要精微論; in *Su wen* treatise 18, "Ping ren qi xiang lun" 平人氣象論; and elsewhere.

Li Jiong: Whenever one examines the [movement in the] vessels [associated with] the liver, he should exert a pressure with his hand that is slightly heavier [than that used to examine the spleen movement].

Liao Ping: The two terms *fu* 浮 ("to float at the surface") and *shen* 沈 ("to sink to the depth") were chosen by the [*Nei*] *jing* because it referred, [in explaining the different levels of the movement in the vessels,] to the image of items floating on water. That was quite intelligible. To discuss [these levels] in terms of "heavy" and "light" according to the number of beans, however, causes the people only to be confused. Questions are bound to arise. Who would experiment with beans to diagnose surface and depth?!

(6) *Lü Guang:* The kidneys rule the bones. Their [movement in the] vessels is deep, near the bones.

Hua Shou: The kidneys are located below the liver; they rule the bones. Hence, one reaches their [movement in the] vessels by pressing down to the bones and by subsequently lifting the fingers so that [the qi may] come [back] and supplement [the area squeezed before]. With regard to the kidneys, [the *Nan jing*] does not speak of beans. In analogy [to the amounts mentioned earlier] the pressure exerted here should be as heavy as fifteen beans.

Zhang Shixian: [The *Nan jing*] does not speak of "fifteen beans" with regard to the kidneys but states "down to the bones" because "down to the bones" is more intelligible than "fifteen beans."

(7) *Yu Shu:* The light or heavy [pressure to be exerted in examining the movements in the] vessels is outlined, by the [*Nan*] *jing*, in great detail. If one relies on the [*Nan*] *jing* to find the location [of the respective movements] and investigate them, the significance [of this paragraph] should become obvious. [The *Nan jing*] provides an example to demonstrate the underlying pattern. If, for instance, one gets hold [of a movement] in the inch opening of the left hand [by exerting a pressure as heavy as] three beans, he knows that lung qi have arrived. If one gets hold [of a movement with a pressure as heavy as] six beans, he knows that qi of that particular conduit have arrived. If one gets hold [of a movement with a pressure as heavy as] nine beans, he knows that qi of the spleen have arrived. If one gets hold [of a movement with a pressure as heavy as] twelve beans, he knows that qi of the liver have arrived. If one presses [one's fingers down] to the bones and gets hold of a movement there, he knows that kidneys' qi have arrived. Obviously, the qi of each of the five long-term depots flow through all [the conduits] and, consequently, the six [possible movements in the] vessels display specific patterns. These [patterns] can be used to determine good or evil auspices,

and to speak about [a person's] disease. All other [possibilities] correspond to [the examples given] here. Hence, [the text] speaks of "light" and "heavy."

Hua Shou: [This difficult issue] talks about "light" and "heavy" in the sense of "surface," "center," and "depth." But [the terms "light" and "heavy"] do not appear in either the [*Nei*] *jing* or the *Su* [*wen*]. It could be an ancient method [to examine the] vessels that was handed down [through generations], but it may also have originated from Yueren's personal perspective.

Li Jiong: The heart and the lung are located above the diaphragm; they constitute the yang [category of the] long-term depots. Yang [qi] float above near the surface. They should be felt by light pressure. Liver and kidneys are located below the diaphragm; they constitute the yin [category of the] long-term depots. Yin [qi] are deep at the bottom. They should be felt by heavy pressure.

Xu Dachun: In the [paragraph] "Ping mai fa" 平脈法, the *Shang han lun* 傷寒論 quotes these sentences, referring to a "scripture" (*jing* 經). This is probably the *Nan jing*. I do not know from what source the *Nan jing* took these [statements].

Ye Lin: Why did [the *Nan jing*] pick just beans [to explain the] light and heavy [pressure to be exerted when examining the movement in the] vessels? Also, it did not refer to "three beans," "four beans," and "five beans"; the amounts must increase by three respectively. Well, beans come in pods where always a number of them are linked together. This is quite similar to the movement of the vessels under the fingers. From this idea we may infer that the statement "as heavy as three beans" does not mean that three beans should be heaped upon each other in one particular [diagnostic] section. Rather, one single finger should be lowered by the pressure of one bean. For [all three fingers covering] all three sections, this [adds up to] three beans. The location of the lung is high [in the body], and it rules the skin [and its] hair. Hence, light [pressure is adequate]. "As heavy as six beans" [indicates that] each of the three sections should receive [a pressure] as heavy as two beans. The heart is located below the lung. It rules the [movement in the] blood vessels. Hence, [the pressure exerted should be] slightly heavier. "As heavy as nine beans" [indicates that] each of the three sections should receive [a pressure] as heavy as three beans. The spleen is located below the heart. It rules the flesh. Hence, [the pressure should be] slightly heavier again. "As heavy as twelve beans" [indicates that] each of the three sections should receive [a pressure] as heavy as four beans. The liver is located below the spleen; it controls the muscles. Thus, a pressure heavier by one bean – in comparison to the spleen – should be exerted here. The kidneys are located below the liver; they rule the bones. Hence, one feels their [movement in the] vessels by pressing down to the bones. That is as deep as one can go. Why is it that a "swift movement" [can be felt] upon lifting [the fingers]? Now, the substance of the [movement in the] vessels is blood; that which [causes the blood to] move are the qi. The kidneys unite water and fire. When fire is brought into water, it is changed into [steam] qi. When one presses right down to the bones, the qi in the vessel have no [space left] to pass below the fingers. Upon slightly lifting the fingers, [the qi] come quickly forward. In this way, the steam[-like] movement of the qi of the kidneys becomes apparent.

六難曰：（一）脈有陰盛陽虛，陽盛陰虛，何謂也？

（二）然：浮之損小，沉之實大，故曰陰盛陽虛。（三）沉之損小，浮之實大，故曰陽盛陰虛，（四）是陰陽虛實意也。

The sixth difficult issue: (1) The [movement in the] vessels may display "yin abundance, yang depletion," or "yang abundance, yin depletion." What does that mean?

(2) It is like this. A diminished and minor [movement] at the surface, together with a replete and strong [movement] in the depth, indicate, of course, "yin abundance, yang depletion." (3) A diminished and minor [movement] in the depth, together with a replete and strong [movement] at the surface, indicate, of course, "yang abundance, yin depletion." (4) The meaning [referred to by these terms] is that of a repletion or depletion of yin and yang [qi].

COMMENTARIES

(1) *Liao Ping*: This difficult issue presents a method of diagnosing the long-term depots and short-term repositories on the basis of an association of "at the surface" and "in the depth" with the long-term depots and short-term repositories. This book already established numerous contradictory doctrines. Later on the *Mai jing*, however, created a real monster by distinguishing – in its apocryphal chapters[1] – forty-eight groupings [of symptomatic vessel movements]!

(2) *Lü Guang*: The yang [movement in the] vessels appears at the inch opening; normally it is at the surface and replete. But if one can feel, with light [pressure of one's] hand, a diminished and minor [movement] at the surface, that is [a condition] called "yang depletion." If one presses with a heavy hand and feels, in the depth, a strong and replete [movement] which is contrary [to what would be normal], that is [a condition] called "yin repletion," because the yin [movements proceed] in the depth.

Ding Deyong: The yang [movement in the] vessels is normally at the surface. If one presses the vessel with a light hand [and feels that the qi] arrive diminished and [with] minor [strength, that indicates that] the yang [qi are] depleted or not enough. The yin [movement in the] vessels is normally in the depth and soft. If one presses the [vessel] with a heavy hand [and feels that the qi] arrive diminished and weak, [that indicates that] the yin [qi are] depleted or not enough.

Yu Shu: Man is endowed with yin and yang [qi]; when his yin and yang [qi] are in a normal state and balanced, then no evidence exists for a change toward de-

---

1   It is not clear whether Liao Ping referred to any specific chapter of the *Mai jing* 脈經 here.

pletion or toward repletion. Here, though, [the *Nan jing*] speaks of "abundance" and "depletion"; these are [conditions of the movement in the] vessels indicating disease. In the [treatise] "Mai yao jing wei lun" 脈要精微論 [of the *Su wen*] it is said: "When the yin [qi] abound, then one dreams of wading through a big water and is in fear. When the yang [qi] abound, then one dreams of big fires burning. When both yin and yang [qi] abound, then one dreams of mutual killings and harmings." In this way, one may examine the meaning of yin and yang depletion and repletion. [2]

Li Jiong: "At the surface" indicates the [movement of the] yang [qi in the] vessels; "at the surface, diminished, and minor" indicates a depletion of yang [qi in the] vessels. The [movement of the] yang [qi in the] vessels appears at the inch opening; normally, it is at the surface and replete. Now, if one gets hold of it at the surface with a light hand and if it has changed into a diminished and minor [movement], that means that the yang [qi] are depleted or not enough. "In the depth" indicates the [movement of the] yin [qi in the] vessels; "in the depth, replete, and strong" indicates an abundance of yin [qi in the] vessels. The [movement of the] yin [qi in the] vessels appears in the foot section; it is normally in the depth and soft. If one presses [the foot section] with a heavy hand, and perceives, in contrast [to what is normal], a replete and strong [movement], that is an abundance or an excessive [presence] of yin [qi].

Liao Ping: If the [movement that can be felt at the] *ren ying* 人迎 is stronger than that at the inch opening, that is called "yang abundance." If the [movement that can be felt at the] inch opening is stronger than that at the *ren ying*, that is called "yin abundance." For details see the treatise "Jing mai" [of the *Ling shu*]. [3]

(3) *Ding Deyong*: The [movement of the] yang [qi in the] vessels is normally at the surface. If it appears even more replete and even stronger [than usual], that is a [situation of] "yang abundance, yin depletion." The *Su wen* states: "All [movements] at the surface indicate that [the qi of] the kidneys are not enough."

Liao Ping: The term *sun* 損 (literally, "to destroy"; here, "diminished") does not represent the opposite of *shi* 實 ("replete").

(1)–(4) *Zhang Shixian*: This [difficult issue] talks about [movements in the] vessels [indicating a] "greatly excessive" or "insufficient" [condition of] yin and yang [qi]. The yin [qi] are responsible for the [movement that can be felt at the] foot [section]; the yang [qi] are responsible for the [movement that can be felt at the] inch [section]. The [qi appear in the] inch [section] at the surface and in the foot

---

2 Water is categorized as yin; fire is categorized as yang.

3 The left hand where the *ren ying* 人迎 is situated is categorized as yang; the right hand where the inch opening is situated is categorized as yin.

[section] in the depth. "Diminished and minor" [means] "not enough" and/or "depletion"; "replete and strong" [means] "greatly excessive" and/or "repletion."[4] The [latter terms] refer to an abundance [of qi] in the vessels. Whenever[5] the yin and the yang [qi] are in balance, this means good fortune. If only one of them is present in abundance, [this indicates disease]. In the case of an abundance of yin [qi together with] a depletion of yang [qi], the [movement] at the surface in the inch [section] will be diminished and minor, while [the movement] in the depth in the foot [section] will be replete and strong. In the case of an abundance of yang [qi together with] a depletion of yin [qi], the [movement] at the surface in the inch [section] will be replete and strong, while [the movement] in the depth in the foot [section] will be diminished and minor. These are depletion and re-pletion of yin and yang [qi as they appear] in the foot and inch [sections]. If one talks about this in terms of the individual conduits, then [it should be pointed out that] each section itself [may display conditions of] repletion or depletion of the yin and yang [qi]. However, if by [exerting] light [pressure with one's] hand one gets hold – at the surface – of a diminished and minor [movement], and if by [exerting] heavy [pressure with one's] hand one gets hold – in the depth – of a replete and strong [movement], that is [always] called "yin abundance, yang repletion." Or, if by [exerting] heavy [pressure with one's] hand one gets hold – in the depth – of a diminished and minor [movement], and if by [exerting] light [pressure with one's] hand one gets hold – at the surface – of a replete and strong [movement], that is [always] called "yang abundance, yin depletion." The language of the [*Nan*] *jing* here is not clear. Anybody [interested in] extended studies should occupy himself with this [issue] in more detail.

Xu Dachun: This [discussion] here differs from the text above [where it was stat-ed]: "The [movement in the] vessels may display patterns of yin and yang."[6] The text above talks about vessel [movements] associated with yin and yang [catego-ries] as normal [movements in the] vessels. Here are discussed the [movements of] yin and yang [qi in the] vessels together with greatly excessive or insufficient vessel [movements] in the [yin and] yang sections, and these are vessel [move-ments indicating] disease.

Katō Bankei: This paragraph appears similar to the third section of the fifty-eighth difficult issue. However, the meaning is different. There, "yang depletion, yin abundance" and "yang abundance, yin depletion" indicate internal or external damage caused by cold. Here, the [concepts of] "at the surface" and "in the

4   *Wei* 謂 must be a mistake here for *shi* 實

5   *Zhe* 者 must be a mistake here for *chu* 諸.

6   Cf. difficult issue 4, sentence 1.

depth" of the preceding text are taken up again in order to establish a method of diagnosing depletion or repletion of yin and yang [qi]. Readers must not mix up these [issues] because of an accidental similarity.

七難曰：(一)經言少陽之至，乍小乍大，乍短乍長；(二)陽明之至，浮大而短；(三)太陽之至，洪大而長；(四)太陰之至，緊大而長；(五)少陰之至，緊細而微；(六)厥陰之至，沉短而敦。(七)此六者，是平脈邪？將病脈邪？

(八)然：皆王脈也。

(九)其氣以何月，各王幾日？

(十)然：冬至之後，得甲子少陽王，(十一)復得甲子陽明王，(十二)復得甲子太陽王，(十三)復得甲子太陰王，(十四)復得甲子少陰王，(十五)復得甲子厥陰王。(十六)王各六十日，六六三百六十日，以成一歲。(十七)此三陽三陰之王時日大要也。

The seventh difficult issue: (1) The scripture states: The arrival of the minor yang [qi] is at times strong, at times minor, at times short, at times extended. (2) The arrival of the yang brilliance [qi] is at the surface, strong, and short. (3) The arrival of the major yang [qi] is vast, strong, and extended. (4) The arrival of the major yin [qi] is tight, strong, and extended. (5) The arrival of the minor yin [qi] is restricted, fine, and feeble. (6) The arrival of the ceasing yin [qi] is in the depth, short, and generous. (7) Are these six normal [movements in the] vessels? Or are these [movements in the] vessels indicative of diseases?

(8) It is like this. All these are [indications of] governing [qi moving through the] vessels.

(9) For how many days, and during which months, do the respective qi govern?

(10) It is like this. After winter solstice, during the [first subsequent] *jia zi* [term],[1] the minor yang [qi] govern. (11) During the following *jia zi* [term], the yang brilliance [qi] govern. (12) During the following *jia zi* [term], the major yang [qi] govern. (13) During the following *jia zi* [term], the major yin [qi] govern. (14) During the following *jia zi* [term], the minor yin [qi] govern. (15) During the following *jia zi* [term], the ceasing yin [qi] govern. (16) All these [qi] govern for 60 days each. Six times six [*jia zi* terms] add up to 360 days, completing one year. (17) These are the essential points of the three yin and three yang [qi] governing at [specific] seasons and [for a specific number of] days.[2]

---

1   A *jia zi* term represents a period of sixty days. *Jia* is the first of the Ten Celestial Stems, and *zi* is the first of the Twelve Earth Branches. By matching each of the former with each of the latter, a counting is possible from one through sixty. It was applied to days and years.

2   The wording of sentences 1 through 6 reminds one of the *Su wen* treatise "Zhi zhen yao da lun," which provides one of the most detailed accounts of the *wu yun liu qi* 五運六

COMMENTARIES

(1) *Lü Guang*: The minor yang [qi] govern during the first and second months. [At that time the yang] qi are still feeble and few. Hence, their arrival in the vessels is marked by irregular approach and withdrawal.

Hua Shou: At the begin of this paragraph, [the *Nan jing*] says: "The scripture states." I have checked the [*Ling*] *shu* and the *Su* [*wen*] but could not find [there the ideas outlined subsequently]. In the treatise "Ping ren qi xiang lun" 平人 氣象論 [of the *Su wen*], such theories are briefly referred to but not in any detail. Perhaps at the time of Yueren another text existed, allegedly dating from high antiquity. It may have been incorporated into the *Nei jing*, where it may have been abridged by later generations. It is impossible to be sure about this. Whenever [the *Nan jing*] says "the scripture states," and whenever [we find] no [corresponding statement in the *Ling shu* or *Su wen*] to check [this quotation], the same interpretation applies.

Xu Dachun: For the statement from the scripture quoted here, see the [treatise] "Zhi zhen yao da lun" 至真要大論 of the *Su wen* where it says: "Qi Bo: 'When ceasing yin [qi] arrive, the [movement in the] vessels is string-like. When minor yin [qi] arrive, the [movement in the] vessels is hook-like. When major yin [qi] arrive, the [movement in the] vessels is in the depth. When minor yang [qi] arrive, the [movement in the vessels] is big and at the surface. When yang brilliance [qi] arrive, the [movement in the vessels] is short and rough. When major yang [qi] arrive, the [movement in the vessels] is big and extended." And in the treatise "Ping ren qi xiang lun" 平人氣象論 [the *Su wen*] states: "The arrival of a major yang [movement in the] vessels, it is vast, big, and extended. The arrival of a minor yang movement in the] vessels, it is at times frequent, at times spaced, at times short, at times extended. The arrival of a yang brilliance [movement in the] vessels, it is at the surface, big, and short." With only a few differences, these [passages] highly correspond to [the statements of the *Nan jing*] here.

氣 ("five periods and six qi") concepts in the *Nei jing* and which may, therefore, be a Tang addition. We do not have to assume, accordingly, that the present difficult issue represents a later amendment to the *Nan jing*, although this possibility exists, especially if we recall Liao Ping's claim that the Lü Guang commentary does not predate the Tang era (see above, section I.E.). My rendering here of sentences 1 through 6 corresponds to three sentences in the *Su wen* treatise, "Ping ren qi xiang lun" 平人氣象論. The meaning of these three sentences appears isolated; it does not follow the flow of the argumentation in that treatise. This short passage may, therefore, be either a later addition or an abridged remainder of a formerly lengthy statement.

Liao Ping: Minor yang should be yang-brilliance.[3] The treatise "Liu ji zheng lun"[4] 六紀正論 lists the term *zhi* 至 ("arrival") seventy-two times, each time related to an assessment of the patterns of the qi. ["At times strong, at times weak, at times short, at times extended"] is the pattern of [a movement in] the vessels [associated with the] spleen. Yang brilliance and major yin are related to each other like outside and inside. Hence this [pattern] develops.

(2) *Lü Guang*: The yang brilliance [qi] govern during the third and fourth months. [At that time the yang] qi begin to sprout, but they are not yet present in abundance. Hence, their arrival in the vessels is located at the surface, and appears strong and short.

Liao Ping: ["Yang brilliance"] should be "major yang."[5] Qi and blood are present in small quantities only. Hence, [the movement is] "short."

(3) *Lü Guang*: The major yang [qi] govern during the fifth and sixth months. [At that time the yang] qi are present in great abundance. Hence, the arrival in the vessels appears vast, strong, and extended.

Ye Lin: A "vast [movement in the] vessels" appears at the surface and is strong. Furthermore, it is powerful. When one presses [the vessel] with lifted fingers, [the movement perceived] comes drifting, supplementing all three sections. It appears like a vast flow of water, with waves bubbling and rising. That [movement in the] vessels comes strong and [resembles the beating of a] drum.

Liao Ping: [The "major yang"] is related to the minor yin like outside to inside. One part minor yang [qi] and two parts major yang [qi move joined together here. Hence, the movement] should be extended .... When the scripture mentions, first, the conduits and their [respective] qi, and talks, then, about "arrivals" (*zhi* 至), this represents, in each case, a [method of] checking the [presence of specific] qi, not a method of carrying out a diagnosis.[6] One cannot speak of "arrivals" or of "coming/going" (*lai/qu* 來去) with respect to the diagnosis of the [movement in the] vessels .... The three yang [categories outlined here] are quoted from the [*Su wen* treatise] "Ping ren qi xiang lun" 平人氣象論. [That treatise, though, contains] no reference to the three [corresponding] yin [categories].

(4) *Lü Guang*: The major yin [qi] govern during the seventh and eighth months. They avail themselves of the remaining yang [qi] of summer. [At that time, the] yin qi are not yet present in abundance. Hence, their arrival in the vessels appears tight, strong, and extended.

---

3   The reason for this statement is unclear.

4   An identification of this treatise has not been possible.

5   See note 3.

6   It is not clear to which *Nei jing* treatise(s) Liao Ping may have referred here.

Ye Lin: A "tight [movement in the] vessels" is sometimes tardy and sometimes frequent; it feels like a rope, like a revolving rope. [Zhu] Danxi 朱丹溪 said that it is like a thread - that is, like a rope, strung together, for instance, from two or three [lines]. They must be twisted and turned around; when they begin to get tight, the rope is completed.

Liao Ping: From here on [the text] was added by the *Nan jing.*

(5) *Lü Guang:* The minor yin [qi] govern during the ninth and tenth months. [At that time] the yang qi are debilitated while the yin qi are present in abundance. Hence, the arrival of [the latter in] the vessels appears restricted, fine, and feeble.

Ye Lin: A "fine [movement in the] vessels" resembles a thread. It is extremely fine and is never interrupted at any of the three indicator [levels].[7] A "feeble [movement in the] vessels" appears to be there and then it appears not to be there. It is at the surface and soft, like powder. Under heavy pressure [by one's fingers], it tends to be cut off.

(6) *Lü Guang:* The ceasing yin [qi] govern during the eleventh and twelfth months. [At that time] the yin qi have reached the peak of abundance. Therefore, one speaks of "ceasing yin."[8] The arrival of [the ceasing yin qi in] the vessels appears deep, short, and generous. *Dun* 敦 ("generous") means *chen* 沈 ("in the depth") and *zhong* 重 ("heavy"). [Each of] the four seasons passes through one yin and one yang [phase, respectively, accounting for] eight governing [periods]. Here, the *Nan jing* places three yang [periods] in the earlier and three yin [periods] in the later [half of one year]. The governing [periods of yin and yang qi] are, therefore, different; the entire process is not the same. The *Nan jing* states that the first through the sixth months – that is, in spring and summer, during [the first] half of a year – the yang [qi] at the surface carry the responsibility for all affairs. Hence, it is said: "The three yang [qi] rule the earlier [half]." From the seventh through the twelfth months – that is, in autumn and winter, during the [second] half of a year – the yin [qi] in the depth carry the responsibility for all affairs. Hence, it is said: "The three yin [qi] rule the later [half]." That means that the four seasons [are divided into the two] governing periods of yin and yang, like husband and wife.

Liao Ping: The term *dun* 敦 ("generous") is particularly weird. The [*Su wen* treatise] "Zhi zhen yao da lun" 至真要大論 refers to "three yin" and "three yang," but [the meaning implied there] is different [from that here].

---

7   For the concept of "indicator levels," see difficult issue 18.

8   This statement contradicts our rendering of *jue yin* 厥陰 as "ceasing yin." One could translate this term here, following Lü Guang's interpretation, as "top yin."

(8) *Liao Ping*: This kind of talk belongs in a section on the [Five] Periods [and Six] Qi; it has nothing to do with diagnosing the [movements in the] conduit vessels.[9]

(17) *Liao Ping*: It is, already, a mistake to apply the doctrine of the [Five] Periods [and Six] Qi to the treatment of diseases. If, however, the [Five] Periods [and Six] Qi are referred to in connection with a mistaken diagnosis of the [movement in the] vessels, that means heaping mistake upon mistake. For details see Tamba's *Su wen shi* 素問識.

(1)–(17) *Ding Deyong*: The governing [periods] of the three yin and three yang qi are elucidated here on the basis of the six *jia* [terms]. This pattern follows the treatise "Liu jie zang xiang lun" 六節藏象論 of the *Huang Di* [*Nei jing Su wen*],where it is stated that the six [*jia* terms] multiplied by six form one year. If one selects the *jia zi* [term] after winter solstice, that is the first qi period of a full year. This *jia zi* [term begins] either early in "minor cold" or late in "massive cold."[10] Because [at that time of the year] the qi of minor yang have not yet emerged from the yin period, their [appearance in the] vessels is at times strong, at times weak, at times short, at times extended. When the next *jia zi* [term begins], the yang brilliance [qi] govern. "The arrival of the yang brilliance [qi] is at the surface, strong, and short": They constitute the second [category of] qi [in the course of the year]. Subsequently, [the climate] begins to warm up. But the [yang] qi are not yet present in abundance. Hence, when the yang brilliance [qi] have reached [their season, their movement in the vessels] is at the surface, strong, and short. "The arrival of the major yang [qi] is vast, strong, and extended": [With them] the next *jia zi* [term] begins; they constitute the third [category of] qi [in the course of the year]. This is the division of abundant yang. Hence, when the major yang [qi have reached their season, their movement in the vessels] is vast, strong, and extended. "The arrival of the major yin [qi] is restricted, strong, and extended": [With them] the next *jia zi* [term] begins; they constitute the fourth [category of] qi [in the course of the year]. This is the division of heat and moisture; the qi of autumn begin to emerge. They avail themselves of the remaining yang [qi] of summer. Hence, when the major yin [qi] have reached [their season, the movement in the vessels] appears restricted, strong, and extended. "The arrival of the minor yin [qi] is restricted, fine, and feeble": [With them] the next *jia zi* [term] begins; they constitute the fifth [category of] qi [in the course of the year]. This is the division of coolness. Hence, when the minor yin [qi] have

---

9   See note 2.

10   "Minor cold" and "massive cold" are the two last solar terms of the year. Their approximate dates according to the Western calendar are early and late in January.

reached [their season, their movement in the vessels] appears restricted, fine, and feeble. "The arrival of the ceasing yin [qi] is in the depth, short, and heavy": [With them] the next *jia zi* [term] begins; they constitute the final [category of] qi [in the course of the year]. This is the division of abundant yin. The water hardens and resembles stones. Hence, when the ceasing yin [qi] have reached [their season, their movement in the vessels] appears in the depth, short, and heavy. These are the governing [periods] of the three yin and three yang [qi] in the vessels. In correspondence to the six *jia* terms, one consequently has these six appearances of the [movements in the] vessels. They are called the "normal [movements in the] vessels."

Hua Shou: In the preceding paragraphs it was outlined how the three yin and three yang [qi] govern the [movements in the] vessels. Here it is outlined how the three yin and three yang [qi] govern the seasons. The appearance of the [movements in the] vessels should correspond to the seasons. The calendar experts say that in high antiquity the *jia zi* term of the eleventh month, with the conjunction of sun and moon, was the calendrical beginning [of the year], and consequently they employ [for their purposes] the regular division [of the year] into qi [terms] and new moon [dates]. But the course of nature may be slower or faster than the movement of sun and moon; they are not identical. Differences occur each year. When Yueren refers to the "*jia zi* [term] after winter solstice," this is perhaps exactly because of these [irregularities]. Thus, the uneven [distribution of] qi [terms] and of new moon [dates], as well as the earlier or later occurrence of seasonal terms, cannot follow any regularity. Hence, Mr. Ding, in his commentary, has stated: "this *jia zi* [date occurs] either early in 'minor cold' or late in 'massive cold'."[11] That is the beginning [of the season] when the minor yang [qi] arrive [in the vessels. The qi associated with] all the remaining conduits follow successively.

Zhang Shixian: "Normal" is a [movement in the] vessels without disease; affected by "disease" is a [movement in the] vessels that is not normal. "Governing" is a [movement in the] vessels that occupies the leading position. A year has twelve months; man has twelve conduits. In ancient times the people linked them to the twelve diagrams of the *Yi* [*jing*] 易經, because everything follows the principle of the rise and fall of yin and yang. That applies to the months of the year, to the conduits of man, and to the diagrams of the *Yi* [*jing*]. They all fit each other like [the tallies of] stamped official documents. Now, the twelve months are

---

11 Katō Bankei, in his commentary to difficult issue 7, pointed out that Hua Shou misinterpreted the term *jia zi* 甲子 as referring only to a particular day, rather than – as would be correct – to an entire period of sixty days. Hence, Hua Shou may also have misinterpreted Ding Deyong's statement, which is therefore rendered slightly differently here.

divided into six *jia zi* [terms]. During these terms the respective seasons govern, each of them lasting sixty days, adding up to one year. The *jia zi* [term] following winter solstice is the first *jia zi* [term]. Winter solstice is a date in the middle of the eleventh month. Because the months vary in their duration and because there are intercalary months, the [bi-]monthly dividing lines between the qi terms vary [with respect to their exact dates]; they may occur earlier or later. The date of the first *jia zi* [term] lies in the eleventh month; it is determined in accordance with the [actual] beginning of that qi term. One should not be confused by an earlier or later beginning. The remaining five *jia zi* [terms] take their turns accordingly .... The yin and yang [aspects] of all the months and diagrams move from below upward. Hence, man's governing [qi in the] vessels move also from the feet to the hands. For example, the minor yang [qi display the following pattern]: The first thirty days of the sixty days of the first *jia zi* [term] are governed by the foot minor yang [qi]. The latter thirty days show a flourishing of the hand minor yang [qi. The qi of] all the remaining conduits follow the same rule. This is related to the fixed pattern of [the interrelationship between] yin and yang; it is a doctrine which has changed never since remote antiquity. If he has understood this [pattern] and if [the interrelations of] yin and yang, and of the Five Phases, are clearly in his breast, a physician upon lowering his hand to examine the vessels feels [a movement in] the vessels corresponding to the season, and he immediately knows that it is neither a normal [movement] nor one affected by a disease, but [a movement of] governing [qi through the] vessels.

Liao Ping: The [movement in the] vessels does not change in accordance with the four seasons. For details, see the [treatise] "Si fang yi lun" 四方異論.[12] [The *Nan jing*] draws here on the patterns of the [Five] Periods [and Six] Qi in the [treatise] "Yin yang da lun" 陰陽大論 in order to discuss the [movements in the] vessels. That is a mistake.

---

12   An identification of this treatise has not been possible.

八難曰：（一）寸口脈平而死者，何謂也？

（二）然：諸十二經脈者，皆係於生氣之原。（三）所謂生氣之原者，謂十二經之根本也，謂腎間動氣也。（四）此五藏六府之本，十二經脈之根，呼吸之門，三焦之原。（五）一名守邪之神。（六）故氣者，人之根本也，（七）根絕則莖葉枯矣。（八）寸口脈平而死者，生氣獨絕於內也。

The eighth difficult issue: (1) The [movement of the qi in the] vessel at the inch opening [displays a condition of] normal balance, and yet [the respective person] dies. What does that mean?

(2) It is like this. All the twelve conduit vessels are linked with the origin of the vital qi.(3) The "origin of the vital qi" refers to the root and foundation of all the twelve conduits – that is, to the "moving qi" between the kidneys. (4) These [qi] are the foundation of the [body's] five long-term depots and six short-term repositories; they are the root of the twelve conduit vessels; they are the gate of exhalation and inhalation, and they are the origin of the Triple Burner. (5) They are also called "the spirit guarding against the evil." (6) Hence, the [moving] qi [between the kidneys] constitute a person's root and foundation. (7) Once the root is cut, the stalk and the leaves wither. (8) In case the vessel [movement] at the inch opening displays a condition of normal balance and yet [the respective person] dies, that is due only to an internal[1] cutting off of the vital qi.[2]

COMMENTARIES

(1) *Lü Guang*: When the [movement of the qi in the] vessel at the inch opening [displays a condition of] normal balance and yet [the respective person] dies, [that indicates that the movement of the qi in] the vessels does not correspond to the [governing qi of the] four seasons. The appearance of the [qi in the] vessels is in a state of normal balance.

---

1 "Internal" (*nei* 內) refers here to the internal section of the organism – that is, the region below the diaphragm where liver and kidneys are located.

2 In this difficult issue, the author(s) appear to have limited the all encompassing validity of the vessel movement at the inch opening as a reliable diagnostic indicator (as propagated in the first difficult issue). The ensuing discussion of its contents by commentators of later centuries mirrors, once again, historical differences in the interpretation of one and the same term or concept. The fact that this difficult issue combines, in its wording, a rather large number of hard-to-define concepts may have contributed to the extraordinarily contradictory nature of the commentaries.

Yang: When the [movement of the qi in the] vessel at the inch opening [displays a condition of] normal balance, [that indicates that the movement of the qi] corresponds to the four seasons.

Liao Ping: [This difficult issue] emphasizes the [role of the] kidneys. It establishes designations for the gate of life which are all alike based in the doctrines of the alchemists. They were appropriated there and applied here to a medical doctrine. The *Nei jing* emphasizes the [role of the] stomach. This book replaced the [role of the stomach] by that of the kidneys, thereby introducing an error which has outlived thousands of years by now .... The [*Nei*] *jing* has no such text and it has no such principle. [Above, the *Nan jing* propagated] the use only of the inch [openings] of the two [hands] for diagnosis; here now it [states] that they are unrelated to [the signs of] life and death. What [does that mean]?

(2)–(8) *Lü Guang*: [The *Nan jing*] states further: "All the twelve conduits are linked with the origin of the vital qi. The 'origin of the vital qi' refers to the root and foundation of all the twelve conduits." Now, the [movement of the] qi in the throughway vessel³ emerges from between the two kidneys. [The latter] are responsible for the [movement of the] qi. Hence, it is said that the "moving qi" of the kidneys ascend on both sides of the "controller vessel"⁴ to the throat. [The throat serves to] pass the breath and is, therefore, called the "gate of exhalation and inhalation." Above, [the throughway vessel] is linked with the three yin and three yang [conduits] of the hands; they form the branches. Below, [the throughway vessel] is linked with the three yin and three yang [conduits] of the feet; they form the root. This is why the sages [of antiquity] referred to the image of a tree as a metaphor. The "origin of the Triple Burner" means the "short-term repository of the Triple Burner."⁵ It distributes the camp and guard [qi], and it bars evil [qi] from entering at will. Hence, it is called the "spirit guarding against the evil." In man, the vessel in the foot [section] constitutes "root and foundation"; the vessel in the inch [section] constitutes "stalk and leaves." Even though the [movement of the qi in the] inch [section may appear in] normal balance, the [movement in the] vessel in the foot [section may have been] cut off already. [That is to say,] the upper section displays [a movement in the] vessel, the lower section does not. Such a situation indicates death.

(2) *Li Jiong*: All the twelve conduits are linked with the kidneys. The kidneys are the source which emits the vital qi [moving through the] vessels.

---

3   For the concept of the "throughway vessel," see difficult issue 27.

4   For the concept of the "controller vessel," see difficult issue 23.

5   The Triple Burner is counted among the six short-term repositories. See difficult issue 38.

(3) *Li Jiong*: The kidneys are the source of the vital qi; they are the root and the foundation of the twelve conduit vessels.

    Ye Lin: The "moving qi" between the kidneys are the origin of the vital qi of the twelve conduits; they control the camp [qi] and the guard [qi]. The moving up and down of the qi and of the blood in the human body depend on exhalation and inhalation to maintain their circulation. Through inhalation the yang [qi] of heaven enter; through exhalation the yin [qi] of the earth leave [the body]. The heart controls the ruler fire. The qi that enter [the body] due to inhalation are the yang [qi] of heaven. They, too, are associated with fire. These qi enter the lung through the nose; afterwards they pass the heart, [from which] they lead the heart fire through the heart duct and following the "supervisor vessel"[6] into the kidneys. Then they proceed further, moving downward from the kidneys to the Lower Burner into the uterus chamber. On both sides of the urinary bladder they descend to the lower opening [of the bladder]. Thus, inhalation draws in the yang qi of heaven. Together with the fire of the heart, these [yang qi] cause the water of the bladder to rise as steam. [Hence, the water] is transformed into qi. These ascend via the throughway and "employer [vessels]." They pass the diaphragm and enter the lung whence, in turn, they leave [the body] through mouth and nose. [Some of the] qi which ascend in order to leave [the body] are transformed into liquids in the mouth and by the tongue and in the long-term depots and short-term repositories. These [liquids] leave [the body] through the skin [and its] hair by way of the "qi streets"[7] (*qi jie* 氣街). They serve to steam the skin and to soften the flesh. They constitute the sweat. [All of] this occurs [in accordance with] the principle that fire is transformed into qi when brought into water.

(4) *Li Jiong*: The moving qi between the two kidneys are the original qi which man has received from father and mother. Furthermore, the [movement of the] qi in the throughway vessel emerges from between the kidneys. The body's five long-term depots and six short-term repositories have twelve separate conduits. Their root and foundation are, indeed, the kidneys. The [qi of the] kidneys ascend, on both sides of the employer vessel, toward the throat. [The throat is responsible

---

6   For the concept of the "supervisor vessel," see difficult issue 38.

7   The term "qi streets" denotes several meanings; it may refer here to certain shortcuts in the passage of the qi through the conduits and network vessels. Altogether, the body has four such paths. They are referred to briefly in the treatise "Wei qi" 衛氣 of the *Ling shu*, where they are identified as located in the head, in the chest, in the abdomen, and in the legs. Specific holes are associated with these paths and can be pierced in case of certain symptoms indicating an undue accumulation of qi. It is not quite clear whether Ye Lin intends to imply here that sweat can leave the body only through the holes associated with the four qi streets.

for] passing the breath; it serves as the gate of exhalation and inhalation. The Triple Burner of man is patterned after the three original qi of heaven and earth;[8] the kidneys are the basic origin [of the Triple Burner].

Hua Shou: Man receives the moving qi between the kidneys from heaven as his vital qi. The kidneys are [associated with the first of the Twelve Celestial Branches, i.e.,] *zi* 子, they are the seat of water; [they are associated, furthermore, with] *kan* 坎 the diagram [in the *Yi jing* 易經] for the Northern regions. They are [associated with] the number one of heaven and they are [associated with the first of the Five Phases, i.e., water], preceding fire, wood, metal, and soil. Hence, they are the origin of the vital qi; they constitute root and foundation of all the conduits.

(5) *Li Jiong*: To the left is the kidney, to the right is the gate of life. A spirit holds guard at the gate of life and does not allow any evil to enter the "home of the mind" (*zhi shi* 志室).[9] If any evil [qi] enter the home of the mind, the person will die. "Home of the mind" is the name of a hole.

Hua Shou: [The kidneys] are, furthermore, the spirit guarding against evil [qi]. When the original qi prevail, evil [qi] cannot enter. When the original qi are cut off, death follows. Similarly, when the roots of a tree are cut off, the stalk and the leaves wither.

(6) *Liao Ping*: These are the "stem qi" (*zong qi* 宗氣),[10] not the qi [that are named] qi and blood .... The *Nei jing* considered the stomach as the sea of water and grains. [Accordingly,] all fourteen conduits[11] receive their supplies from the stomach.

---

8   This sentence should read: "... is patterned after the three original qi of heaven, earth, and man."

9   "Home of the mind" refers to two holes on the foot-major yang conduit, which is associated with the bladder. They are located on the back below the fourteenth vertebra on both sides of the spine, at a distance of three inches each.

10 "Stem qi" refers to qi which are formed by a union of (1) guard and camp qi produced in the body from the essence of beverages and food, and (2) the qi that enter the body through inhalation. They accumulate in the chest and are considered to fulfill two important functions. On the one hand, they may leave the body through the throat and are closely related to one's speaking and breathing capabilities. On the other hand, they pass through the vessel associated with the heart and are here closely related to the circulation of the guard qi and of the blood, as well as to the temperature and moving capabilities of the body and its extremities. The term *zong* 宗, rendered here as "stem," should not imply that these qi have been inherited from one's parents; rather, the term might indicate that these qi are of a more important nature than some other qi in the body. *Zong* carries also the meaning of "distinguished" or "honorable." However, Liao Ping may have used the term *zong qi* here in the same sense with which Li Jiong applied it to the "moving qi" in his comments on sentence 4.

11 This may be a misprint for "twelve conduits." A concept of "fourteen conduits" also existed, however. It was introduced by Hua Shou in his work *Shi si jing fa hui* 十四經發

[Li] Dongyuan 李東垣, in his *Pi wei lun* 脾胃論 [discusses this] correctly. Furthermore, [the *Nei jing*] considered the throughway vessel to be the sea for the twelve conduits;[12] [it did] not [consider] the kidneys to be the ruler.

(7) *Li Jiong*: The three yin and the three yang [conduits] of the hands are the branches; the three yin and the three yang [conduits] of the feet are the root. The foot section is man's root and foundation; the inch opening represents man's stalk and leaves. When a tree's roots are cut off, that tree will die. When a person's kidney [qi] are cut off, that person will die.

(8) *Yang*: When [the *Nan jing*] speaks of "dying," that is because no vessel [movement appears] in the foot [section]. The vessel [movement] in the foot [section] is man's root and foundation. When root and foundation are cut off, stalk and leaves must wither. By taking the vessel in the foot [section] as root and foundation and the vessel in the inch [section] as stalk and leaves, [the *Nan jing*] refers to the image of a tree as a metaphor.

Ding Deyong: The "moving qi between the kidneys" means [the following]. To the left is the kidney; to the right is the gate of life. The gate of life is the domicile of the essence spirit; the original qi are tied to it. It is also named the "spirit guarding against the evil." When the spirit of the gate of life holds guard firmly, evil qi cannot enter at will. If they enter, [the person] will die. In this case, the kidney qi will be cut off internally first. The respective person does not yet appear ill. When he falls ill, he will die.[13]

Li Jiong: The moving qi between the kidneys are normally hidden in the interior. [In this case] now, qi [generated out of the grains consumed] are transmitted to and received at the inch opening. Although [the movement in] the vessel appears in normal balance, [that] person's vital qi have been cut off between the kidneys already. The twelve conduits have nothing to submit to each other. The [movement that can be felt at] the ten [locations on the] employer [vessel][14] and at the inch opening appears normal, and yet [the respective person] will die.

Hua Shou: The meaning of this paragraph seems to contradict what was said in [the discussion of] the first difficult issue; still, both are significant. The first difficult issue started with [a statement that by checking] the inch opening, [one may] determine [whether a person will] survive or die; [it went on to say] that the inch opening is the great meeting point of the vessels where changes

揮 and included, in addition to the twelve regular conduits, the employer vessel and the supervisor vessel.

12 See *Su wen* treatise 44, "Wei lun" 痿論, and *Ling shu* treatise 65, "Wu yin wu wei" 五音五味

13 This is to say, as soon as the respective person becomes aware of his illness, he will die.

14 The *shi ren* 十任 are ten locations on the employer vessel where the movement in the vessels can be felt.

in the [movement of the] qi [generated in the body] from the grains become apparent. This paragraph here talks about the original qi. When man's original qi are abundant, [that means] life. When man's original qi are cut off, [that means] death, even if the vessel [movement] at the inch opening appears normal. The original qi refer to the substance (*ti* 体); the qi [produced in the body] from the grains refer to the functioning [of the substance] (*yong* 用).

Xu Dachun: The flowing movement in the vessels is, indeed, governed by the qi. It cannot be that the vital qi have already been cut off while the [movement of the qi in the] vessel at the inch opening still appears in normal balance. Whether the vital qi have been cut off or not must become apparent through an examination of the [movement in the] vessels. If the vital qi were cut off while the [movement in the] vessels still appears to be normal, then the vital qi would be independent vital qi and the [movement in the] vessels would be [an independent movement in the] vessels, the two being without mutual relationship. Is there such a principle? Obviously, such a slip of the tongue appears nowhere in the *Nei jing*!

Ye Lin: [When the *Nan jing*] states: "The [movement of the qi in the] vessel at the inch opening [displays a condition of] normal balance and yet [the respective person] dies," that has nothing to do with the changes [in the movement] of the qi [produced in the body] from the grains as they become apparent at the inch opening, permitting a decision [whether a person will] survive or die. [The *Nan jing*] here talks about the substance.

Liao Ping: It is quite possible to reject the [doctrine of conducting a diagnosis solely at the] inch opening [and to exchange it with the doctrine of the] three sections and nine indicator [levels]. However, if [at first] special emphasis is placed on examining the inch opening while it is stated here that the inch opening is unrelated to [the signs of] life and death, is this not a case of a fox burying something and then digging it up again?

Nan jing 1962: Inch opening refers only to the vessel in the inch section among the three sections, inch, gate, and foot. "The [movement of the qi in the] vessel at the inch opening is even"[15] indicates – on the basis of the meaning of the words *Cun kou mai ping* 寸口脈平 – that the [movement in the] vessel at the inch opening still appears normal, but it is not really as if no disease were present. One can say only that it is not very different from the appearance of the [movement in the] vessels of a person of normal [health]. However, as far as the [movement in the]

---

15 Obviously the authors of this commentary did not interpret the character *ping* 平 in the same sense as earlier commentators had. The meaning "even" refers here to the movement perceived in the foot section.

vessel in the foot section is concerned, that is clearly very different. Hence, it is called an "even [movement in the] vessel" (*mai ping* 脈平). This statement refers to the foot section; it explains the importance of the vessel [movement] in the foot section for prognosis and diagnosis.

(1)–(8) *Tamba Genkan*: The moving qi between the kidneys are identified, [in the commentaries beginning with Ding Deyong's *Nan jing*] *bu zhu* 補註 [to Xu Dachun's *Nan jing*] *jing shi* 經釋, as the qi of the gate of life - that is to say, as the qi on which man's life depends. [Such explanations are] not as comprehensive as Lü [Guang's] commentary. Mr. Lü lived close to antiquity; he must have received [his ideas] from a teacher. If one tests [his commentary] against the text of the scripture, [it becomes evident that] it is completely reliable. Now, between the kidneys is the place from where the throughway vessel emerges. In addition, it is the *guan yuan* 關元 section[16] and also the origin for the transformation of qi by the Triple Burner. Why would one speak here of "moving qi"? That which is at rest is [categorized as] yin; that which moves is [categorized as] yang. "Moving qi," then, means "yang qi." ... The sixty-sixth difficult issue states: "The moving qi below the navel and between the kidneys constitute man's life; they are root and foundation of the twelve conduits. Hence, they are called 'origin'. The Triple Burner is a special envoy [transmitting] the original qi. It is responsible for the passage of the three qi and for their procession through the [body's] five long-term depots and six short-term repositories. 'Origin' is an honorable designation for the Triple Burner." The meanings [of the sixty-sixth difficult issue] and of the present [paragraph] explain each other. Obviously, the moving qi are the qi controlled by the throughway vessel. They are genuinely yang; they are the origin of the transformation of qi by the Triple Burner. Life is tied to them .... The inch opening referred to at the beginning of this paragraph includes all three sections.[17] It does mean that [in the case discussed here] the upper section displays a vessel movement while the lower section does not. The commentaries by Lü [Guang] and Yang [Xuancao] are too punctilious in this regard.

---

16 "*Guan yuan* section" may refer here to a place in the body where the semen (in males) and the blood (in females) is stored. In the thirty-sixth difficult issue, similar functions were assigned to the *ming men* 命門 (gate of life), which is defined here as the right of the two kidneys. *Guan yuan* is also the name of a hole on the employer vessel located three inches below the navel. This hole is also named *dan tian* 丹田, a term which has, in turn, been applied to the moving qi between the kidneys (among other entities). See also Yang Xuancao's commentary on sentence 16 of difficult issue 66.

17 These are inch, gate, and foot.

Katō Bankei: All the preceding [paragraphs][18] continued the discussion of the meaning outlined in difficult issues 1 and 2 – namely, how to utilize the vessel location in a section of one inch and nine *fen* of the hand major yin [conduit] below the fish-line in order to determine [a person's] death or survival in the case of disease. When the *Nei jing* states that beverages and food enter the stomach where their essence is transformed into qi, [the movement of which] becomes apparent in the qi opening, that is correct. However, while all the preceding paragraphs have focused their discussions on [these] qi [that are produced] by the stomach, this difficult issue emphasizes a very different question. At the very beginning of the fetal [development], the true qi of heaven take their residence in the gate of life mansion between the kidneys. This is called the "origin of the vital qi." The mystery on which all beginnings depend, on which all life depends, works from here. This applies even to [living beings] where one would not expect it – not only to humans! It is the same for all species! As soon as the young come to life they are fed with liquid or solid nourishment which leads to the formation of the long-term depots and short-term repositories, the conduits and network [vessels], the four limbs and hundred bones; all this depends on the foundation provided by those [original] qi. Hence, they are called "the gate of exhalation and inhalation" or "the origin of the Triple Burner." Now, it has been pointed out [in the first difficult issue] that the [movement in the] vessel at the inch opening [can be utilized to] determine [a person's impending] death or his survival [as it is indicated by the conditions] of the long-term depots and short-term repositories. Why would anybody search for an alternative [indicator? In the case referred to] here, the [movement in the] vessels appears to be in a condition of normal balance, and yet [the respective person] dies. Why is that? This may be compared to herbs or branches in a vase supplemented with water. Their flowers and leaves may still be fresh, but their roots have already been cut off. How could they continue to flourish all the time? They are bound to wither and they will lose their original colors. [Humans] should rub their eyes and look at themselves [to see whether their situation is any different].

---

18   Katō Bankei has placed the eighth difficult issue at the end of the first section of the *Nan jing*, which is devoted to diagnosis. Hence, he speaks here of the remaining twenty-one difficult issues of this section as "all the preceding [paragraphs]."

九難曰：（一）何以別知藏府之病耶？

（二）然：數者府也，（三）遲者藏也。（四）數則為熱，遲則為寒。（五）諸陽為熱，諸陰為寒。（六）故以別知藏府之病也。

The ninth difficult issue: (1) How can the diseases in the [body's] long-term depots and short-term repositories be distinguished?

(2) It is like this. A frequent [movement in the vessels indicates a disease] in the short-term repositories. (3) A slow [movement in the vessels indicates a disease] in the long-term depots. (4) Frequency indicates heat; slowness indicates cold. (5) All yang [symptoms] are [caused by] heat; all yin [symptoms] are [caused by] cold. (6) Hence, [these principles] can be employed to distinguish diseases in the long-term depots and short-term repositories.

COMMENTARIES

(1) *Liao Ping*: The method for conducting an examination of the *ren* [*ying*] 人迎 and inch [opening] has been outlined in the [*Nei*] *jing* in sufficient detail. Why would anybody voice such a question?

(2) *Yang*: When the coming and going [of the movement in the vessels] is speedy and urgent, exceeding five arrivals per breathing [period], that is called a "frequent" [movement].

    Li Jiong: Whenever a frequent [movement] appears in the vessels, [one of] the six short-term repositories has fallen ill.

(3) *Yang*: When [the movement in the vessels] arrives three times during one exhalation and inhalation [period], the coming and going [of the qi] is extremely slow. Hence, it is called a "slow" [movement].

    Li Jiong: Whenever a slow [movement] appears in the vessels, [one of] the five long-term depots has fallen ill.

(4) *Ding Deyong*: The [movement in the] vessels should be counted against the clepsydra's dripping. During the two seasons of spring and autumn, [the clepsydra's water] passes by fifty markings both during day and night. During these seasons yin and yang [qi] are present to the same degree. Hence, [the movement of the qi] that can be felt [in the vessels] is in normal balance. At the solstices of both winter and summer, day and night are not equally long. Before summer solstice, the day is sixty [clepsydra] markings long; consequently, six arrivals [of the movement in the vessels] indicate a frequent [movement]. Hence, frequency occurs because of heat. Before winter solstice, the length of the nights is extended to sixty [clepsydra] markings; thus, many yin [qi] are present and few

yang [qi]. This is because of the cold. Then the [degree of the presence of] yin and yang [qi] can be determined from the [number of the] markings [passed by the clepsydra's] dripping [water]. If man's [qi are] diminished or if they have been boosted, their [normal] frequency or slowness [due to the seasons] will be increased. Hence, the [*Nan*] *jing* states: "All yang [symptoms] are [caused by] heat; all yin [symptoms] are [caused by] cold."

Yu Shu: When the yang qi are in disorder, [their movement] will be frequent. When the yin qi are depleted, [their movement] will be slow. From that one understands the symptoms of the presence of heat or cold in the long-term depots and short-term repositories.

(5) *Li Jiong*: When the yang qi are in disorder, [their movement in] the vessels is frequent. Hence, [the *Nan jing* states]: "All yang [symptoms] are [caused by] heat." When the yin qi are depleted, [their movement in the vessels] will be slow. Hence, [the *Nan jing* states]: "All yin [symptoms] are [caused by] cold."

(6) *Li Jiong*: On the basis of frequent or slow [movements in the] vessels, one can differentiate the diseases of the long-term depots and short-term repositories.

(1)–(6) *Hua Shou*: In general [the following can be said about the movement in] man's vessels. One exhalation and one inhalation constitute one breathing [period]. During one breathing [period, the movement in] the vessels arrives four times. [There may be] an extra [arrival] in the vessels, constituting a "great breathing [period]" with five arrivals. [Anybody in that state] is called a "normal" person. Normal persons have [movements in their] vessels that are free from disease. If, during one breathing [period], six arrivals occur, that is called a "frequent" or "excessive" [movement in the] vessels. The long-term depots are associated with yin; the short-term repositories are associated with yang. Frequent vessel [movements] belong to the short-term repositories; they are yang [symptoms] and indicate heat. Slow vessel [movements] belong to the long-term depots; they are yin [symptoms] and they indicate cold. That is quite normal. All yang [movements in the] vessels indicate heat; all yin [movements in the] vessels indicate cold. Starting from these [principles], the diseases in the long-term depots and short-term repositories can be distinguished.

Zhang Shixian: The entire statement here is concerned with diseases of the long-term depots and short-term repositories [as they affect the movement of the qi] in the vessels. When the long-term depots and short-term repositories are not in a state of disease, [the movement of their qi in] the vessels appears in normal balance. [The qi of] the six short-term repositories arrive just five times [per breathing period; that is] neither slow nor frequent. When the short-term repositories have a disease, [the movement of the qi] will be diminished. "Frequency" [indicates] a surplus of yang [qi moving through the] vessels, with six arrivals [per breathing period]. "Slowness" [indicates] an insufficient amount of yin [qi moving through the] vessels, with three arrivals [per breathing period]. If the vessel [movement is marked by] frequency, the disease is in the short-term repositories; if the vessel [movement is marked by] slowness, the disease is in the long-term depots. If the [movement in the] vessels is fast, the yang [qi] are present in surplus and the short-term repositories suffer from heat. If the [movement in the] vessels is slow, the yin [qi are] deficient and the long-term depots suffer from cold. Whenever the yang [qi in the] vessels have a surplus, that is because of heat; whenever the yin [qi in the] vessels are deficient, that is because of cold.

Xu Dachun: To distinguish [the diseases of] the long-term depots and short-term repositories solely on the basis of slowness and frequency [of the movements in the vessels] is not entirely correct. [A movement may be] slow also in the case of a disease in the short-term repositories; and it may be frequent also in the case of a disease in the long-term depots. In general one may say that the one [phenomenon] is associated with yin and [the other] with yang [qi]; but on the whole we encounter an erroneous statement here.

Ding Jin: This paragraph emphasizes the differentiation of the diseases of the long-term depots and short-term repositories. It says that a frequent [movement in the] vessels [points to the] short-term repositories, while a slow [movement in the] vessels [points to the] long-term depots. If [the movement is] frequent, the short-term repositories suffer from heat; if it is slow, the long-term depots suffer from cold. All yang [movements] are related to the short-term repositories; they indicate heat. All yin [movements] are related to the long-term depots; they indicate cold. If one distinguishes the diseases of the long-term depots and of the short-term repositories on these grounds, no further [information] is needed. People in later times have criticized the sentence "frequency indicates heat" as if it were not quite correct. Each time they encountered a disease of depletion of yang [qi] with a rapid and frequent [movement in the] vessels, they just dumped cinnamon and aconite[1] [into the patient] to bring his condition back to normal. Obviously, they did not know that a frequent [movement] indicates heat. The word "frequency" stands for the word "short-term repository." Similarly, a slow [movement] indicates cold; the word "slowness" stands for "depot." That is very

1   Both cinnamon and aconite have been described in Chinese pharmaceutical literature as "hot" or "very hot" substances. Hence, their application would be appropriate only in case of an insufficiency of heat, or yang qi, in the organism.

true! If one reads the writings of ancient authors without taking the greatest pains to comprehend their ideas, how can one light-mindedly criticized them?

Ye Lin: The [paragraph] refers only to yin and yang [associations] in general; one should not stick [to these statements too closely] .... Some diseases in the short-term repositories may also result in slow [movements in the] vessels; some diseases in the long-term depots may also result in frequent [movements in the] vessels. It is definitely impossible to rely solely on slowness or frequency [of the movement in the vessels] in order to distinguish [diseases in the] long-term depots and short-term repositories. And it is equally incorrect to rely solely on slowness or frequency in order to distinguish [whether a disease was caused by] cold or heat. Slowness is a [characteristic feature of the movement of] yin [qi in the] vessels. While the physician exhales once and inhales once, the [movement of the qi in the] vessels of the patient arrives three times – that is, the coming and going [of the qi] are extremely slow. A slow [movement in the] vessels indicates disease. [Such a disease is] always due either to a harm caused by raw, cold, or cool items internally, or to passing through water, ice, or cold qi [which cause harm from the] exterior. These [qi of cold] hit mostly the long-term depots, but some may hit the short-term repositories and some may enter the pores, with the effect of delaying and obstructing the flow of the qi and of the blood. Hence, [this kind of harm] is responsible for a depletion of yang [qi]. When the qi and the blood congeal, that is an indication of an abundance of yin [qi] and of a debility of yang [qi. In such cases it is essential] to investigate whether the slowness [of the movement in the vessels] is mild or severe, and whether the cold has penetrated deeply or remains near the surface. In this way, one may recognize whether it is a case of regular [slowness due to cold]. If, however, [the movement is] retarded and powerful and, at the same time, rough and marked by blockages, no matter whether [it is perceived with the fingers] lifted or firmly pressed, that is a case of heat evil blocking the hidden passages and causing their impassability, with the effect that [the movement in them] loses its regular pace. Hence, the [movement in the] vessels manifests a retardation, although this is contrary [to what one would expect in the case of harm caused by heat]. This [demonstrates] that one should never [arrive at a decision] hurriedly; it is essential to examine a [disease in all its] manifestations. For example, when the chest and the stomach[2] are full and give one a feeling of pressure, when the stool fails to appear and when the urine is red, that goes along with a retarded [movement in the] vessels that was caused by heat!

---

2   Strictly speaking, the term *wan* 脘 denotes the stomach cavity.

Katō Bankei: This difficult issue takes up the two vessel [movements called] "frequent" and "slow" in order to distinguish between diseases in the long-term depots and short-term repositories. Earlier paragraphs have called attention to the two vessel [movements called] "at the surface" and "in the depth," and have associated them with the four long-term depots.[3] When this paragraph now focuses on frequent and slow [movements in the vessels as indicators permitting the physician] to determine whether the long-term depots or short-term repositories have been affected by cold or heat, we have to match these two vessel [movements] with the four expressions "at the surface" and "in the depth," "depletion" and "repletion." This should serve to amplify their meaning. Consequently, the hidden message of this difficult issue will become clear by itself. The four-sentence statement [in the *Nan jing*], "A frequent [movement in the vessels points to a disease in the] short-term repositories. A slow [movement in the vessels points to a disease in the] long-term depots. Frequency indicates heat; slowness indicates cold," was not explained intelligibly in Hua [Shou's] commentary. Actually, all the authors [who have commented on it seem to] have been quite confused. Maybe they were not able to reach a final conclusion [on the meaning of these four sentences] because they did not approach them with sufficient interest! What is [their meaning]? A frequent [movement in the vessels] does not necessarily indicate a disease in the short-term repositories; a slow [movement in the vessels] does not necessarily indicate a disease in the long-term depots. The presence of heat may cause the [movements in the] vessels of the short-term repositories as well as the long-term depots to be frequent; the presence of cold may cause the [movements in the] vessels of the short-term repositories as well as the long-term depots to be slow. This is why the final [two sentences merely] state: "Frequency indicates heat; slowness indicates cold." Now, if we look at it from this point of view, a [movement in the vessels] that is at the surface and frequent indicates external heat; a [movement] that is in the depth and frequent indicates internal heat.[4] A [movement in the vessels] that is depleted and frequent indicates a depletion of yin [qi] and internal heat; a [movement] that is replete and frequent points to a repletion of yang [qi] and external heat. Similarly, a slow [movement in the] vessels may also appear in fourfold modification – that is, at the surface, in the depth, depleted, and replete. Through these [modified appearances] it becomes completely obvious whether cold [qi] have affected the long-term depots or the short-term repositories.

---

3   The spleen, as the fifth long-term depot, was associated with the "center" and is, therefore, not mentioned here. See difficult issue 4, sentence 2.

4   "External" and "internal" refer to the areas above and below the diaphragm, respectively.

Liao Ping: [In the *Nei jing*] the four expressions "at the surface," "in the depth," "slow," and "frequent" are important terms for the examination of the conduit vessels. They have been introduced to recognize [conditions of] internal and external depletion and repletion. [In the *Nan jing*] now, these four expressions were supposed to refer to specific locations [of a disease], so that they could serve no longer as the standard terms in the examination of the conduit vessels. Hence, the necessity arose to draw on all kinds of alternative terms, [a fact] which has obfuscated the [entire affair].

Nan jing 1962: This difficult issue is concerned with the retarded or frequent appearances of the [movements in the] vessels as criteria [permitting the physician] to distinguish the diseases in the long-term depots and short-term repositories. One could say also [that it is concerned with] the general law of the correspondence between vessel [movements] and diseases. However, we should not understand this in a mechanical fashion. For instance, symptoms of repletion in the yang brilliance short-term repositories[5] are also associated with a retarded [movement in the] vessels, and symptoms of leftover heat [when there should be cold] in the ceasing yin [conduits] are also associated with a frequent [movement in the] vessels. It is just as Xu Dachun has said: "A movement may be retarded also in the case of a disease in the short-term repositories, and it may be frequent also in the case of a disease in the long-term depots." Furthermore, in cases such as "true cold" and "false heat" – [that is to say,] when the appearance of the [movement in the] vessels is contrary [to what one would expect] – the situation may differ from that [general statement in the *Nan jing*].

---

5   That is, the stomach.

十難曰：（一）一脈為十變者，何謂也？

（二）然：五邪剛柔相逢之意也。（三）假令心脈急甚者，肝邪干心也；（四）心脈微急者，膽邪干小腸也；（五）心脈大甚者，心邪自干心也；（六）心脈微大者，小腸邪自干小腸也；（七）心脈緩甚者，脾邪干心也；（八）心脈微緩者，胃邪干小腸也；（九）心脈濇甚者，肺邪干心也；（十）心脈微濇者，大腸邪干小腸也；（十一）心脈沉甚者，腎邪干心也；（十二）心脈微沉者，膀胱邪干小腸也。（十三）五藏各有剛柔邪，故令一脈輒變為十也。

The tenth difficult issue: (1) One [specific movement in the] vessels may undergo ten variations. What does that mean?

(2) It is like this. It refers to the five evils[1] – that means, to the mutual interference of hard [evil qi] and of soft [evil qi]. (3) For example, if the [movement in the] heart [section of the] vessels is very tense, evil [qi] from the liver have attacked the heart. (4) If the [movement in the] heart [section of the] vessels is slightly tense, evil [qi] from the gall bladder have attacked the small intestine. (5) If the [movement in the] heart [section of the] vessels is very strong, evil [qi] from the heart itself have attacked the heart. (6) If the movement in the] heart [section of the] vessels is slightly strong, evil [qi] from the small intestine itself have attacked the small intestine. (7) If the [movement in the] heart [section of the] vessels is very relaxed, evil [qi] from the spleen have attacked the heart. (8) If the [movement in the] heart

---

1   The term "five evils" encompasses the five evil qi, originating from five different sources within the organism, that may be responsible for disease in one specific long-term depot or short-term repository. According to the Five Phases paradigm, a depot – for instance, the heart – may fall ill by itself, that is, generate its own evil qi. This would be called a "regular evil" (*zheng xie* 正邪). If qi from the "mother" phase – in the mutual generation order – invade a depot, this is called a "depletion evil" (*xu xie* 虛邪). Such qi are considered as coming "from behind." In case of the heart, which represents the phase of fire, the mother long-term depot "behind" is the liver, which is associated with the phase of wood. Wood generates fire. If qi from the child phase invade a depot, this is called a "repletion evil" (*shi xie* 實邪). Such qi are considered as "returning," as coming "from ahead." In case of the heart, the child long-term depot is the spleen, which is associated with the phase of soil. Fire generates soil. If qi from a long-term depot associated – in the mutual destruction order – with the phase that can be overcome invade a depot, this is called a "weakness evil" (*wei xie* 微邪); the resulting disease will not be serious. In case of the heart, this would be qi from the lung, since the latter is associated with the phase of metal. Fire destroys metal. If qi from a long-term depot associated with the phase that cannot be overcome invade a depot, this is called a "robber evil" (*zei xie* 賊邪); the resulting disease is considered to be serious. In case of the heart, this would be qi from the kidneys, since the latter represent the phase of water. Water destroys fire. The same pattern applies to the individual short-term repositories, as they are associated with the long-term depots.

[section of the] vessels is slightly relaxed, evil [qi] from the stomach have attacked the small intestine. (9) If the [movement in the] heart [section of the] vessels is very rough, evil [qi] from the lung have attacked the heart. (10) If the [movement in the] heart [section of the] vessels is slightly rough, evil [qi] from the large intestine have attacked the small intestine. (11) If the [movement in the] heart [section of the] vessels is very deep, evil [qi] from the kidneys have attacked the heart. (12) If the [movement in the] heart [section of the] vessels is slightly deep, evil [qi] from the bladder have attacked the small intestine.(13) The body's five long-term depots [and their respective short-term repositories] may all [be attacked by] hardness or softness evil [qi], and that may cause [the movement on] one [specific level of the] vessels to undergo ten variations.[2]

---

2   Although this difficult issue appears to impart straightforward data, it has, nevertheless, caused considerable confusion among commentators. In my own view, the answer to the question of sentence 1 considers each of the five long-term depots to encompass two functional units – namely, the long-term depot itself and, as its extension, the respective short-term repository. On the basis of the Five Phases paradigm, each of the two subunits is considered to be vulnerable to five different kinds of evil qi, originating from five different sources. For a single depot – including the long-term depot itself and its respective short-term repository – this adds up to ten different variations in the movement of the vessels associated with this particular depot. This concept of a differentiation of long-term depot and short-term repository as subunits of a long-term depot was not recognized or accepted by some later commentators. This appears to be one reason for discrepancies in their statements. Another reason may be found in the vagueness of the diagnostic pattern applied here. In view of the contents of difficult issue 3, we may infer that the cross-sectional diagnostic pattern was implied here. That is, the left hand is categorized as yang; its inch section—which is located "above" and, hence, represents yang – would be associated with the heart, both being categorized as yang-in-yang. Accordingly, the foot section of the left hand would be associated with the lung (yin-in-yang); the inch section of the right hand would be associated with the liver (yang-in-yin); and the foot section of the right hand would be associated with the kidneys (yin-in-yin). The gate sections of the left and right hands could be associated with the heart-enclosing network and with the spleen, respectively, but this is nowhere outlined in detail. Other interpretations of the locations where the respective movements can be felt are possible, too. Thus, one might think of the movements on the three (or even five) longitudinal levels associated with the five long-term depots, respectively, as they were outlined in difficult issues 4 and 5. Even an interpretation neglecting the emphasis that has been placed thus far on wrist diagnosis could – at least theoretically – be supported by the text of this difficult issue. The wording would have to be understood literally, referring to examinations of the individual conduit vessels themselves in order to find out whether they have been invaded by the evil qi in question. In this case, the hand minor yin and the hand major yang conduits – the former associated with the heart and the latter associated with the small intestine – would have to be considered as one conduit. Such an interpretation has not been offered explicitly by any of the commentators, but it could be inferred from Ding Deyong's commentary (see his comments on sentences 1 through 13 and note 15), in which two conduits are mentioned as passing through each section at the wrist. My own rendering of the text, however, follows the cross-sectional pattern.

(1) *Liao Ping*: In view of the absurd creation of such false doctrines, which are both empty and chaotic, one might wish to ask whether the person who trumped up this book had even the slightest understanding of the facts and principles involved! The [*Nei*] *jing* does not have the two words "ten variations"; it has the diagnostic concept of "ten measurements" (*shi duo* 十度),[3] but that is something different.

(2) *Li Jiong*: The "five evils" include the "depletion evil" (*xu xie* 虛邪), the "repletion evil" (*shi xie* 實邪), the "regular evil" (*zheng xie* 正邪), the "weakness evil" (*wei xie* 微邪), and the "robber evil" (*zei xie* 賊邪). "Hard" and "soft" stand for yin and yang. "Mutual interference" means that at a specific location a vessel [movement] appears [that is characteristic of] another [location].

Hua Shou: The "five evils" means that the qi of the five long-term depots and of the five short-term repositories have deviated from their proper [course], turning into evil [qi that invade territories where they do not belong]. As to "hard" and "soft," yang [qi] are hard [qi] and yin [qi] are soft [qi]. "The mutual interference of hard [evil qi] and of soft [evil qi]" means that [the qi of one] long-term depot interfere with [another] depot, or that [the qi of one] short-term repository interfere with [another] short-term repository. Both the five long-term depots and the five short-term repositories [may be attacked by] the five evils. If the arrival of the [irregular movement in the] vessels is very pronounced, the long-term depots are affected; [if the arrival of such a movement] is only slightly pronounced, the short-term repositories are affected. Here, the heart long-term depot has been selected as an example. [The respective patterns of] all the other [long-term depots and short-term repositories] can be inferred by analogy. Hence, [the text] states: "[The movement in] each [section of the] vessels may undergo ten variations."

Ye Lin: The "five evils" refers to the evil [qi originating] from the five long-term depots and six short-term repositories. As to "hard" and "soft," the five long-term depots represent the soft and the six short-term repositories represent the hard [aspect]. "Mutual interference" means that evil [qi] from one long-term depot attack another depot, or that evil [qi] from one short-term repository attack another short-term repository. When [evil qi from] one long-term depot attack another depot, the [resulting] vessel [movement will be one of] abun-

---

3   The 'ten estimates' refers to an examination method mentioned in the *Su wen* treatise "Fang sheng shuai lun" 方盛衰論. Accordingly, the vessels, the long-term depots, the flesh, the muscles, and the transportation holes had to be examined to estimate whether they were in a state of repletion or depletion. Five times two adds up to ten possible estimates, *shi duo* 十度.

dance; when [evil qi from] one short-term repository attack another short-term repository, the [resulting] vessel [movement will be] feeble.

Katō Bankei: Each of the sections – inch, gate, and foot – may display vessel [movements] indicating that [the qi of one] short-term repository have interfered with [another] short-term repository, or that [the qi of one] long-term depot have interfered with [another] depot. "Variation" refers to the mutual interferences of hard [evil qi from the long-term depots] and of soft [evil qi from the short-term repositories]. The five so-called relaxed, tense, strong, smooth,[4] and rough [movements in the] vessels may each appear very [pronounced] or slightly [pronounced], which accounts for ten variations. Consequently, altogether sixty variations [of the movement in the vessels] may occur in the three sections of the left and of the right [hand]. If we were to talk about the long-term depots individually, each of them [may be subjected to] five kinds of evil [qi]. Five [times] five [adds up to] twenty-five diseases. Hence, the *Su wen* states: "Five [times] five [adds up to] twenty-five variations."[5] And it speaks further of "twenty-five yang."[6] The same applies to diseases in the short-term repositories. If we were to talk about [long-term depots and short-term repositories] summarily, then [altogether] fifty variations are possible. In my own view, the long-term depots and the short-term repositories together may [be responsible for] fifty variations [of the movement in the vessels] as symptoms of disease. According to the *Ling shu*, the [six kinds of movement in the vessels, – namely] relaxed, tense, strong, small, smooth, and rough – may appear very [pronounced] or only slightly [pronounced], which adds up to sixty variations.

Liao Ping: When the [*Nei*] *jing* talks about "evil," it always refers to "evil [qi originating from] outside." Here now, the five long-term depots themselves [transmit] evil [qi] to each other. "One [specific movement in the] vessels may undergo ten variations." If we were to talk this over in terms of the five long-term depots, there should be fifty variations. If we talk this over in terms of the 12 conduits, there should be altogether 144 [*sic*][variations]. If one adds the eight extraordinary conduit vessels, there should be altogether 200 [variations]. If we were to extend this search for the pattern [of variations imagined by the author of the *Nan jing*] to even the most subtle [of all the vessels], ten [sheets of] paper

---

4   The *Nan jing* does not speak of a "smooth" movement here; it mentions a "deep" movement. "Deep" may be a mistake, though, since it is the only term referring to a level.

5   The "twenty-five variations" referred to in the *Ling shu* treatise "Ben zang" 本藏 denote a meaning different from what is implied here. They describe twenty-five variations in the physical condition of the short-term repositories and long-term depots, respectively.

6   Katō Bankei may have thought here of the *Ling shu* treatise "Yin yang er shi wu ren" 陰陽二十五人, where mankind is classified into twenty-five yin and twenty-five yang types.

would not be sufficient [to list all the possibilities]. And one should not hope
that [the entire list] could be as telling as the plan [of the Yellow] River [and the
book of the River] Lo,[7] or [the series of ancient] pitch pipes! The study of the
[movements in the] vessels is truly difficult!

(3) *Lü Guang*: In summer, the heart is the ruler. The vessel [movement associated
with the heart] appears at the surface, strong, and intermittent. Here now, [this
movement is] – contrary [to what would be in accordance with the season] –
thread-like. A thread-like [movement, however, indicates that] evil [qi] from
the liver have attacked the heart.

Yang: *Gan* 干 ("to attack") stands for *cheng* 乘 ("to seize").[8]

Yu Shu: When the mother has seized the child, that is called "depletion evil."

Li Jiong: The liver is the mother, the heart is the child. Wood generates fire. When
the mother has seized the child, that is called "depletion evil."

Liao Ping: I do not know what this is supposed to refer to. Suddenly [such a
concept] is brought forth here! Maybe it refers to the inch [section] of the left
[hand]. The association of "tense" with the [movement of the qi of the] liver is
strange. To distinguish between long-term depots and short-term repositories
on the basis of very [pronounced] or slightly [pronounced movements] represents an erroneous appropriation of the text of the [*Ling shu*] treatise "Xie qi
[zang fu] bing xing" 邪氣藏府病形.[9]

(4) *Lü Guang*: The small intestine is the short-term repository [associated] with the
heart; [the movement of] its [qi in the] vessels should be at the surface, strong,
and vast. When it is extended and slightly thread-like, it is a vessel [movement
characteristic of the] gall bladder.

Yu Shu: Yang [qi] attack yang [long-term depots]; yin [qi] attack yin [short-term
repositories]. Qi of equal kind seek each other.

(5) *Lü Guang*: Although the [movement in the] vessels [of the qi associated with
the] heart is vast and strong, it relies on the qi of the stomach as its basis. Here,
no stomach qi are available; therefore, the [movement in the] vessels of the
[qi associated with the] heart is very strong. That indicates that a disease has
emerged from the heart itself. Hence, [the text] states: "[Qi from the heart] itself
have attacked [the heart]."

---

7 Ancient mystic diagrams said to have been supranaturally revealed.

8 One might want to keep in mind that this term includes, in addition to "seize," the concepts of "to avail oneself of," and "to take passage," "to ride."

9 This *Ling shu* treatise lists a number of diseases and symptoms associated with the heavily
   or slightly pronounced occurrence of the six kinds of movement (tense, relaxed, strong,
   weak, smooth, and rough) in the vessels associated with the five long-term depots.

Yu Shu: That is [a movement in] the vessels that is not in accordance with the season.

Liao Ping: A "self-attack" is particularly strange!

(6) *Lü Guang*: The small intestine is the short-term repository [associated] with the heart. If [the movement of its qi is] slightly strong, [that is to say, if it is] weak, the small intestine has fallen ill by itself. Hence, [the text] states: "[Qi from the small intestine] itself have attacked [the small intestine]."

Yu Shu: The small intestine is [responsible for] the major yang vessel [movement]. It dominates during the fifth and sixth months. This vessel [movement should be] vast, strong, and extended. Here now, it is perceived to be slightly strong. This shows that evil [qi] of the small intestine have attacked the small intestine itself, [creating a situation which] is called "the proper conduits have fallen ill by themselves." According to the rules this is called a "proper evil."[10] Hence, the [text] states: "[Qi from the small intestine] itself have attacked [the small intestine]."

(7) *Lü Guang*: A relaxed [movement indicates that the qi of] the spleen vessel have seized the heart. They cause the [movement in the] vessels of the [qi associated with] the heart to be relaxed.

Yu Shu: When the [movement in the] vessels of the [qi associated with the] heart appears very relaxed, that is called "the child has seized the mother." According to the rules this is called a "repletion evil."

Li Jiong: A relaxed [movement in the] vessels is [characteristic of] the spleen. Here now, the vessel [movement associated with the] heart is very relaxed. That means that, with fire being the mother and soil being the child, the child has seized the mother. This is called "repletion evil." It is a vessel [movement indicating that] evil [qi from the] spleen have attacked the heart.

(8) *Lü Guang*: When a slightly relaxed[11] [movement in the] vessels [that is characteristic] of the stomach appears in the heart-section,[12] [that indicates that] the small intestine – that is, the short-term repository [associated] with the heart – [has been attacked]. Hence, [the text] states: "[Evil qi from the stomach] have attacked [the small intestine]."

---

10 No book title is known that might correspond to the phrase *fa yue*. Hence, I render as "the rule calls it."

11 I interpret *xiao* 小 here as a mistake to be replaced by *wei* 微.

12 Lü Guang employs here the term *bu* 部 ("section"). This may imply that he interpreted the tenth difficult issue on the basis of the cross-sectional diagnostic pattern.

Yu Shu: That is a slightly relaxed [movement that is] felt in the heart section with light [pressure of the] hand.[13]

(9) *Lü Guang*: A rough [movement in the] vessels is [characteristic of the] lung: Hence, [the text] states: "[Evil qi from the lung] have attacked [the heart]."

Yu Shu: When the metal turns back to abuse the fire, that is called a vessel [movement indicating] "slight evil."

Liao Ping: To twist the Five Phases [doctrine] like this is both unreasonable and mistaken. Later people have honored such [ideas] as "classic." [The authors of this book] should really be blamed [for having misled later generations].

(10) *Lü Guang*: A slightly rough [movement in the] vessels is [characteristic of the] large intestine. The small intestine is the short-term repository [associated] with the heart. Hence, [the text] states: "[Evil qi from the large intestine] have attacked [the small intestine]."

(11) *Lü Guang*: A deep [movement in the] vessels is [characteristic of the] kidneys. Hence, [the text] states: "[Evil qi from the kidneys] have attacked [the heart]."

Yu Shu: The flames of the fire in the heart ascend; the respective vessel [movement] should be at the surface. Here now it appears in the depth, [indicating that] water has overcome fire. According to the rules this is called a "robber evil."

(12) *Lü Guang*: A slightly deep [movement in the] vessels is [characteristic of the] bladder. The small intestine is the short-term repository [associated] with the heart. Hence, [the text] states: "[Evil qi from the bladder] have attacked [the small intestine]."

(13) *Lü Guang*: All this refers to the season when [the qi of] summer rule. When [during that period the movement in the] vessels [associated with the] heart appears in any of these [variations,] that indicates a loss of [correspondence to] the season.

Yang: "Hard" and "soft" are yin and yang. "Evil" is a term for what is not proper. When qi that [are supposed to] rule the body [in accordance with the season] are absent, and when, instead, [qi of the phase of] water arrive to attack the body, causing a disease, the [latter] are always called "evil"[qi].

(1)–(13) *Ding Deyong*: When [the *Nan jing*] states that "evil [qi] from the liver have attacked the heart" or "evil [qi] from the gall bladder have attacked the small intestine," then in both cases, a depletion evil has attacked the heart. When [the text] states that "evil [qi] from the heart attack the heart itself" or "evil [qi] from the small intestine attack the small intestine itself," then in both cases, a proper evil is involved. When [it states that] "evil [qi] from the spleen have attacked

---

13 Yu Shu also uses the term *bu* 部, but then he speaks of a "light hand." He may have thought of the diagnostic pattern of longitudinal levels.

the heart" or "evil [qi] from the stomach have attacked the small intestine," then this is, in both cases, a repletion evil. When [the text] states that "evil [qi] from the lung have attacked the heart" or "evil [qi] from the large intestine have attacked the small intestine," then this is, in both cases, a slight evil. When [the text] states that "evil [qi] from the kidneys have attacked the heart" or "evil [qi] from the bladder have attacked the small intestine," then this is, in both cases, a robber evil. When [the *Nan jing*] speaks of a "mutual interference of hard [qi] and of soft [qi]," this refers to the ten variations [of the movements that can be felt in the vessels]. Thus, *jia* 甲 and *ji* 己 form a dual combination; *jia* stands for "hard," *ji* stands for "soft." *Wu* 戊 and *gui* 癸 form a combination; *wu* stands for "hard," *gui* stands for "soft." *Ding* 丁 and *ren* 壬 form a combination; *ding* stands for "hard," *ren* stands for "soft." *Bing* 丙 and *xin* 辛 form a combination; *bing* stands for "hard," *xin* stands for "soft." *Yi* 乙, and *geng* 庚 form a combination; *yi* stands for "hard," *geng* stands for "soft."[14] Whenever hard [qi] or soft [qi] attack each other, the resulting disease will be serious, when the hard [qi] are very [pronounced]; it will be light, when the soft [qi] are very [pronounced]. When soft [qi] interfere with [the long-term depots of] hard [qi], that means that [the disease] originates from [a position] that cannot overcome the hard [qi]; hence, the disease will be serious. If hard [qi] interfere with soft [qi], that means that [the disease] originates from [a position] that can overcome the soft [qi]. Hence, the disease will be light. As for the pattern of the ten variations of one [specific movement in the] vessels, the teacher [who wrote the *Nan jing*] drew only on what happens in the two conduits of this one section of the heart in order to elucidate the [entire system]. The [five long-term depots and five short-term repositories may] attack each other with five kinds of evil [qi]. That may result in the ten variations. Each hand has the three sections [inch, gate, and foot], and each of them has two conduits.[15] If each of these six sections [may display] ten

---

14 The Ten Celestial Stems are used here to illustrate an interpretation that is different from those of other commentators. Ding Deyong may have separated "five evils" and "mutual interference of hard and soft" as two distinct concepts, the first denoting the interference of long-term depots with long-term depots, and of short-term repositories with short-term repositories, the second referring to the interference of yang units with yin units – that is, of long-term depots (yin) with short-term repositories (yang). He has associated the first five Celestial Stems (i.e., *jia, yi, bing, ding, wu*) as lower values with yin, and the second five Stems (i.e., *ji, geng, xin, ren, gui*) with yang, combining *jia* (value = 1) with *ji* (value = 6), *wu* (value = 5) with *gui* (value = 10), *ding* (value = 4) with *ren* (value = 9), and so forth.

15 Ding Deyong may have assumed that each of the six sections reflects the movement in the vessels of a long-term depot and of its respective short-term repository. Hence, he spoke of "two conduits" per section. Whether he believed that two tangible conduits passed through each section (for instance, the hand minor yin conduit of the heart from

variations due to five kinds of evil [qi], which adds up to sixty if each of them is counted separately – that is, if one multiplies six sections with ten variations. That was meant by the Yellow Thearch when he stated: "First take a hold of the yin and yang [qi], then check for the sixty [variations]."

Yu Shu: From the manifestation of these ten variations one may infer the [dynamics between the] Five Phases, in that they overcome [each other], return [against each other], or strengthen each other. That is why the sages spoke of the "five evils." Each of the five long-term depots has an external [extension, which is the short-term repository], and an internal [basis, which is the long-term depot itself]. They all may seize each other. [Hence, the movement of the qi in] one vessel [section] may undergo ten variations. There are yin and yang [long-term depots and short-term repositories, respectively]; hence, [the text] speaks of "hard" and of "soft" [qi]. If at a specific location [qi movements characteristic of] another vessel [section] appear, that is called "mutual attack." The sages [who wrote the *Nan jing*] took the one long-term depot of the heart as an example from which [the variations in] all the remaining [movements] can be derived.

Xu Dachun: This pattern is extremely subtle. It was not yet developed in the text of the [*Nei*] *jing*.

---

the chest to the hand, and the hand major yang conduit of the small intestine back from the hand to the head) cannot be inferred from this short statement.

十一難曰：（一）經言脈不滿五十動而一止，一藏無氣者，何藏也？
（二）然：人吸者隨陰入，呼者因陽出。（三）今吸不能至腎，至肝而還，故
知一藏無氣者，腎氣先盡也。

The eleventh difficult issue: (1) The scripture states: If the movement in the vessels stops once in less than fifty [arrivals], this is because one long-term depot is void of qi.[1] Which long-term depot is it?

(2) It is like this. [The qi] a person inhales enter [the organism] through yin [long-term depots; the qi a person] exhales leave [the organism] through yang [long-term depots. (3) In this case] now, [the qi] inhaled cannot reach the kidneys; they return after they have reached the liver. Hence, the long-term depots which will be void of qi are, obviously, the kidneys; their qi will be depleted first.[2]

COMMENTARIES

(1) *Yang:* The scripture states:[3] "Feel the vessel opening and count the arrivals of the [movement in the vessels]. When fifty movements occur without any inter-mittence in between, [that indicates that] all the five long-term depots receive [their necessary amounts of] qi. Such a person would be called in normal bal-ance and free of disease. When one intermittence occurs after forty movements, one long-term depot has no qi. [That person will] die after four years. When one intermittence occurs after thirty movements, two long-term depots have no qi. [That person will] die after three years. When one intermittence occurs after twenty movements, three long-term depots have no qi. [That person will]

---

1   This quotation may refer to *Ling shu* treatise 5, "Gen jie" 根結. The wording of the cor-responding sentence there is *si shi dong yi dai zhe yi zang wu qi* 四十動一代者一藏無氣 ("If within 40 movements there is one intermittence, one long-term depot is without qi.").

2   The eleventh difficult issue presents a further method for assessing the condition of the body's functional units on the basis of examining the movement in the vessels at – pre-sumably – the inch opening near the wrist. The idea outlined here implies that the normal circulation of qi through the body can be shortened – in case of an illness – so that at least one long-term depot may be skipped. The underlying concept was, obviously, borrowed from the *Ling shu* (see note 1), where it is stated that one, two, three, four, or even all five long-term depots may be skipped by the circulation. The naming of the kidneys here, in the *Nan jing*, as the first long-term depot to be avoided by the circulating qi caused some later commentators to attempt explanations on the basis of various analogies, while the more critical conservatives rejected this innovation altogether because its conceptual consequences are difficult to reconcile with various other ideas concerning the supply of the organism with qi.

3   Cf. *Ling shu*, treatise 5, "Gen jie 根結."

die after two years. When one intermittence occurs after ten movements, four long-term depots have no qi. [That person will] die after one year. If one inter-mittence occurs within less than ten movements, [all] the five long-term depots have no qi. [That person will] die after seven days." The *Nan jing* uses the term *zhi* 止 ("stop"). The original scripture spoke of *dai* 代 ("intermittence"). "Stop" indicates that one has a perception below his fingers, when pressing [the vessel opening], as if [the movement] came to a stop. That is called *zhi*. [The term] "intermittence" indicates [the perception that the movement] returns to the foot [section], where it stays for a while before it comes [back to the vessel opening]. That is called *dai*. Although the two scriptures use the two different [terms] "stop" and "intermittence," the appearances of the respective [movements in the] vessels are not really different. Hence, both [terms] are kept [in use].

Ding Deyong: "Fifty movements" [refers to the dynamics of the] yin and yang [qi of] heaven and earth, as they are measured systematically by the clepsy-dra's markings.[4] When the breathing [movement] in man's vessels amounts to less or more [than fifty movements before an intermittence occurs], that is an abnormal number. It amounts to more when it exceeds sixty [movements be-fore it stops. In this case] the heart and the lung have a surplus [of qi]. When the heart and the lung have a surplus, then the kidneys and the liver have not enough [qi. When the movement amounts to] less, that means that it does not reach the number of forty [movements before it stops. In this case] the heart and the lung have not enough, while the kidneys and the lung have a surplus. Here now, the yang qi are depleted or present only in a small quantity. Hence, [the movement stops once in] less than fifty [arrivals]. When [the *Nan jing*] speaks of "movement" and "stop," that means that the inhaled [qi] cannot reach the kidneys and return after they have reached the liver. That is, the yang [qi] do not circulate through the lower [parts of the body]. Hence, the kidney qi are cut off first. When they are cut off, [their movement] stops. This pattern is the same as that [behind the statement that "a person dies] only because of an internal interruption of the vital qi."

Yu Shu: This [paragraph] is somewhat similar to the meaning of the eighth diffi-cult issue [where it was stated that "a person dies] only because of an interrup-tion of the vital qi." The eighth difficult issue discussed [a situation in which] the source of one's vital qi, which are [inherited from one's] parents, is cut off between the two kidneys. Hence, it spoke of "death." Here, [the *Nan jing*] dis-

---

4   The clepsydra had one hundred markings to be passed by the dripping water within a twenty-four-hour period. Hence, fifty markings correspond to the periods of yin and yang dominance, (i.e., nighttime and daytime, respectively).

cusses [a situation in which] "one long-term depot is void of qi." That is to say, in the course of exhalation and inhalation, the lung [normally] processes the qi [produced out] of the grains [to the remaining long-term depots and also to the source of the vital qi]. If, now, the original qi between the kidneys, [originally endowed] by father and mother, no longer receive nourishment through the qi of the grains, they will diminish gradually, and one knows that [the respective patient] must die within four years, Hence, [the text] states: "The qi of the kidneys will be depleted first."

Liao Ping: This [difficult issue] presents some [aspects of the contents of the *Ling shu*] treatise "Gen jie 根結." In the *Nei jing*, seven treatises are devoted to the movement of the camp and guard [qi through the body. Thus the process of circulation] has already been elucidated there quite clearly. No need existed to raise this issue again. What is raised as an issue [here] is not even of great importance.

(2) *Li Jiong*: [The qi that are] inhaled enter the kidneys and the liver. Hence, [the qi a person] inhales enter through liver and kidneys. Liver and kidneys are located below the diaphragm. Hence, [the text] speaks of "yin." [The qi that are] exhaled leave from the heart and from the lung. Hence, [the qi a person] exhales leave through the heart and the lung. Heart and lung are located above the diaphragm; hence [the text] speaks of "yang."

(3) *Li Jiong*: In general, yin and yang [qi] follow each other moving up and down [in the body in the process of] exhalation and inhalation, and they pass through the five long-term depots.⁵ That is [the situation in] a normal person. Here now, [the qi that are] exhaled leave from the heart and lung, but the [qi that are] inhaled [and should reach the] kidneys [only] reach the liver before they return. They never get through to reach the kidneys. That means that the original qi which were received by the kidneys from father and mother diminish. Hence, when the movement in the vessels stops once in less than fifty [arrivals], one can be sure that [the respective patient] must die.

Hua Shou: Of the five long-term depots, the kidneys are located lowest [in the body]; they are the most distant [long-term depot to be reached] by the qi inhaled. If the movement stops in less than fifty [arrivals], one knows that the kidneys do not receive any supplies; their qi will be depleted first. *Jin* 盡 ("depleted") means *shuai jie* 衰竭 ("exhausted"). If they are exhausted, they cannot follow the qi of all the other long-term depots and move upward.

---

5 "Kidneys" is a mistake to be replaced by "lung."

(1)–(3) *Zhang Shixian*: "Movement" means "arrival" [of the qi in the] vessels. [The amount of] fifty movements corresponds to the *da yan* 大衍 number.[6] The *Nei jing* states: "In man, during one exhalation, the vessels exhibit two movements. During one inhalation, the vessels exhibit two movements too. Exhalation and inhalation constitute one standard breathing period.."[7] Of these five movements, the first [comes from] the lung and the second [comes from] the heart; the third [comes from] the spleen, the fourth [comes from] the liver, and the fifth [comes from] the kidneys. The five movements during one breathing [period are caused by qi] from all the five long-term depots. One through ten are the numbers of creation and formation in heaven and on earth. In ten breathing [periods, the qi of] the five long-term depots have moved through ten cycles. If they appear not to stop before fifty movements [are completed, this indicates that] all the five long-term depots are in normal [state]. When the number of the breathing [periods] corresponds to that of the [movement in the] vessels, what disease could be present? If [the two] do not [correspond], stops [will occur in the movement of the qi through the] vessels. Although it cannot yet be perceived otherwise, a disease has emerged. If a stop can be noticed once in less than fifty movements, that is because [of the following]. Inhaled [qi] constitute the yang; they enter through yin [long-term depots]. Exhaled [qi] constitute the yin; they leave from yang [long-term depots]. When the yang [qi] cannot circulate through the lower [section of the body], they reach only the liver before they return. When they do not reach the kidneys, the qi of the kidneys will be cut off first. That is the reason why the movement stops once in less than fifty [arrivals].

Xu Dachun: In the treatise "Gen jie" 根結 of the *Ling shu* [it is outlined that] In the case of one intermittence after forty movements one long-term depot has no qi, and so forth until in the case of one intermittence within less than ten movements, none of the five long-term depots has any qi, and so on. But there is definitely no clear indication [in the *Ling shu*] as to which depot's [qi] have been cut off first. Thus, one must investigate which of the long-term depots has contracted a disease, and then [one may know] which depot's [qi] have been cut off first. That is a definite principle. According to what is said here, the first [long-term depot to be cut off] are the kidneys, the second is the liver, the third is the spleen, the fourth is the heart, and the fifth is the lung. [This implies that] the long-term depot which contracted the disease [first] is not necessarily the

---

6   The designation *da yan* 大衍 may have been used first to denote a divination method based on a manipulation of fifty stalks of plants. In this connection, and in other usages of the term, the number fifty was supposed to encompass various important aspects – or phenomena – of heaven and earth.

7   Cf. *Su wen* treatise 18, "Ping ren qi xiang lun" 平人氣象論.

one [whose qi are] cut off [first]. I fear that such a principle does not exist. Also, the significance of determining the absence of qi on the basis of [the pattern of] exhalation and inhalation is not established. If the inhaled [qi] cannot reach the kidneys, the fifth [movement] should stop. How can it continue to forty movements before an intermittence occurs?

Katō Bankei: When the [movement in the] vessels arrives five times during one breathing [period], and when it is neither strong nor weak, then this is a normal [movement indicating that] the five long-term depots are in [a state of] normal balance, free from disease. However, [the arrivals that occur] within one breathing [period] are extremely feeble and minute; they have no shape and leave no impression. Hence, one starts from fifty movements within ten breathing [periods] in order to examine whether the qi of [any of] the long-term depots are exhausted [or not] .... The *Ling shu* discusses [the consequences for the movement in the vessels in the case of an exhaustion of a depot's qi for] all five long-term depots. This paragraph talks only about one depot. This, of course, means [the same as the teaching method introduced by Confucius, namely] to raise one [corner of a subject and expect the pupil to] infer the remaining three. Also, the *Ling shu* says only "one depot, two long-term depots," and one still does not know which long-term depots are meant. Hence, Bian Que raised this issue in order to substantiate [the abstract statement in the *Ling shu*]. He let later people know that the so-called first long-term depot is calculated from below. Thus, one knows also that the "lack of qi" starts from the kidneys.

Liao Ping: This dragging in of [the concepts of] exhalation and inhalation belongs to the trumped up [sections of the *Nan jing*]. The talk [about a flow of qi] from the liver to the kidneys represents particular ignorance. [Obviously, the author of this difficult issue] has not read the [*Nei jing*] paragraphs on the movement of the camp and guard [qi]. If he had been induced to take only a little time for reading through the *Nei jing*, he would not have arrived at such statements. The doctrine of highly valuing the kidneys began with Wei Boyang 魏伯陽.[8] Afterwards, each single long-term depot had to be associated with ten circulations. That, already, represented a mistaken interpretation of the text of the [*Nei*]*jing*. [When] now the kidneys are considered to be the first depot, this means heaping mistake upon mistake.

---

8   Daoist philosopher and alchemist of the second century CE; author of the *Can tong qi* 參同契.

十二難曰：（一）經言五藏脈已絕於內，用鍼者反實其外；（二）五藏脈已絕
於外，用鍼者反實其內。（三）內外之絕，何以別之？

（四）然：五藏脈已絕於內者，腎肝氣已絕於內也，而醫反補其心肺；（五）
五藏脈已絕於外者，其心肺脈已絕於外也，而醫反補其腎肝。（六）陽絕補
陰，陰絕補陽，是謂實實虛虛，損不足益有餘。（七）如此死者，醫殺之耳。

The twelfth difficult issue: (1) The scripture states: If the flow of qi of the five long-term depots has already been interrupted internally and one then employs the needles, he will, contrary to his intentions, cause an external repletion. (2) If the flow of qi of the five long-term depots has already been interrupted externally and one then employs the needles, he will, contrary to his intentions, cause an internal repletion.[1] (3) How can one distinguish whether the [movement through the] internal or external [long-term depots] is cut off?

(4) It is like this. "[The movement of qi through] the vessels of the five long-term depots has been cut off from the internal [part of the organism]" means that the vessels associated with the kidneys and with the liver, located in the internal [part of the organism], are cut off from the [movement of the] qi. [In this case] a physician acts contrary to the requirements if he supplements the respective [person's] heart and lungs. (5) "[The movement of qi through] the vessels of the five long-term depots is cut off from the external [part of the organism]" means that the vessels associated with the heart and with the lung, located in the external [part of the organism], are cut off from the [movement of the] qi. [In this case] a physician acts contrary to the requirements if he supplements the respective [person's] kidneys and liver. (6) To supplement the yin [long-term depots] when the yang [long-term depots] are cut off, or to supplement the yang [long-term depots] when the yin [long-term depots] are cut off, means to replenish what is replete already, and to deplete what is depleted already, to diminish what is not enough, and to add where a surplus exists already. (7) If anybody dies due to such [therapies], the physician has killed the respective [patient].[2]

---

1   This is a slightly modified quotation, excerpted from treatise 1, "Jiu zhen shi er yuan" 九鍼十二原 of the *Ling shu*. The original passage in the *Ling shu* speaks of *wu zang zhi qi* 五藏之氣 rather than of *wu zang mai* 五藏脈. Cf. Xu Dachun's commentary. The separation of this quote from its original context gives it a slightly different emphasis.

2   This difficult issue was removed, by Katō Bankei and other *Nan jing* editors, from its twelfth position to become the eighty-first difficult issue. It seems to fit better in the final section of the *Nan jing*, which is devoted to needle therapy, than in the first section, which focuses on diagnosis. Although my rendering of this paragraph follows this therapeutic interpretation, it should be noted that a diagnostic rendering would have been

COMMENTARIES

(1) *Liao Ping*: This difficult issue divides the lung, the heart, the liver, and the kidneys into an internal and an external [category]. This corresponds to the earlier differentiation of the four long-term depots according to [the concepts of] "at the surface" and "in the depth." Whoever wrote this book cannot have had the slightest perspective in his mind. He desired to create regulations not bound by any conventionality. He must really have been a mean man. He incited killings that did not diminish over thousands of years! How could his crime be halted; how could he ever emerge free [from guilt]?

(3) *Liao Ping*: The text of the [*Nei*] *jing* itself is extremely intelligible; no need existed to raise this question. Here, [the author] intends to make use of the [*Nei*] *jing* in order to elucidate his apocryphal doctrine of heart and lung being external and of liver and kidneys being internal. The [*Nei*] *jing* distinguishes the shoulders with the chest and the four limbs as internal and external, respectively. This apocryphal doctrine categorizes the four long-term depots as yin and yang, and as internal and external, on the basis of their being located high or below [in the body].

(7) *Liao Ping*: The persons killed because of this book are as numerous as the sands of the Ganges.

(1)–(7) *Lü Guang*: Heart and lung are [considered to be in the] external [part of the organism] because these long-term depots are located above the diaphragm. The qi that are [related to the] upper [long-term depots of the organism are categorized as] "external"; these are the camp and guard [qi]. They move at the surface in the skin and in the blood vessels, respectively. Hence, [the *Nan jing*] says "cut off from the external [part of the organism]." Kidneys and liver are [considered to be located in the] internal [part of the organism] because these long-term depots are located below the diaphragm. The qi that are [related to the] lower [long-term depots of the organism are categorized as] "internal"; they provide

---

possible, too. Such an understanding is indicated in the *Ling shu* treatise 3, "Xiao zhen jie" 小鍼解, and was referred to by Hua Shou in his commentary. The innovation presented by this difficult issue appears to have been the categorization of the two long-term depots (heart and lung) located above the diaphragm as external, and of the two long-term depots (kidneys and liver) located below the diaphragm as internal. While some commentators faithfully adopted this idea and attempted to integrate it into the general framework of systematic correspondence, it was rejected by the critical conservatives who did not find it in the *Nei jing*. The therapeutic principle of supplementing a depletion and draining a repletion did not create any controversies because it is propagated also by the *Nei jing*. The phrase *sun bu zu yi you yu* 損不足益有餘 in sentence 6 was quoted literally from *Ling shu* treatise 1, "Jiu zhen shi er yuan" 九鍼十二原.

nourishment to the muscles and to the bones. Hence, [the *Nan jing*] says "cut off from the internal [part of the organism]."

Ding Deyong: The "internal" and "external" location of the five long-term depots refers [to the following]. Heart and lung are located above the diaphragm; they are passed by the qi of heaven. The heart rules the [movement in the] vessels; the lung rules the [flow of the] qi. [Together] they provide splendor externally to the skin. Hence, [the *Nan jing*] speaks of "external" [long-term depots]. The kidneys and the liver are located below the diaphragm; they are passed by the qi of the earth. They store the essence and the blood, and they are most closely related to the bones and to the marrow. "Heart and lung, located in the external [part of the organism], are cut off" means that because [heart and lung] are cut off [from the movement of the qi through the organism], the skin shrinks and the hair falls out. "Kidneys and liver, located in the internal [part of the organism], are cut off" means that because [kidneys and liver] are cut off [from the movement of the qi through the organism], the bones weaken and the muscles become flabby. If a student, in checking the [movement in the] vessels, is unable to understand whether [a disease is located] internally or externally, and whether it is a [case of] depletion or repletion, and if he, then, mistakenly dumps his needles or drugs [into the patient], he will but replenish what is replete already, and he will deplete what is depleted already; he will diminish what is not enough, and he will add where a surplus exists. If anybody dies due to such [therapies], the physician has killed the respective [patient].

Hua Shou: In the first treatise of the *Ling shu* it is stated: "Whenever one is about to apply the needles, he must first check the [movement in the] vessels and see whether there are any changes in the [flow of the] qi. Only then may the treatment begin." In its third treatise, [the *Ling shu*] states: "When it says: 'the [flow of the] qi of the five long-term depots has already been interrupted internally', [then that is to say:] the [flow of the] qi in the interior has been interrupted and hence they fail to arrive at the qi opening. If now, against the rules, one removes an illness from a location in the exterior and lets a needle remain at the confluence [opening]³ of the yang conduits to have yang qi arrive, then this will cause a double exhaustion in the interior as soon as the qi arrive. A double exhaustion results in death. Such a death results when the qi no longer move. Hence it is a calm [death]. When it says: 'the [flow of the] qi of the five long-term depots has already been interrupted in the exterior', [then that is to say:] the [flow of the] qi in the exterior has been interrupted and hence they fail to

---

3 The concepts of "confluence" holes and "transportation" holes are outlined in detail in the final section of the *Nan jing;* cf. difficult issues 62 ff.

arrive at the vessel opening. If now, against the rules, one removes [the disease] through the transport [openings] on the four limbs, and lets the needle remain there to have yin qi arrive, then, once the yin qi have arrived, the yang qi in response will move and enter [where the yin qi have left]. When they enter, this is a movement contrary to the norms. Such a movement contrary to the norms results in death. Such a death results because too many yin qi are present. Hence [this death] is fierce." [The *Ling shu*] uses the interior and exterior [sections] of the vessel opening to discuss the [condition of the] yin and yang [long-term depots]. Yueren uses the internal and external [location] of heart and lung and of the kidneys and of the liver, respectively, to differentiate between yin and yang [long-term depots]. The underlying principle is the same.

Zhang Shixian: The *Nei jing* states: "The lung rules the skin; the heart rules the [movement in the] vessels; the liver rules the muscles; the kidneys rule the bones. Skin and vessels are located in the external [parts of the body]; muscles and bones are located in the internal [parts]."[4] [The *Nan jing* states:] "The vessels associated with the kidneys and with the liver, located in the internal [part of the organism], are cut off from [the movement of the qi]." This means that the yang [qi are] depleted and cannot[5] circulate through the lower [part of the body where the kidneys and the liver are located. This has the result that] the yin [long-term depots] are cut off [from the movement of the qi]. If, in this case, anybody, in contrast to the requirements, supplements heart and lung, that would be a supplementing of the yang [long-term depots] while the yin [long-term depots] remain cut off. [The *Nan jing* states further:] "The vessels associated with the heart and with the lung, located in the external [part of the organism] are cut off from [the movement of the qi]." This means that the yin [qi are] depleted and cannot circulate through the upper [sections of the body where heart and lung are located. This has the result that] the yang [long-term depots] are cut off [from the movement of the qi]. If, in this case, anybody, in contrast [to the requirements], supplements the kidneys and the liver, that would be a supplementing of the yin [long-term depots] while the yang [long-term depots] remain cut off. Well, they are truly those who are generally called blind physicians, who do not know medicine, and who practice medicine recklessly. Obviously, they do not realize that the goal of creating a normal balance [of qi in the organism] is the principle of needling. [This implies that] depletions have to be supplemented while repletions have to be drained. If there is too much, it must be diminished; if there is not enough, one must add to it. In the case [described] here, depletion is

---

4   Cf. *Su wen* treatise 23, "Xuan ming wu qi lun" 宣明五氣論, and others.

5   The reiteration of the characters *xu bu* 虛不 is a mistake.

added to depletion, and what is not enough is diminished even further; repletion is added to repletion, and further supplies are added where there is too much already. That is not [the appropriate method] to raise the dead; in contrast, it will kill the living! If anybody dies because of such [therapies], his existence was cut off not because of his disease; the physician killed him.

Xu Dachun: The treatise "Jiu zhen shi er yuan" 九鍼十二原 of the *Ling* [*shu*] states: "If the flow of qi of the five long-term depots has already been interrupted internally and one then employs the needles, and this way, contrary to his intentions, causes an external repletion, that is called 'doubling an exhaustion'. A doubled exhaustion must result in death. That is a quiet death. The one who has treated this [patient], he has inadvertently acted against the [requirements of the status of the patient's] qi. He has chosen [to pierce] the armpits and the chest. If the flow of qi of the five long-term depots has already been interrupted externally and one then employs the needles, and this way, contrary to his intentions, causes an internal repletion, that is called 'movement contrary to the norms, with recession'. A movement contrary to the norms, with recession, must result in death. That is a violent death. The one who has treated this [patient], he has inadvertently acted against the [requirements of the status of the patient's qi]. He has chosen [to pierce] the four extremities." If the internal [long-term depots] are cut off [from the movement of the qi], this implies a depletion of [the qi in] the yin [long-term depots]. Hence, one supplements at armpits and chest because these are [locations] where the qi of the long-term depots originate. If the external [long-term depots] are cut off [from the movement of the qi], this implies a depletion of [the qi in] the yang [long-term depots]. Hence, one supplements at the four limbs because they constitute the source of all yang [vessels]. This therapeutic method is clearly understandable. Here now, [in the *Nan jing*], the word *qi* 氣 [in the sentence "the qi are cut off"] has been replaced by the word *mai* 脈 ("movement in the vessels"). That alone is a deviation. In addition, [the *Nan jing*] considers the heart and the lung to be external, and the kidneys and the liver to be internal. But it also speaks of "the [movement in the] vessels of the five-long-term depots," which include heart, lung, kidneys, and liver.[6] Now, when [the text says that] heart and lung are supposed to be affected when the internal [long-term depots] are cut off [from the movement of the qi], while the kidneys and the liver are supposed to be affected when the external [long-term depots] are cut off, how could the meaning of that text be clear? Yin and yang, internal and external are all [categories that] have their respective [associations]. One cannot stick firmly to a statement that heart and lung are

---

6   The spleen is not mentioned here; it was categorized as being neither yin nor yang.

external, while the kidneys and the liver are internal. One should know that one may speak, in specific situations, of kidneys and liver as internal, and of heart and lung as external, but that, generally speaking, each of the five long-term depots has an external and an internal [aspect] as well.

Nan jing 1962: Depletion and repletion in the five long-term depots can be diagnosed through feeling the vessels. When this difficult issue speaks of "internal" and "external" [sections of the] vessels of the five long-term depots, the "external" points to heart and lung, while the "internal" refers to the kidneys and to the liver. Zhang Jingyue 張景岳[7] has said: "When [the movement felt at] the vessel opening is at the surface and depleted, and disappears if one presses [one's fingers down], that is called '[the qi are] cut off from the internal [part] and do not arrive'. [It signals] depletion of yin qi. When the [movement felt at the] vessel opening is in the depth and feeble, and disappears if one lifts [the finger to apply only a] light touch, that is called '[the qi are] cut off from the external [part] and do not arrive'. [It signals] depletion of yang qi." This is a method to determine, on the basis of the appearance of the [movement in the] vessels, whether·the qi in the five long-term depots are depleted. To diagnose whether [a condition of] depletion or repletion has resulted from a disease, and – in treatment – to supplement what is depleted and to drain what is replete, that is the general therapeutic principle.

---

7   Zhang Jiebin 張介賓, *zi:* Jingyue, is a famed medical author of the seventeenth century. His writings were published as *Jing yue quan shu* 景岳全書.

十三難曰：（一）經言見其色而不得其脈，反得相勝之脈者即死，（二）得相生之脈者，病即自已。（三）色之與脈當參相應，為之奈何？

（四）然：五藏有五色，皆見於面，（五）亦當與寸口、尺內相應。（六）假令色青，其脈當弦而急；（七）色赤，其脈浮大而散；（八）色黃，其脈中緩而大；（九）色白，其脈浮濇而短；（十）色黑，其脈沉濇而滑。（十一）此所謂五色之與脈，當參相應也。（十二）脈數，尺之皮膚亦數；（十三）脈急，尺之皮膚亦急；（十四）脈緩，尺之皮膚亦緩；（十五）脈濇，尺之皮膚亦濇；（十六）脈滑，尺之皮膚亦滑。（十七）五藏各有聲、色、臭、味，當與寸口、尺內相應，（十八）其不相應者病也。（十九）假令色青，其脈浮濇而短，若大而緩為相勝；（二十）浮大而散，若小而滑為相生也。（二十一）經言知一為下工，知二為中工，知三為上工。上工者十全九，中工者十全八，下工者十全六，此之謂也。

The thirteenth difficult issue: (1) The scripture states: If one sees a [person's] complexion and cannot feel the corresponding [movement in the] vessels, but rather feels a [movement in the] vessels [indicating dominance of a superior phase according to the order of] mutual destruction, the [respective person] will die.[1] (2) If one feels a [movement in the] vessels [indicating dominance of a superior phase according to the order of] mutual generation, the disease will come to an end by itself.[2] (3) Complexion and [movement in the] vessels must be compared as to their mutual correspondence, but how is that done?

(4) It is like this. The body's five long-term depots have five [corresponding] complexions[3] which can be seen on the face. (5) They must also correspond to the [movement felt at the] inch opening and to [the condition of the skin of the] foot-interior [section]. (6) For example, [if one sees] a virid complexion, the respective [movement in the] vessels should be like a string and tense. (7) In the case of a red complexion, the respective [movement in the] vessels should be at the surface, strong, and dispersed. (8) In the case of a yellow complexion, the respective [movement in the] vessels should be in the center, relaxed, and strong. (9) In the case of a

---

1   The order of "mutual destruction" or "mutual control" of the Five Phases is wood, soil, water, fire, metal, since wood (for instance, a spade) controls soil; soil (for instance, a dike) controls water; water destroys fire; fire destroys metal; and metal destroys wood.

2   The order of "mutual generation" of the Five Phases is wood, fire, soil, metal, water, wood, since metal generates water; water generates wood; wood generates fire; fire generates soil; and soil generates metal.

3   In this context, the term *se* 色 ("complexion") does not denote the color of the entire face but that of specific sections of the face. See Yu Shu's commentaries to sentences 6 through 10.

white complexion, the respective [movement in the] vessels should be at the surface, rough, and short. (10) In the case of a black complexion, the respective [movement in the] vessels should be in the depth, soft, and smooth. (11) This is meant by the requirement to compare the five complexions with the [movements in the] vessels as to their mutual correspondence. (12) If the [movement in the] vessels is frequent, the skin of the foot[-interior section between elbow and gate should] also be marked by frequency. (13) If the [movement in the] vessels is tense, the skin of the foot[-interior section should] also be tense. (14) If the [movement in the] vessels is relaxed, the skin of the foot[-interior section should] also be relaxed. (15) If the [movement in the] vessels is rough, the skin of the foot[-interior section should] also be rough. (16) If the [movement in the] vessels is smooth, the skin of the foot[-interior section] should also be smooth. (17) Each of the body's five long-term depots has its [corresponding] pitch, complexion, odor, and flavor; they all should correspond to the [movement felt at the] inch opening [and to the condition of the skin of the] foot-interior [section]. (18) No correspondence is [a sign of] disease. (19) For example, [if in case of] a virid complexion the respective [movement in the] vessels is at the surface, rough, and short, or if [the movement is] strong and relaxed, that indicates [dominance of a superior phase in the order of] mutual destruction. (20) If [the movement] is at the surface, strong, and dispersed, or if it is minor[4] and smooth, that indicates [dominance of a superior phase in the order of] mutual generation. (21) The scripture states: The inferior craftsman knows one [diagnostic sign];[5] the mediocre craftsman knows two [diagnostic signs]; the superior craftsman knows [all] three [diagnostic signs]. That is to say, the superior craftsman cures nine out of ten [patients]; the mediocre craftsman cures eight out of ten [patients]; and the inferior craftsman cures six out of ten [patients].[6]

---

4   Katō Bankei and some other *Nan jing* editors have exchanged *xiao* 小 ("minor") here for *ju* 濡 ("soft"); *xiao* may, indeed, be a mistake here. See sentence 10.

5   Later commentators have offered various explanations as to the meaning of "knows one, knows two, knows three." I have preferred a rather neutral phrasing – namely, "diagnostic sign" – because "one," "two," "three" might refer, if we stay closest to the preceding discourse, to vessel movement, pitch, odor, and flavor, or to a knowledge of the number of long-term depots involved in a disease. See also note 11.

6   This difficult issue further widens the scope of diagnostic techniques to be applied within the theoretical framework of systematic correspondence. Its emphasis is twofold. On the one hand, it outlines a series of physiological signs and processes that correspond to each other and, hence, should change simultaneously in case one specific long-term depot develops a disease. On the other hand, this difficult issue demonstrates how the two major sequences of the Five Phases (see notes 1 and 2) may be utilized to understand clinical pictures characterized by an absence of correspondence between the physiological signs and processes regarded as perceivable manifestations of internal conditions. The pattern

COMMENTARIES

(1) *Hua Shou*: In the fourth treatise of the *Ling shu* it is stated: "Someone who looks at the [patient's] complexion and knows his disease, he is called enlightened". Someone who presses the [patient's] vessels and knows his disease, he is called „divine". Someone who asks the [patient] about his disease and knows the location of the disease, he is called „practitioner." Complexion, the [movement in the] vessels, the shape [of the body], and the flesh must not lose their mutual [correspondence]. When the complexion is virid, the corresponding [movement in the] vessels is like a string. Red corresponds to a hook-like [movement in the] vessels. Yellow corresponds to an intermittent [movement in the] vessels. White corresponds to a hair-like [movement in the] vessels. Black corresponds to a stone-like [movement in the] vessels.[7] When one sees a specific complexion but cannot feel the corresponding [movement in the] vessels, that indicates that complexion and [movement in the] vessels do not belong to each other. When complexion and [movement in the] vessels do not belong to each other, one should look which vessel [movement] he has perceived. If he has felt a vessel [movement resulting from qi of a long-term depot associated with a phase that] overcomes [the phase of the long-term depot indicated by the complexion, the

of correspondences followed by this difficult issue and by its commentators can be tabulated as follows:

Five Phases		Wood	Fire	Soil	Metal	Water
Five Depots		Liver	Heart	Spleen	Lung	Kidneys
Correspondence Between	Color	Virid	Red	Yellow	White	Black
	Vessel Movement	(In the Depth) Tense, String-like	At the Surface Strong Dispersed Vast	In the Center Relaxed Intermittent	At the Surface Rough Hair-like Short	In the Depth Soft Stone-like Smooth
Correspondence Between	Vessel Movement	Tense	Frequent	Relaxed	Rough	Smooth
	Skin	Tense	Frequent	Relaxed	Rough	Smooth
Five Pitches		Shouting	Laughing	Singing	Wailing	Groaning
Five Odors		Rank	Burnt	Aromatic	Frowzy	Foul
Five Flavors		Sour	Bitter	Sweet	Acrid	Salty

The *Nei jing* statements referred to by this difficult issue can be found in *Ling shu* treatise 4, "Xie qi zang fu bing xing" 邪氣藏府病形. The differences in the wording and in the underlying concepts were pointed out by some of the commentators.

7 For a more detailed discussion of the movement qualities string-like, hook-like, intermittent, hair-like, and stone-like, see difficult issue 15.

patient] will die. If he has felt a vessel [movement resulting from qi of a long-term depot associated with a phase that] generates [the phase of the long-term depot indicated by the patient's complexion], the disease will come to an end by itself.

Xu Dachun: In the treatise ["Xie qi zang fu bing xing lun" 邪氣藏府病形論], the *Ling shu* states: "The complexion and the [movement in the] vessels in the foot-long section, they correspond to each other in the same manner as the beating and the sound of a drum correspond to each other." [The term] *mai* 脈 ("vessel") [is used here] to indicate diagnosis [through feeling the vessel with one's fingers; the term] *chi* 尺 ("foot") [is used here] to indicate the skin [of the foot-interior section of the arm]. This language is quite reliable. Here now, [in the *Nan jing*, the term] *mai* has been replaced by *cun kou* 寸口 ("inch opening"). Hence, the meaning of these terms has become confused and is difficult to understand. This shows that the text of the [*Nei*] *jing* must not be altered.

Liao Ping: The word *mai* 脈, as used in the *Nei jing*, serves both as a comprehensive and as a specific term. As a comprehensive term, the [word] *mai* 脈 encompasses complexion, skin, qi, blood, conduits, network [vessels], muscles, and bones. This book discards the ancient diagnostic methods completely and no matter which kind of [technical] terms associated with them, everything is moved to the inch [sections near the wrists of the] two [hands. The *Nan jing*] introduces all kinds of false methods in order to justify its own lies. Through a careful analysis of the [*Nei*] *jing* text, the apocryphal [character of the *Nan jing*] will become obvious by itself.

(5) *Zhang Shixian*: The skin of the foot-long section is the skin from the gate up to the foot-marsh [hole].

Liao Ping: The term *pi* 皮 ("skin") of the [*Nei*] *jing* has been replaced here by *chi* 尺 ("foot").

(6) *Lü Guang*: A virid color, that is the liver. A string-like and tense [movement] is [characteristic of the movement of the qi of the] liver [in the] vessels. [When such a color and such a movement in the vessels are present,] that is called mutual correspondence.

Yu Shu: When the color is virid and when the [movement in the] vessels is like a string, [that indicates that] center and external [manifestation] correspond to each other. The *Su wen* states: "The liver section [of the face] is located below the eyes. Look there for the color and compare it with the manifestation of the [movement of the qi in the] vessels."

(7) *Lü Guang*: A red color, that is the heart. A [movement which is] at the surface, strong, and dispersed is [characteristic of the movement in the] vessels [that is

associated with the] heart. [When such a color and such a movement in the vessels are present,] that is called mutual correspondence.

Yu Shu: When the color is red and when the [movement in the] vessels is strong, color and vessel [movement] correspond to each other. The *Su wen* states: "The heart section [of the face] is at the mouth. Look there for the color and compare it with the [movement in the] vessels."

(8) *Lü Guang*: A yellow color, that is the spleen. A [movement which is] in the center, relaxed, and strong is [characteristic of the movement in the] vessels [that is associated with the] spleen.

Yu Shu: [When such a color and such a movement are present,] that represents a mutual correspondence of color and vessel [movement]. The *Su wen* states: "The spleen section [of the face] is at the lips. Look at their center for the color, [and see] whether it corresponds to the shape of the [movement in the] vessels."

(9) *Lü Guang*: A white color, that is the lung. A [movement which is] at the surface, rough, and short is [characteristic of the movement in the] vessels [that is associated with the] lung.[8]

Yu Shu: The lung section [of the face] appears at the *que ting* 闕庭,[9] which is located above the eyebrows.

(10) *Lü Guang*: A black color, that is the kidneys. The kidneys control the water. The nature of water is [to seek the] depth. The kidneys, accordingly, are the lowest of the five long-term depots. Hence, [the movement of their qi in the] vessels is in the depth, soft, and smooth.

Yu Shu: The color of the kidneys appears in the flesh and on the skin. Pick the *di ge* 地閣 in the face[10] [to examine the color].

(11) *Lü Guang*: [Such correspondences occur] because the proper conduits have fallen ill by themselves. They have not been struck by evil [qi] from somewhere else.

Yu Shu: That is to say, these are symptoms corresponding to [conditions of] depletion and repletion in the original conduits.

(12) *Ding Deyong*: "Frequent," that is the heart. Hence, the skin of the inner side of the arm is hot.

Xu Dachun: "Frequent" means that [the qi in the vessels] arrive six, seven times during one breathing [period]. How can any skin be frequent? A mistake must

---

8　See also *Ling shu* treatise 49, "Wu se" 五色, for correspondences between facial color sections and the five long-term depots.

9　The term *que* 闕 is used, in *Ling shu* treatise 49, "Wu se," 五色 to denote the space between the two eyebrows. The character *shang* 上 ("above") in Yu Shu's commentary may be a mistake.

10　This is a designation for the chin.

have been made when this was written down. Hence, the meaning of the text is even more difficult to understand.

(13) *Ding Deyong*: "Tense" indicates that the [main] conduits and the network [vessels] are overly supplemented. Hence, they are hard and tense.

(14) *Ding Deyong*: "Relaxed" indicates that the flesh wanes. Hence, the skin is also relaxed and weak.

(15) *Ding Deyong*: The lung controls dryness. Hence, the skin of the inner side of the arm is rough too.

(16) *Ding Deyong*: The kidneys control the water. [The movement of their qi in] the vessels is smooth. Hence, the skin of the inner side of the arm is smooth too. In all the five situations [mentioned above] one should compare whether a smooth, rough, tense, relaxed, or frequent skin corresponds to a [respective] complexion and to the [movement in the] vessels.

(17) *Ding Deyong*: These so-called correspondences [are as follows]. A frequent [movement in the] vessels, a red color, and a hot skin indicate correspondence of the [movement in the] vessels, the color, and the skin for the one long-term depot of the heart. A tense [movement in the] vessels, a virid color, and a hard and tense skin, as well as [hard and tense] conduits and network [vessels], indicate correspondence of the [movement in the] vessels, the color, and the skin for the one long-term depot of the liver. A relaxed [movement in the] vessels, a yellow color, and a relaxed skin indicate correspondence of the [movement in the] vessels, the color, and the skin for the one long-term depot of the spleen. A rough [movement in the] vessels, a white color, and a rough skin indicate correspondence of the [movement in the] vessels, the color, and the skin for the one long-term depot of the lung. A smooth [movement in the] vessels, a black color, and a smooth skin indicate correspondence of the [movement in the] vessels, the color, and the skin for the one long-term depot of the kidneys. Whenever one examines the [movement in the] vessels, he should first proceed [with his investigation] to the inner and outer parts of the arm, and only then should he check the [movement in the] vessels and take a look at the [patient's] complexion.

Yu Shu: The [movement in the] vessels of the [qi of the] liver is like a string; the respective color is virid, the respective pitch is shouting, the respective odor is rank, the respective flavor [one longs for] is sour. The [movement in the] vessels of the [qi of the] heart is vast: the respective color is red, the respective pitch is laughing, the respective odor is burnt, the respective flavor [one longs for] is bitter. The [movement in the] vessels of the [qi of the] spleen is relaxed, the respective color is yellow, the respective pitch is singing, the respective odor is aromatic, the respective flavor [one longs for] is sweet. The [movement in the] vessels of the [qi of the] lung is rough; the respective color is white, the respective pitch is wailing, the respective odor is frowzy, the respective flavor [one longs for] is acrid. The [movement in the] vessels of the [qi of the] kidneys is deep; the respective color is black, the respective pitch is groaning, the respective odor is foul, the respective flavor [one longs for] is salty. These are the so-called correspondences.

(18) *Yu Shu*: "Correspondence" indicates that the proper conduits have fallen ill by themselves. If, for instance, in the case of a liver disease, the [movement in the] vessels is like a string, the complexion is virid, [the patient] shouts often, loves rank odors, and longs for [items with] sour flavor, that would be called "a disease that has arisen from [the affected long-term depot and its conduits] themselves." "No correspondence" refers to the following. If, for instance, in the case of a liver disease, the [movement in the] vessels is rough, the complexion is white, [the patient] wails often, loves frowzy odors, and longs for [items with] acrid flavor, that would be called a "reversed [situation." That is to say,] in [the patient's] pitch, in his complexion, in the odor, and in the flavor [he prefers], manifestations of the [qi of the] lung are apparent. Metal destroys wood; hence, one speaks here of a robber evil [which has arisen in the lung, i.e., in the phase of metal, and has overcome the liver, i.e., the phase of wood]. That is [a situation of] "no correspondence"; death is inevitable.

(19) *Lü Guang*: A virid color, that is the liver. A [movement in the vessels which is] at the surface, rough, and short is [characteristic of the qi of] the lung. When [qi from] the lung overcome the liver, that is a robber evil. If [the movement is] at the surface, strong, and dispersed, that is a [movement in the] vessels of the [qi of the] heart. The heart is the child [depot] of the liver. If [the movement is] minor and smooth, that is a [movement in the] vessels of the [qi of the] kidneys. The kidneys are the mother [depot] of the liver. The liver is the child [depot] of the kidneys. [The Five Phases are related among themselves like] mother and child; they give life to each other. Hence, one speaks of mutual generation.

Ding Deyong: The [*Nan*]*jing* refers to the one long-term depot of the liver. [The movement of] its [qi in the] vessels should be like a string and tense; the respective color should be virid. That would indicate compliance. When the color is virid and the [movement in the] vessels is rough, that indicates opposition. When the [movement in the] vessels is strong and relaxed, the [qi of the] liver have overcome the spleen. That is a serious disease. Hence, one speaks of mutual destruction. When the [movement in the] vessels is at the surface, strong, and dispersed, or when it is minor and smooth, that indicates [a dominance of qi from the long-term depot related to the liver in the order of] mutual generation.

Xu Dachun: These sentences explain the meaning of the word "mutual" with such great perfection that it is not even reached by the text of the [*Nei*] *jing*.

(21) *Lü Guang*: When the five long-term depots have a disease, it may, in each case, have [originated from] five [different sources].[11] Here now, the [*Nan*] *jing* refers only to the one long-term depot of the liver as an example. Anybody who is able to interpret [the condition of] but one long-term depot is an inferior practitioner. Anybody who can interpret [the conditions of] two long-term depots is a mediocre practitioner. Anybody who can interpret [the conditions of all] five long-term depots [as they relate to the long-term depot with the disease], is a superior practitioner.

Ding Deyong: A "superior practitioner" means that someone knows the principles of the three [symptomatic] patterns which appear in the complexion, in the [movement in the] vessels, and in the [condition of the] skin, of mutual generation and of mutual destruction. Hence, when [such a person] treats diseases, he will cure nine out of ten. The mediocre practitioner knows two [of the diagnostic patterns]. He cannot take all [the information offered by the organism]. Hence, when [such a person] treats diseases, he will cure eight out of ten. An inferior practitioner knows one [diagnostic pattern]; that is to say, he does not know how to interpret the complete [symptomatic] pattern. He devotes himself entirely to treating the [depot] which has already fallen ill [but does not know how to relate it to the remaining long-term depots]. Hence, out of ten [cases] he will cure only six.

Yu Shu: As to "practitioner," someone who studies ten thousand [patients] and cures ten thousand [patients] is then called a practitioner. Whoever practices medicine must thoroughly study the *Nan jing*. [There he learns how] to investigate whether the [movement in the] vessels is at the surface or in the depth, and whether the long-term depots and short-term repositories are in a [condition of] depletion or repletion. He must penetrate the *Su wen* [in order to understand] the passage of the conduit vessels. He must thoroughly study the *Ben cao* 本草 in order to know about the cold and warm [nature of] drugs, and [in order to understand] where qi and flavors turn to [in the organism]. When someone controls these three schools completely and then treats diseases, one may say that he "knows three [medical disciplines] and is a superior practitioner." If a

---

11 Evil qi may originate from the sick long-term depot itself, from mother or child depot, or from the two long-term depots preceding and following the sick long-term depot in the order of mutual destruction. See difficult issue 10, note 1.

physician is not [well versed] in these three areas, do not take any of his drugs.[12] That means he is not a practitioner. The *Su wen* states: "Anybody who knows how to draw conclusions from the manifestations of the five long-term depots, and anybody who can reflect about and understand [what has happened] when the [qi of the] five long-term depots are in a state of mutual confusion, can be called a practitioner."

(12)–(21) *Hua Shou:* In the fourth treatise of the *Ling shu*, the Yellow Thearch states: "Once the complexions and the [movement in the] vessels are determined, how are the [diseases] distinguished? Qi Bo: Examine whether the [movements in the] vessels are relaxed or tight, diminished or increased, smooth or rough, and the pathological changes can be determined. Huang Di: How is such an examination to be conducted? Qi Bo replied: If the [movement in the] vessels is tight, the skin in the foot-long section will be tight too. If the [movement in the] vessels is relaxed, the skin in the foot-long section will be relaxed too. If the [movement in the] vessels is diminished], the skin in the foot-long section will be diminished too. //Qi//. If the [movement in the] vessels is increased, the skin in the foot-long section will be thick and elevated too. If the [movement in the] vessels is smooth, the skin in the foot-long section will be smooth too. If the [movement in the] vessels is rough, the skin in the foot-long section will be rough too. All these changes may be subtle or extreme. The fact is: those who know how to examine [the condition of the skin in] the foot-long section, they do not take into account the [movement in the vessels at the] inch[-opening]. Those who know how to examine the [movement in the] vessels, they do not take into account [the patient's] complexion. Those who in their practice are able to consider everything together, they may be regarded as superior practitioners. A superior practitioner cures nine out of ten [patients]. Those who bring together in their practice two [of these approaches], they are mediocre practitioner. A mediocre practitioner cures seven out of ten cases. Those who rely in the practice on only one [approach], they are inferior practitioners. An inferior practitioner cures six out of ten cases."

(21) *Xu Dachun:* In the treatise "Xie qi zang fu bing xing" 邪氣藏府病形 of the *Ling* [*shu*] it is stated: "Those who know how to examine [the condition of the skin in] the foot-long section, they do not take into account the [movement in

---

12 *Yi bu san shi bu fu qi yao* 醫不三世不服其藥 has become a proverb based on several interpretations of *san shi*. Chapter 2 of the Neo-Confucian compilation *Xiao xue* 孝學 (by Zhu Xi 朱熹, 1130-1200) presents two explanations: (1) "Do not take drugs from a physician who does not carry out his occupation in [at least] the third generation," and (2) "Do not take drugs from a physician who is not well versed in the [scriptures] *Huang di zhen jiu* 黃帝鍼灸, *Shen nong ben jing* 神農本經, and *Su nü mai jue* 素女脈訣."

the vessels at the] inch[-opening], ... [For the entire length of this quote, see preceding paragraph, Hua Shou's commentary] ... cures six out of ten cases." That is very clear. This paragraph [of the *Nan jing*] here takes up that threefold [categorization of practitioners], but does so in complete disorder. Suddenly it speaks of "knows one, knows two," and if the text of the [*Nei*] *jing* did not exist today, this statement would be quite difficult to interpret! Furthermore, this response-paragraph – in its entirety – represents a text from the [*Nei*] *jing;* it does not explain anything! On the contrary, it turns the text of the [*Nei*] *jing* upside down and confuses it completely, often interrupting the stylistic sequence of the [original] text. The reader should examine the treatise "Xie qi zang fu bing xing" of the *Ling shu* for comparison. The mistaken wording [of the *Nan jing*] will become quite obvious to him.

Katō Bankei: The *Zhou li* 周禮, [in its chapter] "Tian guan"天官, says about the physicians: "Those who cure ten [patients out of ten] are superior practitioners; those who miss one out of ten are next [in standing]; those who miss two are next [in standing]; those who miss three are next [in standing]; those who miss four are inferior practitioners." Both this [*Nan jing*] paragraph and the *Ling shu* say "the superior practitioner cures nine out of ten [patients]," marking [the success rate] down by one degree. A sense of caution is obvious here. This [curing nine out of ten patients] corresponds to the rank "miss one" of the *Zhou li*. The "cures eight" corresponds to the "miss two" of the *Zhou li*. The "cures seven" of the *Ling shu* corresponds to the "miss three" of the *Zhou li*. This [*Nan jing*] treatise [skips this rank and] advances – again for educational purposes – one degree. Those [who cure] seven or eight [out of ten patients] are ranked together in the *Zhou li* as mediocre practitioners. There are no differences in the meaning [of these passages in the *Nan jing* and in the *Zhou li*]. "Those who cure six [out of ten patients] are inferior practitioners." The *Zhou li* and the *Ling shu* [as well as the *Nan jing*] all agree on this.

十四難曰：（一）脈有損至，何謂也？

（二）然：至之脈，一呼再至曰平，（三）三至曰離經，（四）四至曰奪精，（五）五至曰死，（六）六至曰命絕，（七）此死之脈。（八）何謂損？（九）一呼一至曰離經，（十）二呼一至曰奪精，（十一）三呼一至曰死，（十二）四呼一至曰命絕。（十三）此謂損之脈也。（十四）至脈從下上，損脈從上下也。（十五）損脈之為病奈何？

（十六）然：一損損於皮毛，皮聚而毛落；（十七）二損損於血脈，血脈虛少，不能榮於五藏六府也；（十八）三損損於肌肉，肌肉消瘦，飲食不為肌膚；（十九）四損損於筋，筋緩不能自收持；（二十）五損損於骨，骨痿不能起於床。（二十一）反此者，至於收病也。（二十二）從上下者，骨痿不能起於床者死；（二十三）從下上者，皮聚而毛落者死。

（二十四）治損之法奈何？

（二十五）然：損其肺者，益其氣；（二十六）損其心者，調其榮衛；（二十七）損其脾者，調其飲食，適寒溫；（二十八）損其肝者，緩其中；（二十九）損其腎者，益其精，（三十）此治損之法也。（三十一）脈有一呼再至，一吸再至；（三十二）有一呼三至，一吸三至；（三十三）有一呼四至，一吸四至；（三十四）有一呼五至，一吸五至；（三十五）有一呼六至，一吸六至；（三十六）有一呼一至，一吸一至；（三十七）有再呼一至，再吸一至；（三十八）有呼吸再至。（三十九）脈來如此，何以別知其病也？

（四十）然：脈來一呼再至，一吸再至，不大不小曰平。（四十一）一呼三至，一吸三至，為適得病，（四十二）前大後小，即頭痛目眩，（四十三）前小後大，即胸滿短氣。（四十四）一呼四至，一吸四至，病欲甚，（四十五）脈洪大者，苦煩滿，（四十六）沉細者，胸中痛，（四十七）滑者傷熱，（四十八）濇者中霧露。（四十九）一呼五至，一吸五至，其人當困，（五十）沉細夜加，（五十一）浮大晝加，（五十二）不大不小，雖困可治，其有大小者為難治。（五十三）一呼六至，一吸六至，為死脈也，（五十四）沉細夜死，（五十五）浮大晝死。（五十六）一呼一至，一吸一至，名曰損，（五十七）人雖能行，猶當著床，（五十八）所以然者，血氣皆不足故也。（五十九）再呼一至，呼吸再至，名曰無魂，（六十）無魂者當死也，（六十一）人雖能行，名曰行尸。（六十二）上部有脈，下部無脈，其人當吐，不吐者死。（六十三）上部無脈，下部有脈，雖困無能為害也。（六十四）所以然者，譬如人之有尺，樹之有根，枝葉雖枯槁，根本將自生。（六十五）脈有根本，人有元氣，故知不死。

The fourteenth difficult issue: (1) The [movement in the] vessels may be "injured" or "arriving." What does that mean?

(2) It is like this. An "arriving" [movement in the] vessel [implies the following. If during a period of] one exhalation two [movements] arrive, that is called "normal." (3) If three arrive, that is called "departure from the regular." (4) If four arrive, that is called "loss of essence." (5) If five arrive, that is called "death." (6) If six arrive, that is called "severance of fate." (7) These are the arriving¹ [movements in the] vessels.

(8) What does "injured" [movement in the] vessels mean?

(9) If one [movement] arrives [during the period of] one exhalation, that is called "departure from the regular." (10) One arrival during two exhalations is called "loss of essence." (11) One arrival during three exhalations is called "death." (12) One arrival during four exhalations is called "severance of fate." (13) These are injured [movements in the] vessels. (14) In the case of arriving [movements in the] vessels, [the disease] proceeds from the lower [long-term depots] to the upper [long-term depots]; in the case of injured [movements in the] vessels, [the disease] proceeds from the upper [long-term depots] to the lower [long-term depots].

(15) What [course of a] disease is signaled by injured [movements in the] vessels?

(16) It is like this. The first [stage of an] injured [movement in the vessels corresponds to an] injury of the skin [and of its] hair. The skin contracts and the hair falls out. (17) The second [stage of an] injured [movement in the vessels corresponds to an] injury of the blood vessels. Hence, the blood vessels have little or no contents which could circulate through the [body's] five long-term depots and six short-term repositories. (18) The third [stage of an] injured [movement in the vessels corresponds to an] injury of the flesh. The flesh grows lean; food and beverages can no longer create flesh and skin. (19) The fourth [stage of an] injured [movement in the vessels corresponds to an] injury of the muscles. The muscles relax and are unable to support one's stature. (20) The fifth [stage of an] injured [movement in the vessels corresponds to an] injury of the bones. The bones become powerless, and [one is] no longer able to rise from bed. (21) Opposite to this is the [course of a] disease [corresponding to] arriving [movements in the vessels].² (22) Thus, if [the disease, as happens in the case of an injured movement,] proceeds from the upper [long-term depots] to the lower [long-term depots, the patient will] die when the bones have become powerless so that he is unable to rise from bed. (23) If, however, [the disease] proceeds from the lower [long-term depots] to the upper [long-term depots, as happens In the case of

---

1   The text says *si mai* 死脈 ("deadly movement in the vessels"). All editions consulted, except for the *Nan jing ji zhu*, have replaced the character *si* 死 by *zhi* 至 ("arriving"). In analogy to sentence 13, such a correction seems justified, so I have adopted it in my rendering.

2   The characters *yu shou* 於收 appear to be superfluous here: see the commentaries.

an arriving movement in the vessels, the patient] will die when the skin contracts and when the hair falls out.

(24) What methods exist to treat injury?

(25) It is like this. If the injury has affected the respective [patient's] lung, supplement his qi. (26) If the injury has affected his heart, balance his guard and camp [qi]. (27) If the injury has affected his spleen, balance his food and beverages, and see to it that [his exposure to] cold and warmth is appropriate. (28) If the injury has affected his liver, relax his center. (29) If the injury has affected his kidneys, supplement his essence. (30) These are the methods to treat injury.

(31) [Consider the following situations. The movement in the] vessels arrives twice during one exhalation and twice during one inhalation; (32) it arrives three times during one exhalation and three times during one inhalation; (33) it arrives four times during one exhalation and four times during one inhalation; (34) it arrives five times during one exhalation and five times during one inhalation; (35) it arrives six times during one exhalation and six times during one inhalation. (36) Or it arrives once during one exhalation and once during one inhalation; (37) it arrives once during two exhalations and once during two inhalations; (38) or it arrives twice during exhalation and inhalation. (39) If the [movement in the] vessels comes like any of these [situations], how can the respective diseases be distinguished?

(40) It is like this. If the [movement in the] vessels comes in such a way that it arrives twice during one exhalation and twice during one inhalation, and if it is neither strong nor minor, that is called "normal." (41) Three arrivals during one exhalation and three arrivals during one inhalation indicate that one just happens to contract a disease. (42) If the [movement in the vessels is felt to be] strong in front [of the gate and] minor behind [the gate, that is accompanied by] headache and dizziness. (43) If the [movement in the vessels is felt to be] minor in front [of the gate] and strong behind [the gate, that is accompanied by a perception of] fullness in one's chest and by short breath. (44) Four arrivals during one exhalation and four arrivals during one inhalation indicate that the disease tends to become serious. (45) If the [movement in the] vessels is vast and strong, one suffers from uneasiness and has [a perception of] fullness [in his chest]. (46) If the [movement in the] vessels is deep and fine, one suffers from abdominal pain. (47) A smooth [movement indicates] harm due to heat. (48) A rough [movement indicates] mist and dew in one's center. (49) Five arrivals during one exhalation and five arrivals during one inhalation indicate that the [situation of that] person is critical. (50) If [in this case the movement in the] vessels is deep, and fine, [the seriousness of the disease] will increase during the night. (51) If it is at the surface and strong, [the seriousness of the disease] will increase during

the day. (52) If it is neither strong nor minor, [the disease] can be cured, although [the situation of the patient] is critical. [If the movement is] either strong or minor, a cure will be difficult. (52) Six arrivals during one exhalation and six arrivals during one inhalation indicate a deadly [movement in the] vessels. (53) If it is deep and fine, death will occur during the night. (54) If it is at the surface and strong, death will occur during the day. (55) One arrival during one exhalation and one arrival during one inhalation is called "injury." (56) The [afflicted] person may still be able to walk, but should stay in bed. (57) The reason for such [a condition] lies in a depletion of blood and of qi.(58) One arrival during two exhalations [and one arrival during two inhalations] or two arrivals during exhalation and inhalation are called "absence of *hun*."³(59) If one's *hun* is absent, he must die. (60) The [afflicted] person may still be able to walk, but one speaks here of a "walking corpse." (61) If [a movement in the] vessels is [perceivable] in the upper section, while no [movement in the] vessels is [perceivable] in the lower section, the respective person should vomit; if he does not vomit, he will die. (62) If no [movement in the] vessels is [perceivable] in the upper section, while [a movement in the vessels is perceivable] in the lower section, the [respective person] will not suffer any harm, although [his situation] is critical. (63) The reason for this lies in the fact that just as a person has feet, a tree has roots. Even though branches and leaves may wither, the roots can live by themselves. (64) [Similarly,] the vessels have their root, [and that is where] man has his primordial qi. Hence, one knows that [the respective patient] will not die.⁴

---

3 The term *hun* 魂 may have been used here in an ancient metaphysical sense, referring to a *hun* soul which enters the body some time after its birth and leaves it upon its death (also during unconsciousness). In the context of the medicine of systematic correspondence, this concept was modified and the *hun* was considered to be one of several spirit-qi stored in the body's long-term depots.

4 The tenth difficult issue discussed the transmission of diseases (i.e., evil qi) from one long-term depot to the next in the context of the Five Phases doctrine. As outlined there, evil qi can develop in a long-term depot and cause it itself to be ill, or they may be transmitted – in accordance with the orders of mutual generation and of mutual destruction – from child phase to mother phase, from mother to child, from inferior phase to superior phase, and from superior phase to inferior phase. Here in the fourteenth difficult issue, a different mode of transmission is introduced which is not recorded in the *Nei jing*, together with a method for diagnosing the resulting diseases. The *Nan jing* points out that diseases may descend from the lung – via the heart, spleen, and liver – to the kidneys; or they may be transmitted from the kidneys upward – via the liver, spleen, and heart – to the lung. The first of these two courses of transmission is considered to be paralleled by – and thus perceivable through – a decreasing frequency of the movement in the vessels, while the second course is supposed to be accompanied by an increasing frequency of this movement. The author(s) of this difficult issue introduced two new terms to denote these innovative concepts – namely, "injury" for the transmission downward, and "arrival" for the transmission upward. The discussion of this difficult issue by the commentators followed the usual path; some adopted the new ideas and attempted to reconcile them as

(1) *Ding Jin*: An injured [movement in the] vessels is a slow [movement in the] vessels. An arriving [movement in the] vessels is a frequent [movement in the] vessels. However, [this question] does not refer to slow or frequent [movements in the] vessels, but talks about "injury" and "arrival," because if [it had referred to] "slow" and "frequent" [movements in the] vessels, those would have been all-encompassing terms, including symptoms of depletion and symptoms of repletion, external symptoms and internal symptoms - [in other words,] including each and every [diagnostic] pattern.

Katō Bankei: *Zhi* 至 ("arriving") stands for *jin* 進 ("approaching"). *Sun* 損 ("injured") stands for *tui* 退 ("withdrawing"). When [the text here] speaks of "injured" and "arriving," that means "frequent" and "slow." The seventh difficult issue has already discussed [the terms] "frequent" and "slow." However, that discussion emphasized the differentiation of [harm due to] cold or heat in the long-term depots and short-term repositories. Here, [the *Nan jing*] calls a depletion of the yin [qi] in the [body's] lower section and an ascension of the yang-in-yin [qi] an "arriving" [movement in the vessels], and [it calls] a depletion of the yang [qi] in the upper section and a descent of the yin-in-yang [qi] an "injured" [movement in the vessels]. What is meant in both cases is that [a disease] progresses from a gradual [beginning] to extreme [seriousness].

Liao Ping: To change "slow" and "frequent" into "injured" and "arriving" is one of the greatest errors to be committed! But all the five apocryphal writings[5] have followed [the *Nan jing* in this regard]. The apocryphal chapters of the *Mai jing* 脈經 even invented [a story] that "injured" and "arriving" are the language of the Yellow Thearch and Qi Bo 岐伯.[6] This is another shamelessness. [The terms] "slow" and "frequent" of the [*Nei*] *jing* are clearly intelligible; also, they have been in use for a long time. Why should one change them? These terms have conveyed textual meanings with satisfying [clarity]; they have permitted differ-

---

best as they could with other concepts of systematic correspondence, while the conservatives ridiculed any innovation and focused their comments on contradictions with terms and concepts recorded by the *Nei jing*.

5   In Liao Ping's view, the "five apocryphal writings" include the chapter "Ping mai fa" 平脈法 of the *Shang han lun* 傷寒論 by Zhang Ji 張機 (142-220?); chapter 4 of the *Mai jing* 脈經 by Wang Xi 王熙 (218-285); chapter 28, "Ping mai" 平脈, of the *Qian jin fang* 千金方, and chapter 25, "Se mai" 色脈, of the *Qian jin yi fang* 千金翼方 – both by Sun Simiao 孫思邈 (581-682); and the *Mai jue* 脈訣, a work of uncertain authorship compiled under the name of Wang Xi. All these writings have adopted the terminology and concepts of the *Nan jing*.

6   Most of the treatises in the *Nei jing* are structured as discussions between the Yellow Thearch and his adviser Qi Bo.

entiating discussions. The two words "injured" and "arriving" do not represent opposites in their meanings. Why did [the author of the *Nan jing*] not select *yi* 益 ("well-being") to follow *sun* 損 ("injured")? Why did he use two terms that do not correspond to "slow" and "frequent"? Also, the word "arriving" by no means contrasts with the word "frequent." Even if I were to turn gold into iron[7] I would not be sufficiently equipped to illustrate [the meaning of these new terms]. One could truly call all this ignorant and incoherent work.

(2) *Lü Guang*: "Normal" refers to a normally balanced [movement in the] vessels.

Ding Deyong: "Normal" is a [movement in the] vessels without excesses.

Yu Shu: Man's exhalation and inhalation are called yin and yang. One exhalation and one inhalation are called one breathing [period]. The [*Nan*] *jing* states: "[If during a period of] one exhalation two [movements] arrive, that is called a 'normal' [movement in the] vessels." Man's exhalation and inhalation reflect the pattern of yin and yang. One breathing [period] reflects one year. During one breathing [period] the vessels' movement arrives four times. These four arrivals reflect the pattern of the four seasons. During one exhalation the [qi in the] vessels proceed by three inches, reflecting the three yang. During one inhalation the [qi in the] vessels proceed three inches, reflecting the three yin. Hence, that is called "normal."

Li Jiong: "Normal" means a [movement in the] vessels that is in normal balance, without exceeding or falling short [of its regular appearance].

(3) *Lü Guang*: The [*Nan*] *jing* states: "Two arrivals, that is called normal; three arrivals, that is called departure from the regular." It is not as the [*Nan*] *jing* states; such a person must be sick.

Yu Shu: "Regular" (*jing* 經) stands for "usual" (*chang* 常). This means that the [movement in the] vessels leaves its regular and usual place. To explain in detail, when a person exhales once, the [qi in the] vessels proceed by three inches, and when he inhales, the [qi in the] vessels proceed by three inches [too]. Exhalation and inhalation determine one breathing [period], during which the [qi in the] vessels proceed by six inches. During one day and one night, that is, during 13,500 breathing [periods], the [qi in the] vessels proceed by 810 *zhang*. That constitutes one cycle.[8] Then they continue again proceeding from the conduit at which they initially began [their movement]. Consider, now, that during one exhalation, when the [qi in the] vessels arrive three times, [these qi in] the vessels would proceed four and a half inches, and during one inhalation, with three arrivals, the

---

7   "I turn gold into iron" is a polite phrase indicating that one has made corrections in a writing of someone else.

8   Cf. the first difficult issue.

[qi in the] vessels would [again] proceed by four and a half inches. [That would mean that the qi in the] vessels would proceed by nine inches during one breathing [period]. One day and one night include 13,500 breathing [periods] during which [the qi in] the vessels would proceed by 1,215 *zhang*. That would exceed the [entire length of the] vessels by one half, and the movement could not start again from that conduit where it started from orginally. Hence, that is called "departure from the regular." Let me give an example for comparison. If a person makes daily rounds of 100 *li* 里[Chinese miles], he will [always] proceed again from the same location at which he first started. That would be called "normal." If one day he goes further [than usual and] travels 150 *li* , he would exceed [his regular distance] by 50 *li*, and he would not again proceed from the same location in the circle where he [used to] start. Hence, that is called "departure from the regular."

(4) *Lü Guang*: That a person is in a critical situation and [suffers from] a loss of essence can be diagnosed from the color at the nose, the eyes, the lips, and the mouth, where the loss of essence is perceivable.

Yu Shu: A normal [movement in the] vessels proceeds by six inches during one breathing [period]. Here now, a "loss of essence" [movement in the] vessels proceeds by one foot and six inches during one breathing [period]. Thus, in the course of the breathing [periods] of one day and one night, [the qi in] the vessels move as far as they are supposed to move within two days and two nights. [In such a case,] the vessels at the foot and inch [sections] display a frequent [movement], and the yang qi are in disorder. Furthermore, when the yang [long-term depots] have a disease, [the respective person] talks wildly and his complexion is indistinct. Mr. Lü says that [this situation can be diagnosed by] the color at the nose, the eyes, the lips, and the mouth, where the loss of essence is perceivable. That is wrong. Man consumes the five flavors. The flavors return to form. Form returns to qi. Qi return to essence. If, now, four arrivals occur during one breathing [period], that [indicates that] the yang qi are in disorder. Hence, the vessels' [movement] is frequent. When [the movement in the] vessels is frequent, the qi are diminished. When they are diminished, there is nothing that could return to essence: it is as if it had been lost. Hence, [this condition] is called "loss of essence." This is similar to a man who [usually] walks 100 *li* per day. Now if he walks 200 *li* on one day, his qi will be exhausted and, therefore, diminished.

(5) *Yu Shu*: Compared with a normal [movement in the] vessels, these are two and a half times more [arrivals per breathing period]. When four arrivals [occur during one breathing period], that already means loss of the essence. In the case of five arrivals, it is obvious that death will follow.

(6) *Lü Guang*: [The patient will] die before the next morning.

Yu Shu: In the case of five arrivals, death comes slowly; in the case of six arrivals, death will occur the same day.

(7) *Li Jiong*: The original text said: "That is the vessels' [movement of] death." Some ignoramus has changed that into "these are the arriving [movements in the] vessels," because the entire passage is concerned with arriving [movements in the] vessels.

(9) *Yu Shu*: Earlier, the "departure from the regular" [was discussed in connection with accelerated] arrivals of the [qi in the] vessels; that is to say, the [qi in the] vessels exceed their [regular] course by one half. Here the departure from the regular [is discussed in connection with] an injured [movement in the] vessels; that is to say, the [qi in the] vessels fall short of [proceeding according to] their [regular] course by one half. That is so because exhalation supports inhalation.[9]

(10) *Yu Shu*: The [qi in the] vessels of a normal person circulate 50 times through the body in the course of one day and one night. Here the [qi in the] vessels arrive once during two exhalations. That is, during one day and one night, they circulate through the body not even 13 times. The [qi in the] vessels proceed only by 202 *zhang* and five feet. The qi of a person in such a [condition] are diminished and his blood has decayed. His spirit is grieved. It is as if he had lost his fresh-looking complexion and his essential splendor.

(11) *Yu Shu*: The [movement in the] vessels of a normal person is such that six arrivals occur in the course of three exhalations; [the qi in] the vessels proceed during one day and one night by 810 *zhang*. No danger is present. Here the [qi in the] vessels arrive once during three exhalations at the vessel opening, and they proceed only one and a half inches. During one day and one night, they move only 67 *zhang* and five feet. They do not even complete five circulations of the body.[10] When such a condition appears, death can be expected.

(12) *Yu Shu*: During four exhalations, eight arrivals should occur. Here now, in the course of four exhalations, the [qi in the] vessels arrive once. In the course of one day and one night they do not even complete four circulations of the body.[11] qi and blood have been exhausted entirely; the long-term depots are ruined; the spirit has left. Thus, the fate has been severed.

(13) *Lü Guang*: "In the case of arriving [movements in the] vessels, [the disease] proceeds from the lower [long-term depots] to the upper [long-term depots]": This

---

9   This last sentence may be corrupt.

10   Qian Xizuo 錢熙祚, the editor of the *Nan jing ji zhu*, commented: "These figures are wrong. They should read: 'They move 135 *zhang*. They do not even complete nine circulations of the body'."

11   Qian Xizuo 錢熙祚: "This should read: 'They do not even complete seven circulations of the body'."

means that the movement in the vessels increases gradually. It moves up until six arrivals occur. The arrivals are many while the exhalations are few. "In the case of injured [movements in the] vessels, [the disease] proceeds from the upper [long-term depots] to the lower [long-term depots]": This means that the movement in the vessels diminishes gradually to one arrival [only during four exhalations]. The exhalations are many while the arrivals are few.

(1)–(14) *Ding Jin*: When it is stated, in the first section [of this difficult issue, that an arriving [movement in the] vessels begins with four arrivals during one breathing [period] and extends up to twelve arrivals, or that an injured [movement in the] vessels begins with two arrivals during one breathing [period] and extends up to one arrival during two breathing [periods], these are references to the leading principles of but the basic symptoms [of arriving and injured movements in the vessels]. "In the case of arriving [movements in the] vessels, [the disease] proceeds from the lower [long-term depots] to the upper [long-term depots]": [This sentence] illustrates that an arriving [movement in the] vessels starts from a depletion of the yin [qi] of the kidneys and proceeds to a depletion of the qi of the lung. An injured [movement in the] vessels starts from a depletion and cooling of the qi of the lung and proceeds to an exhaustion of the yang [qi] of the kidneys.

(14) *Liao Ping*: Here, the two words "arriving" and "injured" are employed to replace the words *shun* 順 ("in accordance with a proper course") and *ni* 逆 ("contrary to a proper course") of the [*Nei*] *jing*. The meaning of the text is not at all intelligible. This reminds one, really, of kindergarten language used to analyze the classics!

(15) *Liao Ping*: Here, the [term] *sun* is used as the *sun* in *sun shang* 損傷 ("injury"). Thus, within one difficult issue the [meaning of the] language changes three times! This doctrine certainly represents strange talk!

(16) *Yu Shu*: In a first [stage of an] injured [movement in the vessels], the lung is injured. The lung controls skin and hair. Hence, the skin contracts and the hair falls out.

Tamba Genkan: *Pi ju* 皮聚 means the skin wrinkles, dries out, and loses its glossiness.

(17) *Yu Shu*: In a second [stage of an] injured [movement in the vessels], the blood vessels are injured. Hence, one knows that the heart has got it. The heart controls the blood. Here, then, heart and blood decay, and [the latter is] no longer able to circulate through the five long-term depots and the six short-term repositories.

Tamba Genkan: The character *rong* 榮, in the sentence *bu neng rong yu wu zang liu fu* 不能榮於五藏六府 was used in ancient times with the same [meaning] as *ying* 營. That meaning is "to circulate" (*zhou yun* 周運).

(18) *Yu Shu*: In a third [stage of an] injured [movement in the vessels], the spleen is injured. The spleen takes in the five flavors. It transforms them to produce the five qi [for the] long-term depots and short-term repositories, and to make flesh and skin grow. Here now, because of the injury, the flavors are not transformed and, hence, the flesh becomes emaciated.

(19) *Yu Shu*: "The fourth [stage of an] injured [movement in the vessels corresponds to an] injury of the liver." The disease [manifests itself] as is described here. The *Su wen* states: "If there is harm to the sinews and they slacken, they appear unable to function." *Bu rong* 不容 ("unable to function") stands for *bu chi* 不持 ("unable to hold").

(20) *Yu Shu*: "The fifth [stage of an] injured [movement in the vessels corresponds to an] injury of the kidneys." The kidneys control the bones. Hence, the bones lose their strength and one is no longer able to rise from bed. The *Su wen* states: "When the kidney qi are hot, the lower back and the spine cannot be raised. The bones dry and the marrow decreases. That develops into bone limpness." *Wei* means lack of strength.

(21) *Lü Guang*: *Shou* 收 ("to contract") means *qu* 取 ("to pick up"). The [*Nan*] *jing* records [here only an example of] an injury disease; it does not record [an example of] an arrival disease. Arrival diseases are all yang [diseases, i.e.,] diseases of the six short-term repositories. In the case of diseases in the six short-term repositories, one suffers from headache and from heat in the body. Suddenly, [the short-term repositories] do not function any longer. The injury diseases are different. Here now, in contrast [to the symptoms of arrival diseases], the symptoms of injury diseases are recorded. Hence, the injured [movement in the] vessels in case one has contracted an [injury] disease is different from [the arriving movement in the vessels in case one has contracted an] arrival disease.

Hua Shou: [The sentence] *fan ci zhe zhi yu shou bing ye* should read *fan ci zhe zhi bing ye*. The two characters *yu shou* 於收 are a mistake.

Tamba Genkan: [Hua Shou in his *Nan jing*] *ben yi* was right when he pointed out that [the sentence] *zhi yu shou bing* was marred by an error. However, the *Mai jing* and the text of the [*Nan*] *jing* agree on this; hence, this mistake must be quite old already. Lü [Guang's] commentary ... is muddled.

(23) *Lü Guang*: When the injury has proceeded from the lung to the bones, [the qi of] all the five long-term depots have become depleted. Hence, one dies. The lung is the upper [depot].

Yu Shu: Up to here, all the symptoms of injury diseases have been pointed out. The first [stage of an] injury [affects] the lung; the second [stage of an] injury [affects] the heart; the third [stage of an] injury [affects] the spleen; the fourth [stage of an] injury [affects] the liver; the fifth [stage of an] injury [affects] the kidneys. This is similar to the [examination of the] vessels with light or heavy pressure – [increasing like the weight of a] number of peas – [to follow] the downward movement of an injury until it has reached the kidneys, [which was outlined in] the fifth difficult issue.

(23) *Lü Guang*: When the injury has proceeded from the kidneys to the lung, the [qi of] all five long-term depots are equally depleted. Hence, one dies. These are the symptoms of the injury diseases. These are not the symptoms of the arrival diseases. [The text] speaks of "proceeding from the lower [long-term depots] to the upper [long-term depots]," because the kidneys are located below.

(15)–(23) *Zhang Shixian*: The lung rules the skin [and its] hair; the heart rules the [movement in the] blood vessels; the spleen rules the flesh; the liver rules the muscles; the kidneys rule the bones. When the skin contracts and the hair falls out, the injury is in the lung. When the [contents of the] blood vessels are depleted or few, the injury is in the heart. When the flesh is emaciated, the injury is in the spleen. When the muscles are relaxed, the injury is in the liver. When the bones lack strength, the injury is in the kidneys. Among the five long-term depots generated in the human [body], the lung occupies the top position. Next come the heart, the spleen, the liver, and the kidneys. Hence, if [the disease] proceeds from the upper [long-term depots] to the lower [long-term depots], the lung will be affected first, while the kidneys are reached last. That is called "injury." If [the disease] proceeds from the lower [long-term depots] to the upper [long-term depots], the kidneys will be affected first; while the lung is reached last. That is called "arrival." The fifth [stage of an] injury is an extreme injury, and the fifth [stage of an] arrival constitutes an extremely [accelerated] arrival. Hence, both [stages] mean death.

(22)–(23) *Xu Dachun*: That is how to determine the time of death in the case of an arriving or injured [movement of the qi in the] vessels. [The argument is based on the following considerations.] "Injury" means a slowing down [of the movement in the vessels]. A slowing down is associated with cold. Hence, the external [long-term depots] are hit first. "Arrival" means an acceleration [of the movement in the vessels]. An acceleration is associated with heat. Hence, the internal [long-term depots] are hit first. If [heat and cold] are exchanged over a long period, reaching inner and outer [regions of the organism, respectively], then all the internal and external [long-term depots] are affected alike and there is no way of achieving a cure.

(15)–(23) *Ding Jin*: This second section [of the fourteenth difficult issue] elucidates [the concept] that the basic symptoms of an injured [movement of the qi in the] vessels start from the lung. If one fails to treat [at this stage, the injury] will be transmitted to heart, spleen, liver and kidneys. The injured [movement in the] vessels will [finally] turn into its opposite and become an arriving [movement in the] vessels. Because the kidneys are empty, scorched by the fire, [the disease] starts again from the kidneys and is transmitted to liver, spleen, heart, and lung, leading to death. Hence, [the text] states: "When this turns around, it is a disease of an arriving [movement in the] vessels."

Katō Bankei: Here an example of an injury disease is given; it applies also to diseases [corresponding to an] arriving [movement in the] vessels. In each case one should examine the sections [of the body] ruled [by the individual organs] in order to recognize which long-term depot has been affected by the disease. Now, in the case of an injury disease, a skin contraction is the beginning of the disease. A lack of strength in the bones is a sign of the apex of such a disease. Here, the apex of an injury is considered to be the beginning of an arrival disease, while the beginning of an injury disease is the apex of an arrival disease. This is not explained clearly enough in Hua [Shou's] commentary. The beginning student cannot avoid some doubts. Mr. Cao 曹 says in his poem on the [movement in the] vessels:[12] "If an injury disease exceeds the third [depot, the patient] will die. The same applies to an arriving [movement in the] vessels." One may say that he has grasped the meaning of the discussion in this difficult issue. Now, the so-called third [depot] refers to an injury of the spleen. As soon as the disease exceeds the spleen and moves down to affect the liver and the kidneys, [the patient] will die. Also, if an arrival disease exceeds the spleen and moves further upward, [the patient] will die when it reaches the heart and the lung. Hence, one realizes that the most important rule in the treatment of injury and arrival [diseases] is [to start therapy] before the spleen has been affected.

(25) *Lü Guang*: The lung controls the qi. When an injury has occurred here, one must supplement its qi by means of needles and/or drugs.

Ding Deyong: The lung controls the qi. Hence, in the case of its injury, one supplements them with needles. The supplementation should occur at the transportation [hole] of the hand major yin conduit – namely, the *da yuan* 大淵 hole.[13] With acrid flavor one can assist that which is not enough. That constitutes a "supplementation of his qi."

(26) *Lü Guang*: The heart is the origin of camp and guard [qi]. When an injury has occurred here, one must regulate it by means of needles and/or drugs.

---

12 I have not been able to identify this work.

13 See difficult issue 68, especially Li Jiong's commentary on sentence 1.

Ding Deyong: The heart controls the camp and guard [qi]. Hence, in the case of its injury, one supplements them with needles. The supplementation should occur at the "well"[hole] of the hand minor yin conduit and/or at the well [hole] of the hand ceasing yin conduit, which is [the former's] mother. The hand minor throughway and the hand medium throughway [holes][14] also constitute its mother. One assists with bitter flavor. That is a presentation of how to regulate the [patient's] camp and guard [qi].

Yu Shu: The heart controls the blood. If the blood carries sadness, grievance, pondering, and considering, it will harm the heart. Hence, an injury results. In each person the flow of the blood depends on the [movement of the] qi, and the movement of the qi depends on the [movement of the] blood. To "balance the camp and guard [qi" means that] in order to treat such [a condition successfully], one should be moderate in his sadness, grievance, pondering, and considering.

(27) *Lü Guang*: The spleen controls food and beverages. Here now, its qi are diminished and [consequently] the grains are not transformed through digestion. Hence, one must regulate [this situation] by means of balancing with the appropriate amounts of cold and warmth.

Ding Deyong: When the spleen [suffers from an] injury, one must balance the [patient's intake of] food and beverages, and one must provide the appropriate [amounts of] cold and heat. It is said that the spleen controls intellect and thought. Hence, one must bring the [patient's] intellect and thought, as well as his food and beverages, into compliance [with the requirements], and one must provide the appropriate amounts of cold and warmth.

Yu Shu: The spleen transforms water and grains to generate qi and blood. Here now, the spleen seems to have suffered an injury; food and beverages are not turned into flesh. Thus, one must balance [the situation through] moderation in drinking and eating, so as not to cause any harm to the spleen. As to the appropriate exposure to cold and warmth, Qixuan zi has stated: "In spring the food should be cool; in summer the food should be cold; in autumn the food should be warm; in winter the food should be hot." The *Ben jing* 本經[15] states: "Food and beverages, as well as exhaustion and fatigue, harm the spleen."

---

14 The hand-minor throughway hole (*shou shao chong* 手少衝) is the well hole of the hand major yin conduit, which is associated with the heart. The hand-medium throughway hole (*shou zhong chong* 手中衝) is the well hole of the hand-ceasing-yin conduit, which is associated with the heart-enclosing network. (For the concept of „well" holes see difficult issues 62 ff.)

15 Namely, the *Ben cao jing* 本草經, the earliest known Chinese materia medica compiled during the later Han dynasty.

Tamba Genkan: *Shi qi han wen*[16] 使其寒溫 refers to clothing, rising and resting. It does not repeat the meaning of food and beverages.

(28) *Lü Guang*: The liver controls the anger; its qi are tense. Hence, one uses needles and/or drugs to relax the [patient's] center.

Ding Deyong: The liver controls the anger. With sweet [flavor] one relaxes the [patient's] center. With the flavor [associated with the] earth one harmonizes the [patient's] liver. One must supplement at the confluence hole of the foot ceasing yin [conduit]. That is the *qu quan* 曲泉 hole.

Yu Shu: In the case of anger, the qi move contrary to their proper direction. Hence, the [movement in the] vessels is like a string and tense. In relying on the prescription art, one relaxes the [patient's] center. The *Su wen* states: "When the liver suffers from tensions, quickly consume sweet [items] to relax [these tensions]." It states further: "When it is suitable to eat sweet [items], non-glutinous rice, beef, dates, and *kui* 葵[17] all have sweet [flavor]." The nature of sweet [flavor] is to relax.

(29) *Lü Guang*: The kidneys control the essence. Here now, they are affected by an injury. Hence, one employs needles and/or drugs in order to supplement their essence qi.

Ding Deyong: "To supplement their essence" one uses salty flavor in order to replenish them. It is necessary to provide replenishment [with a needle] at the *fu liu* 復溜 hole of the foot minor yin-conduit. That is the mother.

Yu Shu: [The essence] is diminished because too much of it was used. This has resulted in an injury of the kidneys. It is suitable to utilize salty flavor in order to replenish the essential splendor.

(24)–(30) *Ding Jin*: The third section [of this difficult issue] elucidates all the basic methods for regulating and treating [such conditions]. It states: "If the injury has affected the respective [patient's] lung, supplement his qi." Now, an injury of the lung means an injury of the qi. These qi are the true qi of the gate of life. When the true qi are injured, the skin cracks and the hair withers. Hence, [the text] says: "The skin contracts and the hair falls out." For treatment one must supplement the [respective patient's] qi. To supplement means to replenish. When the qi are depleted, [that means] the yang [qi are] depleted. Through replenishment of the yang qi, skin and hair can be supplemented to become replete.

(42) *Yu Shu*: The disease is in the three yang [conduits].

---

16   Tamba Genkan's edition and some others have added a *qi* 其 to sentence 27.

17   Various herbal drugs carry the designation *kui;* an identification of the substance referred to here is problematic. One possible identification is "Seeds of *Malva verticillata* L.," *dong kui zi* 冬葵子 These are seeds already described in the *Ben jing* 本經 as having a sweet flavor.

(43) *Ding Deyong*: "Strong in front" means that it is strong outside of the inch [section]. "Minor behind" means that it is minor inside the inch [section]. When it is strong in front of the inch [section], one suffers from headache and dizziness. When it is strong behind the inch [section], one has a feeling of fullness in his chest, together [with a feeling of] short breath. The scripture states: "The inch section reflects the pattern of heaven. Hence, it is in control when the region from the chest upward to the head has a disease."

Yu Shu: The disease is in the three yin [conduits].

(44) *Yu Shu*: The [movement in the] vessels suffers from irregularity. The rules call that "a loss of the essence [movement in the] vessels." The [movement in the] vessels is strong. The rules call that a "turbid torrent." [The qi] arrive like a bubbling spring. The principle of the disease's tendency to become serious is obvious.

(45) *Yu Shu*: The disease is in the three yang [conduits]. When the yang [qi] are present in abundance, uneasiness and [a sensation of] fullness [result].

(46) *Yu Shu*: The disease is in the three yin [conduits]. The yin [conduits] control the internal [long-term depots]. Hence, the disease is located in the abdomen.

(47) *Yu Shu*: The [qi in the] vessels move like taking slow steps forward, flowing gently at the same time. Heat abounds among the qi. The [movement in the] vessels is smooth.

(48) *Yu Shu*: The appearance of a rough [movement in the] vessels resembles a knife cutting bamboo. Cold abounds in the blood. Hence, the [movement in the] vessels is rough.

Tamba Genkan: "Rough" [means] that the vessels are hardly passable. How can such a [movement] appear if eight arrivals occur per breathing [period]? The term "rough" in this paragraph is explained in the *Mai jing* 脈經 as "one stop and then coming again." That is an occasional knotted [movement] in an otherwise frequent [movement]. Yu [Shu's] commentary says that it resembles a knife cutting bamboo. [Such an explanation] is not satisfactory.

Liao Ping: There is absolutely no reason [to assume] that a rough [movement in the vessels] indicates harm caused by moisture.

(49) *Yu Shu*: The [movement in the] vessels arrives ten times during one breathing [period]. Qi and blood rush in great haste, and yet the [situation] is not critical. To contract [such a disease may] result in survival or death, just as is outlined below.

Xu Dachun: "Critical" means "close to death."

(50) *Yu Shu*: The yin [movement in the] vessels is fine and deep. Hence, it is evident that it increases during the night. The yang [movement in. the] vessels is at the

surface and strong. Hence, one knows that it will be even more so during the daytime.

(51) *Yu Shu*: If [the movement in the vessels] is extremely strong, yang [qi] are present in great abundance. They will, out of necessity, diminish to an extremely minor [movement]. Yin [qi] are weak, like water. Their depletion is inevitable. Hence, [the text] states: "A cure will be difficult."

Xu Dachun: "Strong" means "at the surface and strong"; "minor" means "deep and fine." If it is neither strong nor minor, [the disease] will not increase during day or night. Hence, it can be cured. If [the movement is] either strong or minor, the disease advances during day and night, and thus it will be difficult to achieve a cure.

(52) *Yu Shu*: That is three times more than normal. The yang qi are in extreme disorder. Hence, [the *Nan jing*] speaks of "death."

(53) *Yu Shu*: That is so because the [flow of the] yin qi is cut off.

Xu Dachun: Deep and fine [movements in the vessels] belong to the yin. Hence, [the disease] increases at night.

(54) *Yu Shu*: That is so because the [flow of the] yang qi is cut off.

Xu Dachun: [A movement which is] at the surface and strong belongs to the yang. Hence, [the disease] increases during the daytime.

(55) *Yu Shu*: That is the symptom of a departure from the regular [movement in the] vessels [corresponding either] to an injury or to an arrival [disease].

(56) *Katō Bankei*: The literary style of the text following [the sentence] "one arrival during one exhalation" does not fit [the preceding text]. It seems as if something is missing. Hence, one should not force an explanation on it.

(56)–(60) *Yu Shu*: If one takes a close look at this [last] frequency of arrivals, [one will notice] that it contradicts the meaning of earlier [statements]. I fear that this is due to either an error or an omission .... The *hun* 魂 belongs to the yang. The yang rules life-generation. Here now, the appearance of the [movement in the] vessels seems to indicate an injury. Hence, one knows that the yang [qi have been] cut off. When the yang [qi] are cut off, the *hun* leaves. Hence, that person will die.

Zhang Shixian: The *hun* 魂 belongs to the yang; the *po* 魄 belongs to the yin. In the case of one arrival per breathing [period], the yang [qi] are already ruined and [their movement is] cut off. If the yang [qi] are ruined, [with their movement being] cut off, the *hun* is gone while the *po* stays.[18] Hence, [the text] states: "If one's *hun* is absent, he must die." That person may still be able to walk, but this is

---

18 Zhang Shixian's understanding of *hun* may be that of a vital spirit, while he may have interpreted *po* 魄 – considered in antiquity to be a soul which appears and disappears with the body – as the material body itself.

only because some lingering qi have not yet been ruined; they keep the corpse *po* still moving. That is it. Hence, such a person is called a "walking corpse."

(58) *Xu Dachun*: "Absence of *hun*" means that the *hun* qi have already departed.

(61) *Yang*: The "upper section" is the inch opening; the "lower section" is in the foot [section].

Xu Dachun: Vomiting causes the qi to flow contrary to their proper course and to move upward. Hence, the [movement in the] vessels follows and proceeds upward, too. Then, the fact that no [movement in the] vessels is present in the lower section is caused by the vomiting. It is not so that [the qi] have really left the respective [patient's] root. If no [movement in the] vessels is present and if no vomiting [can be induced], then the [movement in the] vessels [of the lower section] is truly absent without this being caused by a reversed flow of the qi. Hence, [the text] speaks of "death."

Ding Jin: If [a movement] is present in the upper [section], and if no [movement] is present in the lower [section], that means that [a movement] is present in the inch [section] while no [movement] is present in the foot [section]. Because a repletion evil at one time blocks [the movement in the vessels], it obstructs [the flow of] the vital qi. Through vomiting, this evil can be overcome and the qi are allowed to rise. If one does not apply the [therapeutic] method of vomiting here, death will occur.

十五難曰：(一)經言春脈弦，夏脈鉤，秋脈毛，冬脈石，是王脈耶？將病脈也？

(二)然：弦、鉤、毛、石者，四時之脈也。(三)春脈弦者，肝，東方木也，萬物始生，未有枝葉。故其脈之來，濡弱而長，故曰弦。(四)夏脈鉤者，心，南方火也，萬物之所盛，垂枝布葉，皆下曲如鉤。故其脈之，來疾去遲，故曰鉤。(五)秋脈毛者，肺，西方金也，萬物之所終，草木華葉，皆秋而落，其枝獨在，若毫毛也。故其脈之來，輕虛以浮，故曰毛。(六)冬脈石者，腎，北方水也，萬物之所藏也，盛冬之時，水凝如石。故其脈之來，沉濡而滑，故曰石。(七)此四時之脈也。

(八)如有變奈何？

(九)然：春脈弦，反者為病。

(十)何謂反？

(十一)然：其氣來實強，是謂太過，病在外；(十二)氣來虛微，是謂不及，病在內。(十三)氣來厭厭聶聶，如循榆葉曰平；(十四)益實而滑，如循長竿曰病；(十五)急而勁益強，如新張弓弦曰死。(十六)春脈微弦曰平，弦多胃氣少曰病，(十七)但弦無胃氣曰死，(十八)春以胃氣為本。

(十九)夏脈鉤，反者為病。何謂反？

(二十)然：其氣來實強，是謂太過，病在外；(二十一)氣來虛微，是謂不及，病在內。(二十二)其脈來累累如環，如循琅玕曰平；(二十三)來而益數，如雞舉足者曰病；(二十四)前曲後居，如操帶鉤曰死。(二十五)夏脈微鉤曰平，(二十六)鉤多胃氣少曰病，(二十七)但鉤無胃氣曰死，夏以胃氣為本。

(二十八)秋脈微毛，反者為病。何謂反？

(二十九)然：氣來實強，是謂太過，病在外；(三十)氣來虛微，是謂不及，病在內。(三十一)其脈來藹藹如車蓋，按之益大曰平；(三十二)不上不下，如循雞羽曰病；(三十三)按之消索，如風吹毛曰死。(三十四)秋脈微毛為平，(三十五)毛多胃氣少曰病，(三十六)但毛無胃氣曰死，秋以胃氣為本。

(三十七)冬脈石，反者為病。何謂反？

(三十八)然：其氣來實強，是謂太過，病在外；(三十九)氣來虛微，是謂不及，病在內。(四十)脈來上大下兌，濡滑如雀之啄曰平；(四十一)啄啄連屬，其中微曲曰病；(四十二)來如解索，去如彈石曰死。(四十三)冬脈微石曰平，(四十四)石多胃氣少曰病，(四十五)但石無胃氣曰死，冬以胃氣為本。(四十六)胃者，水穀之海也，主稟四時。故皆以胃氣為本，(四十七)是謂四時之變病，死生之要會也。(四十八)脾者，中州也，其平和不可得見，衰乃見耳。來如雀之，如水之下漏，是脾之衰見也。

The fifteenth difficult issue: (1) In spring the [movement in the] vessels is string-like; in summer the [movement in the] vessels is hook-like; in autumn the [movement in the] vessels is hair-like; in winter the [movement in the] vessels is stone-like. Do these [movements in the] vessels [indicate the normal presence of the] governing [qi of the respective seasons], or do these [movements in the] vessels [indicate] disease?

(2) It is like this. String-like, hook-like, hair-like, and stone-like [movements in the] vessels are [those in accordance with] the four seasons. (3) In spring [the movement in] the vessels is like a string because [it corresponds to] the liver, the Eastern region, [and to the phase of] wood. [During that season] all things come to life; [trees] have no branches and leaves yet. Hence, the respective [movement in the] vessels is soft, weak, and extended. Hence, it is called "like a string." (4) In summer the [movement in the] vessels is hook-like because [it corresponds to] the heart, the Southern region, [and to the phase of] fire. [During that season] all things flourish; the branches and the leaves are spread out, and they all point downward and are curved like hooks. Hence, the [respective movement in the] vessels comes swiftly and goes slowly. Hence, it is called "hook-like." (5) In autumn [the movement in] the vessels is hair-like because [it corresponds to] the lung, the Western region, [and to the phase of] metal. [During that season] all things come to an end. All the blossoms and leaves of herbs and trees fall in autumn. Only the branches remain, resembling fine hair. Hence, [the movement in] the vessels comes light, depleted, and is at the surface. Hence, it is called "hair-like." (6) In winter [the movement in] the vessels is stone-like because [it corresponds to] the kidneys, the Northern region, [and to the phase of] water. [During that season] all things are stored. When winter is at its peak, the water congeals to resemble stones. Hence, [the movement in] the vessels comes in the depth, is soft, and smooth. Hence, it is called "stone-like." (7) These are the [movements in the] vessels [in accordance with] the four seasons.

(8) What about variations?

(9) It is like this. In spring the [normal movement in the] vessels is like a string. [A movement] contrary [to this] indicates disease.

(10) What does "contrary" mean?

(11) It is like this. If the qi come replete and vigorous, that is called "greatly excessive"; [in this case] a disease is located in the external [sections of the organism]. (12) If the qi come depleted and slight, that is called "insufficient"; [in this case] a disease is located in the internal [sections of the organism]. (13) If the qi come serene and whispering, as if they followed [the movement of] elm-leaves [in a spring

breeze], that implies a normal state. (14) [If they come] increasingly replete, as if they followed [the movement of] long canes, that implies disease. (15) [If the qi come] tense and are unyielding and increasingly vigorous, like a new bowstring, that implies death. (16) [If the movement in] the vessels in spring is slightly like a string, that implies a normal state; if it is mostly like a string, and if few qi of the stomach are present, that implies disease. (17) But if it is like a string in the absence of qi of the stomach, that implies death. (18) In spring [the organism needs] the qi of the stomach as its basis.

(19) In summer the [normal movement in the] vessels is hook-like. [A movement] contrary [to this] indicates disease. What does "contrary" mean [in this case]?

(20) It is like this. If the qi come replete and vigorous, that is called "greatly excessive"; [in this case] a disease is located in the external [sections of the organism]. (21) If the qi come depleted and slight, that is called "insufficient"; [in this case] a disease is located in the internal [sections of the organism]. (22) [If the qi in] the vessels come tied together like rings, or as if they were following [in their movement a chain of] *lang gan* stones, that implies a normal state. (23) [If they come] in increasing frequency, resembling chickens lifting their feet, that implies disease.(24) [If the movement is felt to be] curved in front [of the gate and] settled behind [the gate], like a hook holding a belt, that means death. (25) [If the movement in] the vessels in summer is slightly hook-like, that implies a normal state. (26) If it is mostly hook-like, and if few qi of the stomach are present, that implies disease. (27) But if it is hook-like in the absence of qi of the stomach, that implies death, [because in] summer [the organism needs] the qi of the stomach as its basis.

(28) In autumn the [normal movement in the] vessels is hair-like. [A movement] contrary [to this] indicates disease. What does "contrary" mean [in this case]?

(29) It is like this. If the qi come replete and vigorous, that is called "greatly excessive"; [in this case] a disease is located in the external [sections of the organism]. (30) If the qi come depleted and slight, that is called "insufficient"; [in this case] a disease is located in the internal [sections of the organism]. (31) [If the qi in] the vessels come luxuriously, resembling the canopy on a carriage, and if their strength increases under pressure, that implies a normal state. (32) [If the qi remain] neither above nor below [the gate, but flap up and down] as if they followed [the movement of] chicken wings, that implies disease. (33) If under pressure [the movement feels like] a loose rope, resembling hair blown by the wind, that implies death. (34) [If the movement in] the vessels in autumn is slightly hair-like, that implies a normal state. (35) If it is mostly hair-like, and if few qi of the stomach are present, that implies

disease.(36) But if it is hair-like in the absence of qi of the stomach, that implies death, [because in] autumn [the organism needs] the qi of the stomach as its basis.

(37) In winter the [normal movement in the] vessels is stone-like. [A movement] contrary [to this] indicates disease. What does "contrary" mean [in this case]?

(38) It is like this. If the qi come replete and vigorous, that is called "greatly excessive"; [in this case] a disease is located in the external [sections of the organism]. (39) If the qi come depleted and slight, that is called "insufficient"; [in this case] a disease is located in the internal [sections of the organism]. (40) [If the qi in] the vessels come strongly above [the gate and] sharply below [the gate], and if they are soft and smooth, resembling a bird's beak, that implies a normal state. (41) [If the movement in the vessels resembles] continuous pecking, and if it is slightly curved in between, that implies disease.(42) [If the movement in the vessels] comes like a loose rope, and if it goes like a stone ball, that implies death. (43) [If the movement in] the vessels in winter is slightly stone-like, that implies a normal state. (44) If it is mostly stone-like, and if few qi of the stomach are present, that implies disease. (45) But if it is stone-like in the absence of qi of the stomach, that implies death, [because in] winter [the organism needs] the qi of the stomach as its basis. (46) The stomach is the sea of water and grains; it is responsible for supplying [the long-term depots during all] four seasons. Hence, the qi of the stomach constitute the basis for all [the long-term depots]. (47) This is [what is] meant by variations [in the movements in the vessels] and by diseases related to the four seasons; these are the essential criteria [for recognizing a person's impending] death or survival. (48) The spleen is the central region. Its balanced and normal state cannot be recognized [through feeling the movement in the vessels. Only its] exhaustion can be recognized. [In this case, the movement in the vessels] comes like the pecking of birds, like the dripping of water. This is how one may recognize exhaustion of the spleen.[1]

---

1   In this difficult issue, the author of the *Nan jing* once again modified the meaning of certain terms and concepts of the *Nei jing* in order to introduce innovative diagnostic criteria. As the commentators pointed out, the *Neijing* treatises thus "misused" were the two *Su wen* treatises, "Ping ren qi xiang lun" 平人氣象論 and "Yu ji zhen zang lun" 玉機真藏論. Two basic concepts are presented in this difficult issue. The first is the idea of normal changes in the movement in the vessels in accordance with the changing dominant qi during the four seasons, and the idea of the diagnostic significance of aberrations from this pattern. This first concept was somewhat modified by a second, which emphasized the importance of the stomach qi as accompanying the proper qi of the respective long-term depots. A diagnostic pattern is offered, outlining guidelines for diagnosing the partial or complete absence of stomach qi and for drawing the appropriate prognostic conclusions. The entire scheme is clear and logical if regarded in its own right, but conservative commentators evaluated its contents against the contents of the *Su wen*. They obviously failed to appreciate the attempt of the *Nan jing* author(s) to replace the often

(1) *Li Jiong*: In spring the breathing[2] in the vessels resembles the string-like tightness of a bowstring or of a kite string. In summer the breathing in the vessels resembles the curved shape of a hook. In autumn the breathing in the vessels resembles the lightness and the floating of hair. In winter the breathing in the vessels resembles the [tendency to fall] deep and the weight of stones.

Xu Dachun: [The remark] "the scripture states" refers to the *Su wen* [treatises] "Ping ren qi xiang lun" 平人氣象論 and "Yu ji zhen zang lun" 玉機真藏論.

Liao Ping: This [difficult issue] discusses the appearances of the [movements in the vessels] in accordance with the four seasons. All earlier commentaries are wrong. For details, see the treatise "Si fang yi zhen" 四方異診.[3] [The term] *mai* 脈 originally referred to some extended, straight [item]. It goes without saying that the [term] "string" cannot [describe] the appearance of the [movement in the] vessels. Hence, further down [in the text] a "like" is added. When the people in later generations talked about a "string-like" [movement in the] vessels, this should be read either as "vigorous" (*qiang* 強) or as "weak" (*ruo* 弱). For details see the *Mai xue ji yao ping* 脈學輯要評 ["string-like," "hook-like," "hair-like," and "stone-like"] refer to four truly opposite [movements in the vessels. These terms] are symbolic of the four [cardinal] directions; they are not proper terms

---

incoherent and contradictory presentation of concepts in the *Nei jing* with a set of ideas designed to serve as a concise and coherent guide to practice (a function which the *Nei jing* could hardly fulfill). The correspondences alluded to in this difficult issue and by later commentators can be put into tabular form for easier reference as follows:

Phases	Seasons	Celestial stems	Long-term depots and associated conduits (internal)	Short-term repositories and associated conduits (external)	Ruled units	Seasonal vessel movement	Complexion	Mental tendency
Fire	Summer	*bing ding* 丙丁	heart hand minor yin	small intestine hand major yang	blood vessels	hook-like	red	joy/laughing
Metal	Autumn	*geng xin* 庚辛	lung hand major yin	large intestine hand yang brilliance	skin, hair	hair-like	white	grief
Soil	Late summer		spleen foot major yin	stomach foot yang brilliance				
Wood	Spring	*jia yi* 甲乙	liver foot ceasing yin	gall bladder foot minor yang	muscles	string-like	virid	anger
Water	Winter	*ren gui* 壬癸	kidneys foot minor yin	urinary bladder foot major yang	water, bones	stone-like	black	fear

2 The term *xi* 吸, ("breathing") was employed here by Li Jiong possibly in reference to the "throbbing" character of the movement in the vessels.

3 This treatise could not be identified.

[for describing the movement in the] vessels. The *Mai xue ji yao ping* contains a special section discussing this [issue] .... The character *wang* 王 ("governing") should be *ping* 平 ("normal"). The form [of the two characters] is similar, and this could be an accidental mistake. A literal reading would be wrong.

(2) *Liao Ping*: The four [terms, "string," "hook," "hair," and "stone"] use the contrasts between the curved and straight, light and heavy [nature] of the four [cardinal] directions as symbols; they do not really describe the appearance of the [movement in the] vessels. It is correct to say "a hook-like [movement in the] vessels."

(3) *Lü Guang*: In spring all things come to life; [the trees] have no branches and leaves yet. Their shape is straight like the string [of a bow]. Hence, the [movement in the] vessels is patterned accordingly.

Li Jiong: The spring is associated with the eastern region, with [the dual combination] *jia yi* 甲乙 [of the Ten Celestial Stems], with the liver, and with [the phase of] wood. The corresponding [movement in the] vessels is like a string. "Extended" describes the string[-like nature of the movement in the] vessels. "Soft, weak, and extended" describes that the [movement in the] vessels is slightly like a string. If it is slightly like a string, that indicates that stomach qi are present.

(4) *Lü Guang*: The [movement in the] vessels [associated with the] heart is patterned after the fire. It is curved like a hook. Also, if yang [qi are present in] abundance, the [movement in the] vessels comes swiftly; if the yin [qi are de-]pleted, the [movement in the] vessels goes slowly. [That is to say, the movement in] the vessels proceeds swiftly from below upward to the inch opening; it returns slowly to the foot-interior [section]. The [movement that can be felt at the] inch opening is smooth and tight. Hence, [the movement in] the vessels turns around in a curve like a hook.

Li Jiong: The summer is associated with the southern region, with [the dual combination] *bing ding* 丙丁 [of the Ten Celestial Stems], with the heart, and with [the phase of] fire. The corresponding [movement in the] vessels is hook-like. "Comes swiftly" indicates that yang [qi are present in] abundance; a swift [movement can be felt] at the inch opening. "Goes slowly" indicates that the yin [qi] are depleted; a slow [movement can be felt] at the foot-interior [section]. "Comes swiftly" describes [the idea] that the [movement in the] vessels is vast. "Comes swiftly and goes slowly" describes [the idea] that it is slightly vast. That is to say, qi of the stomach are present.

Liao Ping: When the [*Nei*] *jing* [talks about] "comes swiftly, goes slowly" or "comes slowly, goes swiftly," these are always [references to] the method of using a needle to examine the qi. By observing whether the qi arrive or do not arrive immediately upon the application of a needle, one can distinguish their slow or frequent coming and going. Beginning with this book, these terms have been employed for examinations at the inch opening. A vessel displays a movement, but how could one add [the distinction between] a "coming" and a "going" [of that movement], and furthermore, how could one add [the distinction that the one is] swift and [the other is] tardy? The text of the [*Nei*] *jing* is transformed here not just into something useless, but into a narcotic drug that harms people! ... "Swift" and "tardy" cannot be [equated with] "hook-like."

(5) *Lü Guang*: The lung floats above; its qi rule the skin [and its] hair. Hence, [the movement of these qi in] the vessels [come floating] at the surface like hair.

Li Jiong: The autumn [is associated with] the western region, [with the dual combination] *geng xin* 庚辛 [of the Ten Celestial Stems, with] the lung, and [with the phase of] metal. The corresponding [movement in the] vessels is hair-like.

Liao Ping: This interpretation [of the remaining branches as "resembling fine hair"] is forced and ridiculous .... This book often changes the character *qi* 氣 ("qi") of the [*Nei*] *jing* into *mai* 脈 ("[movement in the] vessels"), thereby transforming a method to examine the qi into [a method to] diagnose the conduits.[4] Hence, it is difficult to comprehend .... A single person's [movement in the] vessels does not change in accordance with the four seasons. But there are many who cling to such a doctrine and kill other people. This must be pointed out.[5]

(6) *Lü Guang*: The [movement in the] vessels [associated with the] kidneys is patterned after the water. Water congeals to resemble stones. Also, [the qi of the kidneys] move hidden, providing warmth to the bones and their marrow. Hence, [the movement of] their [qi in the] vessels is replete and firm, like a stone.

Li Jiong: The winter [is associated with] the northern region, [with the dual combination] *ren gui* 任癸 [of the Ten Celestial Stems, with] the kidneys, and [with the phase of] water. The corresponding [movement in the] vessels is stone-like. At the time when winter is at its peak, heaven is cold and the earth freezes, and water congeals to become like stones. "In the depth" is the proper appearance of a winter [movement in the] vessels. "In the depth, soft, and smooth" means that it is slightly in the depth. That is to say, stomach qi are present.

---

4   At times, Liao Ping appears to have interpreted the term *mai* 脈 literally – that is, as "vessel" – when its usage in the *Nan jing* in fact suggested the meaning "movement in the vessels."

5   Liao Ping stated elsewhere in his commentary on the fifteenth difficult issue that the concept of the *si shi* 四時 ("four seasons") had originated from a concept of the *si fang* 四方 ("four cardinal directions"). Hence, his remark here may express his understanding (1) that the people who live in different cardinal directions are marked by characteristic movements in their vessels, and (2) that this ancient concept was later modified to include the seasonal change of the movement in the vessels.

(1)–(7) *Ding Deyong*: "In spring the [movement in the] vessels is like a string": if it is slightly like a string, that indicates that it is normal. If it is normal, that is to say that qi of the stomach are present. The stomach is [associated with the] soil; [soil is] formed in all cardinal directions, and it supplements the space at the four sides. Hence, the string-like, hook-like, hair-like, and stone-like [movement in the] vessels that can be felt during the four seasons should always be felt as slightly [string-like, hook-like, etc.]. That would indicate that qi of the stomach are present. However, if one perceives nothing but the [movement in the] vessels [characteristic] of any of the four seasons, that always indicates that no qi of the stomach are present.

Hua Shou: This paragraph is the result of a blending – marred by mistakes – of the [two *Su wen* treatises,] "Ping ren qi xiang lun" 平人氣象論 and "Yu ji zhen zang lun" 玉機真藏論. "In spring the [movement in the] vessels is string-like" because the liver governs the muscles, and [hence the movement of its qi] reflects the image of the muscles. "In summer the [movement in the] vessels is hook-like" because the heart rules the blood vessels, and [hence, the movement of its qi] reflects the image of the coming and going of the blood vessels. "In autumn the [movement in the] vessels is hair-like" because the lung rules the skin [and its] hair. "In winter the [movement in the] vessels is stone-like" because the kidneys rule the bones. In each case the respective image is reflected. The meaning [of the terms "string-like," "hook-like," etc.] is taken from the images of both the seasons and the items.[6] As to "comes swiftly and goes slowly," Liu Lizhi 劉立之[7] has stated: "The 'comes swiftly' refers to the ascension of those qi which emerge from the section of bones and flesh and come out to the borderline of the skin. The 'goes' refers to the descending of those qi which emerge from the borderline of the skin and return to the section of bones and flesh."

(8) *Xu Dachun*: Bian 變 ("variations") is to say *shi chang* 失常; ("out of their usual order").

(9) *Li Jiong*: In spring the [movement in the] vessels should be like a string. If [the movement that is actually felt is] in contrast to a string-like [movement in the] vessels, that indicates a disease in the liver.

(10) *Ding Deyong*: "Contrary" means that [in spring one feels an] autumn [movement, i.e., a] hair-like [movement in the] vessels. That indicates a disease in the liver.

---

6 *Wu* 物 ("items") appears to refer here to the functional characteristics of the four long-term depots, as already pointed out.

7 Liu Kai 劉開, *Zi*-name Lizhi, was a Yuan dynasty author of medical works, including the *Shang han zhi ge* 傷寒直格 and the *Fang mai ju yao* 方脈舉要. The remarks quoted here may have been taken from the latter.

Liao Ping: *Fan* 反 ("contrary") should be *bing* 病 ("disease"). [The phrase] should read *wei he bing* 謂何病 ("indicates which disease?").

(11) *Lü Guang*: "Replete and vigorous" [indicates] an abundance of yang qi. The [movement associated with the foot] minor yang [vessel][8] should be weak and slight.[9] Here it has changed to be replete and vigorous. That means that it greatly exceeds [its normal level]. The yang [qi] rule the external [sections of the organism].

Ding Deyong: When a disease is located in the external [sections of the organism], that is a minor yang [problem]. The respective [movement in the] vessels [should be] slightly string-like. Here it is replete and vigorous. That indicates a surplus in the gall bladder. The face is virid, and one has a tendency to become angry. Anger is an external manifestation of the liver and [of the phase of] wood.

Li Jiong: Spring is the season when the minor yang [qi] are in charge. The respective [movement in the] vessels is slightly string-like. If this is so, stomach qi are present. Here the arrival of the qi in the vessels is replete and vigorous, indicating that it greatly exceeds [its normal level]. Repletion and vigor indicate great abundance of yang [qi]. The respective disease is located in the external [section of the organism]. External manifestations [of this disease include] an inclination to cleanse [oneself], a virid face, and a tendency to become angry.

(12) *Lü Guang*: The ceasing yin [qi] provide nourishment to the muscles; the respective [movement in the] vessels is string-like. Here it is depleted and slight. Hence, [the text] speaks of "insufficiency." The yin [qi] are situated in the center;[10] hence, the disease is located in the internal [section of the organism].

Ding Deyong: "A disease is located in the internal [section of the organism" means that the qi in] the liver are not enough. The liver harbors the blood and nourishes the muscles. If [its qi are] not enough, the muscles relax; urination and stools are difficult [to control]. These are internal manifestations of [a disease in] the liver.

(11)–(12) *Xu Dachun*: Anything "greatly excessive" is categorized as yang; [such conditions are always] displayed externally. Hence, such a disease is located in the external [sections of the organism]. Anything "insufficient" is categorized as yin; [such conditions are always] hidden inside with embarrassment. Hence, such a disease is located in the internal [sections of the organism].

---

8 The foot minor yang conduit is, in turn, associated with the gall bladder, which represents the short-term repository – or external extension – of the liver.

9 I read *wei ruo* 微弱 here as *ruo wei* 弱微.

10 *Zhong*, 中, ("center") may be a mistake here for *nei* 內 ("interior").

(13) *Lü Guang*: In spring the minor yin[11] and the ceasing yin [qi] rule jointly. Their [movement in the] vessels comes like a spring breeze blowing through elm leaves. It is soft, weak, and balanced. Hence, it is called a normal [movement in the] vessels.

(1)–(13) *Xu Dachun*: In the treatise "Ping ren qi xiang lun" 平人氣象論 of the *Su [wen]* it is stated: "The arrival of a normal liver [movement in the] vessels is soft and weak and waving, as if one were raising the tip of a long bamboo cane. That is called 'the liver is normal'." It states further: "The arrival of a normal lung [movement in the] vessels is faded, like the murmur [of trees], resembling falling elm seeds. That is called 'the lung is normal'." This [latter metaphor] is used [in the *Su wen*] to illustrate the meaning that the [movement in the] vessels [associated with the] lung resembles [the floating of] hair. Here now, [in the *Nan jing*,] it is quoted to describe a normal state of the liver. I fear that does not fit.

(14) *Lü Guang*: That is to say that it is mostly like a string, and that few qi of the stomach are present.

Ding Deyong: It is extended but not tender, thus it seems as if it followed [the movement of long] canes. That indicates disease.

(15) *Lü Guang*: That is to say that it is just like a string, and that no qi of the stomach are present.

Ding Deyong: That is to say, it is vigorous and tense, and also restricted and fine. Hence, it is called "like a new bowstring."

(16) *Li Jiong*: "Slightly string-like" means that it slightly resembles a string-like [movement). It does not mean that [the movement] is slight and like a string. When it is slightly like a string, one part stomach qi and two parts string-like qi move together, making [the movement] slightly string-like.

(17) *Li Jiong*: All three parts [of the qi moving through the] vessels are like a string and no stomach qi are present. That causes the true [qi of] the respective long-term depot to appear;[12] death is inevitable.

(18) *Ding Deyong*: The stomach is the sea of water and grains. All the five long-term depots receive qi from the grains. The stomach controls the supply of the four directions; hence, the [long-term depots depend] on the qi of the stomach as their basis.

Li Jiong: The qi of the five long-term depots are all balanced by the stomach qi. It cannot be allowed that just one single [depot] makes use [of the stomach qi]. That is like something that is extremely hard; it, too, cannot be used at one single

---

11 Minor yin may be a mistake for minor yang.

12 For the concept of the "true [qi of the] long-term depots," see difficult issue 3, sentence 17, and its commentaries.

[spot]. If it were used at one single [spot only], it would break. If the utilization is balanced and gentle, it will remain firm. The stomach is the sea of water and grains. Man receives his qi from the grains. The grains enter the stomach and are further transmitted to the five long-term depots and to the six short-term repositories. Hence, the stomach qi constitute the basis of the liver. The same applies to the remaining four long-term depots.

(19) *Ding Deyong*: That is to say, the [movement in the] vessels becomes stone-like and smooth, resembling a winter [movement in the] vessels. Hence, it is called "contrary."

Li Jiong: In summer the [movement in the] vessels should be hook-like. If [the movement actually felt] is in contrast to [a] hook-like [movement], this indicates a disease in the heart.

(20) *Lü Guang*: "Replete and vigorous" [means here that] the major yang [vessels] receive qi in abundance. The major yang [movement in the vessels] is at the surface and dispersed. Here it is replete and vigorous. Hence, it is called "greatly excessive."

Ding Deyong: An "external [location]" is the major yang [conduit with the] small intestine as its short-term repository.[13] Hence, when the disease is located in the external [section of the organism], the respective [person's] facial complexion is red and he has a tendency to laugh. That is an external manifestation of the [phase of] fire [that is associated with the] heart.

Li Jiong: The [movement in the vessels associated with the] heart is at the surface, strong, and dispersed. Here, on the contrary, it is replete and vigorous. That means that it is greatly excessive. External manifestations are a red face, a dry mouth, and an inclination to laugh.

Liao Ping: [Here the *Nan jing*] has appropriated the doctrine of investigating the [condition of the] short-term repositories at the *ren ying* 人迎.[14]

(21) *Lü Guang*: The hand minor yin [long-term depot, i.e., the heart] rules the [movement in the] blood vessels. Its qi are balanced and replete. Here, in contrast, they appear depleted and slight. Hence, [the text] speaks of "insufficiency."

Ding Deyong: The minor yin [movement of qi in the vessels associated with the] heart [is marked] in summer by abundance and prosperity. Here, in contrast, it is depleted and slight. That is [what is] meant by "insufficiency." In the case of such an insufficiency, the disease is located in the internal [section of the organism].

13　The short-term repository small intestine is the external extension of the long-term depot heart.

14　The left is categorized as yang; hence, the condition of the short-term repositories (which are categorized as external and yang) was examined, in the *Nei jing*, at the qi opening of the left hand, which is called *ren ying* 人迎. See also difficult issue 2, note 6.

One has a tendency to laugh; the respective spirit does not [fulfill its function as a] guardian.

Liao Ping: [Here the *Nan jing*] has appropriated the doctrine of investigating the [condition of the long-term depots] at the inch opening.[15] Actually, both the internal and the external [sections of the body] may be marked by depletion or repletion. One cannot base his decision about whether a depletion or a repletion is present on an internal or external [location of the disease].

(22) *Lü Guang*: The [vessels associated with the] heart are full and replete [with qi that come] tied together, [creating a feeling which is] as if someone would follow, with his fingers, [a chain of] *lang gan* stones. It is the stiffness of items such as metal bracelets made from gold or silver. All these are examples of repletion;[16] Hence, [such a condition] is called "normal."

Ding Deyong: That is to say, the vessels [associated with] the heart are supplemented and replete; [the arrival of the movement in these vessels is] tied together like a string of pearls. As to the statement "as if they were following *lang gan* stones," that refers to the image of an annular string of jade- or pearl-like items.

Xu Dachun: "Like a ring": the *Su wen* says "like pearls strung together" in order to describe the fullness and abundance of this [movement in the vessels]. *Lang gan* stones resemble pearls.

(23) *Lü Guang*: The [movement in the] vessels [associated with the] heart should only be at the surface and dispersed; it should not be frequent. [The expression] "chicken lifting their feet" is used to illustrate frequency.

(14)–(23) *Xu Dachun*: In the treatise "Ping ren qi xiang lun" 平人氣象論 of the *Su* [*wen*] it is stated: "When [a movement in the] vessels arrives [that is characteristic] of a disease in the heart, it resembles continuous panting, and is slightly curved in between. That indicates a disease in the heart." It states further: "If it is replete, abundant, and frequent, resembling chicken lifting their feet, that indicates a disease in the spleen." [The same metaphor is] quoted here [in the *Nan jing*] to indicate the [movement in the] vessels [associated with] a disease in the heart. That is another error.

(24) *Lü Guang*: "Settled behind" means that [the movement is] straight behind [the gate]; it is like the hook of a person's leather belt, namely, curved in front and straight behind. That is to say, only hook-like [qi] but no stomach qi are present.

Liao Ping: *Ju* 居 ("settled") should be read as *ju* 倨 ("haughty").

---

15 The right is categorized as yin; hence, the condition of the long-term depots (which are categorized as internal and yin) was examined, in the *Nei jing*, at the qi opening of the left hand, where this location is called inch opening.

16 The term *shi* 實 ("repletion") also evokes the image of "solid," "substantial".

(25) *Li Jiong*: In summer the [movement in the] vessels slightly resembles a hook. It is not [meant to be] slight and hook-like. Happily, stomach qi are present [if the movement is slightly hook-like]. Hence, it is called a normal [movement in the] vessels.

(28)–(29) *Lü Guang*: The [movement in the] vessels [associated] with the lung should be slightly hair-like. Here it is changed to be replete and vigorous. Hence, [the text] states "a disease is located in the external [section of the organism]."

Ding Deyong: "External [sections]" refers to the hand yang brilliance and [hand] major yin [conduits]. Hence, the external manifestations are a white facial complexion and an inclination to have a running nose. One is sad and grieved, without joy; skin and hair are dry. These are the external manifestations of the metal [phase that is associated with the] lung.

(30) *Lü Guang*: The [movement in the] vessels [associated with the] lung is light, depleted, and floats at the surface like hair. Here, under pressure, it is even more depleted and slight. This is [a situation where] no qi of the stomach are present. Hence, the disease is in the internal [sections of the organism].

Ding Deyong: "A disease is located in the internal [sections of the organism" refers to] the hand major yin [conduit] of the lung. Its internal manifestations are panting, coughing, shivering, and coughing with [fits of] cold and heat. These are the internal manifestations of the [phase of] metal [that is associated] with the lung.

(31) *Lü Guang*: "The canopy on a carriage" is the canopy of a small carriage. Light and floating, that is [what is meant by] *ai ai* 藹藹 ("luxuriously"). When the strength [of the movement] increases under pressure, qi of the stomach are present. Hence, that is called normal.

Xu Dachun: The [treatise] "Ping ren qi xiang lun" 平人氣象論 [of the *Su wen* states:] "The arrival of a normal lung [movement in the] vessels is faded, like the murmur [of trees], resembling falling elm seeds." What is called a normal lung [movement] has erroneously been considered as a normal heart [movement in the] vessels above already. The two sentences used here [to describe a normal movement associated with the lung] do not appear in the [*Nei*] *jing*.

Liao Ping: [Here the *Nan jing*] mistakenly considers the examination of the qi to be diagnosis of the conduits; it makes the *Nei jing* appear like a [Chinese transliteration of a] Sanskrit text where all the characters [if taken literally] have no meaning at all.

(32) *Lü Guang*: "As if they followed [the movement of] chicken wings" – that is to say, the qi are depleted and [their movement is] slight, and there are few stomach qi present. Hence, this is called [a state of] disease.

Li Jiong: The [qi associated with the] metal of the lung [may] seize, in summer, additional yang [positions]. Hence, the respective [movement in the] vessels would be above [the gate]. The qi [associated with the] metal of the lung belong to the yin; the [movement in the] vessels is [perceivable] below [the gate]. Here now, the [movement perceived remains] neither above nor below [the gate; the arrival of the qi] appears to follow [the movement of] chicken wings and is rough. Hence, [the text] speaks of disease.

(33) *Lü Guang*: In this case no qi of the stomach are present.

Ding Deyong: "Hair blown by the wind" implies the image of whirlingly soaring up with no fixed direction and without return. Hence, [the text] states: "Resembling hair blown by the wind, that implies death."

(34) *Li Jiong*: The [movement in the] vessels slightly resembles [the floating of] hair; it is not meant to be slight and hair-like. One part [of the qi] consists of stomach qi, two parts consist of hair-like qi. When they move jointly, that is a slightly hair-like [movement].

(36) *Li Jiong*: If all three parts [of the qi moving through the vessels] are hair-like, and if no stomach qi are present, that causes the true [qi of the respective] long-term depot to appear, [indicating imminent] death. All the five long-term depots are supplied with qi by the stomach. The stomach is the basis of the five long-term depots. The qi of the long-term depots cannot by themselves proceed to the hand major yin [conduit]; they must be guided by the stomach qi, only then can they reach the hand major yin [conduit]. If they cannot reach the hand major yin [conduit] together with the stomach qi, the true qi of the [respective] long-term depot alone will appear. If they appear alone, a disease has overcome that depot. Hence, [the text] speaks of death.

(37)–(38) *Lü Guang*: In winter the [movement in the] vessels should be deep and soft. Here it is, on the contrary, replete and vigorous. Hence, it is called "greatly excessive." Greatly excessive is a yang disease. Hence, [the text] states: "A disease is located in the external [sections of the organism]."

Ding Deyong: "Contrary" means that in winter one feels a vessel [movement characteristic] of late summer. Late summer is [associated with] soil. The [movement in the] vessels of the [qi of] the stomach, [which is associated with] soil, is relaxed and slightly curved. Hence, that is a state of disease. By "it is located in the external [sections of the organism]," the foot major yang conduit [is meant]. The face is black and one has an inclination to be fearful and to yawn. These are the external manifestations of the [phase of] water [that is associated with] the kidneys.

(39) *Lü Guang*: In winter the vessel [movement] is deep and soft. Here, in contrast, it is depleted and slight. Hence, [the text] speaks of "insufficiency." If [the move-

ment] is insufficient, that is a yin disease; it is located in the internal [sections of the organism].

Ding Deyong: That is the foot minor yin [movement in the] vessels [which is associated with the] kidneys; it controls the water and it prospers in winter. This [movement in the] vessels is deep, soft, and smooth. Here it is depleted and slight, with few qi [moving]; this is called "insufficient." The disease is located in the interior [sections of the organism]. Its internal manifestations are qi moving against their proper course, and a tense lower abdomen, as well as painful diarrhea [giving a feeling] as if something heavy were moving downward. These are the internal manifestations of the [phase of] water [that is associated with] the kidneys.

(40) *Lü Guang*: "Strong above" is [a movement associated with] the foot major yang [conduit]; "sharp below" is [a movement associated with] the foot minor yin [conduit]. If both yin and yang [qi] are felt at their proper locations, this indicates that the qi of the stomach are vigorous. Hence, [the text] calls such a [situation] normal. A bird's beak is strong at its basis and sharp at its end.

Ding Deyong: The kidney vessel [movement] is basically smooth and soft. Here now, upon examination, it responds with a strong [arrival] to the [pressure exerted by one's] hand. Upon lifting [the hand] it is minor. Hence, [the text] states: "Strong above and sharp below."

(41) *Lü Guang*: "Pecking" goes on without break; hence, [the text] calls it "continuous." "Slightly curved in between" refers to a situation where the [qi of the] spleen arrive and seize the kidneys. The [resulting movement in the] vessels is relaxed and curved. Hence, [this is a state of] disease.

(32)–(41) *Xu Dachun*: The [treatise] "Ping ren qi xiang lun" 平人氣象論 of the *Su [wen]* states: "Panting and strung together, and like a hook, and hardening under pressure, that is called: 'the kidneys are normal'." [And it states further:] "If [the movement] comes as if one pulled a creeper, and increasing in firmness under pressure, that is called 'the kidneys are [in a state of] disease'." The [image] of a crow's beak, furthermore, [refers in the same treatise] to a deadly [movement in the] vessels [associated with the] spleen, while [the phrase] "continuously pecking and slightly curved in between" [is used to describe a movement in the] vessels [indicating a] disease in the heart. I do not know how all these errors could occur.

(42) *Lü Guang*: A "loose rope" – that is to say, [the qi are] depleted and thread-like; they have no root or basis. They come slowly and they go swiftly. Hence, [the text] speaks of a "stone ball."

(46) *Li Jiong*: The diameter of the stomach is one foot and five inches; its length is two feet and six inches. It lies horizontally and is curved. It receives three pecks and five pints of water and grains. Two pecks of grains and one peck and five pints of water remain in it permanently.

(48) *Lü Guang*: The spleen prospers during [all] four seasons. Hence, [the text] does not speak of "prospering" but of a "normal and balanced" state. Its [normal movement in the] vessels cannot be recognized; only its suffering from exhaustion can be recognized. When the respective [movement in the] vessels is perceived to resemble the leaking of a [roof on a] house, the pecking of birds, or the dripping of water, then in all these cases the [qi of the] kidneys have come to seize the spleen, Hence, they cause [the spleen] to suffer from exhaustion. If the [qi of the] liver seize the spleen, that means death. The kidneys, [however, are associated with a phase that] cannot overcome the spleen, Hence, [if their qi seize the spleen] only a disease [but not death will result].

Yu Shu: "Like the dripping of water" means that the [movement in the] vessels [associated with the] spleen is greatly excessive. "Like the pecking of birds" is to say that the [movement in the] vessels [associated with the] spleen is insufficient, In case it is greatly excessive, the [respective] person will not be able to lift his four limbs; in case it is insufficient, the [respective] person's nine orifices will be impassable. Hence, a normal and balanced [state of the spleen] cannot be perceived; only its exhaustion can be perceived.

Xu Dachun: The [treatise] "Ping ren qi xiang lun" 平人氣象論" states: "The normal spleen [movement in the] vessels comes harmonious, soft and distanced, resembling the [feet of] chicken stepping on the earth." This indicates that the spleen is in normal state. Thus, a normal [movement in the] vessels [associated with the] spleen can also be perceived. Only the *Su* [*wen* treatise] "Yu ji zhen zang lun" 玉機真藏論 states: "The spleen [movement in the] is [associated with the phase] soil. It is the one single long-term depot serving to pour [its qi] to [all] four sides. .. A good [condition] cannot be seen: a bad [condition] can be seen." The statement in the [*Nan jing*] may be based on these [words].

(1)–(48) *Xu Dachun*: This difficult issue is nothing but a quotation of the two *Su wen* treatises "Ping ren qi xiang lun" 平人氣象論" and "Yu ji zhen zang lun," marred by mistakes. It not only fails to elucidate anything but also has some passages contradicting the [*Nei*] *jing*. Contrary to [the intention to explain difficult issues, this paragraph] is appropriate only for creating doubts in students of later times. I do not know how all these errors could have been brought into this [paragraph].

十六難曰：（一）脈有三部九候，（二）有陰陽，（三）有輕重，（四）有六十
首，（五）一脈變為四時，（六）離聖久遠，（七）各自是其法，何以別之？
（八）然：是其病，有內外證。
（九）其病為之奈何？
（十）然：假令得肝脈，（十一）其外證：善潔，面青，善怒；（十二）其內
證：齊左有動氣，按之牢若痛；（十三）其病：四肢滿，（十四）閉癃，溲便
難，轉筋。（十五）有是者肝也，無是者非也。（十六）假令得心脈，（十七）
其外證：面赤，口乾，喜笑；（十八）其內證：齊上有動氣，按之牢若痛；（
十九）其病：煩心，心痛，掌中熱而啘。（二十）有是者心也，無是者非
也。（二十一）假令得脾脈，（二十二）其外證：面黃，善噫，善思，善味；（
二十三）其內證：當齊有動氣，按之牢若痛；（二十四）其病：腹脹滿，食
不消，體重節痛，怠墮嗜臥，四肢不收。（二十五）有是者脾也，無是者非
也。（二十六）假令得肺脈，（二十七）其外證：面白，善嚏，悲愁不樂，欲
哭；（二十八）其內證：齊右有動氣，按之牢若痛；（二十九）其病：喘欬，
洒淅寒熱。（三十）有是者肺也，無是者非也。（三十一）假令得腎脈，（三
十二）其外證：面黑，喜恐欠；（三十三）其內證：齊下有動氣，按之牢若
痛；（三十四）其病：逆氣，少腹急痛，泄如下重，足脛寒而逆。（三十五）
有是者腎也，無是者非也。

The sixteenth difficult issue: (1) The [movement in the] vessels can be [examined at the] three sections and nine indicator [levels], (2) as well as through its yin or yang [nature]. (3) [One may, further, examine it by exerting] light or heavy [pressure, (4) or by taking into regard the] sixty informants, (5) or one single [movement in the] vessels as it varies in accordance with the four seasons. (6) The distance from the sages is long and far. (7) [Today,] everybody [selects but one of these methods and] considers his [choice] to be correct. How can one distinguish [what are correct and incorrect diagnostic techniques]?

(8) It is like this. Any verification of a disease should be based on the presence of certain internal and external evidence.

(9) What kind of [evidence] do diseases create?

(10) It is like this. Consider feeling a [movement in the] vessels [that is associated with a disease in the] liver. (11) External evidence of such [a disease includes] a tendency towards tidy appearance, a virid face, and an inclination to become angry. (12) Internal evidence of such [a disease is the presence of] moving qi to the left of the navel which, if pressed, respond with firmness and pain. (13) The disease, as perceived by the [patient], consists of four swollen limbs, (14) closure and protu-

berance-illness, difficult urination and defecation, as well as twisted muscles. (15) If this [evidence] is present, the liver is [afflicted]. If it is not present, [the liver] is not [afflicted]. (16) Consider feeling a [movement in the] vessels [that is associated with a disease in the] heart. (17) External evidence of such [a disease includes] a red face, a dry mouth, and a tendency to laugh. (18) Internal evidence of such [a disease is the presence of] moving qi above the navel which, if pressed, respond with firmness and pain. (19) The disease, as perceived by the [patient], consists of uneasiness of the heart and of pain in the heart. The center of the palms is hot, and dry vomiting occurs. (20) If this [evidence] is present, the heart is [afflicted]. If it is not present, [the heart] is not [afflicted). (21) Consider feeling a [movement in the] vessels [that is associated with a disease in the] spleen. (22) External evidence of such [a disease includes] a yellow face, a tendency to belch, a tendency to ponder, and a fondness of tasty [food]. (23) Internal evidence of such [a disease is the presence of] moving qi right at the navel which, if pressed, respond with firmness and pain. (24) The disease, as perceived by the [patient], consists of a swollen and full abdomen; his food is not digested; his body feels heavy and the joints ache. He is tired and weary, desires to lie down, and is unable to pull his four limbs together. (25) If this [evidence] is present, the spleen is [afflicted]. If it is not present, [the spleen] is not [afflicted]. (26) Consider feeling a [movement in the] vessels [that is associated with a disease in the] lung. (27) External evidence of such [a disease includes] a white face, a tendency to sneeze, grief without joy, and an inclination to cry. (28) Internal evidence of such [a disease is the presence of] moving qi to the right of the navel which, if pressed, respond with firmness and pain. (29) The disease, as perceived by the [patient], consists of panting and coughing, and of shivering from [fits of] cold and heat. (30) If this [evidence] is present, the lung is [afflicted]. If it is not present, [the lung] is not [afflicted]. (31) Consider feeling a [movement in the] vessels [that is associated with a disease in the] kidneys. (32) External evidence of such [a disease includes] a black face and a tendency to be fearful, as well as yawning. (33) Internal evidence of such [a disease is the presence of] moving qi below the navel which, if pressed, respond with firmness and pain. (34) The disease, as perceived by the [patient], consists of qi moving contrary to their proper course, tensions and pain in the lower abdomen, and diarrhea [linked with a feeling] as if something heavy was moving down, as well as [a feeling] of cold and reversed [moving qi] in the feet and shinbones. (35) If this [evidence] is present, the kidneys are [afflicted]. If this [evidence] is not present, [the kidneys] are not [afflicted].[1]

---

1   Various commentators have argued that the question voiced in sentences 1 through to 7 is unrelated to the answer given in sentences 10 through 35, and they have reached the conclusion that the text of this difficult issue is corrupt. This may be so, but one could also support a different interpretation. In the preceding difficult issues, several diagnostic

COMMENTARIES:

(1) *Lü Guang*: The "three sections" are the inch, the gate, and the foot. The "nine indicator [levels]" are the three indicator [levels] in the upper section, the three indicator [levels] in the middle section, and the three indicator [levels] in the lower section. Three times three makes nine.

Ding Deyong: The "nine indicator [levels]" refer to [the three levels] at the surface, in the center, and in the depth. That has been elucidated in the first difficult issue.

Yu Shu: The three sections reflect the pattern of the Three Powers. Just as there are heaven, earth, and man [in nature], each of the three sections also has a heaven, earth, and man, respectively. Hence, that adds up to nine indicator [levels]. The heaven [level] of the upper section is used to inquire about head and temples. The man [level] of the upper section is used to inquire about ears and eyes. The earth [level] of the upper section is used to inquire about mouth and teeth. The heaven [level] of the middle section is used to inquire about the lung. The man [level] of the middle section is to used to inquire about the heart. The earth [level] of the middle section is used to inquire about the qi in the chest. The heaven [level] of the lower section is used to inquire about the liver. The man [level] of the lower section is used to inquire about spleen and stomach. The earth [lev-

---

patterns have been outlined which, although based on the same fundamental paradigms of yinyang and of the Five Phases, cannot be reconciled entirely with each other. The quest for one general, coherent system, supposedly encompassing all acknowledged facts and concepts, has characterized Western science for centuries. Yet such an all-embracing system may be elusive to the human mind, at least for the time being. As developments in modern physics demonstrate (for instance, the renewed recognition of contemporaneous phenomena and of the singularity of certain events), man's desire for knowledge may have to be satisfied with a series of rather distinct explanatory models, often linked only by a common acknowledgment of some basic paradigms of science. Such was also the case with the knowledge in the medicine of systematic correspondence. Evidence obtained through experience and insights derived from theoretical conclusions appear to have suggested various distinct explanatory models for an understanding of diseases and their symptoms. The question raised in sentences 1 through 7 may express the concern that individuals would select one or another of these models and proclaim that their choice alone represents the truth, while neglecting or even denouncing the other models. The response to this complaint avoids a decision as to which of the diagnostic patterns mentioned is "correct," because there is no point in making such a decision. Instead, a general survey is given which considers the examination of the movement in the vessels – regardless of which pattern one relies on to determine it – as but one facet of a comprehensive assessment of the patient's state. Such a comprehensive assessment, it is pointed out, has to take into account much more than the condition of the qi in the conduits. The "holistic" schema of diagnosis actually outlined in this difficult issue appears, however, merely as a hint; the scope is pointed out, but only a few selected details are offered. For a tabular illustration of this schema see figure 7:

el] of the lower section is used to inquire about the kidneys. Hence, [the text] speaks of "three sections and nine indicator [levels]."

Liao Ping: This book has completely discarded all the ancient diagnostic methods. Even if one finds the terms [used here] in the *Nei jing*, in the [works of Zhang] Zhongjing 張仲景, and in the *Mai jing* 脈經, they should not be confused [because their meanings are different]. All the terms have been transferred [in the *Nan jing*] to the two inch [openings]. Later on the [diagnostic system developed in the *Nan jing*] was changed further and additional [terms] were ground, including *qi biao* 八表 (the "seven externals"), *ba li* 八裏 (the "eight internals"), and *jiu dao* 九道 (the "nine paths") – altogether, twenty-four terms.[2] Then, Li Binhu[3] once again took the twenty-seven vessels into regard, and father and

Phases		Wood	Fire	Soil	Metal	Water
Long-term depot		Liver	Heart	Spleen	Lung	Kidneys
Conduit		foot ceasing yin	hand mirror yin	foot major yin	hand major yin	foot minor yin
Internal Evidence	Moving qi	to the left of navel	above the navel	right at the navel	to the right of the navel	below the navel
Short-term repository		gall bladder	small intestine	stomach	large intestine	bladder
Conduit		foot minor yin	hand major yang	foot yang brilliance	hand yang brilliance	foot major yang
External Evidence	Com-plexion	virid	red	yellow	white	black
	State of mind	angry	joy (laughing)	pondering	grief	feat
	Other	tidiness	dry mouth	fondness for tasty food	sneezing, crying	yawning
Illness as perceived by the patient		swollen and stiff limbs, dripping urine, difficult stools, twisted muscels	uneasiness in the heart, heartache	swollen and full abdomen, food is not digested, body feels heavy, joints ache, tired and weary, desire to lie down, unable to pull four limbs together	panting and coughing, shivering from (fits of) cold and heat	qi moving contrary to proper course, tension and pain in the lower abdomen, diarrhea, cold and reversed (moving) qi in feet and shinbones

2   This critique is directed at the *Mai jue* 脈訣 (see difficult issue 14, note 5), which distinguished movements identified as at the surface, hollow, smooth, frequent, string-like, tight, and vast as the "seven external movements in the vessels"; slight, in the depth, relaxed, rough, slow, subdued, soft, and weak as the "eight internal movements in the vessels"; and extended, short, depleted, urgent, knotted, intermittent, firm, excited, and fine as the "nine paths' movements in the vessels."

3   Li Shizhen 李時珍 (1518-1593], *hao* Binhu 濱湖, was author of the famous materia medica *Ben cao gang mu* 本草綱目, and of works on pulse diagnosis. See difficult issue 27.

son Tamba⁴ were able to dismiss the erroneous [concept of the] "three sections" and to make use, also, of the twenty-seven vessels in their *Mai xue ji yao* 脈學輯要. It is necessary to root out everything perverted, and to strictly adhere to the diagnostic methods of antiquity. Each [term] must be returned to its [proper] location. Once this is done, a success is achieved.

(2) *Lü Guang*: The yang [movement in the] vessels appears at the inch opening for a length of nine *fen* 分 at the surface. The yin [movement in the] vessels appears in the foot section for a length of one inch in the depth.

Yu Shu: In each of the three sections there are yin and yang [aspects], respectively. The coming [movement in the vessels] is yang; the leaving [movement in the] vessels is yin. From an examination of the yang [movement], one recognizes where a disease is located. From an examination of the yin [movement], one recognizes the dates of death or survival.

(3) *Lü Guang*: The [movement in the vessels associated with the] lung [can be felt with a pressure] as heavy as three beans. That is called "light." [To check the movement in] the vessels [associated with the] kidneys, one must press down to the bones, [exerting a pressure] as heavy as fifteen beans. That is called "heavy."

Yu Shu: Whenever one feels for the yang [movement in the] vessels, one gets hold of it with a light hand. That is to say, the yang [movement in the] vessels is at the surface. The yin [movement in the] vessels is felt with a heavy hand. That is to say, the yin [movement in the] vessels is in the depth. Hence, [the text] speaks of "light and heavy."

(4) *Lü Guang*: *Shou* 首 ("informant") means *tou shou* 頭首 ("head"). The three sections originate from the head; the [movement in the] vessels has "sixty heads."⁵

Ding Deyong: The "sixty informants" were [discussed as] the tenth difficult issue. Each single [movement in the] vessels may undergo ten variations.

Yu Shu: The "sixty informants" refers to the variations which each single [movement in the] vessels may undergo during the four seasons. That is to say, in spring [the movement in the] vessels is string-like; in summer it is hook-like; in autumn it is hair-like; in winter it is stone-like. During [the season of] late summer and during the [remaining] four seasons, these dominant [movements in the] vessels relax [successively] in accordance with the retirement from rule of the [dominant qi of each of the] four seasons. Thus, each single [movement in the] vessels may undergo five variations [during the five seasons]; since there are twelve conduits, this adds up to sixty informants.

---

4   These are Tamba Genkan 丹波元胤 (alias Taki Mototane 多紀元胤) and his father, Tamba Motohiro 丹波元簡.

5   The meaning of this statement is unclear.

Ding Jin: The "sixty informants" is the title of an ancient scripture.

Liao Ping: Liu shi shou 六十首 ("sixty informants") is a mistake for *zhi qu* 直曲 ("straight and curved"). If light and heavy, straight and curved are put together, they represent the listing of the seasonal variations [of the movement in the vessels which were called, in the preceding difficult issue,] hair-like, stone-like, string-like, and hook-like.

(5) *Lü Guang:* This refers to the [examination of the] movement in the hand major yin [conduit, which is carried out] to determine [whether the condition of the qi follows] the four seasons, [whether the qi] move contrary to or in accordance with their proper course, and [whether the outcome of a disease will be] good or bad.

Ding Deyong: The fifteenth difficult issue stated correctly that the four seasons have the stomach qi as their basis. Furthermore, there are twelve conduit vessels. When the [*Nan*] *jing* states that the [movement in the] vessels varies in accordance with the four seasons, it does not [just refer to] the hand major yin [conduit].

Yu Shu: Whenever one feels the [movement in the] vessels, he begins by determining [the presence of any of] the six [possible kinds of movement in the] vessels. That is to say, [he examines whether a movement is] at the surface or in the depth, extended or short, smooth or rough. These are the three yin and the three yang [movements in the] vessels. [Each of] these six [movements in the] vessels reflects the changing [dominance of qi during the] four seasons. Hence, there are twenty-four different appearances of the [movement in the] vessels. Here now, [the text speaks of] "sixty informants." That is an all-embracing reference to the three yin and three yang [conduits] of the hands and feet, respectively, adding up to twelve vessels. [The movement in these twelve vessels] varies with "seasonal [movements in the] conduits" from string-like to hook-like to hair-like and to stone-like. This amounts, altogether, to sixty [different movements in the] vessels. Hence, [the text] states: "Each single [movement in the] vessels varies in accordance with the four seasons."

(6) *Ding Deyong:* "The distance from the sages is long and far" means that the time of Yueren was already far removed from the [time of the] sages [of antiquity].

(7) *Lü Guang:* That is to say, the three sections [reveal] a specific pattern; the nine indicator [levels reveal] a specific pattern; the yin and yang [nature of the movement in vessels reveals] a specific pattern; light and heavy [pressure reveals] a specific pattern; the sixty informants [reveal] a specific pattern. That is to say, the images revealed by these patterns are not very many, and it is difficult to

distinguish [different diseases on their basis]. Hence, they are discussed as the present difficult issue.

(1)–(7) *Xie Jinsun*: This paragraph inquires about the three sections, the nine indicator [levels], and so on – six items altogether – but the subsequent text of the [*Nan*] *jing* itself does not answer these questions at all. It appears that some portion of the text was missing here. If we look at this [issue] closely, the three sections and the nine indicator [levels] are discussed in the third section of the eighteenth difficult issue. [That section] should belong to this paragraph here; it is mistakenly abridged there. [For a discussion of] the yin and yang [nature of the movement in the vessels, see] the fourth difficult issue; [for a discussion of] light and heavy [pressure, see] the fifth difficult issue. The variations of each [movement in the] vessels according to the four seasons include the string-like [movement] in spring, the hook-like [movement] in summer, the hair-like [movement] in autumn, and the stone-like [movement] in winter, [as dealt with] in the fifteenth difficult issue. [A reference to] the sixty informants [may be found] in the [treatise] "Fang sheng shuai" 方盛衰 of the *Nei jing* [*Su wen*], where it is stated: "The path followed by the sages in conducting an examination by feeling [the movement in the vessels] with their fingers consisted in investigating the sequence and the yin and yang [nature of the movement in the vessels]. Strange and regular circumstances [were examined by checking the] sixty informants." Wang [Bing] 王冰[6] said in his comment: "[Knowledge about these] strange and regular [circumstances as well as about the] sixty informants no longer exists these days." Thus, these traditions have been lost for a long time.

Zhang Shixian: That many diagnostic methods exist! Yueren himself has stated that his time was removed from that of the sages of high antiquity Xian [Yuan] and Qi [Bo] by many years. After him, through the ages, scores of renowned physicians came forward, each of them clinging to his own experience and establishing it as a perfect [diagnostic] method. They were separated from the sages by an even longer time and they had lost the truth of the [ancients] to an even greater degree. Finally, how should one distinguish who was right and who was wrong? Alas! Obviously, there are a number of different diagnostic methods, and they appear to enable one to examine the evidence created by the diseases with regard to the presence of this disease or that ailment. And if one also gets hold of a specific [movement in the] vessels, it may even be that one is not far [from the truth].

---

6   Wang Bing 王冰 (eighth century) compiled an amended version of the *Su wen* by adding text and comments.

Ding Jin: Here Yueren says that a long time has already elapsed since Xian [Yuan] and Qi [Bo] in antiquity, and that all the physicians [who lived in the meantime] have clung to their own experience. Each of them established his own perfect method, but how could one distinguish which one is right and which one is wrong? From "the three sections" down to "varies in accordance with the four seasons," these are all those individually established methods. [The text] says that it is not necessary to decide who was right and who was wrong; rather, one should rely on the internal and external evidence of diseases as elucidated in the text further down, in order to distinguish what is present or absent in the [movement of the] vessels. These are instructions by Xian [Yuan] and Qi [Bo] that can be trusted word by word!

(8) *Lü Guang*: The images revealed by the patterns [of the movement in the vessels] are not very many; some of them change to account for [the course of the] four seasons. It is difficult to distinguish [different diseases influencing these patterns]. Hence, one distinguishes the diseases according to their location in the internal or external [sections of the organism].

Ding Deyong: The character *shi* 是 ("verification") should be *shi* 視 ("observation"), as in *shi wu* 視物 ("observation of things"). The first segment of this text refers to the method of [examining] a disease by observation; that is different from the method of examination [by feeling the movement in the vessels]. Hence, [the text] speaks of "distinguishing" [these different methods].

Yu Shu: One long-term depot and one short-term repository constitute one external and one internal [section, respectively]. The diseases of the short-term repositories dominate in the external [sections]; hence, external evidence appears. The diseases of the long-term depots dominate in the internal [sections]; hence, internal evidence appears.

Xu Dachun: Whenever a person receives harm, that represents a disease. These diseases are diagnosed by means of the evidence [which they generate]. Now, [various] diseases may appear together, but the respective evidence [they produce] remains separated.

(10) *Yu Shu*: [A movement in] the vessels associated with the liver is like a string, tender, and extended.

(11) *Lü Guang*: The short-term repository is the indicator of "external evidence." [In this case] it is the gall bladder, which is the short-term repository of tidiness. Hence, the face is virid and one has a tendency toward a tidy appearance. When his clothes are worn-out, or if food and beverages are unclean, the respective person will easily become angry. The color of the gall bladder is virid. Hence, the [complexion of the] face is virid.

Yu Shu: The gall bladder, [associated with the] foot minor yang [conduit], is a short-term repository. Hence, if it has a disease, that will become apparent externally. The gall bladder is the short-term repository of tidiness. Hence, one has a tendency towards a tidy appearance. Its external domination [in the case of a disease] becomes apparent in a virid face. Also, the gall bladder is the officer [whose duty it is to maintain the golden] mean and to enforce what is proper. It is responsible for decisions and judgments. Hence, [it is associated with] an inclination to become angry.

Hua Shou: The liver is the general among the officials; hence, it has a tendency to become angry.

(12) *Lü Guang*: The "internal evidence" is the evidence provided by the liver [itself]. The liver is [associated with] the Eastern region; it represents the virid dragon.[7] It is located on the left side. Hence, [internal] evidence of [a disease in] the liver appears to the left of the navel.

Yu Shu: This is an indication of one of the "five accumulations" (*wu ji* 五積).[8] The specific accumulation [associated with] the liver is called *fei qi* 肥氣 ("fat qi").

Zhang Shixian: The liver rules in the left side. Hence, its moving qi appear to the left of the navel.

(13) *Yu Shu*: The liver is [associated with the phase of] wood; the spleen is [associated with] soil. The spleen controls the four limbs. When the wood is affected by a disease, the soil has nothing to fear. Hence, the four limbs turn stiff and are swollen.

(14) *Yu Shu*: "Dripping urine" indicates that the "small short-term repository" [i.e., the urinary bladder] is rough. "Difficult stools" [indicates that] difficulties exist in the outflow from the "large short-term repository" [i.e., the large intestine]. That is to say, the liver vessel follows the genital organs. Hence, [in the case of a liver disease] dripping urine results. Liver and kidneys control the lower section [of the organism]. When the liver is ill, the qi move contrary to their proper course and fail to descend downward. Hence, the stools are difficult [to pass]. The liver belongs to the wood, which means being curved and straight. This image is reflected by the muscles. Here, the liver has a disease. Hence, the muscles are twisted.

Zhang Shixian: "Twisted muscles" means that the muscles are tense.

(16) *Yu Shu*: The [movement in the] vessels associated with the heart is at the surface, strong and dispersed.

---

7   The virid dragon, the white tiger, the scarlet bird, and the black warrior are four celestial spirits supposed to rule the eastern, western, southern, and northern regions, respectively.

8   See difficult issue 56.

(17) *Ding Deyong*: The "external evidence" [appears in] the hand major yang vessel [because this] is an external conduit. Hence, when it has a disease, that will become apparent externally. It corresponds to the fire. Hence, in the case of a disease there will be external heat, a dry mouth, and a tendency to laugh. These [phenomena] constitute its external evidence.

Lü Guang: As "external evidence," the hand major yang vessel of the small intestine creates heat. Hence, it causes the mouth to be dry. Yang [qi] are responsible for dryness. Hence, one has a tendency to laugh.

Yu Shu: The heart belongs to the fire. The nature of the fire is to flame up. Hence, the face is red and the mouth is dry. The heart represents itself in the pitches as laughing.

Xu Dachun: The qi of the heart pass through the tongue. When the fire [of the heart] sends its flame up, [the mouth will be] dry.

(18) *Lü Guang*: The "internal evidence" is [provided by] the heart [itself]. The heart is located in the front; [it represents the] scarlet bird. Hence, [internal] evidence [of a disease in the heart] appears above the navel.

Yu Shu: The specific accumulation [of qi associated with] the heart is called *fu liang* 伏梁 ("hidden beam"). It occurs above the navel. Fire generates heat.

Zhang Shixian: The position of the heart is in the upper [section of the body]; hence, its moving qi appear above the navel.

(19) *Yu Shu*: The heart is the lord of the five long-term depots. If any of the [remaining] four long-term depots has a disease, the heart as their master knows about it and develops pain. That is all the more so when its own conduit has a disease. When the [heart] is marked by constant pain, the heart enclosing [network] vessel is [affected]; the heart itself does not contract a disease. If it were to contract a disease in the morning, one could predict death for the coming night, or at night one could predict death for the coming day. That should make it doubly clear that if [the heart] contracts a disease, the heart enclosing [network is affected in reality]. The hand ceasing yin vessels originate from the end of the middle finger of both hands. They do not enter the center of the palms. One can get hold of these [vessels in the bend of] a curved third finger. The name of the hole there is *lao gong* 勞宮 hole. When the heart enclosing [network] is ill, the center of the palms is hot and dry vomiting occurs.

Zhang Shixian: "Dry vomiting" is [a vomiting] that creates sounds but does not [throw up] substance.

(21) *Yu Shu*: The [movement in the] vessels [associated with the] spleen is in the center, relaxed, and strong.

(22) *Lü Guang*: "External evidence" is the evidence provided by the foot yang brilliance vessel of the stomach. When the stomach is replete with qi, the qi of the grains will be digested. [A person can] ponder about many [things] and has the desire to consume beverages and food. When [someone's] stomach qi are depleted, his food will remain undigested. The strength [provided to that person by the] qi will be depleted [before long] and he will become thin. This person will then be affected by his own pondering and planning.

Ding Deyong: Its "external evidence includes a yellow face" [because] the [foot] yang brilliance [vessel] is the conduit of the stomach. Hence, when a yellow complexion appears, this is external evidence.

Yu Shu: The spleen is [associated with] the soil; when it moves, it causes belching. The mental attitude [associated with the] spleen is to ponder. The spleen is responsible for sweetness; [it rules] the intake of the [different] flavors. Hence, [the text speaks of] "a fondness for tasty [food]."

Zhang Shixian: Belching results when the qi of the spleen fail to move along their proper course. The *Ling shu* states: "When cold qi lodge in the stomach, they will move contrary to their proper direction, move upward, and disperse from there, leaving the stomach repeatedly. That leads to belching." The statement here [in the *Nan jing*] does not agree with the discourse on spleen and stomach in the *Ling shu*. Now, the stomach is the short-term repository of the spleen, and for that reason they were discussed here as one entity.

Xu Dachun: In the [treatise] "Kou wen" 口問 of the *Ling* [*shu*] it is stated: "When cold qi lodge in the stomach, they move contrary to their proper direction. They ascend from below and disperse, leaving the stomach repeatedly. That leads to belching." Spleen and stomach are united. Hence, their diseases are identical.

(23) *Yu Shu*: The specific accumulation [associated with the] spleen is called *pi qi* 痞氣 ("blocked qi"). It occurs exactly in the navel.

(24) *Lü Guang*: "Internal evidence" is provided by the spleen [itself]. The spleen is located in the center. Hence, [internal] evidence [of its disease] appears exactly in the navel. Furthermore, the navel lies in the center between the yin and yang [sections of the organism]. Hence, the [movement in the] vessels [that can be felt there] is associated with the spleen.

Ding Deyong: The "internal evidence" is manifested in the foot major yin [conduit associated with the] spleen. "Moving qi right at the navel" become apparent [at that location] because the spleen controls the central region. "The disease, as perceived by the [patient], consists of a [swollen and] full abdomen; his food is not digested; his body feels heavy and the joints ache. He is tired and weary and desires to lie down, and is unable to pull his four limbs together," – all that refers to [the phase of] soil. The soil is quiet; hence, such evidence occurs. Earlier, I have commented on the yellow face as an external evidence, but I did not explain the remaining [phenomena], including what was called a "tendency to belch" and a "fondness for tasty [food]." These are [indeed associated with] the spleen. Here, a swollen and full abdomen and a lack of digestion of food [are named as symptoms of a disease in the spleen, while they are, in fact, associated with] the stomach. The stomach is the sea of water and grains. When it is affected by a disease, the food is not digested. The body [feels] heavy, and the joints ache. One is tired and weary and desires to lie down. One is unable to pull his four limbs together. All these [phenomena] appear as external evidence. Here they are mentioned as internal evidence. The statements made here by the [*Nan*] *jing* are extremely unclear. I do not dare to fully explain them. I would rather wait for some sage in future time [to do this].

Yu Shu: A dominance of humid qi causes swelling in man. The yang qi are located in the lower [section of the organism; a condition which is irregular]. As a consequence, the food remains undigested, and it comes to dominate the internal [sections]. The [resulting] disease [manifests itself] as is described here. The spleen belongs to the [phase of] soil. The nature of soil is to be quiet and motionless. Hence, it is obvious that if the soil assumes control over the four limbs, the disease [as perceived by the patient will consist of his] inability to pull his four limbs together.

Zhang Shixian: When the spleen is sick, it cannot function. Hence, the abdomen will be swollen and full, and water and grains cannot be digested.

Xu Dachun: In the [treatise] "Jin kui zhen yan lun" 金匱眞言論 of the *Su* [*wen*] it is stated: "The abdomen is yin. The extreme yin in the yin is the spleen." Hence, the diseases [of the spleen] appear in the abdomen. The spleen is responsible for the grinding of food.

(26) *Yu Shu*: The [movement in the] vessels [associated with the] lung is at the surface, short, and rough.

(27) *Lü Guang*: "External evidence" is [provided by] the vessel of the large intestine – namely, the hand yang brilliance vessel – which is the short-term repository of the lung. The qi [of the lung] pass through the nose. Hence, [in the case of a disease one has] a tendency to sneeze. The lung [qi] rule in autumn. *Qiu* 秋 ("autumn") stands for *chou* 愁 ("grief"). Hence, [a person with such a] disease [displays] grief and [has a tendency to] cry.

Ding Deyong: The "external evidence" appears in the hand yang brilliance conduit [because] the large intestine is the short-term repository of the lung. Hence, [anybody with a disease here] has a tendency to sneeze. "Grief without joy, and an inclination to cry" are its external evidence.

Yu Shu: If the face is white, that is the color of metal. The lung rules the skin [and its] hair. If skin and hair are affected by cold from outside, they relate this [cold] internally to the lung. Hence, one sneezes. Grief is the state of mind [associated with the] lung. The spleen is soil; the lung is metal. The spleen is the mother of the lung. The spleen is responsible for singing. When a child is sick, a mother is sad. Hence, there is no joy. The resulting sound is crying.

(28) *Lü Guang*: "Internal evidence" is evidence [provided by] the lung. The lung rules the skin [and its] hair. When [the lung is affected by] cold, shivering, coughing, and sneezing develop. The lung is located in the Western region. This is [the region of] the white tiger. It rules the right side. Hence, the evidence appears to the right of the navel.

Ding Deyong: This "internal evidence" discussed here [is provided by] the hand major yin conduit, which corresponds to the Western region. Metal is [associated with the diagram] *dui* 兌. Hence, [the text] states: "Moving qi are present to the right of the navel."

Yu Shu: The specific accumulation [of qi associated with the] lung is called *xi ben* 息賁 ("hasty breath"). It occurs on the right side, below the ribs.

Zhang Shixian: The lung rules in the right [side of the body]. Hence, its moving qi appear to the right of the navel.

(29) *Ding Deyong*: The "panting and coughing, as well as the shivering from [fits of] cold and heat" represent, obviously, internal evidence.

Yu Shu: The lung rules the skin [and its] hair. Here now, cold qi have affected skin and hair from outside and have been related to the lung internally. As a consequence, the paths of the [breathing] qi become uneven. Hence, panting and coughing result. The lung controls the qi; external indicators [of its condition] are the skin [and its] hair. When the lung [suffers from] a depletion [of qi], one shivers from cold. When the lung is replete, one feels hot and perceives a pressure in his chest. Hence, [the text] speaks of "cold and heat."

(31) *Yu Shu*: The [movement in the] vessels [associated with the] kidneys is in the depth, soft, and smooth.

(32) *Ding Deyong*: The "external evidence" appears in the [foot] major yang conduit of the urinary bladder [because] this is an external conduit. Hence, In the case of a disease here, black color [develops]. The face will be black; one has a tendency to be fearful and to yawn.

Yu Shu: The color black is the color of the kidneys. The [associated] state of mind is called "fearful." When the [foot] major yang [conduit] is depleted, one must yawn.

(33) *Lü Guang*: The "internal evidence" appears below the navel [because] the [qi of the] kidneys dominate in winter. They rule the Northern region [where] the "black warrior" [resides].

Ding Deyong: The "internal evidence" appears below the navel [because the qi of] the kidneys dominate in winter. They correspond to the Northern region.

Yu Shu: The specific accumulation [associated with the] kidneys is called *ben tun* 賁豚 ("running piglet"). It occurs below the navel. Hence, [the text] says "below the navel."

Zhang Shixian: The kidneys are located in the lower [section of the body]; hence, their moving qi appear below the navel.

(34) *Ding Deyong*: "The disease [as perceived by the patient] consists of qi moving contrary to their proper course, tensions and pain in the lower abdomen, and a diarrhea [accompanied by a feeling] as if something heavy was moving down" – this kind of diarrhea is called *da jia* 大瘕. It is a diarrhea with internal tensions and a [perception of] heaviness at the behind.

Yu Shu: When the kidneys have not enough qi, the throughway vessel is injured. Hence, the qi move contrary to their proper course. The kidneys are [associated with the] foot minor yin vessel, which follows the lower abdomen and meets there – as one of three yin [vessels] – with the foot ceasing yin and foot major yin [vessels]. Here, [the kidneys are] affected by a disease. Hence, the lower abdomen suffers from tensions and pain. As for indicators of the five kinds of diarrhea, the kidneys are [associated with] a [kind of] diarrhea [that goes along with a feeling of] heaviness at the behind. The kidneys constitute the gate of the stomach. Here, they [suffer from a] depletion of qi. Hence, diarrhea results. That is to say, as soon as one has finished eating, one perceives an urgent drive to go to the latrine .... Five inches above the inner ankle of the feet is the [location where the] movement in the foot minor yin vessel [can be felt]. Hence, when the feet and the shinbones are cold, the qi move contrary to their proper course. [In the treatise] "Tong ping xu shi lun" 通評虛實論 [of the *Su wen*] it is stated: "When the qi move contrary to their proper course, the feet are cold."

Zhang Shixian: The [flow of the] vital qi has its origin in the kidneys. When the latter have a disease, the ways of the qi are blocked and the urine moves upward. Hence, [the text speaks of] "qi moving contrary to their proper course." The kidneys are located near the lower abdomen. Hence, tensions and pain occur in the lower abdomen.

(1)–(35) *Yu Shu*: The [*Nan*] *jing* states: "Any verification of a disease should be based on the presence of certain internal and external evidence." If we follow [the evidence as outlined in this difficult issue] thus far, the external evidence of [a disease in] the vessels [associated with the] liver is [defined as] a "tendency toward a tidy appearance." But these words refer to evidence gained from looking at a patient's external appearance. No external evidence is outlined that might be offered by the hand major yang [conduit in the case of a disease in the] vessels [associated with] the heart. In the [discussion of diseases in the] vessels [associated with] the spleen, a "tendency to belch" is mentioned. This is, indeed, external evidence. For [diseases in] the vessels [associated with] the lung, no evidence that might be offered by the hand yang brilliance [vessel] is mentioned. In the [discussion of diseases in the] vessels [associated with] the kidneys, only the one word "yawning" is mentioned. This is evidence of insufficient [qi] in the foot major yang [conduit]. With regard to all five long-term depots, one may conclude that the *Huang Di Su wen*, together with [the *Nan jing*], discusses [genuine external] evidence only for those long-term depots [that are associated with] foot [conduits]. When Yueren referred to "external evidence," he drew on [phenomena that can be] observed in the external appearance of a [person]. The commentaries by Mr. Lü often fail to reflect the message of the [*Nan*] *jing*.

Katō Bankei: The "internal" and "external" evidence discussed in this paragraph does not refer to symptoms of diseases as they might appear outside or inside [of the body]. What is discussed here is an internal or external diagnosis of [disease] indicators. What does that mean? How could a "virid face," a "tendency toward a tidy appearance," and a "tendency to become angry" simply represent external evidence? And how could "fullness and swelling in the four limbs," "protuberance-illness and difficult stools," as well as "twisted muscles" simply represent internal evidence? [The same] applies to the remaining [phenomena mentioned above]. Now, the so-called external evidence is that which is obtained by a physician when he sits to the side of a patient to observe [his condition] and listen [to his voice]. Internal evidence is [obtained by the physician] through personally [soliciting information by asking or by] touching [the patient. This is done by] pressing his abdomen and by feeling the [movement in the] vessels – [techniques] which are called *wen* 問 ("asking") and *qie* 切 ("cutting") [into the movement in the vessels]. To be more explicit, for the liver a virid face and a tendency toward a tidy appearance are named. For the heart a red face and a dry mouth are named. For the spleen a yellow face, a tendency to ponder, and a fondness for tasty [food] are named. For the lung a white face and grief without joy are named. For the kidneys a black face and a tendency to be fearful are named. This [evidence can be obtained] through observation. For the liver a tendency to become angry is named. For the heart a tendency to laugh is named. For the spleen a tendency to belch is named. For the lung a tendency to sneeze is named. For the kidneys a tendency to yawn is named. This [evidence can be obtained] through listening [to the patient]. For the liver fullness and swelling of the four limbs is named. For the heart uneasiness in the heart and pain in the heart are named. For the spleen a swollen and full abdomen is named. For the lung panting and coughing as well as [perceptions of] cold and heat are named. For the kidneys qi moving contrary to their proper course as well as tensions and pain in the lower abdomen are named. This [evidence is obtained] by asking [the patient]. For the liver moving qi to the left of the navel are named. For the heart [moving qi] above the navel are named. For the spleen [moving qi at] the navel itself are named. For the lung [moving qi to] the right of the navel are named. For the kidneys [moving qi] below the navel are named. This [evidence can be obtained] through cutting [with one's fingers into the movement in the vessels]. The meaning of *wang* 望 ("observation"), *wen* 聞 ("listening/smelling"), *wen* 問 ("asking"), and *qie* 切 ("cutting") is elucidated, in detail, in the sixty-first difficult issue. However, the discussion there focuses on an explanation of the meaning [of these approaches] for the physician. Here, the actual confrontation with the patient [is emphasized] in order to substantiate the practical [application of these approaches]. If one looks at it from this point, what is called *zheng* 證 ("evidence") here is the *zheng* of *zheng ju* 證據 ("proof", "to prove"); it is not the *zheng* 證 of *bing zheng* 病證 ("signs of disease"). That should be clear now.

THE SEVENTEENTH DIFFICULT ISSUE

十七難曰：（一）經言病或有死，或有不治自愈，或連年月不已。其死生存
亡，可切脈而知之耶？
（二）然：可盡知也。診病若閉目不欲見人者，脈當得肝脈強急而
長，（三）而反得肺脈浮短而濇者，死也。（四）病若開目而渴，心下牢者，
脈當得緊實而數，反得沉濡而微者，死也。（五）病若吐血，復鼽衄血者，
脈當沉細，而反浮大而牢者，死也。（六）病若譫言妄語，身當有熱，脈當
洪大，而手足厥逆，脈沉細而微者，死也。（七）病若大腹而洩者，脈當微
細而濇，反緊大而滑者，死也。

The seventeenth difficult issue: (1) The scripture states: In the case of a disease one
may die, or a cure will occur by itself without any treatment, or [the disease] will
continue for years and months without remission. Is it possible, by feeling¹ the
[movement in the] vessels, to know whether the respective [person] will die or
survive, will continue to exist or will perish?

(2) It is like this. This can be known entirely. If one examines a patient who keeps his
eyes closed and does not wish to look at anybody, one should feel a liver [movement
in his] vessels that is vigorous, tense, and extended. (3) If one feels, in contrast to
this, a lung [movement in the] vessels, which is short, rough, and at the surface, that
[signals] death. (4) If the patient has his eyes open and is thirsty, and if there is a
firm [area] below his heart, the [movement in the] vessels should be tight, replete,
and frequent. If it is, in contrast, in the depth, rough, and slight, that [signals] death.
(5) If the patient spits blood, and [if he suffers] repeatedly from a stuffy nose and
nosebleed, the [movement in the] vessels should be deep and fine. If it is, in contrast,
at the surface, strong, and firm, that is [a sign of] death. (6) If the patient speaks
incoherently and utters nonsense, his body should be hot, and the [movement in
the] vessels should be vast and strong. If, in contrast, hands and feet are marked by
reversed [moving qi], and if the [movement in the] vessels is deep, fine, and slight,
that is [a sign of] death. (7) If the patient has a large abdomen and [suffers from]
diarrhea, the [movement in the] vessels should be slight, fine, and rough. If it is, in
contrast, tight, strong, and smooth, that is [a sign of] death.²

---

1   The term 切 alludes to the image of "cutting" into the vessels with the tip of one's fingers.
In Katō Bankei's commentary to difficult issue 16 (sentences 1 through 35), I have translated qie in this literal meaning. In the text of the Nan jing, however, I render qie as "to
feel [the movement in the vessels]" to avoid misinterpretations that might be evoked by
a literal translation.

2   Various commentators have expressed the opinion that the text of this difficult issue is
corrupt. This may be indeed the case because the structure of the response in sentences 2
through 7 is unusually unsystematic. Sentences 4 and 6 are both devoted to the appear-

(1) *Hua Shou*: In this paragraph three questions are raised, and the [initial] response indicates that [the answers to them] "can be known entirely." However, the response is then limited to [an outline of] the symptoms of [imminent] death; [answers to] the remaining [points at issue] do not appear. Something must be missing here.

 Xu Dachun: This is another erroneous quotation of a statement from the [*Nei*] *jing*. The [*Nei*] *jing* does not contain such a passage in full.

 Ding Jin: Here [the text] says "one may die." This [issue is dealt with] below [on the basis of the movement in] the vessels [indicating] mutual destruction. [The statement] "or a cure will occur by itself without any treatment" refers to the thirteenth difficult issue [where this topic is discussed on the basis of movements in] the vessels [indicating] mutual generation. [The final statement] "or it will continue for years and months without remission" refers to the fifty-fifth difficult issue [where it is discussed on the basis of] the mutual correspondence between accumulations and diseases. Hence, [the text here] says: "This can be known entirely."

 Ye Lin: This [paragraph] quotes statements from the *Su wen* [treatises], "Mai yao jing wei lun" 脈要精微論 and "Ping ren qi xiang lun" 平人氣象論, mistakenly confusing them in its discussion here. The [*Nei*] *jing* does not contain such a passage in full.

 Katō Bankei: This does not appear in the *Nei jing*.

 Liao Ping: The [*Nei*] *jing* says: "Live or die." That is all. This difficult issue adds a useless repetition.

(2) *Ding Deyong*: These are symptoms of a disease in the liver. Hence, the [movement in the] vessels [to be expected] is vigorous, tense, and extended.

 Yang: "Vigorous and tense" is the same as "like a string and tense."[3]

 Hua Shou: The orifices kept open by the liver are the eyes. If someone has his eyes closed and does not wish to look at anybody, he has a disease in his liver. In the case of a disease in the liver, a lung [movement in the] vessels appears because metal subdues wood.

---

ance of kidney symptoms in case of a disease in the heart; a disease in the kidneys is not mentioned at all. Some authors have assumed that the question in sentence 1 raises three issues, while the answer responds to only one of them. I do not agree with this argument because, in my opinion, the question begins – after a general introductory statement – with *qi si sheng* 其死生. The fragmentary character of this difficult issue has lead Katō Bankei to believe that sentences 12 through 19 of difficult issue 18 actually belong to this difficult issue. In his edition of the *Nan jing* he has, therefore, moved them here to follow sentence 7.

3 Yang may have implied here that *qiang* 強 ("vigorous") is a mistake for *xian* 弦 ("string-like") because the two characters resemble each other closely.

Xu Dachun: These are manifestations of a disease in the liver. The liver and the gall bladder represent one unit. In the case of a disease in the liver, the gall bladder suffers from depletion. Hence, [the patient] keeps his eyes closed and does not wish to look at anybody.

Liao Ping: When the [*Nei*] *jing* speaks of *gan mai* 肝脈 ("liver movement in the vessels"), these two characters linked together often refer to [the movement of the] qi [in the vessels] and to the color [that appears in the face] .... The creation of designations for the [movement in the] vessels is one of the great crimes of this book.

(3) *Ding Deyong*: "At the surface, short, and rough" are the [characteristics of a movement in the] vessels [associated with the] lung. In this situation here the metal must have overcome the wood. Hence, one knows that death [is imminent].

Yang: The liver is wood; the lung is metal. If in the case of a disease in the liver one feels a lung [movement in the] vessels, that is really [as if] a demon had come to cause destruction. Metal overcomes wood. Hence, death is inevitable.

(4) *Ding Deyong*: These are symptoms of a disease in the heart. Here now, however, in contrast [to what one should expect], a kidney [movement in the] vessels appears. The heart is fire; the kidneys are water. Water has come to destroy fire. Hence, one knows that death [is imminent].

Yang: If one perceives a short, replete, and frequent [movement in the vessels], as if one felt a [moving] rope, that is called "tight." If one feels a short and weak [movement], lacking any agitated motion, [and if this movement] is sometimes present, sometimes absent, [and if it] can be felt by a light hand, but not by a heavy hand, that is called "slight."

Yu Shu: If a disease [is associated] with open eyes, thirst, and a firm [area] below the heart, and if the [movement in the] vessels is tight, replete, and frequent, that would be called "feeling a yang [movement in the] vessels in the case of a yang disease." [In such a case the disease and the movement in] the vessels are not in contrast to each other. Here now, one perceives a soft and slight [movement] in the depth. That is called "feeling a yin [movement in the] vessels in the case of a yang disease." Hence, [the text] speaks of [imminent] death.

Hua Shou: The disease is repletion but the [movement in the] vessels [signals] depletion.

Xu Dachun: These are manifestations of a disease in the heart. The heart controls the heat. If the heat is extreme, [the patient] will keep his eyes open and be thirsty.

(5) *Ding Deyong*: These are symptoms of a disease in the lung. Here now, however, in contrast [to what one should expect], a heart [movement in the] vessels appears.

The heart is fire; the lung is metal. Fire has come to overpower the metal. Hence, one knows that death [must follow].

Yu Shu: The blood is associated with yin. If in the case of spitting blood and nosebleed the [movement in the] vessels is in the depth and fine, this is called "mutual correspondence between [movement in the] vessels and disease." Here now, [the movement in the vessels] is at the surface, strong, and firm. These [are symptoms] in contrast to the disease. Hence, death [must follow].

Hua Shou: Loss of blood and a replete [movement in the] vessels are [symptoms] in mutual contrast.

Xu Dachun: The meaning implied here differs [from that of the preceding instances]. "The disease is depletion but the [movement in the] vessels is replete, hence death [must follow" syndrome] is not discussed here in terms of the [mutual] generation or destruction [orders of the Five Phases]. The treatise "Yu ban" 玉 版 of the *Ling* [*shu*] states: "When someone [suffers from] unending nosebleed associated with a massive [movement in the] vessels, that is a third [example of a] movement contrary to the norms." This is the meaning implied here.[4]

Ye Lin: These are manifestations of a depletion of blood. The [movement in the] vessels should be in the depth and fine, but a replete [movement in the] vessels appears which is, on the contrary, at the surface, strong, and firm. This is the case of a yin disease where one feels a yang [movement in the] vessels. The disease is depletion while the [movement in the] vessels [signals] repletion. Hence, death must follow.

Liao Ping: The use of [the term] "firm" as a designation for a [movement in the] vessels originated with the *Nan jing*.

(6) *Ding Deyong*: These are symptoms of a disease in the heart. Here, however, in contrast [to what one would expect,] hands and feet are marked by reversed

---

4   The entire passage alluded to here reads: Huang Di: All diseases are either movements contrary to or movements in accordance with the norms. Can I be informed of that? Qi Bo: When the abdomen is bloated, the body is hot, and the [movement in the] vessels is massive, that is a first [example of] a movement contrary to the norms. When there are noises in the abdomen associated with a feeling of fullness, when the four limbs are cool and [the patient suffers from] outflow, associated with a massive [movement in the] vessels, that is a second [example of a] movement contrary to the norms. When someone [suffers from] unending nosebleed associated with a massive [movement in the] vessels, that is a third [example of a] movement contrary to the norms. When someone coughs and discharges blood with his urine and loses weight, associated with a minimal [movement in the] vessels, that is a fourth [example of a] movement contrary to the norms. When someone coughs, loses weight, and his body is hot, associated with a minimal and accelerated [movement in the] vessels, that is called a fifth [example of a] movement contrary to the norms. Those with such states [of health] will die within 15 days.

[moving qi, and the movement in the] vessels is fine, slight, and in the depth. This means that water has overcome fire. Hence, one knows that death [must follow].

Yang: If one feels a slow but weak [movement], that is called "fine."

Yu Shu: The lung controls the sounds; the heart controls the [way of] speaking. [In the case of the disease indicated] here, the [movement in the] vessels should be vast and strong. If this were so, one would know that heat has seized the heart, and that evil [qi from the] lung have been received here. Hence, [the patient] would speak incoherently and utter nonsense. The lung controls the skin [and its] hair. [In the case of the disease indicated] here, evil [qi] have taken residence among the guard qi. [The latter] are no longer able to proceed, and the body is hot. Hence, if it were like that, disease and [movement in the] vessels would correspond. Here, [however, the qi in the patient's] hands and feet move contrary to their proper course; the movement is in the depth, fine, and slight. In the case of a yang disease one perceives a yin [movement in the] vessels. Hence; [the text] says death is inevitable.

Hua Shou: If in the case of a yang disease a yin [movement in the] vessels appears, [disease and symptoms] are in mutual contrast.

Ye Lin: Incoherent talk and [the uttering of] nonsense are manifestations of heat. The body should be hot and the [movement in the] vessels should be vast and strong. Here, on the contrary, hands and feet appear cold because of reversed [moving qi]. The [movement in the] vessels comes in the depth, is fine and slight. This is a case where the disease is repletion while the [movement in the] vessels [signals] depletion. Hence, death [must follow].

(7) *Ding Deyong:* These are symptoms of a disease in the spleen, that is, earth. A tight, strong, and smooth [movement is associated with] the liver. The wood has come to overpower the earth. Hence, one knows that death [must follow]. The [*Nan*] *jing* does not discuss here symptoms of [a disease in the] kidneys, that is, [the phase of] water. This particular long-term depot is omitted here.

Yang: In all these five cases, the disease and the [movement in the] vessels are in contrast to each other. Hence, death is inevitable. The [*Nei*] *jing* states: "The five [movements in the vessels] contrary to the norms are fatal."[5] That is meant here.

Yu Shu: Wherever humid qi gain the upper hand, swellings occur. The spleen has lost its inhibitive [function]; hence, diarrhea occurs. If the [movement in the] vessels were slight, fine, and rough, [the movement in] the vessels and the disease would correspond to each other. Since it is tight, strong, and smooth, [the text] speaks of mutual contrast. It should be clear that death must follow if such symptoms occur.

---

5   See note 4.

十八難曰：（一）脈有三部，部有四經，手有太陰、陽明，足有太陽、少陰，為上下部，何謂也？

（二）然：手太陰，陽明金也；足少陰，太陽水也。金生水，水流下行而不能上，故在下部也。（三）足厥陰，少陽木也，生手太陽、少陰火，火炎上行而不能下，故為上部。（四）手心主，少陽火，生足太陰、陽明土，土主中宮，故在中部也。（五）此皆五行子母更相生養者也。

（六）脈有三部九候，各何所主之？

（七）然：三部者，寸、關、尺。九候者，浮、中、沉也。（八）上部法天，主胸以上至頭之有疾也；（九）中部法人，主膈以下至齊之有疾也；（十）下部法地，主齊以下至足之有疾也。（十一）審而刺之者也。

（十二）人病有沉滯久積聚，可切脈而知之耶？

（十三）然：診在右脅有積氣，得肺脈結，脈結甚則積甚，結微則氣微。

（十四）診不得肺脈，而右脅有積氣者，何也？

（十五）然：肺脈雖不見，右手脈當沉伏。

（十六）其外痼疾同法耶？將異也？

（十七）然：結者，脈來去時一止，無常數，名曰結也。伏者，脈行筋下也。浮者，脈在肉上行也。（十八）左右表裏，法皆如此。（十九）假令脈結伏者，內無積聚；脈浮結者，外無痼疾；（二十）有積聚脈不結伏，有痼疾脈不浮結。為脈不應病，病不應脈，是為死病也。

The eighteenth difficult issue: (1) The [movement in the] vessels appears in three sections; [each] section has four conduits, with the major yin and the yang brilliance [conduits] of the hands, and the major yang and the minor yin [conduits] of the feet constituting the upper and the lower sections. What does that mean?

(2) It is like this. The hand major yin and the [hand] yang brilliance [conduits] are [associated with the phase of] metal; the foot minor yin and the [foot] major yang [conduits] are [associated with the phase of] water. Metal generates water. Water flows downward and is unable to ascend. Therefore, [the foot minor yin and the foot major yang conduits can be felt] at the section below [the gate]. (3) The foot ceasing yin and the [foot] minor yang [conduits] are [associated with the phase of] wood; it generates the [phase of] fire, [which is associated with the] hand major yang and the [hand minor yin [conduits]. The flames of fire ascend; they are unable to move downward. Hence, [the hand major yang and the hand minor yin conduits can be felt] at the section above [the gate]. (4) The hand heart ruler and the [hand] minor yang [conduits are associated with the phase of] fire; it generates the [phase of] soil, [which is associated with the] foot major yin and with the [foot] yang brilliance [conduits]. The soil rules the central short-term repository and is, therefore, situated

in the central section. (5) All of this is [in accordance with] the mutual generation and nourishment of the Five Phases [as in a] child–mother [relationship].

(6) The [movement in the] vessels appears in three sections and on nine indicator [levels]. By which diseases are the [movements in these sections and on these levels] governed, respectively?

(7) It is like this. The three sections concerned are the inch [section], the gate [section], and the foot [section]. The nine indicator [levels] refer to surface, center, and depth [of each of the three sections]. (8) The upper section is patterned after heaven; it is governed by diseases located from the chest upward to the head. (9) The central section is patterned after man; it is governed by diseases located below the diaphragm to the navel. (10) The lower section is patterned after earth; it is governed by diseases located below the navel to the feet. (11) [For a treatment, one should first] conduct a careful examination [as to which section displays which movement in the vessels] and only then apply the needles.

(12) When a person suffers from deep, stagnant, and long-term accumulations and collections [of qi], can this be known by feeling the vessels?

(13) It is like this. Consider that an examination reveals an accumulation of qi in the right side of the human body, and furthermore, that one feels a knotted [movement in the conduit] vessel [associated with the] lung. [In this case] the accumulation is extensive if the knotted [character of the movement in the] vessels is extensive; the [accumulation of] qi is slight if the knotted [character of the movement is] slight.

(14) What is the matter, though, if one feels nothing in the [conduit] vessel [associated with the] lung, and if there is still an accumulation of qi in the right side of the body?

(15) It is like this. Although a [movement in the conduit] vessel [associated with the] lung is not apparent, a deep and subdued [movement in the] vessels must be present in the right hand.

(16) Does the same pattern apply to chronic diseases in the outer [sections of the body], or should different [considerations be applied here]?

(17) It is like this. "Knotted" [means that the movement in the] vessels stops once in a while in the process of coming and going, and that this does not occur with regular frequency. That is called "knotted." To be "subdued" [means that] the movement in the vessels occurs below the muscles. "At the surface" [means that] the movement

in the vessels occurs above the flesh.[1](18) No matter whether [a disease is situated in the] left or right side, in the external or internal parts [of the body], the pattern is always like this. (19) If, for instance, the [movement in the] vessels is knotted and subdued, no accumulation exists internally; if the [movement in the] vessels is at the surface and knotted, no chronic disease exists in the external [sections of the body]. (20) If, however, in the case of accumulations, the [movement in the] vessels is not knotted and subdued, or if, in the case of a chronic disease, the [movement in the] vessels is not at the surface and knotted, that means that the [movement in the] vessels does not correspond to the disease, and that the disease does not correspond to the [movement in the] vessels. Such diseases are fatal.[2]

COMMENTARIES

(1) *Ding Deyong*: "The [movement in the] vessels appears in three sections": These are the inch, the gate, and the foot [sections]. Speaking of both hands together, these are six sections. Within each section there are two conduits; within the six sections this adds up to a total of twelve conduits. When this paragraph here speaks of "four conduits," it refers to the hand major yin and [hand] yang brilliance, as well as to the foot major yang and [foot] minor yin [conduits]. These four conduits reflect the nature of water and fire. Each of them is controlled by a specific principle; they cannot change [their whereabouts] and penetrate higher or lower [sections at will]. The remaining eight conduits are situated in the hands where they generate [those in] the feet, or in the feet where they gen-

---

1 The Chinese wording here could indicate a belief in the passage (*xing* 行) of individual vessels through the wrist. Thus, the last sentence could also be translated as: "'At the surface' [means that] the vessel passes above the flesh." However, in accordance with the preceding and following passages, I have preferred a rendering indicating a concept of one vessel with several levels and sections. This, of course, should not exclude the concept of various conduits passing through the arms and wrists. The question (to which I shall return in note 2) is whether the movement in a single vessel was investigated for diagnostic purposes, or whether separate vessels were pressed to assess the movement of the qi through each of them. It is rather difficult to assume that the author(s) thought that a single vessel could change its position from the depth below the muscles to the surface above the flesh, or that the movement could cease in one vessel for some extended period and appear in another vessel. These would be logical consequences if one were to apply the multi-vessel concept here. See also difficult issue 1.

2 The first section of this difficult issue (sentences 1 through 5) once again offers an innovative diagnostic pattern using terms from the *Nei jing* but supplying them with a very different meaning. A comparison with the *Su wen* treatise "San bu jiu hou lun" 三部九候 論 appears in Xu Dachun's commentary on sentence 6 and needs not be repeated here. Yet the pattern developed in the first section of this difficult issue is only hinted at. If Yu Shu is correct in his commentary on sentence 4, the data provided can be put into tabular form as follows:

erate [those in] the hands. This is why the [*Nan*] *jing* states "has four conduits." That is [to say], at the inch opening of the right hand the [conduits of the] lung

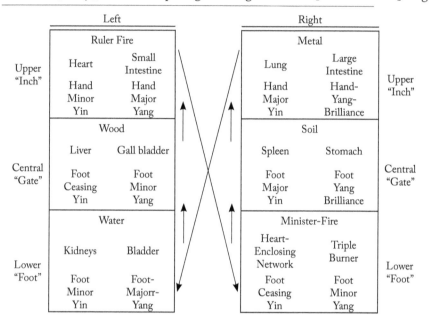

	Left				Right		
	Ruler Fire				**Metal**		
Upper "Inch"	Heart	Small Intestine			Lung	Large Intestine	Upper "Inch"
	Hand Minor Yin	Hand Major Yang			Hand Major Yin	Hand-Yang-Brilliance	
	Wood				**Soil**		
Central "Gate"	Liver	Gall bladder			Spleen	Stomach	Central "Gate"
	Foot Ceasing Yin	Foot Minor Yang			Foot Major Yin	Foot Yang Brilliance	
	Water				**Minister-Fire**		
Lower "Foot"	Kidneys	Bladder			Heart-Enclosing Network	Triple Burner	Lower "Foot"
	Foot Minor Yin	Foot-Majorr-Yang			Foot Ceasing Yin	Foot Minor Yang	

This pattern displays a relatively high level of theorization, and it is not clear whether the author(s) believed in the actual presence of the individual conduits in the respective sections or whether – on the basis of systematic correspondence – the terms "major yang," "minor yin," and so on indicate the kinds of movement in one single vessel (as outlined in difficult issue 7, sentences 1 through 6). With this schema, which appears to transcend all previous patterns, an apex was reached in the process of supplying vessel diagnosis at the wrist with a theoretical foundation. Both the yinyang associations of the six long-term depots and six short-term repositories and their mutual relationships on the basis of the Five Phases doctrine appear to have been taken into account. Although not stated explicitly by the text of the *Nan jing*, here for the first time it may have been realized that the left hand and the right hand offer different information. The rationale given for the allocation of the individual conduits in one of the six sections followed the mutual generation order of the Five Phases; the latter was abstracted here to such a degree that Liao Ping, the conservative commentator in favor of what he considered the more down-to-earth argumentation in the *Nei jing*, denounced this first section as "empty talk" (see his commentary on sentence 3).

The second section appears to integrate the patterns outlined in difficult issues 1 through 4. After reading the question in sentence 6 one might expect, as an answer, a complicated summary of all the diagnostic data that can be obtained from the three cross-sections and nine longitudinal levels (as outlined in the early difficult issues). Yet the response that actually follows could be called incomplete. It may have been intended merely as a concluding statement, omitting the details which any interested reader could supplement in by himself. Katō Bankei concluded that this section should be considered as difficult issue 3. The third section, finally, appears out of place here. Various commentators have suggested that it originally may have been part of difficult issue 17 or some other treatise.

and of the large intestine, both corresponding to metal, generate the water of the left foot [section]. The foot major yang and the [foot] minor yin [conduits correspond to the] water. Its nature is to moisten that what is below. Hence, they cannot move upward to generate the [conduits in the] hands; rather, they generate the ceasing yin and minor yang [conduits associated with the] wood of the left foot. Both these two sections regulate the transactions in the feet. Hence, [the text] speaks of a "lower section." That is, the water of the left foot [section] generates the wood of the left gate [section].

Hua Shou: The "three sections" are the upper, central, and lower [sections] which are distinguished according to the [differentiation between] inch, gate, and foot [sections]. As to the "four conduits," if the two [corresponding inch, gate, and foot sections of the two hands] are collated respectively, then each [pair] has four conduits. As to "the major yin and the yang brilliance [conduits] of the hands and the major yang and the minor-yin [conduits] of the feet constitute the upper and the lower [sections, respectively]," the lung [vessel] is located at the inch [section] of the right [hand, while] the kidney [vessel] is located at the foot [section] of the left [hand]. In a circular movement they nourish each other. The lung is on high, the kidneys are below; they look at each other like mother and child. This is [what is] meant when the scripture states: "The long-term depots are truly on high with the lung; they are truly below with the kidneys."

Zhang Shixian: The "three sections" are the inch, the gate, and the foot [sections] in both hands. In each [pair of these] sections there are four conduits. Thus, for example, the inch [section] of the left [hand] contains the [conduits associated with the] heart and with the small intestine, [while the inch section of] the right [hand] contains [the conduits of the] lung and of the large intestine. [With all three sections] this adds up to twelve conduits. The upper section is the "inch"; the lower section is the "foot."

Liao Ping: The [*Nei*] *jing* does not distinguish between an upper and a lower [section] according to hands and feet.

(2) *Yang*: The hand major yin [conduit] is the vessel of the lung. The lung constitutes the cover above all the remaining long-term depots; its place of rule is in the right side [of the body]. Hence, [its vessel movement appears] in the upper section of the right hand. The hand yang brilliance [conduit] is the vessel of the large intestine which, in turn, constitutes the short-term repository associated with the lung. Like the lung, it is located in the upper section. The foot minor yin [conduit] is the vessel of the kidneys. The kidneys represent the water. This is the child of the [metal of the] lung. The water flows quickly to the kidneys, and [the latter] are located at the lowest position [in the body]. Hence, [the vessel

movement associated with the kidneys appears] in the lower section of the left hand. The foot major yang [conduit is the vessel of the] bladder, [the latter] constituting the short-term repository of the kidneys. Hence, like the kidneys, it resides in the lower section [of the body]. The [*Nan*] *jing* states: "The [movement in the] vessels appears in three sections and each section has four conduits." This is an all-encompassing reference to both hands. Each of the two hands has three sections and each section has two conduits. Thus, both hands together have four [conduits] in the upper section. The same applies to the central and to the lower sections. Three times four is twelve. Hence, these are the twelve conduits. The metal of the lung resides above and generates the water of the kidneys below. Hence, lung and kidney [vessels appear] in the upper and lower sections of the right and left hands, respectively.

Liao Ping: The [*Nei*] *jing* contains no statements to the effect that the hand metal [conduits] constitute the upper [section], while the foot water [conduits] constitute the lower [section]. The [respective] question was posed simply because [the author of this difficult issue] wished to develop his personal doctrine of the upper and lower [location] of metal and water. ... If these locations are above and below in the first place, why should one discuss them in terms of the Five Phases?

(3) *Ding Deyong*: The hand major yang and the [hand] minor yin [conduits] correspond to the inch [section] of the left [hand] and to the ruler fire. The nature of fire is to flame upward. It cannot descend to generate [the water in] the feet; rather, it generates the fire of the hand heart ruler and of the [hand] minor yang [conduits associated with the heart enclosing network and with the Triple Burner, respectively]. That is [to say], it generates the minister fire in the foot [section] of the right [hand].

Yang: The foot ceasing yin [conduit] is the vessel of the liver. The liver rules in the left side [of the body]. Hence, [its vessel movement appears] in the lower section of the left hand.³ The foot minor yang [conduit is associated with the] gall bladder, [the latter] constituting the short-term repository of the liver. Hence, like the liver, [the gall bladder] is located in the lower section. The hand major yang [conduit] is the vessel of the small intestine, which is the short-term repository of the heart. Hence, like the heart, it is located in the upper section.

Liao Ping: [The statements in the] *Nei jing* concerning yin yang and the Five Phases represent classic doctrines of the realm of medicine; among the nine streams,⁴ they constitute the specialty of the Yin-Yang and Five Phases schools. When they are employed to discuss the therapy of diseases, the examination

---

3   This statement appears to contradict the same author's commentary on sentence 2.

4   These are the nine classes of ancient Chinese literature or philosophy.

of long-term depots and short-term repositories is considered [to reveal] solid evidence; [the *Nei jing*] does not value empty talk. The lofty and inappropriate [application] of the Five Phases originated from this book. [It resulted from] a mistaken reading of the *Nei jing* which was combined with the [doctrine of the] Five Phases. Consequently, the medical community of subsequent times believed that anybody who could utter empty talk was a competent person. The [actual] structure of the long-term depots and short-term repositories, as well as the [actual] holes and passageways of the [main] conduits and of the network [vessels] were discarded and were no longer taken into consideration. Rather, "generation" and "overcoming," "control" and "changes" were discussed exclusively. This led to an entanglement of medicine with speculations, resembling the teachings of the astrologers. [The former] created "complexions" and "flavors"; [the latter] drew pictures of dogs and horses. It is hard [to imagine that this could] be more appropriate than [a belief in] demons and spirits! But everybody followed these [trends] .... How can liver and gall bladder generate the heart? The generation and destruction among the Five Phases [refers to] qi not to form.

(4) *Ding Deyong*: This is the minister fire; it corresponds to the ruler fire. The central section is the gate of the right [hand]. It generates the inch of the right [hand, which] is [associated with] metal.

Yang: The hand heart ruler [conduit] is the vessel of the heart enclosing [network]. The hand minor yang [conduit] is the vessel of the Triple Burner. Hence, the two together represent the central section of the left hand. The foot major yin [conduit] is the vessel of the spleen. The foot yang brilliance [conduit] is the vessel of the stomach. Hence, the two together represent the central section of the right hand. The way in which the [*Nan*]*jing* distinguishes [the three sections and their respective vessels] here is different from the gouping [of the vessels in but] two sections, as outlined by the *Mai jing*.

Yu Shu: The [*Nan*]*jing* states: "The hand heart ruler and ... situated in the central section" of the right hand. This is a discourse on the meaning of the generation of soil by fire only, it is not a discourse on the hand heart ruler and [hand] minor yang [conduits] in the central section of the left hand. The only item discussed here is the mutual generation [of two of the Five Phases]. Now, the meaning of the mutual generation of the [vessels associated with the] three sections has been elucidated here as follows. The fire of the minor yang [conduit] in the foot [section] of the right hand generates the soil of the yang brilliance [conduit] of the gate [section]. The soil of the yang brilliance [conduit] from above the gate[5]

---

5 "Above the gate" does not refer here to the inch section but to the gate itself. *Guan shang* 關上 could also be rendered here as "on the gate."

then generates the metal of the major yin [conduit] in the inch opening. The
metal of the major yin [conduit] in the inch opening generates the water of the
minor yin [conduit] in the foot [section] of the left hand. The water of the minor
yin [conduit] in the foot [section] of the left hand generates the wood of the
ceasing yin [conduit] above the gate of the left hand. The wood of the ceasing
yin [conduit] above the gate generates the fire of the minor yin [conduit] in the
inch opening of the left hand. [The text] further distinguishes a fire of the heart
ruler [conduit]. Hence, the [fire of the] heart ruler [conduit] generates the soil
of the yang brilliance and of the major yin [conduits] of the feet. This then is the
meaning of the "mutual generation of the Five Phases." Furthermore, why are the
foot ceasing yin and the foot major yin [conduits] located in the gate sections of
the left and right hand, respectively? Stomach and spleen are both major yin. The
vessel associated with the spleen is located in the central section. This is above
the gate of the right hand. Also, the foot ceasing yin [conduit is associated with
the phase of] wood. The roots of wood grow into the earth; branches and leaves
extend toward heaven. Thus, both yin and yang are also represented here. Hence,
[the respective conduit] is located in the central section too.

(5) *Ding Deyong*: When [the text] here states that "all of this is [in accordance with]
the mutual generation and nourishment of the Five Phases [as in a] child-mother [relationship]," that is to say that the metal of the right inch generates the
water of the left foot; that water generates the wood of the left gate; that wood
generates the ruler fire of the left inch; that ruler fire generates the minister fire of
the right foot; that minister fire generates the soil of the right gate; and [that soil]
finally generates the metal of the right inch. Hence, [the text] speaks of "mutual
generation and nourishment [as in a] child-mother [relationship]."

(2)–(5) *Hua Shou*: Because the major yin and the yang brilliance [conduits] of the
hands and the major yang and minor yin [conduits] of the feet constitute the
passageways of the upper and lower sections, respectively, [the author] has ex-
trapolated on the general [system] of mutual generation of the Five Phases.
Yueren also drew his conclusions on the basis of the high or low position of the
respective sections, where the five long-term depots are located after [a person's
birth]. This does not mean that this is so already before [a person] is born; it is so
after birth. [Yueren also] lectured on the three sections. The meaning referred to
here is found in the discussion of the fourth difficult issue, where it is said that
[the movements in the vessels associated with the] heart and [with the] lung are
both at the surface, that [the movement in the vessels associated with the] kidneys and [with the] liver are both in the depth, and that the spleen represents the
central region. However, there [in the fourth difficult issue] this was discussed

with reference to the long-term depots only. Here it is discussed on the basis of the conduits, which are then related to the long-term depots and short-term repositories. The question-and-answer dialogue above elucidates the [relationships among the] conduits. The following two paragraphs are both irrelevant here. I suspect that they constitute mistaken abridgments from other [sections of this] scripture.

(1)–(5) *Katō Bankei*: Each of the three sections is matched with [one of] the long-term depots and short-term repositories, respectively. But in their discussions of this matching, all authors [of the past] have been utterly confused. Apparently, [their interpretations] did not coincide with the meaning of the [*Nan*] *jing*. I have extensively studied the diagnosis of the three sections inch, gate, and foot [as it is related in the *Nan jing*]. Among all the eighty-one discourses, it says only "feel at the left" or "feel at the right." These then are references to the vessels of the right hand, and so on. But I have found nowhere a word on the matching of the long-term depots and short-term repositories with the foot and inch [sections] of the left and right [hand], respectively. Statements such as "the heart [corresponds to] the inch [section] of the left [hand] and the lung [corresponds to] the inch [section] of the right [hand]" were first released like a whirling dart by Wang Shuhe 王叔和 from the Western Jin. All the authors of the Tang, Song, Yuan, and Ming [eras] followed his signal flag. Increasingly, they acted contrary to all reason; increasingly, [their ideas] became more numerous and confused. Finally, they even took the *Su wen* paragraph – which explains that the two sides of the foot-interior [section correspond to] the tender ribs, and so on – and began to believe that it contains the meaning of matching [the long-term depots and short-term repositories, or their respective conduits] with the three sections of the left and right [hand]. Here they greatly missed the meaning of the ancients. But why was it that it was not just a single dog who barked in the void? Why were there tens of thousands of dogs who transmitted his voice? Finally, in the middle of the Ming [era], Zhao Jizong 趙繼宗[6] and Li Shizhen 李時珍 crushed what had become too numerous and disorderly, with the intention to devise a concise [system of diagnosis]. But Mr. Zhao took over only the information that "the soil controls the central short-term repository," and Mr. Li grasped only the meaning of "[each] section has four levels." Wang Chengshu 王誠叔[7] of the Song said that the only thing he considered to be correct was that [movements

---

6 Zhao Jizong's dates are unknown. He is the author of a medical treatise entitled *Ru yi jing yao* 儒醫精要.

7 Chengshu 誠叔 is the *zi* of Wang Zongzheng 王宗正, the author of the *Nan jing shu yi* 難經疏義.

corresponding to] the heart and the lung are at the surface, that [those corresponding to] the kidneys and to the liver are in the depth, while the [movement associated with the] spleen is in the central region. But when he distinguished between sections in both hands and [when he outlined] that the vessels of the long-term depots and short-term repositories at times appear differently in the foot and inch [sections], he, like all the others, believed that the mistakes of Mr. Wang's *Mai jing* could be called exalted views from high antiquity! How regrettable that the mouths of the many, which [are supposed to] melt metal, cause one but to have the talent to drop an awl![8]

(6) *Ding Deyong*: Above, [mutual] generation and nourishment [resulting from a movement of qi through the conduits] in accordance with the Five Phases were discussed. Here [the issue of] a reverse [movement] in the three sections and of an arrival [of qi contrary to their proper course is discussed]. Therefore, the [*Nan*] *jing* asks in an additional question: "By which [diseases] are the [movements in the three sections and on the nine indicator-levels] governed, respectively?"

Yang: The inch opening is yang. The gate is the central section. The foot-interior is yin. Each of these three sections has surface, center, and depth as its three indicator [levels]. Three times three is nine. Hence, it is said: "[Of the qi on the] nine indicator [levels], those at the surface are yang [qi], those in the depth are yin [qi], and those in the center are stomach qi."

Yu Shu: In each section there are three indicator [levels]. Those at the surface represent the short-term repositories. Those in the depth represent the long-term depots. Those in the center represent the [movement in the] vessels of the Central Burner. Take, for example, the inch opening. The surface represents a short-term repository, the depth represents a depot, and the center represents the Central Burner. All the others are used accordingly.

Xu Dachun: According to the *Su* [*wen* treatise], "San bu jiu hou lun" 三部九候論, the "three sections" point to an upper section, a central section, and a lower section [of the entire body]. The "nine indicators" include the vessel movements at the two [sides of the] forehead as "heaven of the upper section," the vessel movements at the two [sides of the] jaws as "earth of the upper section," and the vessel movements in front of the ears as "man of the upper section"; the hand major yin [conduit] as "heaven of the central section," the hand yang brilliance [conduit] as "earth of the central section," and the hand minor yin [conduit] as "man of the central section"; and the foot ceasing yin [conduit] as "heaven of the lower section," the foot minor yin [conduit] as "earth of the lower section," and the

---

8   In the Confucian classic *Guo yu* 國語, chapter "Zhou yu xia" 周語下, it is said: "The hearts of the many may erect city walls; the mouths of the many may melt metal."

foot major yin [conduit] as "man of the lower section." Here [in the *Nan jing*],
the inch, the gate, and the foot constitute the three sections, and the surface,
center, and depth [of each of them] represent the nine indicator [levels]. That
is entirely different. Obviously, in the *Nei jing* various methods [are discussed]
to examine the [movement in the] vessels. But the *Nan jing* focuses on the inch
opening exclusively. Here then seems to be an attempt to completely integrate
the [diversity of] the diagnostic methods of the [*Nei*] *jing*. There must have been
a separate tradition which cannot be criticized as entirely wrong.[9] Thus, [the au-
thor] has taken over the text of the [*Nei*] *jing* in order to elucidate the meaning
of that [separate tradition], because everything is supposed to have its origin in
the [*Nei*] *jing*.

Liao Ping: The following text is identical with that of the [*Nei*] *jing*. But by employing the [idea of the] three sections of the [*Nei*] *jing* and by changing it [to
indicate] inch, gate, and foot, and by employing the [idea of the] nine indicators
and interpreting them as referring to the images of the [movement in the] vessels, the ancient methods have been discarded entirely. The discussion focuses
exclusively on examinations to be carried out at both hands. This is one of the
great crimes of this book.

(8) *Ding Deyong*: The inch openings of both hands constitute the upper section. The
inch-exterior [section] controls the head; the inch-interior [section] controls the
central part of the chest. All [the afflictions of] the head [can be felt] under the
first finger, [with] the front and the back [half of the finger] revealing the [same]
diseases.[10] The pattern is the same for the left and right [hands of the patient].

Yang: The so-called [region] above the diaphragm is the Upper Burner.

(9) *Ding Deyong*: [That] refers to the two gates of the left and right [hands]. The
front half of the second finger tells about [the region] below the diaphragm. The
back half controls [the region] above the navel. The [pattern] is the same for the
left and right [hands of the patient].

Yang: The so-called [region] below the diaphragm is the Central Burner.

---

9   Liao Ping commented on this assumption: "[Diagnosis] was transferred to the two inch
    openings because head and feet of females cannot be examined. There was no ancient
    book [relating such a tradition]. This is selfevident from an analysis of the [*Bei ji*] *qian jin*
    [*yao fang*] 備急千金要方 and from the *Wai tai* [*mi yao*] 外臺秘要."

10 Here and below, Ding Deyong introduces a concept which further complicates vessel
    diagnosis at the wrist by subdividing each of the three sections into one "front" and one
    "back" subsection, respectively, the movements in which can be felt under the front half
    and back half of each of the three fingers used for diagnosis. "Front" indicates the subsec-
    tion facing the palm; "back" indicates the subsection facing the elbow.

(10) *Ding Deyong*: The lower sections are the two foot [sections] of the left and right [hand]. The front half of the third finger controls the diseases below the navel; the back half indicates diseases down to the feet.

Yang: The so-called [region] below the navel to the feet is the Lower Burner.

(11) *Ding Deyong*: The character *ci* 刺 ("to pierce") should be the character *ci* 次 like in *ci di* 次第 ("sequence", "series"). This [line here speaks of] an examination of the three sections, each of which has an interior and an exterior [subsection]. They control the presence of diseases from head to feet. Hence, one knows that the character *ci* 刺 represents a mistaken transmission.

Yang: Anybody who uses needles must carefully examine the nine indicator [levels] in the three sections for the whereabouts of a disease. Only then should he apply the needles according to the origin of the respective [ailment].

(6)–(11) *Xie Jinsun*: This paragraph must be a mistaken abridgment of the words given as an answer to the sixteenth difficult issue. They are superfluous here. The ten characters *mai you san bu jiu hou ge he zhu zhi* 脈有三部九候各何主之 can be omitted. With regard to [the phrase] *shen er ci zhi* 審而刺之, Mr. Ji Tianxi has said: If one is about to investigate the movement in the vessels and [discovers] that it has been hit by a disease, one must conduct a careful examination. Hence, [the *Nan jing*] states *shen er ci zhi*. *Ci* means that the movement has been hit.

Tamba Genkan: Ever since Yang's commentary [was written], the meaning of this paragraph was interpreted as a matching of the three sections of the left and right [hand] with the short-term repositories and long-term depots. However, such a doctrine does appear neither in the *Nan jing* nor in the *Nei jing*. It originated, in fact, from the treatise "Liang shou liu mai suo zhu zang fu yin yang ni shun" 兩手六脈所主藏府陰陽逆順 of the *Mai jing* 脈經.

(12)–(15) *Ding Deyong*: As to [the question,] "when [a person] suffers from long-term accumulations, can this be known by feeling the vessels," all the five long-term depots and six short-term repositories [may] have accumulations. Here, [the text] says that "an accumulation of qi is present in the right side of the body." [In that case] a vessel [movement associated with the] lung should appear. If in that case such a vessel [movement] does not appear, it is nevertheless present, but in the depth and subdued. Let us take a closer look at the meaning of the [*Nan*] *jing* here. [When the movement in] the vessels is at the surface, it proceeds above the flesh. [When the movement in] the vessels is in the depth, it proceeds below the muscles. When it is at the surface and proceeds above the flesh with irregular frequency and [occasional] stops, that is called "knotted." When it is in the depth and proceeds below the muscles, at times coming up, that is called "subdued." A subdued [movement indicates] that the long-term depots suffer from a *ji* 積

accumulation [of qi; a movement that is] at the surface and knotted indicates that the short-term repositories suffer from a *ju* 聚 collection. The three sections of both hands have [vessel movements] appearing at the surface or in the depth, knotted or subdued. Here, the [*Nan*] *jing* refers to the vessel [movement associated with the] lung to discuss this issue.

Yang: [A movement that] is relaxed and repeats its arrival with occasional stops is called "knotted."

Yu Shu: A "knotted" [movement in the] vessels indicates lump-like accumulations. The respective vessel movement stops occasionally; it occurs with low frequency and may return to move backward. Hence, it is called "knotted."

(12) *Hua Shou*: It is not clear where the following questions and answers belong. Some have said they are part of the seventeenth difficult issue. Some have [interpreted them as] answers to the [question] "will continue for years and months without remission."

(20) *Ding Deyong*: If the heart has some [reason to] ponder, [the movement in its] vessel will also be knotted. If the heart has no [reason to] ponder, if no disease is present internally or externally, and if [the movement in] the respective vessel is still subdued and knotted, in that case the form has no disease, but the vessels display a disease. Hence, one knows that death [must follow].

(19)–(20) *Ye Lin*: In the case of a specific disease there must be a specific [movement in the] vessels. If accumulations are present internally, the [movement in the] vessels must be subdued and knotted. If a chronic disease is located in the external [sections of the body, the movement in the] vessels must be at the surface and knotted. If one observes a subdued and knotted [movement in the] vessels or one that is at the surface and knotted, while no symptoms [are present corresponding to movements in the vessels that are] subdued and knotted or at the surface and knotted, respectively – or if one observes symptoms [associated with movements in the vessels that are] subdued and knotted or at the surface and knotted, respectively, while no [movement in the] vessels is present that is subdued and knotted or at the surface and knotted – these are so-called [situations where] the [movement in the] vessels does not correspond to the disease, or where the disease does not correspond to the [movement in the] vessels. Now, if the disease and the [movement in the] vessels do not correspond, the true qi have left [the long-term depots and conduits] already; the blood vessels are no longer linked up with each other. Hence, [the text] speaks of "death." Whenever disease and [movement in the] vessels do not correspond to each other, these are always indications of [imminent] death. One need not wait for accumulations to draw this [conclusion].

十九難曰：（一）經言脈有逆順，男女有常，而反者，何謂也？

（二）然：男子生於寅，寅為木，陽也；（三）女子生於申，申為金，陰也。（四）故男脈在關上，女脈在關下。（五）是以男子尺脈恆弱，女子尺脈恆盛，是其常也。（六）反者，男得女脈，女得男脈也。

（七）其為病何如？

（八）然：男得女脈為不足，病在內；（九）左得之，病則在左；右得之，病則在右，隨脈言之也。（十）女得男脈為太過，病在四肢；（十一）左得之，病則在左；右得之，病則在右，隨脈言之，此之謂也。

The nineteenth difficult issue: (1) The scripture states: The [movement in the] vessels may be contrary to or in accordance with [the proper course of qi]. In males and females it may be regular[1] or in contrast [to what is regular]. What does that mean?

(2) It is like this. A male child is born in a *yin* [month]; a *yin* [month is associated with the phase of] wood, and that is yang. (3) A female child is born in a *shen* [month]; a *shen* [month is associated with the phase of] metal, and that is yin. (4) Hence, in males [a strong movement in] the vessels appears above the gate; in females [a strong movement in the] vessels appears below the gate. (5) Therefore, if in males the [movement in the] vessels is constantly weak in the foot [section], or if in females the [movement in the] vessels is constantly full in the foot [section], that is their regular condition. (6) In a situation that is in contrast to [such a regular condition], a male's vessels display a female [movement, or] a female's vessels display a male [movement].

(7) What kinds of disease does that indicate?

(8) It is like this. If a male's vessels display a female [movement, that indicates that the yang qi are] not enough, and that the disease is situated in the internal [parts of the body]. (9) [In this case] a disease which is felt in the left [hand] is, in fact, located in the left [side of the body], and a disease which is felt in the right [hand] is, in fact, located in the right [side of the body. The disease] can be determined in accordance with the [actual symptoms displayed by the] vessels. (10) If a female's vessels display a male [movement, that indicates that the yang qi] greatly exceed [their normal limits], and that the disease is situated in the four limbs. (11) [In this case, too,] a disease which is felt in the left [hand] is, in fact, located in the left [side of the body], and a disease which is felt in the right [hand] is, in fact, located in the right [side of the body. The disease] can be determined in accordance with the

---

1   Later editions have *heng* 恆 instead of *chang* 常

[actual symptoms displayed by the] vessels. This is [what is] meant by all the [terms mentioned initially].[2]

(1) *Hua Shou*: *Heng* 恆 ("regular") stands for *jing* 經 ("constant"). *Ni shun* 逆順 ("contrary to or in accordance with [the proper course of qi]") means that [a movement in the vessels] that is proper in males is contrary to what is proper in females, and that [a movement] that is proper in females is different from that [which is proper] in males. Still, this [difference] is the normal condition of males and females. *Fan* 反 means "in contrast to what is normal."

Xu Dachun: If one can feel a [movement in the] vessels, that is *shun* 順 ("in accordance with what is regular"). If one cannot feel a [movement in the] vessels, that is *ni* 逆 ("contrary to what is regular"). *Heng* 恆 stands for *chang* 常 ("regular"). That is to say, [the movement in the vessels follows] constantly a specific pattern. "In contrast" means that strength and weakness of the [movement in the vessels in the] upper and lower sections are mutually reversed, as is outlined by the text below. No [corresponding passage] exists in the [*Nei*] *jing* that could be examined [for comparison].

Katō Bankei: The [movement in the] vessels of females is contrary to [the proper course of qi]; the [movement in the] vessels of males is in accordance with [the proper course of qi]. "In accordance with [the proper course of qi]" implies that the qi are generated in spring and summer, and that they move upward from below. "Contrary to [the proper course of qi]" implies that the qi are generated in autumn and winter, and that they move downward from above. This is meant by "in males and females [the movement in the vessels] may be regular." In his commentary, Hua [Shou] does not distinguish between the meanings of *ni shun* 逆順 ("contrary to or in accordance with [the proper course of qi]") and of *fan* 反 ("in contrast to [the regular condition of males and females]"). Thus, he missed the meaning of this dialogue. How is that? In the question of this difficult issue, *ni shun* and *fan* carry two [different] meanings. The answers repeat this differentiation. Students should consider that.

Liao Ping: This difficult issue discusses differences in the [movement in the] vessels of males and females. All the five apocryphal writings have followed its

---

2 This difficult issue is based on the innovative assumption that the movement in the vessels of males and females is different. Hence, these differences have to be taken into account during an examination. The theoretical rationale in sentences 2 and 3 corresponds to the calendrical cycle of the Twelve Earth Branches (*di zhi* 地枝). The application of this pattern is outlined by various commentators below.

[argumentation]. The [movement in the] vessels of males and females are not contrary to each other. This is an erroneous statement.

(2)–(3) *Hua Shou*: This is an investigation of the beginning of living beings which is clad in a discussion of male and female, of yin and yang. Mr. Ji [Tianxi] has said: "All living beings originate in the *zi* 子 [month]."[3] The *zi* [month] is the beginning of all things. From the *zi* [date, the process of generation] is carried on for males to the left for thirty [years] in the [calendrical] cycle, until it reaches the *si* 巳 [date]. For females it is carried on to the right for twenty [years] until it too reaches the *si* [date]. That is the number [of years] at which males and females marry. When pregnancy [begins] in a *si* [month], for males it takes ten months in the cycle to the left; birth occurs in the *yin* 寅 [month]. The *yin* [month is associated with the phase of] wood and with yang. For females, [pregnancy] takes ten months in the cycle to the right. Birth occurs in the *shen* 申 [month]. The *shen* [month is associated with the phase of] metal and with *yin* 陰. Mr. Xie [Jinsun] has said that the *yin* 寅[month] is wood, and wood generates fire. Fire,

---

3   *Zi* 子 is the month of winter solstice. The following calculations are based on the pattern of the cycle of the Twelve Earth Branches:

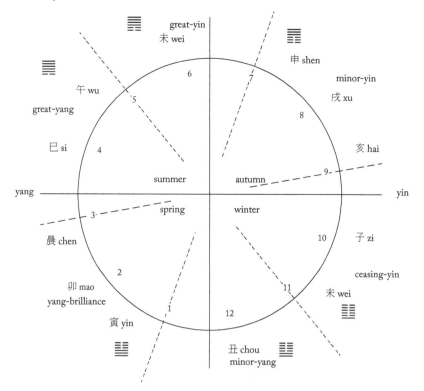

then, is generated in the *yin* 寅 [month] and its nature is to send its flames upward. Hence, in males [a strong movement in] the vessels appears above the gate. The *shen* 申 [month] is metal, and metal generates water. Water, then, is generated in the *shen* [month] and its nature is to flow downward. Hence, in females [a strong movement in] the vessels appears below the gate. My own opinion is that yang bodies are light and clear and that they ascend to the way of heaven. Hence, in males [a strong movement in] the vessels appears above the gate. Yin 陰 bodies are heavy and turbid; they descend to the ways of earth. Hence, in females [a strong movement in] the vessels appears below the gate. That is the normal situation in males and females.

Katō Bankei: This is the answer to the first of the two issues raised. It says that it is natural for males and females to be distinguished by [movements in the vessels that are, in the case of females,] contrary to and, [in the case of males,] in accordance with [the proper course of qi]. The *yin* 寅 [month] is wood; it is yang. That is to say, with the beginning of the *yin* 寅 month, all the qi start to rise from the earth, and the vital qi of all things are in the upper realm. The six branches from *yin* 寅 to *wei* 未 match [the six months of] spring and summer; they are all yang. The *shen* 申 [month] is metal; it is yin 陰. With the beginning of the *shen* [month], the yang qi descend and the yin qi begin to dominate. All the vital qi of the many kinds [of beings] now enter the earth. The six branches from *shen* 申 to *chou* 丑 match [the six months of] autumn and winter; they are all yin 陰. All [earlier] authors have too closely adhered to the statements [in the *Nan jing* referring to] the *yin* 寅 and *shen* 申 [months only]. One should not follow them.

Tamba Genkan: "The [movement in the] vessels may be contrary to or in accordance with [the proper course of qi]" means that there are [movements in the] vessels which are in accordance with [what is proper for] males and contrary to [what is proper for] females, and that there are [movements in the] vessels which are in accordance with [what is proper for] females and contrary to [what is proper for] males .... The [chapter] "Fan lun xun" 凡輪訓 of the *Huai nan zi* 淮南子[4] says: "According to the rites [a man] marries with thirty." And the commentary adds: "[A man] marries at the age of thirty because both [males and females] are born in the *zi* 子 [period] when yin and yang are not yet differentiated. Beginning with the *zi* [period], males count leftward [in the calendrical cycle] and proceed through thirty [years] to reach the *si* 巳 [period]. Females [also] begin with the *zi* 子 [period], count rightward, and proceed until age twenty when they, too, reach the *si* 巳 [period]. Then they enter a union as husband and wife.

---

4 The *Huai nan zi* is supposed to have been compiled in the second century BCE by Liu An 劉安 (d. 122 BCE) or scholars close to him.

Hence, the sages followed this [pattern] when they established the rites. They let males become thirty before they marry, and they let females become twenty before they enter matrimony. For a male child [resulting from their union,] counting starts from the *si* [month] to the left and proceeds through ten [months] until the *yin* 寅 [month]. Hence, a [male] person is born, after ten months, in a *yin* 寅 [month], and the counting of a male's [years of life] starts from *yin* 寅. For a female child, counting starts from the *si* 巳 [month] to the right until the *shen* 申 [month] is reached. [A female person,] too, is born after ten months, but in a *shen* [month]. Hence, the counting of a female's [years of life] starts from *shen*." The *Shuo wen* 說文 states: "*Bao* 包 reflects pregnancy. It has [the character] *si* 巳 in its center. This is the image of a still formless child. The original qi begin to emerge at the *zi* 子 [month]. *Zi* is when man is born. Males proceed to the left for thirty, females proceed to the right for twenty [years]. Both then arrive at *si*. They become husband and wife. Pregnancy begins in a *si* [month]. In the *si* [month] a child [is conceived which] is born after ten months. For males [this process of birth] begins at the *si* 巳 [month] and ends at the *yin* 寅 [month]; for females it begins at the *si* 巳 [month] and ends at the *shen* 申 [month]. Hence, the years of life of males begin with *yin* 寅; the years of life of females begin with *shen* 申."

Liao Ping: These statements originate from the [chapter] "Fan lun xun" 凡輪訓 of the *Huai nan* [*zi*] 淮南子. The *Nei jing* has no such text. From the fact that [the *Nan jing*] quotes many statements from Han Confucians, the *Huai nan* [*zi*], master Dong [Zhongshu] 董仲舒, Xu [Shen] 許慎 and Zheng [Xuan] 鄭玄, Tamba [Genkan] concluded that it appeared rather late.[5] That is correct.

(4)–(5) *Ding Deyong*: When the [text here] speaks of the [movement in the] vessels in the foot [section] of males and females, it [refers to] root and basis of yin and yang. "Contrary to or in accordance with [the proper course of qi]" means that yang [qi] are held while yin [qi] come to life, and that yin [qi] are held while yang [qi] come to life. The three yang start their existence at "spring begins." That is [the date] when the *yin* 寅 [period] commences. Hence, [the text] states: "A male is born in the *yin* 寅 [period], which is wood and yang." The three yin are generated at "autumn begins." In the seventh [month] the *shen* [period] commences. Hence, [the text] states: "A female is born in the *shen* 申 [period], which is metal and yin." The qi of a male child begin [their existence] in the minor yang [period]; they peak in the major yang [period]. That is why in males the [movement in the] vessels in the foot [section] is constantly weak, while the

---

5   Dong Zhongshu (second century BCE); Xu Shen (d. 120 CE); Zheng Xuan (127-200).

[movement in the] vessels in the inch [section] is strong.[6] The qi of a female child begin [their existence] in the major yin [period]; they peak in the ceasing yin [period]. In females the [movement in the] vessels in the foot [section] is at the surface, while it is in the depth in the inch [section]. Hence, [the text] states: "In males [a strong movement in] the vessels appears above the gate; in females [a strong movement in] the vessels appears below the gate."

Yang: In males yang qi abound; hence, the [movement in the] foot [section of the] vessels is weak. In females yin qi abound; hence, the [movement in the] foot [section of their] vessels is strong. That is a normal condition.

Li Jiong: The qi of a male child begin [their existence] in the minor yang [period]; they peak in the major yang [period]: The arrival of minor yang [qi] is at times strong, at times minor, at times short, at times extended. That is [reflected by] the hexagram *fu* 復 ䷗ ("return") of the *Yi* [*jing*] 易經. The first yang resides in the foot section.[7] The arrival of the yang brilliance [qi] is at the surface, strong, and short. That is [reflected by] the hexagram *lin* 臨 ䷒ ("approach") of the *Yi* [*jing*]. The second yang resides in the gate-section. The arrival of the major yang [qi] is vast, strong, and extended. That is [reflected by] the hexagram *tai* 泰 ䷊ ("extreme") of the *Yi* [*jing*]. The third yang resides in the inch section. The three yang grow from the earth; hence, the [movement in the] vessels of a male is [marked by] abundance in the inch [section] and by weakness in the foot [section]. The qi of a female child begin [their existence] in the major yin [period]; they peak in the ceasing yin [period]. The arrival of the major yin [qi] is tight, strong, and extended. That is [reflected by] the hexagram *gou* 姤 ䷫ ("meeting") of the *Yi* [*jing*]. The first yin resides in the inch section. The arrival of the minor yin [qi] is tight, fine, and slight. That is [reflected by] the hexagram *dun* 遯 ䷠ ("retreat") of the *Yi* [*jing*]. The second yin resides in the gate-section. The arrival of the ceasing yin [qi] is in the depth, short, and generous. That is [reflected by] the hexagram *bi* 否 ䷋ ("stoppage") of the *Yi* [*jing*]. The third yin resides in the foot section. The three yin are generated by heaven; hence, the [movement in the] vessels of a female is [marked by] depth in the inch [section] and by abundance in the foot [section].

(6)–(11) *Ding Deyong*: When [the text] states that if a male's vessels display a female [movement,] that is "not enough," it means that the yin [qi] are not enough. Hence, yang [qi] enter and seize [their location]. Hence, the yang [qi] do not appear at the inch opening but, in contrast [to what is proper], they appear in

---

6   The text has *yang* 陽 instead of *qiang* 強.

7   Unbroken lines are categorized as yang; broken lines as yin. The three bottom lines of the hexagrams are considered here to reflect the three sections (i.e., foot, gate, and inch).

the foot-interior [section]. The yin qi control the interior; [here] they are not enough. Hence, one knows that the disease is situated in the internal [parts of the body]. When a female's vessels display a male [movement,] that indicates a [movement] greatly exceeding [its normal limits]. When the disease is situated in the four limbs, the [movement in the] vessels in the foot [section,] which originally is at the surface, is now, in addition, apparent in the inch [section]. That is called "greatly exceeding [its normal limits]." The yang [qi] control the exterior; hence, the disease is situated in the four limbs. If one determines [the location of a disease] according to the [movement in the] vessels [felt] in the left or right [hand], the disease is in the left [side of the body] when one feels the [respective movement] in the left [hand]; the disease is in the right [side of the body] when one feels [the respective movement] in the right [hand].

Zhang Shixian: From the *yin* 寅[month] to the *wu* 午 [month] is the time of spring and summer, when water generates wood. Then, in a normal situation, the inch [section] of males abounds [with qi] while their foot [section is marked by] weakness. From the *shen* 申 [month] to the *zi* 子 [month] is the time of autumn and winter, when metal generates water. Then, in a normal situation, the foot [section] of females abounds [with qi] while their inch [section is marked by] weakness. Thus, if one does not neglect [a lifestyle in] accordance with the ascent and descent of yin and yang, that would be a normal course. If one acts contrary [to the requirements of the seasons], a male's vessels will display a female [movement, that is to say] in spring and summer a [movement appears in the] vessels that [should appear only] in autumn and winter. Or, a female's vessels will display a male [movement, that is to say.] in autumn and winter [a movement appears in] the vessels that [should appear only] in spring and summer. If a male's vessels display a female [movement, this indicates that the yang qi are] not enough. That is, in spring and summer [one feels a movement in the] vessels [which is characteristic] of autumn and winter. In spring and summer all things come to life and grow. Hence, the [movement in the vessels of the] inch [section] should be [marked by] abundance while the [movement in the vessels of the] foot [section should be marked by] weakness. Here, in contrast, abundance marks the foot [section] and weakness marks the inch [section]. This indicates that the water of the kidneys [has become] evil [in that it] has overcome the fire of the heart. The yang qi are not enough. They cannot [stimulate] birth and growth. The disease is in the internal [parts of the body]. If a female's vessels display a male [movement], this means that in autumn and winter one feels [a movement in] the vessels [which is characteristic] of spring and summer. In autumn and winter all things are collected and stored away. Hence, the [movement in the vessels in the] foot [section] should be [marked by] abundance, while the inch [section should be marked by] weakness. Here, in contrast, abundance marks the inch [section] and weakness marks the foot [section]. This indicates that the depletion fire[8] abounds while the water of the kidneys is exhausted. The yang [qi have turned] evil [in that they] greatly exceed [their normal limits]; they cannot be collected and stored away. The disease is in the external [parts of the body].

Liao Ping: A difference in the manifestation of disease in males and females appears only at their reproductive openings. In every other aspect they are identical. The *Nei jing* does not discuss different diagnostic patterns for males and females. With such a theory this book can no longer honor the ancient [diagnostic] patterns. If the examination is to be carried out with but one finger, why should there be the difference between foot and inch section? The overall fabrication intended here is an absorption of the three sections into the two inch [sections of the two hands]; the difference between males and females is used as illustrative material. But if the skin exists no longer, how could the hair remain at its place? The best remedy would be to delete all this with a single stroke of one's pen!

(8)–(11) *Katō Bankei*: This is the second answer. This section discusses how greatly excessive or insufficient [qi] are responsible for [diseases in] heart and lung, as well as in kidneys and liver; it refers to unilateral depletion or repletion of the qi or of the blood. When [the text] says: "A male's vessels display a female [movement]," with a weak [movement appearing] in the inch [section] while the foot [section] is full, that can be compared to the failure of yang qi to rise in spring and summer when they remain, instead, down in the earth. In this case the yin has a surplus while the yang does not have enough. Hence, the disease is located in the internal [section of the body). This is to say that the yin section is stronger [than the yang section]. "If a female's vessels display a male [movement, this indicates that the yang qi] greatly exceed [their normal limits]" – [in this case] the inch [section] is full while the [movement in the] foot [section] is weak. That is to say, the yin does not have enough and the yang has a surplus. This can be compared to the failure of the yang [qi] to descend in autumn and winter when they stay above the earth. Hence, the sections of heart and lung dominate. The first "left" and "right" refer to the position of the [movement in the] vessels; the second "left" and "right" refer to the long-term depot sections.

(10) *Liao Ping*: This kind of talk is not even worth a contradiction.

(11) *Liao Ping*: If such differences did in fact exist between males and females, not a single medical pattern could be [applied to both sexes] alike.

---

8 *Xu huo* 虛火 ("depletion fire") is the term used to indicate a condition in which heat in the body results from a depletion of yin qi.

二十難曰：（一）經言脈有伏匿，伏匿於何藏而言伏匿耶？
（二）然：謂陰陽更相乘，更相伏也。（三）脈居陰部而反陽脈見者，為陽乘
陰也；（四）脈雖時沉濇而短，此謂陽中伏陰也；（五）脈居陽部而反陰脈見
者，為陰乘陽也；（六）脈雖時浮滑而長，此謂陰中伏陽也。（七）重陽者
狂，重陰者癲。（八）脫陽者見鬼，脫陰者目盲。

The twentieth difficult issue: (1) The scripture states: The [movement in the] vessels
may be hidden and concealed. In which long-term depot could [qi] be hidden and
concealed so that one may speak of them as being hidden and concealed?

(2) It is like this. [The statement referred to] implies that yin and yang [qi] seize
each other's [proper section], and that yin and yang [qi may] hide in each other. (3)
A [yin movement in the] vessels resides in the yin section. If, in contrast, a yang
[movement in the] vessels appears here, this indicates that yang [qi] have seized the
yin [section]. (4) But if [that movement in the yin] vessels is at times deep, rough,
and short, this indicates that yin [qi] lie hidden among the yang [qi]. (5) A [yang
movement in the] vessels resides in the yang section. If, in contrast, a yin [move-
ment in the] vessels appears here, this indicates that yin [qi] have seized the yang
[section]. (6) But if [that movement in the yang] vessels is at times at the surface,
smooth, and extended, this implies that yang [qi] lie hidden among the yin [qi]. (7)
A doubling of the yang [qi results in] madness; a doubling of the yin [qi results in]
peak-illness. (8) When the yang [qi] are lost, one sees demons; when the yin [qi] are
lost, one's eyes turn blind.

COMMENTARIES

(1) *Xu Dachun*: No [corresponding text exists in the *Nei jing* that could be] examined [for comparison with] the "statement from the scripture" quoted here.
"Hidden and concealed" means that [a specific movement in the] vessels cannot
be perceived at its proper location but is, in contrast, stored away in another
section and can be perceived there.

(2)–(3) *Ding Deyong*: The [yin and yang] sections referred to here are not simply
the inch [section] as yang and the foot [section] as yin. Speaking in terms of
"in front" and "behind," the inch represents the yang section while the foot represents the yin section. But speaking in terms of "above" and "below," the [sec-
tion] above the flesh constitutes the yang section while the [section] below the
flesh constitutes the yin section. Here, [an example is given of] a depletion of
yin qi, [that is to say, a situation in which yin qi] are not enough, [so that] yang
[qi] enter and seize [their section]. Hence, a yang [movement in the] vessels ap-

pears in the yin section.¹ When this [movement in the] vessels is at times deep, rough, and short, this indicates that yin [qi] lie hidden among the yang [qi].

Yang: That is to say, the [movement to be felt in the] foot [section] is at the surface, smooth, and extended.

Hua Shou: "To seize" is used here in the sense of "to climb on and ride in a car." "To lie hidden" is used here in the sense of "soldiers lying in ambush."

Liao Ping: Here, [on the one hand,] the appearance of the [movement in the] vessels is differentiated according to yin and yang, and [on the other hand,] the sections [where these movements appear] are differentiated according to yin and yang. When a yang [movement in the] vessels appears in the yin section, that is considered to be "hidden and concealed." That is, the yin section has a yin [movement in the] vessels as its resident, and the yang [movement in the] vessels of the yang section is considered as a separate item. When [the latter] leaves the yang section and arrives at the yin section, the yin [movement in the] vessels fears it and retreats. This kind of talk is, indeed, completely ignorant of the principles of the [movement in the] vessels!

(4)–(5) *Ding Deyong*: In the inch opening and above the flesh, [a movement of qi] occurs from time to time that is in the depth, rough, and short.

Yang: [The movement of the qi] in the foot [section] is entirely at the surface, smooth, and extended. However, from time to time it appears in the depth, rough, and short. Hence, [the text] states: "Yin [qi] lie hidden among the yang [qi]." The movement that appears in the] inch opening and in the gate [section is permanently] in the depth, short, and rough.

Xu Dachun: That is to say, even though the yang qi have seized the yin [section], still yin [qi] lie hidden among the yang [qi].

(6) *Ding Deyong*: If the [movement in the] vessels in the inch opening and below the flesh appears occasionally at the surface, smooth, and extended, this indicates that yang [qi] lie hidden among the yin [qi].

Yang: The [movement in the] inch and gate [sections appears] entirely in the depth, short, and rough, But from time to time it is at the surface, smooth, and extended, Hence, [the text] states: "Yang [qi] lie hidden among the yin [qi]."

(7)–(8) *Ding Deyong*: "A doubling of the yang [qi results in] madness" – that is to say, if the [movement in the] vessels is at the surface, smooth, and extended – and if it is, in addition, replete and frequent – [the patient] will talk madly of great affairs. He will perceive himself to be in a high position and to have wisdom like a sage. He will madly overstep [propriety] and he will take off his clothes, The

---

1 Qian Xizuo has commented that the character *cheng* 乘 ("to seize") is a mistaken addition here. It seems to be superfluous and I have omitted it.

[statement,] "when the yin [qi] are lost, one's eyes turn blind," [means] that suddenly one loses his ability to see something. Hence, [the text] speaks of "blindness." Here *mang* 盲 ("blind") equals *huang* 荒 ("empty", "barren"). "A doubling of the yin [qi results in] peak-illness": Here *dian* 癲 ("peak-illness") stands for *jue* 蹶 ("to fall")."When the yang [qi] are lost," the patient will see demons in the dark. That is why the [*Nan*] *jing* says: "A doubling of the yang [qi results in] madness; a doubling of the yin [qi results in] peak-illness. When the yang [qi] are lost, one sees demons; when the yin [qi] are lost, one's eyes turn blind."

Yang: "A doubling of the yang [qi]" indicates a concentration of yang qi in the upper [section]. That is to say, [the movement in the vessels] in front of the gate is at the surface, smooth, and extended, At the same time it is replete and vigorous, In addition, it is panting and frequent. That is called "a doubling of the yang [qi]." "A doubling of the yin [qi]" refers to a [movement] in the foot [section] that is in the depth, short, and rough, and, furthermore, full and replete. That is called "a doubling of the yin [qi]." "When the yang [qi] are lost" [refers to an] absence of yang qi. That is to say, [the movement in the vessels] in front of the gate is very fine and slight. Hence, one's vision is blurred and he sees demonic beings. "When the yin [qi] are lost" refers to a very slight and fine [movement] in the foot [section]. The yin [qi] are the essence qi. When the essence qi are lost, blindness results. The expressions *mang* 盲 ("blind") and *tuo* 脱 ("lost") stand for *shi* 失 ("to lose"). That is to say, one has lost yin or yang qi.

Yu Shu: The inch opening is termed yang. Here, a yang [movement in the] vessels appears that is [increased] more than threefold. Hence, [the text] speaks of a "doubling of yang." The resulting disease is madness and delusion. [The patient] perceives himself to be in a high position and to have wisdom like a sage. He will climb on high locations and start singing. He will take off his clothes and run around [in this condition]. He will use insulting language regardless of whether he meets relatives or strangers. Hence, [the text] speaks of "madness." The foot [section] is termed yin. [Here] a double yin [movement] appears in the foot [section of the] vessels. Hence, [the text] speaks of a "doubling of yin." The resulting disease is called "peak-illness." That is to say, [the patient] falls down on the earth, has his eyes closed, and does not wake up. When the yin peaks, the yang returns. Hence, after a long time [the respective person] will wake up again. Hence, one speaks of *dian* 癲. This [term] corresponds to contemporary expressions like *tian diao* 天弔 ("visitations by heaven"). Man is endowed with yin and yang [qi]. When the yin and yang [qi] are balanced, [his entire organism] is adjusted. Here, the yin qi are lost and only the yang qi are present in abundance. The five long-term depots belong to the yin. The five long-term depots transmit the qi and the blood to pour them [wherever they are needed]. Above, they provide nourishment to the eyes. Here, the yin qi are lost. The qi of the five long-term depots cannot provide nourishment to the eyes. Hence, the eyes turn blind and cannot see anything. Hence, [the text] states: "When the yin [qi] are lost, the eyes turn blind."

Hua Shou: This is a mistaken abridgment of the text of the fifty-ninth difficult issue that has been placed here.

Zhang Shixian: When yang [movements appear] in both the foot and the inch [sections], that is a "double yang [movement]." When yin [movements appear] in both the foot and the inch [sections], that is a "double yin [movement]." Madness is a yang disease; peak-illness is a yin disease. Demons belong to the yin. One sees them when the yang [qi] are lost. The eyes are the essence of yin; they turn blind when the yin [qi] are lost.

Katō Bankei: Hua [Shou] has stated that this text on madness and peak-illness has been mistakenly abridged from the fifty-ninth difficult issue. In my view that is not so. The discussion there is concerned with diseases that originate internally, in that an unbalanced repletion of the qi in the long-term depots emerges. Here, yang and yin symptoms occur because one suffers from harm due to cold or heat. These diseases originate externally. Hence, one sees demons or becomes blind and dies afterwards. Madness and peak-illness as discussed there, [in the fifty-ninth difficult issue, refer to] a loss of the proper qi themselves. Essence and spirit are dispersed; they do not return to their original shelter. Such [a situation] may continue for years without end. How could it [be related to] such dangerous and acute situations as blind eyes or the perception of demons? Students must investigate all this.

(8) *Xu Dachun*: When the eyes are supplied with blood, they can see. When the yin [qi] are lost, no blood is available to nourish the eyes. Hence, they will turn blind.

(1)–(8) *Liao Ping*: In conclusion, the author(s) of this book did not understand the literature, they did not know the principles of the [movement in the] vessels, and when they added a quotation from the text of the [*Nei*] *jing*, their explanations were all wrong and based on erroneous readings. This difficult issue is particularly meaningless.

二十一難曰：（一）經言人形病、脈不病曰生，脈病、形不病曰死，何謂也？（二）然：人形病，脈不病，非有不病者也，謂息數不應脈數也。（三）此大法。

The twenty-first difficult issue: (1) The scripture states: If a person's physical appearance has a disease while the [movement in his] vessels has no disease, that implies life. If the [movement in the] vessels has a disease while the physical appearance has no disease, that implies death. What does that mean?

(2) It is like this. If a person's physical appearance has a disease while the [movement in his] vessels has no disease, that does not mean that [the movement in his vessels has] no disease; it means that one's breathing frequency does not correspond to the [movement in the] vessels. (3) That is a pattern of great [importance]!

COMMENTARIES

(1) *Ding Deyong*: This [question refers to the fact that] each of the five long-term depots has [some other entity in the organism] which it controls. The lung controls the [breathing] qi; the heart controls the vessels; the spleen controls the flesh; the liver controls the muscles; the kidneys control the bones. Heart and lung control the breathing and the vessels; thus, they are responsible for the passage of the qi of heaven [through the body]. They must not be struck by evil [qi]. If they are struck by evil [qi], the [frequencies of the] breathing and of the [movement in the] vessels do no longer correspond to each other. Although the physical appearance has no disease, one should know that death [is imminent]. Kidneys, liver, and spleen control [man's] physical appearance; they all are responsible for the passage of the qi of the earth. If they are struck by evil [qi], the physical appearance will be injured. If the [movement in the] vessels does not yet display a disease, life [will continue]. Once both the physical appearance and the [movement in the] vessels are affected by a disease, nothing can be done. That is [what is] meant by [the statement] that each of the five long-term depots controls either the physical appearance or the [movement in the] vessels. Hence, [the text below] speaks of a "pattern of great [importance]."

Li Jiong: "If the physical appearance has a disease," [means that] the body is thin and emaciated; hands and feet are numb. "If the [movement in the] vessels has no disease," [means that] the movement in the vessels corresponds to the up and down of exhalation and inhalation, neither greatly exceeding nor falling short [of its normal limits]. The [prognostic] judgment is [that the respective person will continue to] live. "If the [movement in the] vessels has a disease" [means that] an examination of the frequency of the arrival [of the qi will reveal a movement] either greatly exceeding or falling short [of its normal limits]. Thus, a person may not yet suffer from ailments such as fits of cold or heat. Even though he [appears] not to have a disease, he will nevertheless die.

(2) *Lü Guang*: "The physical appearance has a disease" means that the five long-term depots are hurt. The physical appearance is emaciated; the [movement of the] qi is slight. The [movement in the] vessels is reversed and slow; it does not correspond to the [frequency of the] breathing. Thus, when the [frequency of the breathing] does not correspond to the [movement in the] vessels, that is a disease of the physical appearance. "The [movement in the] vessels has a disease" means that [the movement of the qi] arrives with [increased] frequency. When the [movement in the] vessels has a disease, the respective person may not yet suffer from headache or from fits of cold or heat. The disease has just [emerged]; it has not yet continued for long. When [the person begins to perceive his] disease, he will [soon] die.

Li Jiong: By "[movement in the] vessels," the blood is meant here. By "breathing," the qi are meant here. The movement in the vessels [i.e., of the blood] does not occur by itself; it is caused by the qi. Here now, the breathing [frequency] of the qi does not correspond to the frequency of the [movement in the] vessels by the blood.

(1)–(2) *Zhang Shixian*: The [movement in the] vessels is most decisive for man. Hence, if [this movement in] the vessels is balanced, that means life. If the [movement in the] vessels has a disease, that means death. The [movement in the] vessels and the physical appearance [should] fit each other like the two halves of a tally. If the [movement in the] vessels has a disease while the physical appearance does not, then the [movement in the] vessels has lost its normal status; it may, for instance, appear intermittent. Hence, one knows that the [respective person] will die. "The [movement in the] vessels has no disease" does not mean that the [movement in the] vessels has no disease; it means that the frequency of the breathing does not correspond to the frequency of the [movement in the] vessels. That is [what is] meant when [the text] says "no disease is present." The [movement in the] vessels may indeed have a disease. The frequency of human breathing through exhalation and inhalation, regardless of [whether one is] male or female, amounts in one day and one night to 13,500 breathing [periods. In this time, the movement in the] vessels proceeds over 810 *zhang* 丈. In the case of a disease, this is different, in that the frequency of the breathing and of the [movement in the] vessels either greatly exceeds or falls short of [their normal limits]. Hence, it is customary to take [the condition of someone who has] no disease [as a standard] for regulating [the condition of] the person with the disease."One's breathing frequency does not correspond to the [movement in the] vessels" means that the physician, in his examination, takes his own breathing frequency [as a standard for measuring the movement in] the vessels of the patient. [He may feel that] with each of his breathing [periods, the movement in the patient's vessels] has five arrivals, thus reaching 810 *zhang*. Still, the patient's breathing frequency may not coincide with the amount of 13,500 [breathing periods per day and night]. Thus, the physician knows only that the frequency [of the arrival of the movement in the patient's] vessels corresponds to his own breathing, and he will tell the [patient] that he has no disease. But [the physician] does not know that the [patient's] breathing frequency does not correspond to his own.

Xu Dachun: In a case where "a person's physical appearance has a disease while the [movement in the] vessels has no disease," [that person] has received, for instance, evil cold which has not penetrated deeply [into the body. The cold] is unable to cause changes and disturbances among the qi and the blood. Hence, life [will continue]. "If the [movement in the] vessels has a disease while the physical appearance has no disease," then the evil qi have already penetrated deeply [into the body]; they lie hidden and will not come out. Blood and qi are disturbed first. Hence, death [results]. That is very straight-forward. The present answer, however, is quite beside the point [of the question]. I fear that something has been left out by mistake. Also, in the treatise "Bian mai fa" 辨脈法 of the *Shang han lun* 傷寒論 [it is said]: If the [movement in the] vessels has a disease while the person has no disease, that is called a "walking corpse" because no "governing qi" are present. [That person] will be dizzy, fall down, and recognize nobody. His life will be shortened and he will die. If the person has a disease while the [movement in the] vessels has no disease, that is called "inner depletion" because no qi from the grains are present. That may be a hardship, but it does not constitute suffering. The meaning of this is clear too.

Ding Jin: This chapter elucidates the meaning of [what happens when] the qi have contracted a disease first and the blood is affected afterwards, and vice versa. Thus it introduces the issue raised in the following chapter. That is to say, when the physical appearance has a disease while the [movement in the] vessels has no disease, that does not mean that the [movement in the] vessels is free from disease. It is just that the frequency of the patient's breathing does not correspond to the frequency of the [movement in his] vessels. Consider, for instance, [a situation in which] evil [qi] have entered his qi. The qi belong to the yang and correspond to the external [parts of the organism]. Hence, the physical appearance will be affected by the disease first, and the breathing, too, will be disturbed first. The [disturbance of the movement in the] vessels will follow later. It is not that the [movement in the] vessels will not be affected by the disease at all. This means that the physical appearance contracts the disease first, and the breathing frequency no longer corresponds to the frequency of the [movement in the] vessels, [which remains normal for some time]. Consider, for example [a situation in which] evil [qi] have entered the blood. The blood belongs to the yin and corresponds to the internal [parts of the organism]. In this case the physical appearance will be affected by the disease only later, and the breathing, too, will be disturbed later, although the [movement in the] vessels has been already affected by the disease. It is not that the physical appearance will not be affected by the disease at all. This means that the [movement in the] vessels is affected by the disease first, and the frequency of the [movement in the] vessels no longer corresponds to the breathing frequency, [which remains normal for some time]. This is a pattern of great [importance that elucidates the consequences of] whether the qi or the blood are affected by a disease first or later. [The text] speaks of "life" because the disease is in the external [parts of the organism, i.e., in the] short-term repositories. [The text] speaks of "death" because the disease is in the internal [parts of the organism, i.e., in the] long-term depots.

Liao Ping: Both question and answer raise no [point] at all. Why was it necessary to establish this difficult issue? For no reason other than to expand the contents [of this book] in order to reach the number of eighty-one [treatises].

Nan jing 1962: This difficult issue states "a [person's] physical appearance has a disease while the [movement in the] vessels has no disease" and "the [movement in the] vessels has a disease while the physical appearance has no disease" in order to elucidate – by comparing a [person's] physical appearance and the [movement in his] vessels – the relationship between various courses a disease may take and prognostic [diagnosis]. The basic meaning of this [difficult issue is to focus attention on] whether the [movement in the] vessels and the [bodily] symptoms correspond to each other, and whether the physical appearance and the [movement of the] qi coincide with each other. Furthermore, it emphasizes the importance of the appearances of the [movement in the] vessels because the appearances of the [movement in the] vessels accurately reflect the [conditions of the] true qi in the human body. For this reason they are of particular importance for prognostic diagnosis. Hence, the original text says: "If a person's physical appearance has a disease while the [movement in the] vessels has no disease, that implies life" and "if the [movement in the] vessels has a disease while the physical appearance has no disease, that implies death." This pattern coincides with a statement in the [treatise] "Fang sheng shuai lun" 方盛衰論 of the *Su wen*: "When the qi of the physical appearance have a surplus while the qi in the vessels are not enough, death [must follow]. When the qi in the vessels have a surplus while the qi of the physical appearance are not enough, life [will continue]."

二十二難曰：（一）經言脈有是動，（二）有所生病。（三）一脈輒變為二病者，何也？

（四）然：經言是動者，氣也；所生病者，血也。（五）邪在氣，氣為是動；（六）邪在血，血為所生病。（七）氣主呴之，（八）血主濡之。（九）氣留而不行者，為氣先病也；（十）血壅而不濡者，為血後病也。故先為是動，後所生病也。

The twenty-second difficult issue: (1) The scripture states: The [movement in the] vessels may be excited, (2) and it may be marked by diseases that are generated. (3) One single [movement in the] vessels may, therefore, be the result of two kinds of disease. How is that?

(4) It is like this. When the scripture speaks of "excitement," the qi are meant; [when the scripture speaks of] diseases "that are generated," the blood is meant. (5) When evil [qi] have entered one's [proper] qi, these qi will be excited. (6) When evil [qi] have entered one's blood, the blood will have a disease that is generated [by the disease that had affected the qi first]. (7) The qi are responsible for providing the [body] with a warm flow; (8) the blood is responsible for providing the [body] with moisture. (9) When the qi stagnate and do not move, the qi were affected by a disease first. (10) When the blood is obstructed [in its movement] and fails to moisten the body, the blood was affected by that disease later on. Thus, first comes an excitement and then, afterwards, [come the diseases] that are generated.[1]

---

1   This difficult issue introduces new meanings for the *Ling shu* terms *shi dong* 是動 and *suo sheng bing* 所生病. It states that when evil qi hit the organism, they affect the guard qi first and the blood afterwards. This is a rather straightforward message, yet the commentaries added by later authors are rather heterogeneous. The reasons for the great degree of conceptual confusion and for the absence of a stringent, technical terminology in the medicine of systematic correspondence are highlighted here most clearly. They are to be seen in the fact that at no time in the first or second millennium did more recent conceptual insights replace older views for good. Instead, later innovative ideas (and the contents of the *Nan jing* are to be counted among them) were interpreted by some commentators on the basis of their understanding of the "original" concepts, while others accepted the innovations for what they were. When an author introduced a new meaning of an ancient term, this meaning did not eventually replace the older meaning(s) but was merely added to the existing range of meanings. This increased the insecurity among the readers as to what a particular author really wanted to say. The terms *shi dong* and *suo sheng bing* can be traced to the *Yin yang shi yi mai jiu jing* 陰陽十一脈灸經, a fragment of which was found among the Ma wang dui scripts in the early 1970s (see Anon., *Wu shi er bing fang* 五十二病方, Beijing, 1979, 10-20). This fragment contains a listing of the then eleven *mai* 脈 which were not yet understood as parts of a circulatory system of conduits, but as individual entities. It is not even clear whether the *Yin yang shi yi mai jiu jing* considered the *mai* – as did for instance the Ma wang dui fragment *Mai fa* 脈法

(1) *Yu Shu*: That is a movement which is in contrast to what is normal.

(2) *Yu Shu*: The movement in the vessels is in contrast to what is normal. Hence, [the text] says: "It may be marked by diseases that are generated."

(3) *Yu Shu*: Diseases of the qi are transmitted to the blood. That is [what is meant by] *yi mai bian wei er bing* (perhaps, "one single vessel may be affected by two diseases").

(1)–(3) *Xu Dachun*: This is not the complete text of the [*Nei*] *jing*. This text here is an abridgment of statements in the [*Nei*] *jing*. The term *mai* refers here to the conduit vessels. For a discussion of the "excitement" and of the "diseases that are generated," see the treatise "Jing mai" 經脈 of the *Ling* [*shu*]. "Two kinds of disease" refers to the diseases listed in the text of the [*Nei*] *jing* under "excitement" and under "diseases that are generated."

Liao Ping: The treatise "Jing mai" 經脈 states for each of the twelve conduit vessels: "In the case of an excitement, the diseases resulting are [etc., etc.]" Further down, [the *Nei jing*] states that this [excitement] is responsible for diseases generated in specific other areas [of the organism]. For example, [once the conduit of] the large intestine [is affected by a disease due to excitement, it] is responsible for the generation [of diseases] among the body's liquids, and the [conduit of the] stomach is said to be responsible for the generation of diseases of the blood. Thus, an initial summarization is followed by specific records [of various manifestations of a disease in the respective conduit vessels]. Strangely enough, those men who have explained the [*Nei*] *jing* up to now have considered [diseases due to] "excitement" as one category and "diseases that are generated" as another

---

– as tube-like entities which could contain too much or not enough *qi* 氣 or whether it still saw them as strings linking various sections of the body. It may have been the string concept of *mai* which led to the terms *shi dong* 是動 and *suo sheng bing* 所生病. *Shi dong* could be interpreted as "set in motion" and *suo sheng bing* as the "illnesses resulting secondarily" from the *mai* motion. Hence, for each of the eleven *mai*, the *Yin yang shi yi mai jiu jing* lists various symptoms indicating the motion itself, and then various symptoms (partly overlapping with the former) indicating the diseases resulting from that motion. In the treatise "Jing mai" of the *Ling shu*, we find an obviously more recent listing of the characteristics of the now twelve conduit vessels. The structure of the descriptions is the same as in the *Yin yang shi yi mai jiu jing*. After an outline of the course a conduit takes in the body, the text says *shi dong* and lists a number of diseases. Since the string concept of the *mai* cannot be applied here, the meaning of the ancient terms must have been changed. Zhang Yin'an 張隱庵 (ca. 1700), in his *Huang Di Nei jing ling shu ji zhu* 黃帝內經靈樞集注, may have been correct when he interpreted *shi dong* as "affected by an external stimulus" and *suo sheng bing* (which replaced *suo chan bing*) as "illnesses generated internally," possibly as a secondary result of the primary affect. The terms appeared again, supplied with a third meaning, in the *Nan jing*.

category. This is different from the meaning of the text. [These commentators] did not know that they followed the lead of the apocryphal *Nan jing*. Whoever has compiled this apocryphal book used the name of Yueren as his pseudonym. That he was unable to read the ancient books is reflected by this [difficult issue,] which is most ridiculous .... Xu [Dachun's] commentary distinguishes between two kinds [of disease] too. [Xu] was not aware that the diseases listed below the initial summarization are specific records [of various manifestations of a disease in the individual conduit vessels]. Hence, his explanation is inadequate.

(4) *Liao Ping*: This is in stark contrast to the original text [of the *Nei jing*].

(5) *Yu Shu*: When the movement in the vessels is in contrast to what is normal, evil [qi] have entered the [proper] qi.

(6) *Yu Shu*: When the [proper] qi have received evil [qi], they transmit them to the blood. Hence, the blood is affected by diseases that are generated [by the qi].

(1)–(6) *Zhang Shixian*: *Yi mai* 一脈 ("one single vessel") refers to the vessel of one specific conduit. "Two kinds of disease" are the diseases of the blood and of the [guard] qi. The [movement in the] vessels is tied to individual conduits; two kinds of disease may result from changes [in that movement]. In man's entire body, the blood constitutes the camp [qi] while the qi constitute the guard [qi]. The camp [qi] move inside the vessels; the guard [qi] move outside of the vessels. Evil [qi] enter from outside; they affect the [guard] qi first and are then transmitted to the blood. The blood corresponds to the [proper] qi. The rise and the descent of the blood coincides with the rise and the descent of the [proper] qi. When the [proper] qi receive evil [qi], the [latter] must be transmitted to the blood. Hence, the diseases of the blood are generated by the [proper] qi.

(7) *Ding Deyong*: "The qi are responsible for providing the [body] with a warm flow." *Xu xu* 呴呴 reflects the image of the arrival of a genial breeze.

    Yu Shu: *Xu zhi* 呴之 ("provide the body with a warm flow") refers to the flow of the qi.

    Hua Shou: *Xu* 呴 stands for *xu* 煦 ("warm"). "The qi are responsible for providing the [body] with a warm flow" means that man's true qi arrive like a genial breeze, steaming through the interspace between skin and flesh. "The blood is responsible for providing the [body] with moisture" means that man's blood vessels moisten his muscles and bones, soften his joints, and nourish his body's long-term depots and short-term repositories. The term *mai* 脈 here is not the *mai* 脈 ("movement in the vessels") of the foot and inch [sections]; it is the *mai* 脈 ("vessel") of the twelve conduit-channels. That is to say, in each vessel of the twelve conduit vessels there may be two kinds of disease – namely, those affecting the division of the qi and those affecting the division of the blood. When evil [qi] reside among the [proper] qi, these qi will be excited as a result. When evil [qi] reside in the blood, the blood has a disease that is generated [as a result of the excitement of the proper qi]. When the [proper] qi stagnate and do not move, that is a disease of the qi; when the blood is obstructed [in its movement] and cannot moisten [the body any longer], that is a disease of the blood. Hence, first comes the excitement and then, afterwards, come the diseases generated [as a consequence of this excitement]. One speaks of "first" and "afterwards" because the [guard] qi are in the external [parts of the body] while the blood is in the internal [parts of the body]. The external [parts] are affected by evil qi first; the internal [parts] follow and are affected by the disease afterwards. However, evil [qi] may also remain among the [proper] qi [without affecting the blood later on], and they may reach the blood directly [without having affected the proper qi first]. One should not adhere to this [doctrine of] "first" and "afterwards" too closely. "Scripture" refers to treatise 10 of the *Ling shu*.

(8) *Ding Deyong*: "The blood is responsible for providing the [body] with moisture." *Ru* 濡 means "to moisten," "to soften." When the qi move, the blood moves; when the qi stop, the blood stops too.

Yu Shu: *Ru* 濡 refers to "moistening." That is to say, the human body is endowed with the qi and with blood. The qi and the blood proceed through [the entire body]. Their diseases are outlined below.

(9)–(10) *Ding Deyong*: Man's conduit vessels pass qi and blood through his entire body. It may occur that [the qi and the blood] settle in one specific conduit vessel. When the qi stagnate and do not move, the blood will, as a result, also be obstructed [in its movement] and cannot moisten [the body any longer]. The qi are affected by a disease first; that is called *shi dong* 是動 ("excitement"). The obstruction [of the movement] of the blood and [the latter's] failure to moisten [the body] constitute a secondary disease. That is called *suo sheng* 所生 ("generated"). That is [what is] meant by *yi mai che bian wei er bing* 一脈輒變爲二病 (here, "one single vessel may develop two kinds of disease").

Yu Shu: The first section of the text states: "The [movement in the] vessels may be excited." *Dong* 動 ("movement," "excitement") is yang. That is to say, at first the qi receive heat. The heat will also be transmitted to the blood. Then, qi and blood have both received heat. As a consequence, the body's liquids will move in a disorderly fashion. Thus, one knows that "the [movement in the] vessels is excited." Here, [the text] says: "The [qi] stagnate and do not move." This means that the qi and the blood as well as the body's liquids move in a disorderly fashion. [Then the] robber wind hits them. Hence, they do not move at all. The qi transmit [the robber wind] to the blood. Hence, the blood is obstructed [in its movement] and does not moisten [the body any longer]. It has also received the robber wind. Hence, the [movement of the] blood comes to a halt and has a disease.

Yang: Man has been endowed with the qi and with the blood to govern his existence. The qi are yang. Yang [qi] are the guard [qi]. The blood is yin. Yin [qi] are the camp [qi]. Normally, these two kinds of qi [i.e., the guard qi and the blood] flow [through the organism]; under this condition no disease is present. Evil [qi] hit the yang [qi]. The yang [qi] are the [guard] qi. Hence, these qi are the first to be affected by a disease. That is because the yang qi are located in the external [parts of the organism]. If no cure is achieved while [the disease is still] in the yang [section], it will enter then the yin [section, i.e., the yin qi]. The yin [qi] are the blood. Hence, the blood is affected by a disease afterwards. That is because the blood is located in the internal [section of the organism]. When the qi are replete, heat results. When the qi are depleted, cold results. When the blood is replete, cold results; when the blood is depleted, heat results. The reason for this lies in the principles of yin and yang. The diseases of each long-term depot include depletion and repletion, cold and heat, and they may be [located or caused] internally or externally. In each case one must know the location of the long-term depots and short-term repositories, and one must be familiar with the [course of the] flow of the [qi through the main] conduits and network [vessels]. diseases must be investigated beginning with their place of origin. Only then can the symptoms of the diseases be differentiated properly so that the application of needles or drugs will not result in failure. If someone is not familiar with these principles, it would be difficult for him to cure diseases even though he knew drugs or inserted needles.

(1)–(10) *Xu Dachun*: In the treatise "Jing mai" [of the *Ling shu*], all diseases due to "excitement" are those of the conduit where [a particular disease] has originated, while all "diseases that are generated" are those that are transmitted, by analogy [to the patterns of the Five Phases, from the original conduit] to neighboring and other conduits. The text of the [*Nei*] *jing* is very clear on this; there is no such statement that these [diseases] correspond to the division between qi and blood.

Chapter Two
The Conduits and the Network vessels

THE TWENTY-THIRD DIFFICULT ISSUE

二十三難曰：（一）手足三陰三陽，脈之度數，可曉以不？

（二）然：手三陽之脈，從手至頭，長五尺，五六合三丈。（三）手三陰之脈，從手至胸中，長三尺五寸，三六一丈八尺，五六三尺，合二丈一尺。（四）足三陽之脈，從足至頭，長八尺，六八四丈八尺。（五）足三陰之脈，從足至胸，長六尺五寸，六六三丈六尺，五六三尺，合三丈九尺。（六）人兩足蹻脈，從足至目，長七尺五寸，二七一丈四尺，二五一尺，合一丈五尺。（七）督脈、任脈，各長四尺五寸，二四八尺，二五一尺，合九尺。（八）凡脈長一十六丈二尺，此所謂十二經脈長短之數也。

（九）經脈十二，絡脈十五，何始何窮也？

（十）然：經脈者，行血氣，通陰陽，以榮於身者也。（十一）其始從中焦，注手太陰、陽明；陽明注足陽明、太陰；太陰注手少陰、太陽；太陽注足太陽、少陰；少陰注手心主、少陽；少陽注足少陽、厥陰；厥陰復還注手太陰。（十二）別絡十五，（十三）皆因其原，如環無端，轉相灌溉，（十四）朝於寸口、人迎，以處百病，而決死生也。

（十五）經曰：明知終始，陰陽定矣，何謂也？

（十六）然：終始者，脈之紀也。（十七）寸口、人迎，陰陽之氣通於朝使，如環無端，故曰始也。（十八）終者，三陰三陽之脈絕，絕則死。死各有形，故曰終也。

The twenty-third difficult issue: (1) Can one be instructed on the measurements of the three yin and three yang vessels of the hands and feet?

(2) It is like this. The vessels of the three hand yang [conduits] extend from the hands to the head. They are five feet long. Five [feet] times six amounts to three *zhang*.(3) The vessels of the three hand yin [conduits] extend from the hands into the chest.[1] They are three feet five inches long. Three [feet] times six amounts to one

---

1   In a corresponding *Nei jing* outline – in *Ling shu* treatise 17, "Mai du" 脈度 – the courses of the conduits take the same direction as is indicated here. It should be pointed out, however, that the conduit directions defined in the present paragraph and in the "Mai du" do not completely coincide with those defined elsewhere in the *Nei jing*, (i.e., in *Ling shu* treatise 10, "Jing mai" 經脈), where the hand yin and foot yang conduits are assigned

zhang eight feet; five [inches] times six amounts to three feet. Together this is two *zhang* and one foot. (4) The vessels of the three foot yang [conduits] extend from the feet to the head. They are eight feet long. Six times eight [feet] amounts to four *zhang* and eight feet. (5) The vessels of the three foot yin [conduits] extend from the feet to the chest. They are six feet five inches long. Six [feet] times six amounts to three *zhang* and six feet; five [inches] times six amounts to three feet. Together this is three *zhang* and nine feet. (6) Man has in both feet the walker vessels; they extend from the feet to the eyes. They are seven feet five inches long. Two times seven [feet] amounts to one *zhang* four feet; two times five [inches] amounts to one foot. Together this is one *zhang* and five feet. (7) The vessel of the supervisor [conduit] and the vessel of the controller [conduit] are both four feet five inches long. Two times four [feet] amounts to eight feet; two times five [inches] amounts to one foot.

---

the opposite direction. That is, the former are said to extend from the chest into the hands, while the latter are said to extend from the head into the feet. Interestingly, the conduit directions outlined here in the *Nan jing* and in the "Mai du" coincide completely with the oldest record extant on conduit therapy – namely, the *Zu bi shi yi mai jiu jing* 足臂十一脈灸經, a fragment of which was unearthed at Ma wang dui in 1973. Another fragment discovered at Ma wang dui, the *Yin yang shi yi mai jiu jing* 陰陽十一脈灸經, relates the same overall structure with but two exceptions, as is illustrated by the following table:

Source		*Zu bi shi yi mai jiu jing*	*Yin yang shi yi mai jiu jing*	*Nei jing* "Jing mai"	*Nan jing*, *Nei jing* "Mai du"
hand / arm	yin	hand → chest	hand → chest (or shoulder)	chest → hand	hand → chest
	yang	hand → head	hand → chest (except major yang; head → hand)	hand → head	hand → head
foot	yin	foot → thighs, or abdomen	foot → abdomen (except major yin; abdomen → foot)	foot → chest	foot → chest
	yang	foot → head	foot → thighs, head	head → foot	foot → head

Together this is nine feet. (8) All vessels together have a length of sixteen *zhang* and two feet. These are the so-called linear measurements of the twelve conduit vessels.

(9) There are twelve conduit vessels and fifteen network vessels. Where does (the movement in these conduits) start and where does it end?

(10) It is like this. The conduit vessels pass the blood and the qi, penetrating the yin and yang [sections of the organism], in order to provide nourishment to the body. (11) The [blood and the qi] start from the Central Burner and flow into the hand major yin and [hand] yang brilliance [conduits. From the hand] yang brilliance [conduit] they flow into the foot yang brilliance and the [foot] major yin [conduits. From the foot] major yin [conduit] they flow into the hand minor yin and the [hand] major yang [conduits. From the [hand] major yang [conduit] they flow into the foot major yang and the [foot] minor yin [conduits. From the foot] minor yin [conduit] they flow into the hand heart ruler and the [hand] minor yang [conduits. From the hand] minor yang [conduit] they flow into the foot minor yang and the [foot] ceasing yin [conduits. From the foot] ceasing yin [conduit] they flow back again into the hand major yin [conduit].[2] (12) There are fifteen secondary network [vessels]. (13) [The movement through] all of them returns [again and again] to its origin, as in a ring without end, with [the qi and the blood] pouring from one [conduit] into the next, thus revolving [through the entire organism]. (14) [All the qi and the blood] appear at the inch opening and at the *ren ying;* therefore, every disease can be located here and judgments can be made concerning [a person's] death or survival.

(15) The scripture states: A clear understanding of end and of beginning can be determined at the yin and yang [locations]. What does that mean?

---

2   This pattern is identical with the sequence of the conduits outlined in the *Nei jing,* for instance in *Ling shu* treatise 15, "Ying qi" 營氣. The circulatory movement through the vessels can be illustrated as follows:

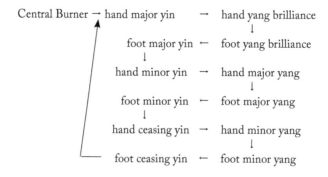

(16) It is like this. End and beginning can be inferred from information provided by the [movement in the] vessels. (17) In the morning, the qi begin their passage at the inch opening and at the *ren ying*, [i.e.,] at the yin and yang [locations, respectively]. They cause [each other to flow through the organism] as in a ring without end. Hence, [the text] speaks of [a continuous] "beginning." (18) In the case of an "end," the [movement in the] three yin and three yang [vessels] is interrupted. Interruption entails death. Each [such situation of imminent] death has its [specific symptoms that appear in the patient's physical appearance. Hence, [the text] speaks of [an imminent] end.³

COMMENTARIES

(2) *Yang:* Each hand has three yang [conduits]. Both hands together have six yang [conduits]. Hence, [the text] says: "Five [feet] times six amounts to three *zhang*."
Yu Shu: The vessels of the hand major yang [conduits] start from the tip of the small fingers of both hands and extend upward along the arms to in front of the pearls of the ears. They are [each] five feet long; for both hands together that adds up to one *zhang*. The vessels of the hand yang brilliance [conduits] start from the outer sides of the fingers adjoining the thumbs of both hands and extend upward along the arms until they reach the nose, [with the vessel coming from the] left [arm connecting with the] right [side of the nose, and the one coming from the] right [arm connecting with the] left [side of the nose]. They are [each] five feet long; for both hands together that adds up to one *zhang*. The vessels of the hand minor yang [conduits] start from the tips of the fingers adjoining the small fingers of both hands. They extend upward along the arms and end in front of the ears. They are [each] five feet long; for both hands together that adds up to one *zhang*. Hence, [the text] states: "Five [feet] times six amounts to three *zhang*."
(3) *Yang:* Both hands have three yin [conduits], respectively; together that amounts to six yin [conduits]. Hence, [the text] says: "Three [feet] times six amounts to one *zhang* and eight feet."

---

3 The twenty-third difficult issue marks the transition from a discussion of the diagnostic significance of the movement in the vessels to a discussion of the structure of the system of these vessels. As the commentaries indicate, it was not at all easy for some later authors to interpret the meaning of this issue – especially of sentences 14 through 18. The idea that it is sufficient to investigate the movement in the vessels at the two hands is expressed in the *Nan jing* as a logical consequence of the recognition of a continuous circulation. It was difficult to assert this new idea, in part because the technical terms used to transmit it were identical to those used in the *Nei jing*; thus conservative authors interpreted them on the basis of their *Nei jing* meanings.

Yu Shu: The vessels of the hand major yin [conduits] start from the Central Burner; they reach downward to the large intestine where they turn around to proceed to the "stomach-opening." They are attached to the lung and emerge below the armpits. They descend [in the arms] to the elbows and enter the inch opening, from which they move upward to the fish-line. They emerge [again] at the tips of the thumbs. They are [each] three feet five inches long. For both hands, that adds up to seven feet. The vessels of the hand minor yin [conduits] start from the heart center. There they emerge to become attached to the heart duct. They move downward until they reach the small intestine. From there they ascend to the lung and emerge below the armpits. They extend along the arms and emerge [again] at the tips of the small fingers. They are [each] three feet five inches long; for both hands, that adds up to seven feet. The vessels of the hand ceasing yin [conduits] start from the center of the chest. They are attached to the heart enclosing [envelope] and to the Triple Burner. They emerge from the ribs below the armpits. They extend along the shoulder blades, enter the elbows, and emerge [again] at the tips of the fingers adjoining the small fingers. They are [each] three feet five inches long; for both hands, that adds up to seven feet. Hence, [the text] speaks of "two *zhang* and one foot."

(4) *Yang*: Both feet have three yang [conduits], respectively; hence, [the text] says: "Six [feet] times eight amounts to four *zhang* and eight feet." The measurement of these vessels is seven feet five inches for the body of a medium-sized person. However, [the text here] speaks of "eight feet." The reason for this is difficult to explain. It is [perhaps] like this. The six yang [conduits] of the feet start from the toes and extend upward. Because they are bent and make curves, [the text] speaks of "eight feet."

Yu Shu: The vessels of the foot major yang [conduits] start from the outer sides of the small toes of both feet. They extend upward to the knees, pass through the popliteal space, and ascend in the center of the back up to the head. Then they descend to enter into the inner corner of the eyes. They are [each] eight feet long; for [the two] ascending both feet, that adds up to one *zhang* eight feet. The vessels of the foot yang brilliance [conduits] start from the tips of the toes adjoining the large toes. They follow the shinbones, extending upward to the navel, [which they pass] to the left and to the right at a distance of two inches, respectively. They end at the hairline of the temples. They are [each] eight feet long; for both feet together, that adds up to one *zhang* six feet. The vessels of the foot minor yang [conduits] start from the tip of the toes adjoining the small toes. They extend upward along the outer corners of the knees. They enter into the tender ribs, extending upward to the outer corners of the eyes. They are

[each] eight feet long; for both feet together, that adds up to one *zhang* six feet. Hence, [the text] speaks of "four *zhang* and eight feet."

(5) *Yang*: Both feet have three yin [conduits], respectively. Hence, [the text] says: "Six [feet] times six amounts to three *zhang* and six feet." The foot major yin and the [foot minor yin [conduits] both extend to below the tongue. The foot ceasing yin [conduits] extend to the top of the head. Here, [the text] says: "They extend to the chest." This [statement] is probably based on the place where [the two foot ceasing yin conduits] meet each other.

Yu Shu: The vessels of the foot major yin [conduits] start from the inner sides of the big toes. They extend upward following the inner ridges of the shinbones. They emerge in front of the [foot] ceasing yin vessels and extend further upward to enter the abdomen. They are attached to the liver and are linked to the stomach; [finally] they connect with the base of the tongue. They are [each] seven feet five inches long. The two together extend over one *zhang* five feet. The vessels of the foot ceasing yin [conduits] start from above the accumulation of hair on the big toes. They extend upward along the ridge of the insteps, passing the inner ankles at a distance of one inch. Eight inches above the ankles, they emerge behind the foot major yin [conduits]. They follow the thighs and enter into the pubic hair. They encircle the genital organs and arrive at the lower abdomen. They pass close to the stomach, they are attached to the liver, and they link up with the gall bladder. They follow the windpipe and enter into the pharynx, connecting with the eye duct and emerging at the forehead. They are [each] six feet five inches long. The two together extend over one *zhang* three feet. The vessels of the foot minor yin [conduits] start from below the small toes. They proceed diagonally toward the center of the feet, from which they extend upward through the inner sides of the calves and thighs. They are linked with the spine, they are attached to the kidneys, and they are tied to the urinary bladder. They are linked with the liver and they enter the lung. They follow the windpipe and approach the base of the tongue. They are [each] six feet five inches long; together, that is one *zhang* three feet. Hence, [the text] speaks of "three *zhang* and nine feet."

(6) *Yang*: Man is seven feet five inches tall. Thus, the walker vessels, extending [only] from the ankles to the eyes, cannot measure seven feet five inches [too]. When the [*Nan*] *jing* speaks here of seven feet five inches, it [appears to consider] the vessels as proceeding from the feet to the [top of the] head. When [the text] says "they extend to the eyes," it refers to [the highest points where they display their] function.

Yu Shu: Man has the two vessels of the yin walker and yang walker [conduit vessels]. For both feet together these are four vessels. The yang walker [conduit vessels] start from the centers of the heels. They extend upward along the outer ankles and enter into the "pond of winds."[4] The yin walker [conduit vessels] also start from the centers of the heels. They are secondary network [vessels] of the foot minor yin [conduits]. From behind the inner metatarsal bones, they extend upward above the inner ankles. They extend upward directly to the inner side of the thighs, from which they enter into the genital [region]. Along the abdomen they extend further upward into the chest and enter into the hollow behind the clavicle. Further up they emerge in front of the *ren ying* 人迎 [holes][5] and enter into the inner ridges of the cheek bones. They are attached to the inner corners of the eyes where they join the major yang vessels. They are [each] seven feet five inches long. The two together extend over one *zhang* five feet. In accordance [with this delineation of the courses of the yin and yang walker conduits], one may conclude that [the statement in the text] "they extend to the eyes" refers only to the extension of the two yin walker vessels from the feet. Hence, the [*Nan*] *jing* states: "They extend from the feet to the eyes. They are seven feet five inches long, adding up to one *zhang* and five feet."

Xu Dachun: One distinguishes between yin and yang walker vessels. To the left and to the right these are altogether four vessels. I do not know where this [fact] is pointed out here [in the *Nan jing*]. Also, the yin walker vessels are secondary [vessels] of the minor yin [conduits]; the yang walker vessels are secondary [vessels] of the major yin [conduits]. In the *Ling shu* treatise "Mai du" 脈度, the start and the end of the walker vessels is outlined, but only the yin walker is mentioned, not the yang walker. This is because its length equals the length of the yin walker. Hence, when Huang Di asked: "Among the walker vessels are those of a yin and of a yang category. How do they fit into the total number [of the vessels]?" Qi Bo replied: "In males the yang [vessels] are counted. In females the yin [vessels] are counted."[6] Although there are differences between the yang walkers and the yin walkers, in that the former are located internally and inside, while the latter are located externally and outside, their lengths are about identical.

Liao Ping: The two walker [vessels] are not necessarily equally long. Their [length] is calculated in the same way as that of the supervisor and controller vessels.

(7) *Yang*: The vessel of the supervisor [conduit] starts from the flesh adjoining the [lower end of the] spine and extends upward to the head. From there it descends into the face where it reaches the [upper] seam of the teeth in the mouth. Cal-

---

4   *Feng chi* 風池 ("pond of winds") is the name of a hole behind the ears at the side of the head shortly above the hairline.

5   These *ren ying* 人迎 holes are the original *ren ying* 人迎 locations to the right and left of the throat. See also below Hua Shou's commentary on sentence 14.

6   Cf. *Ling shu* treatise 17, "Mai du" 脈度.

culating this [course, the vessel should] not be only four feet five inches long. When [the text] here speaks of four feet five inches, it refers to the "wind palace"[7] as the topmost position reached by this conduit. Both the hands and the feet have twelve vessels [each]. That adds up to a total of twenty-four vessels. Together with the supervisor [conduit] and the controller [conduit], as well as with the two walker [conduit vessels], that adds up to twenty-eight vessels, a number corresponding to the twenty-eight zodiacal constellations. The total length [of all twenty-eight vessels together] is sixteen *zhang* two feet. When the camp and the guard [qi] have circulated through this distance, that constitutes one passage.

Yu Shu: The [*Nei*] *jing* states: "The supervisor vessel starts from the bottommost transportation [hole]";[8] it ascends inside the spine up to the wind palace. There it enters into and becomes attached to the brain. It is four feet five inches long. The controller vessel starts from below the *zhong ji* 中極 [hole],[9] from which it ascends to the [pubic] hairline. It extends upward through the abdomen. From the *guan yuan* 關元 [hole],[10] it reaches to the throat. It is four feet five inches long. Calculating the supervisor and the controller [vessels] together, they are nine feet long. The twelve conduits mentioned above represent altogether twenty-four vessels. Their total length is thirteen *zhang* and eight feet. If the [lengths of the] vessels of the supervisor, of the controller, and of the yin walker are added, their total length is two *zhang* and four feet. All in all, these are twenty-seven vessels with a total length of sixteen *zhang* and two feet. They reflect the pattern of the numbers three and nine, corresponding to the [clepsydra's] water dripping down by two markings. Mr. Yang has spoken of twenty-eight vessels. Here he has included the yang walker in his considerations. Two walker [conduit vessels would imply that] four [vessels] pass through [both feet]. That would result in a surplus of feet and inches. When Mr. Yang spoke of twenty-eight vessels he was wrong.

Liao Ping: The supervisor [vessel] is long and the controller [vessel] is short. But just as [in the case of] the two walker [conduit vessels], they are calculated together and then divided up into two vessels of equal length.

---

7 *Feng fu* 風府 ("wind palace") is the name of a hole on the back of the head, one inch above the hairline.

8 This quotation refers to *Su wen* treatise 60, "Gu kong lun" 骨空論. However, the *Nei jing* wording is slightly different; it says: "The supervisor vessel emerges from the lower abdomen and then moves down to the center of the [pubic] bone."

9 The *zhong ji* hole is located shortly above the genital organs.

10 The *guan yuan* hole is located on the abdomen below the navel.

(9)–(14) *Ding Deyong*: This [refers to] the rise and fall of the yin and yang qi of heaven and earth in the course of one year, and to the appearance and disappearance of sun and moon, light and darkness, within twenty-four hours. Similarly, man's camp and guard [qi] proceed through twenty-four sections of conduits and network [vessels] before they meet once again with the inch opening and the *ren ying* 人迎. The so-called inch opening is the vessel opening of the hand major yin [conduit]. This hole is called *tai yuan* 太淵. Hence, the [movement in the] vessels meets with the *tai yuan* [hole]. All the twelve conduits and fifteen network [vessels] are supplied [with qi] by the Triple Burner; [as long as this continues, a person will] live. Hence, [the qi] start from the Central Burner and flow into the hand major yin and [hand] yang brilliance [conduits]. This is, therefore, the place where the diseases can be located and where [prognostic] judgments can be made concerning death or survival.

(11)–(14) *Yang*: The twelve conduit vessels and the fifteen network vessels contain altogether twenty-seven [kinds of] qi. This reflects the pattern of the numbers three and nine. Heaven has the nine stars; earth has the nine geographical regions, and man has the nine orifices. All the [qi] flowing through the conduits and network [vessels] meet with the inch opening and with the *ren ying*. Therefore, if one examines the (movement in the vessels at the) inch opening and at the *ren ying*, he will recognize the diseases of the conduits and network [vessels], and the symptoms of [imminent] death or survival.

(11) *Yu Shu*: When [the text states: "blood and qi] start from the Central Burner," that refers to [a location] directly between the two breasts, called the *dan zhong* 膻中 hole. Another name is *qi hai* 氣海 ("sea of qi"). That is to say, the qi rise from here to flow into the major yin [conduit of the] lung. After they have completed their move through the lung [conduit] they are transmitted to the hand yang brilliance [conduit]. The *Su wen* states: "The *dan zhong* is the official functioning as minister and envoy."[11] That is to say, the stomach transforms the flavor [of food] into qi which are transmitted from here upward to the lung. [The text states further: "From the foot] ceasing yin [conduit] they flow back into the hand major yin [conduit]." If one investigates the [number of] *zhang* and feet [to be passed in one passage] on the basis of this [circuit], then a contradiction emerges between meanings [of statements] in different sections of the [*Nan*] *jing*. The distance from the sages [of antiquity] is far; it is difficult to provide even a rough explanation.

Xu Dachun: The treatise "Ying qi" 營氣 of the *Ling* [*shu*] discusses the same order of the movement of the camp qi, but its discussion focuses on the camp qi, not

---

11 Cf. *Su wen* treatise 8, "Ling lan mi dian lun" 靈蘭祕典論.

on the [course of the] vessels. The text of the [*Nei*] *jing* is much more detailed. Here, there is only a summary on the basis of the end and beginning of the vessels. Because the camp qi proceed inside the vessels, the movement of the camp qi is the movement in the vessels. Thus, the meaning [of the present paragraph] is also understandable.

Hua Shou: *Yin* 因 stands for *sui* 隨 ("to follow"). *Yuan* 原 stands for *shi* 始 ("begin").

Liao Ping: When [the text] says that "[the qi] move in a ring without end," what sense does it make to state further down that they appear only at the inch opening?

(14) *Li Jiong*: The inch opening is the great meeting point of the [movement in the] vessels; it [is the place] where the movement in the hand major yin vessel [can be felt]. Hence, when a disease is present in the five long-term depots and six short-term repositories, it always becomes apparent at the qi opening. Consequently, based on its [examination] one can make judgments concerning auspicious or inauspicious signs, that is, concerning death or survival. Also, the ascent and the descent of yin and yang [qi] in the course of one year has its meeting point at "spring begins." Light and darkness of the yin and yang [sections] in the course of one day have their meeting point in the early morning. The circulation of the camp and guard [qi] through the entire body has its meeting point at the [qi opening of the] hand major yin [conduit]; it follows the passage of heaven and amounts to 13,500 breathing periods [each twenty-four hours]. The original [text of the *Nan*] *jing* states: *zhao yu cun kou ren ying* 朝於寸口人迎 ("[all the qi and the blood] appear at the inch opening and at the *ren ying*"). The *ren ying* is at the left hand; it belongs to the minor yin (conduit). It is a location where [various] conduit vessels meet. In the same way as in the text further down, I have changed [the statement mentioned above] to *zhao yu cun bu qi kou* 朝於寸部氣口 ("they appear in the inch section of the qi opening").

Hua Shou: *zhao* 朝 ("to appear") equals the *zhao* in *zhao hui* 朝會 ("to assemble") .... Those [vessels] passing straight [through the body and its extremities] are the *jing* 經 ("conduits"); [those vessels] emerging sidewise [from the conduits] are the *luo* 絡 ("network vessels") .... As for the inch opening and the *ren ying*, a [diagnostic] method of ancient times considered the [locations] on both sides of the throat where a movement in the vessels [can be perceived] to be the *ren ying* [holes]. Then, Wang Shuhe 王叔和 of the Jin 金 [era] regarded a section in front of the gate of the left hand as the *ren ying* and a section in front of the gate of the right hand as the qi opening. Later generations followed him. I say the reason why the people in old times selected the *ren ying* and the qi opening [for diagnostic purposes] is that the *ren ying* belongs to the foot yang brilliance conduit of the stomach which receives the qi of the grains and nourishes the five long-term depots, while the qi opening belongs to the hand major yin conduit of the lung, [constituting a location] where [the qi of] all the vessels appear and are represented in equal balance.

Xu Dachun: For the "inch opening," see the first difficult issue. *Ren ying* is the inch opening at the left hand. *Zhao* 朝 is used here like the zhao in *zhao jin* 朝 覲 ("to appear at an audience"); that is to say, they come together here. They are supplied with qi once again and leave. *Chu* 處 ("to locate") stands for *kui duo* 揆 度 ("to estimate"). The meaning is that of the first difficult issue where it was stated: "One selects only the inch opening in order to determine life or death."

Liao Ping: The character *zhao* 朝 is a mistake here. The vessels do not *zhao* 朝 ("meet") with each other. This [expression here] results from a mistaken reading of the sentence *fei zhao bai mai* 肺朝百脈. *Bai mai* 百脈 refers to the tertiary network [vessels]. *Fei zhao sun luo* 肺朝孫絡 ("the tertiary network [vessels] meet with the lung") is not the same as *bai mai zhao fei yu cun kou* 百脈朝肺於 寸口 ("all vessels meet with [that of the] lung at the inch opening"). Xu [Da-chun's] commentary is wrong.

(15)–(18) *Hua Shou*: Mr. Xie [Jinsun] has stated that treatise 9 of the *Ling shu* says: "The WAY of all piercing requires an understanding of end and beginning [of the conduits]. [12] To know clearly about end and beginning [of the conduits], the five long-term depots serve as structural elements. [This information] is determined by their yin and yang [association]." It says further: "Not to have a disease is [to say: the movements in the vessels palpable] at the vessel opening and the *ren ying* [opening] correspond to the four seasons." [Later on the same treatise states:] "When someone is short of [breath] qi, [the qi] at both the vessel opening and the *ren ying* [opening] are diminished, and they fail to cover the foot- and inch-long sections." If one considers the present paragraph in light of earlier statements to the effect that every disease can be located at the inch opening and at the *ren ying*, and that judgments can be made [on their basis] concerning death or survival, [the present paragraph contains the] message that if one wishes to know about [imminent] end or [continuous] beginning [of the movement in the vessels], this can be determined by examining the yin and yang [movements in the conduits]. The [condition of the] yang [movement in the] conduits is judged by taking [information] from the *ren ying*; the [condition of

12　　SDY: „*End and Beginning* is the title of an antique text lost long ago. ‚To clearly recognize beginng and end' refers to those locations where the conduit vessels appear and where they end. That is documented in the text *End and Beginning*. One must know this to be able to supplement and drain without problem."

the] yin [movement in the] conduits is judged by taking [information] from the qi opening. As for *chao shi* 朝使, *chao* means that the qi and the blood pour through [the body] in correspondence to the time [of the day] like tides (*chao* 潮) of water. *Shi* means that the yin and yang [qi] activate each other. Here "beginning" refers to the beginning of living beings; "end" refers to the expiration of living beings. If one wishes to know about the [imminent] death or survival [of a person], that can be investigated through [an examination of the condition of the movement in his] vessels. When the yin and yang qi move through the vessels like tides, [alternately] activating [each other], like in a ring without end, then no disease is present. But if they do not move like tides alternately activating each other, then a disease is present.

Zhang Shixian: Yin [refers to] the long-term depots; yang [refers to] the short-term repositories.

(16) *Xu Dachun*: In the treatise "Zhong shi" 終始 of the *Ling* [*shu*], it is stated: "The WAY of all piercing requires an understanding of end and beginning. To know clearly about end and beginning, the five long-term depots serve as structural elements. [This information] is determined by their yin and yang [association]." Further down the text states: "The yang [vessels] receive their qi from the four limbs; the yin [vessels] receive their qi from the five long-term depots. Hence, in order to drain one moves [the needle] against the [regular course of the flow]; in order to supplement one follows, [with the needle, the regular course of the flow]." "Beginning" and "end" obviously refer here to the beginning and end of the twelve conduits. By moving [the needle] against or following [the regular flow], one supplements or drains them. It does not say that the flow of the qi constitutes a [continuous] beginning, while the interruption of the [movement in the] vessels is the end. At the conclusion of the "Zhong shi" treatise, the [appearances of] diseases [in one's physical appearance due to an interruption of the [movement in each of the] twelve conduits is recorded in the same manner as in the *Su wen* [treatise] "Zhen yao jing zhong lun" 診要經終論. Here, ["end"] is used with still another meaning, which is by no means the meaning of "end and beginning." How can anybody commit the error of considering the "end" of "end and beginning" to be the "end" [meant] here, only because at the conclusion of that [*Su wen*] treatise the [appearances of] diseases [in one's physical appearance due to an "end" of the [movement in the] conduits [is discussed for all] twelve conduits? Why did nobody think about this thoroughly?

(17) *Li Jiong*: The yin and yang qi appear, beginning with the early morning, at the qi opening in the inch section, revolving through the vessels like in a ring without end, and continuously beginning [their movement at this location]. Hence, [the

text] speaks of [continuous] "beginning." I have changed the statement *cun kou ren ying* 人迎 ("inch opening and *ren ying*") of the original text to *qi kou* 氣口 ("qi opening").

Liao Ping: The two characters *ren ying* appear here because they were not deleted entirely. The doctrine of [the location of] the *ren ying* at the left [hand] was introduced relatively late; no such doctrine existed in antiquity. Hence, the text of the *Nan jing* is not clear on this .... Xu [Dachun] commented on *zhao shi* 朝 使 (see above). Xu's commentary is wrong. The [meaning of the] two characters *zhao* and *shi* cannot be understood.

(18) *Li Jiong*: The [appearance in the patient's] physical appearance of an interruption [of the flow] of qi through the foot minor yin [conduit] is such that the teeth grow long and decay, while the flesh turns soft and shrinks. The [appearance in the patient's] physical appearance of an interruption [of the flow] of qi through the foot major yin [conduit] is such that the flesh [swells because of] fullness and the lips turn around. The [appearance in the patient's] physical appearance of an interruption [of the flow] of qi through the foot ceasing yin [conduit] is such that the tongue rolls up and the testicles shrink. The [appearance in the patient's] physical appearance of an interruption [of the flow] of qi through the hand major yin [conduit] is such that the skin dries out and the hair breaks off. The [appearance in the patient's] physical appearance of an interruption [of the flow] of qi through the hand minor yin [conduit] is such that the face turns black and resembles a pear. The [appearance in the patient's] physical appearance of an interruption [of the flow] of qi in three yin [conduits] is such that one's vision is dizzy and that he loses the ability to clearly distinguish between black and white. The [appearance in the patient's] physical appearance of an interruption [of the flow] of qi in six yang [conduits] is such that sweat protrudes like pearls. Hence, [the text] says: "Each [such situation of imminent] death has its specific [symptoms that appear in the patient's] physical appearance." "End" stands for death.

Zhang Shixian: "Three yin and three yang" [refers to] the twelve conduits. Changes in the twelve conduits become apparent in the inch opening and in the *ren ying*. If the circulating flow continues without break, that is called [continuous] "beginning"; if it is interrupted or blocked and cannot pass through [the conduits], specific [manifestations of such blockades appear in one's physical appearance corresponding to the specific long-term depot [where the movement] died. That is meant by "the end has its [specific symptoms appearing in the patient's] physical appearance." For an outline [of these symptoms,] see difficult issue 24.

二十四難曰：（一）手足三陰三陽氣已絕，何以為候？可知其吉凶不？
（二）然：足少陰氣絕，即骨枯。少陰者，冬脈也，伏行而溫於骨髓。故骨
髓不溫，即肉不著骨；骨肉不相親，即肉濡而卻；肉濡而卻，故齒長而
枯，髮無潤澤者，骨先死。戊日篤，己日死。（三）足太陰氣絕，則脈不榮
其口唇。口唇者，肌肉之本也。脈不榮，則肌肉不滑澤；肌肉不滑澤，則
肉滿；肉滿，則唇反；唇反，則肉先死。甲日篤，乙日死。（四）足厥陰氣
絕，即筋縮引卵與舌卷。厥陰者，肝脈也。肝者，筋之合也。筋者，聚於
陰器而絡於舌本。故脈不榮，則筋縮急；即引卵與舌；故舌卷卵縮，此筋
先死。庚日篤，辛日死。筋縮急。（五）手太陰氣絕，即皮毛焦。太陰者，
肺也，行氣溫於皮毛者也。氣弗榮則皮毛焦，皮毛焦則津液去，津液去即
皮節傷，皮節傷則皮枯毛折，毛折者則毛先死。丙日篤，丁日死。（六）手
少陰氣絕則脈不通，脈不通則血不流，血不流則色澤去，故面黑如梨，此
血先死。壬日篤，癸日死。（七）三陰氣俱絕者，則目眩轉目瞑。目瞑者，
為失志；失志者，則志先死，死即目瞑也。（八）六陽氣俱絕者，則陰與陽
相離，陰陽相離，則腠理泄，絕汗乃出，大如貫珠，轉出不流，即氣先
死。旦占夕死，夕占旦死。

The twenty-fourth difficult issue: (1) When the [flow of the] qi through the three yin or three yang conduits of the feet and hands has been cut off, what could serve as an indicator [of which conduit is affected]? Is it possible to know whether such [a situation] will have a favorable or unfavorable outcome?

(2) It is like this. When the foot minor yin [conduits] are cut off from the [movement of the] qi, the bones wither. The minor yin [conduit] is a vessel [associated with] winter; its course lies [deeply] hidden, and it provides warmth to the bones and their marrow.[1] Hence, when the bones and the marrow are not supplied with warmth, the flesh will not remain tightly attached to the bones. When the bones and the flesh are no longer close to each other, the flesh will be soft and will shrink. When the flesh is soft and shrinks, the teeth grow long and wither, [and one's hair will lose its glossiness and moisture].[2] When the hair lacks its glossiness and moisture, [that is an indication that] the bones have already died. [Such a disease will be] severe on a *wu* day; death will occur on a *ji* day.[3](3) When the foot major yin

1 *Ti* 体 ("body") appears to be a mistake for *sui* 髓 ("marrow"). Most later editions have corrected this mistake.
2 The passage in brackets corresponds to the general structure of argumentation in this paragraph. It was added by later editions.
3 *Wu* and *ji* are two of the so-called Ten Celestial Stems (*tian gan* 天干). Like the Twelve Earth Branches (*di zhi* 地枝), they represent ancient astronomical patterns. The Celestial Stems are used here, on the basis of their association with the Five Phases, as prognostic

[conduits] are cut off from the [movement of the] qi, the [movement in the] vessels will no longer supply the mouth and the lips of that [person with qi]. Mouth and lips represent the basis of the flesh. When the [movement in the] vessels no longer supplies [mouth and lips], the flesh will no longer retain its smoothness and moisture. When the flesh is no longer smooth and moist, the flesh will be full. When the flesh is full, the lips will curl back. When the lips curl back, this [indicates that] the flesh has died already. [Such a disease will be] severe on a *jia* day; death will occur on an *yi* day. (4) When the foot ceasing yin [conduit] has been cut off from [the movement of] the qi, the muscles will shrink, drawing in the testicles and rolling back one's tongue. The ceasing yin [conduit] is a vessel [associated with] the liver. The liver and the muscles represent one unit. The muscles assemble at the sexual organ and are tied to the base of the tongue. Hence, when they are not supplied by the [movement in the] vessels, the muscles will shrink. When the muscles shrink they draw in the testicles and the tongue. Thus, when the tongue is rolled back and when the testicles are drawn in, [that is an indication that] the muscles have already died. [Such a disease will be] severe on a *geng* day; death will occur on a *xin* day. (5) When the hand major yin [conduits] are cut off from the [movement of the] qi, the skin [and its] hair will be scorched. The major yin [conduit is associated with the] lung. It transports qi and warmth to the skin [and its] hair. When the skin [and its] hair are not supplied with qi, they will be scorched. When the skin [and its] hair are scorched, the liquids leave. When the liquids leave, the skin and the joints will be harmed. When the skin and the joints are harmed, the skin will wither and the hair will break. Hence, when the hair breaks, [that is an indication that] the hair has died already. [Such a disease will be] severe on a *bing* day; death will occur on a *ding* day. (6) When the hand minor yin [conduits] are cut off from the [movement of the] qi, the [blood] vessels are blocked. When these vessels are blocked, the blood does not flow. When the blood does not flow, one's complexion and glossiness fade away. Hence, when the color of one's face has turned black, resembling a pear, [this is an indication that] the blood has died already. [Such a disease will be] severe on a *ren* day; death will occur on a *gui* day. (7) When the three yin [conduits] are cut off from the [movement of the] qi at the same time, one's vision will be dizzy. One's eyes will turn uncontrolled or will be closed. When the eyes are closed one loses his mind. When one has lost his mind the mind has died. When it has died, one's eyes are closed. (8) When the six yang [conduits] are cut off from the [movement of the] qi at the same time, the yin and yang [sections of the organism] are separated from

---

devices to define days on which the patient's condition worsens and turns fatal. Thus, "*wu* day" may indicate here the fifth day after the onset of the illness, since *wu* is the fifth Celestial Stem. The usual sequence of the Celestial Stems is *jia, yi, bing, ding, wu, ji, geng, xin, ren, gui.*

each other. When the yin and yang [sections of the organism] are separated from each other, the pores will be drained. Sweat will appear intermittently, resembling a string of pearls. [These pearls] roll out [of the skin] but there is no flow. [This is an indication that] the qi have already died. If it occurs in the morning, one may foretell death for the night; if it occurs at night, one may foretell death for the morning.[4]

COMMENTARIES

(1) *Xu Dachun*: This treatise repeats exactly the original text of the "Jing mai" 經脈 treatise of the *Ling shu*. Only a few words have been changed. It does not explain anything.

  Ye Lin: This [difficult issue] quotes from the treatise "Jing mai" 經脈 of the *Ling shu,* but the discussion here is confused.

(2) *Ding Deyong*: The foot minor yin conduit is the vessel [associated with] the kidneys; it belongs to [the phase of] water and it reigns in winter. Internally, [the movement of] qi through this [conduit] nourishes the bones and the marrow. Externally, it provides brilliance to the hair. When [the movement of] qi [through this conduit] is cut off, the base of the teeth grows long, the bones wither, and the hair loses its glossiness. Hence, [the text] states: "[Such a disease will be] severe on a *wu* day; death will occur on a *ji* day." This is the [appearance in the patient's] physical appearance of a [situation where the flow of qi through the] foot minor yin [conduit] is cut off.

  Yang: Que 卻 ("to withdraw"; here, "to shrink") stands for *jie suo* 結縮 ("to shrink"). That is to say, the flesh at the roots of the teeth shrinks. Hence, the teeth gradually grow longer and wither. That is to say, the teeth dry out and their color lacks any moisture. The kidneys control the body's liquids. Here now, no liquids are present any more. Hence, that causes the hair to lose its glossiness. [The days] *wu* and *ji* are [associated with the phase of] soil. The kidneys are [associated

---

4 This difficult issue is one of the relatively few that closely adhere to the text of the *Nei jing*, in this case to *Ling shu* treatise 10, "Jing mai" 經脈. Yet it is not clear whether the meaning expressed is identical. The *Nan jing* appears to assign specific physiological functions to the individual conduits – functions which can be fulfilled only if the respective conduits are passed by the circulatory movement of the qi. That is, the *Nan jing* regards the qi themselves as neutral; they serve, for instance, as major yin qi only as a result of being utilized by the major yin section of the circulatory system to fulfill its physiological functions. This concept marks a final departure (1) from the idea that there are eleven unrelated conduits, each supplemented with its own specific contents, as appeared in the Ma wang dui texts of around 200 BCE, and (2) from the transitional idea, expressed in the *Nei jing*, of specific yin and yang qi circulating through a system of yin and yang conduits. As the *Nan jing* states, an individual conduit-section – or groups of conduit-sections – can be cut off from the movement of the qi, which means that smaller cycles of circulation are possible, bypassing those single or grouped conduit-sections.

with the phase of] water. The soil is capable of overcoming water. Hence, [the text] states: ["Such a disease will be] severe on a *wu* day; death will occur on a *ji* day."

Yu Shu: The yin and yang [categories] have weak and strong [subcategories]. Hence, three yin and three yang [conduits] exist to transport the qi and the blood and to nourish the human body. Thus, the three yin [conduits are linked to vessels which] part from them and tie them [to the other yin conduits], The major yin [conduit] is the "opener." The ceasing yin [conduit] is the "cover." The minor yin [conduit] is the "pivot." The opener guards the foundations of movement and rest. The cover holds control over tight sealing. The pivot controls the subtleties of the revolving movement. The three conduits must not lose [contact to] each other. Here, the [flow of the qi through the] foot minor yin vessel of the kidneys is interrupted. Hence, [contact to] one of the conduits has been lost. The minor yin [conduit] cannot act as pivot; the subtleties of the revolving movement are out of control. Hence, [the text] speaks of "death."

Li Jiong: The brain is the sea of the marrow. The kidneys control the bones and the marrow. The hair is nourished by the brain. Hence, the [latter] provides brilliance to the hair. Here, the bones and the marrow wither. Hence, the hair lacks its glossiness.

Xu Dachun: Ru 濡 ("soft") means *zhi* 滯 ("to obstruct"). The [*Nei*] *jing* states: "The flesh softens *(ru* 濡) and recedes." *Que* 卻 ("to recede") stands for *tui suo* 退縮 ("to withdraw and shrink"). For *ku* 枯 ("to wither") the [*Nei*] *jing* has *gou* 垢 ("to become stained"). When the flesh shrinks, the [teeth] have been severed [from their base] and the upper section becomes visible. Hence, [the text states]: "The teeth grow long." "To wither" means that they lack moisture. The teeth are extensions of the bones. Hence, [the condition of the latter] is examined in the [condition of the former].

Ye Lin: The kidneys control the storage of the essence [qi] and the transformation of the blood. The hair is the excess of the blood. When the [movement of the] essence qi of the kidneys is cut off, the hair lacks its glossiness.

(3) *Ding Deyong*: The foot major yin conduit is the vessel [associated with] the spleen; it belongs to [the phase of] soil and it reigns in late summer.[5] Internally, [the movement of] qi through this [conduit] nourishes the flesh; externally, it provides brilliance and protection to mouth and lips. When [the movement of] qi through this [conduit] is cut off, the lips will curl back. Hence, [the disease will be] severe on a *jia* day; death will occur on an *yi* day. This is the [appearance

5   "Late summer" is a fifth season, conceptualized to achieve correspondence between the Five Phases and the seasons of a year.

in the patient's] physical appearance of a [situation where the flow of qi through the] foot minor yin [conduit] is cut off.

Yang: *Jia* and *yi* are [associated with the phase of] wood. The spleen is [associated with the phase of] soil. Wood is capable of overcoming soil. Hence, [the text] states: ["Such a disease will be] severe on a *jia* day; death will occur on an *yi* day."

Yu Shu: Mouth and lips are extensions of the flesh. They are also called "[external] brilliance of the spleen." Here now the lips curl back and the complexion turns virid because the wood [has come to] destroy the soil. In the [system of the] separate and combined [functioning] of the yin and yang [conduits], the major yin [conduits] are considered to be the "openers." That is to say, they watch over the foundation of movement and rest. Here now, [the flow of qi through] these vessels has been cut off. As a consequence, the foundations of movement and rest have lost their overseer. Hence, [the text] speaks of "death."

Xu Dachun: The treatise "Jing mai" 經脈 [of the *Ling shu*] states: "Once the vessels fail to supply nourishment, then the muscles and the flesh soften. Once muscles and flesh have softened, then //the tongue withers// and there is a feeling of fullness in the center of the body. Once a feeling of fullness has set in in the center of the body, then the lips will curl." That is quite clear. Here [in the *Nan jing*, the text] states: "The flesh [is full]." That is difficult to explain.

(4) *Ding Deyong*: The foot ceasing yin conduit is the vessel [associated with] the liver; it belongs to the [phase of] wood and it reigns in spring. Internally [the movement of] qi through this [conduit] nourishes the muscles; externally [this conduit] is tied to the base of the tongue. Below, it circles around the genital organ. When [the movement of] the qi through this [conduit] is cut off, the tongue rolls back and the testicles shrink. Hence, [the disease will be] severe on a *geng* day; death will occur on a *xin* day.

Yang: *Geng* and *xin* are [associated with the phase of] metal. The liver is [associated with the phase of] wood. Metal is capable of overcoming wood. Hence, [the text] states: "[The disease will be] severe on a *geng* day; death will occur on a *xin* day."

Li Jiong: The liver controls the muscles. All the movements of man result from the strength of the muscles.

(5) *Ding Deyong*: The hand major yin conduit is the vessel [associated with] the lung; it belongs to the [phase of] metal and reigns in autumn. Internally, [the movement of] qi through this [conduit] controls the [camp] qi; externally, it nourishes the skin [and its] hair. When the [movement of the] qi through this [conduit] is cut off, the body's liquids leave. Skin and hair burn out. Hence, [such a disease will be] severe on a *bing* day; death will occur on a *ding* day.

Yang: *Bing* and *ding* are [associated with the phase of] fire. The lung belongs to the [phase of] metal. Fire is capable of overcoming metal. Hence, [the text] states: "[Such a disease will be] severe on a *bing* day; death will occur on a *ding* day."

(6) *Ding Deyong*: The hand minor yin conduit is the vessel [associated with] the true heart; it belongs to the [phase of] the ruler fire and it reigns in summer. It controls the transport of the camp [qi] through the vessels. It is not so that the [*Nan*]*jing* does not talk about the hand ceasing yin [conduit which is associated with the] heart enclosing [network] controlling the minister fire. A minister acts but the ruler gives the orders. [Together] they control the passage of the camp qi. Here, the true heart has been cut off from the [movement of the] qi. Consequently, the camp qi do not move [through the organism any longer]. When the camp qi do not move, the blood does not flow. Therefore, one's complexion and moisture fade away. Hence, the face turns black and assumes a sallow color. [Such a disease will be] severe on a *ren* day; death will occur on a *gui* day. This is a disease; it is not [the result of] exhaustion due to old age! The character *li* 梨 ("pear") should be changed here to *li* 黧 ("sallow").

Yang: The [*Nei*]*jing* speaks of three hand yin [conduits]. Here, however, only the major yin and the minor yin [conduits] are referred to. The heart ruler [conduit] is not discussed. Why is that? It is like this. The heart ruler [conduit] is the vessel [associated with] the heart enclosing network. The minor yin [conduit] is the vessel [associated with] the heart [itself]. Both these conduits [generate symptoms that] are indicators of [diseases of] the heart. Hence, when it is stated that the [movement of qi through the] minor yin [conduit] is cut off, then the [movement of qi through the] heart ruler [conduit] is cut off, too. Both [conditions] are examined the same way; hence, they are not distinguished in this explanation here. The [*Nei*]*jing* stated originally: "The face of the [patient] has assumed a black color resembling *qi chai* 漆柴."[6] Here, [the *Nan jing*] states: "It resembles a pear." *Qi chai* grows in the *Heng* 恆 mountains; the color of this herb is yellow-black. It has no glossiness. Hence, it was used here as an illustration. "Pears" are fruits consumed by man. Again, their yellow-black color was used [as an illustration] to explain that a person's complexion turns yellow-black when no blood is present. That resembles the lack of brilliance of both [*qi chai* and pears]. *Ren* and *gui* are [associated with the phase of] water; the heart is [associated with the phase of] fire. Water overcomes fire. Hence, [the text] states: "[Such a disease will be] severe on a *ren* day; death will occur on a *gui* day."

---

6 *Ling shu* treatise 10, "Jing mai" 經脈.

(7) *Ding Deyong*: The so-called three yin [conduits] are just the three yin [conduits] of the feet. The foot minor yin [conduit] is [associated with] the liver. The kidneys store the essence [qi] and the mind. The foot ceasing yin [conduit] is [associated with] the liver. The liver stores the *hun* 魂 and [its spirit] passes through the eyes.[7] Hence, when [the flow of qi through these conduits is] cut off, one loses his mind and becomes disorderly; the *hun* leaves and the eyes will be confused through dizziness.

Yang: The three yin [conduits] are the three yin vessels of the hands and the feet, constituting the vessels of the five long-term depots. The five long-term depots are the root and basis of man. Hence, when all three yin [conduits] are cut off [from the movement of the qi] at the same time, the eyes will be closed. *Ming* 瞑 ("closed eyes") stands for *bi* 閉 ("closed"). That is to say, the root is cut off internally and one's external brilliance is lost. The eyes are man's [external] brilliance. *Xuan* 眩 ("confused vision") stands for *luan* 亂 ("disorder"). That is to say, the eyes are in disorder and cannot recognize anybody. The kidneys store the essence [qi] and the mind. [Here] the essence qi are completely exhausted. Hence, [the text] speaks of a "loss of one's mind." When all three yin [conduits] are cut off [from the movement of the qi at the same time], death follows within one day and a half.

Yu Shu: The vessels of the five long-term depots are the three yin [conduits]. The vessels of all the five long-term depots meet in the eyes. Here, the three yin [conduits] have been cut off [from the movement of the qi through the organism]. Hence, the eyes are confused by dizziness [or] are closed. The five mental [states] of man are all associated with yin. That is to say, the mental [state associated with the] liver is anger; the mental [state associated with the] heart is joy; the mental [state associated with the] spleen is pondering; the mental [state associated with the] lung is grief; and the mental [state associated with the] kidneys is fear. Here, the three yin [conduits] have been cut off [from the movement of the qi]; the five long-term depots have lost their mental [states]. Hence, there is no joy, no anger, no grief, no pondering, no fear. All the five mental [states] have gone. Hence, [the text] speaks of a "loss of one's mind." When Mr. Yang spoke of a "loss of one's mind," he only talked about one depot, that is, the kidneys. In the [*Nei*] *jing* it was stated originally: "when the yin and yang [sections of the organism] are separated from each other, dissatisfaction results and loss of one's mind." That is [what is] meant here.

Ding Deyong: The so-called six yang [conduits] are the three yang [conduits] of the hands and feet, respectively. Then [the text] states: *yin yu yang xiang li* 陰

---

7 See difficult issue 34.

與陽相離. That is to say, the three yang [conduits] of the hands pass the qi of
heaven. Therefore, they are termed yang. The three yang [conduits] of the feet
pass the qi of the earth. Hence, they are termed yin. When the yin and yang [qi]
of heaven and earth are not [mutually exchanged in the organism but remain]
separate from each other, that is meant when [the text] states: *yin yang xiang li*
陰陽相離 ("yin and yang [qi] remain separate from each other"). As a result, the
pores will be drained and sweat will appear intermittently, resembling a string of
pearls. Hence, death will occur before the coming morning or night.

Yang: This [paragraph elucidates the idea that] one will die before one day has
passed if the six yang [conduits] have been cut off from the [movement of the]
qi. The manifestations of such an interruption of the [movement of the]
qi through the six yang [conduits] are summarily delineated here. The [*Nei*]
jing states: "The end [of a movement] in the major yang vessels [shows as fol-
lows].⁸ The eyes are motionless directed upward. The body is bent backward,
with tugging and spasms and relaxation [alternating]. The complexion is white.
[The flow in] the skin is interrupted, and intermittent sweating sets in. Once
intermittent sweating has set in, that is the end. The end [of a movement] in the
minor yang [vessels shows as follows]. The ears are deaf. All joints relax. The
eye connection [to the brain] is interrupted. When the eye connection [to the
brain] is interrupted, [the patient] will die within one and a half days. When he
dies his complexion assumes a greenish-white color. Then he dies. The end in the
yang brilliance [vessels shows as follows]. Mouth and eyes move. [The patient] is
easily frightend and his words are meaningless. His completion is yellow. Once
the conduits above and below abound [with qi] and are numb, then this is the
end."⁹ These are the manifestations of the interruption of the [movement of the
qi through the] three yang [conduits]. Above, [the *Nan jing* text] speaks of "six
yang [conduits]." Here, the [*Nei*] *jing* speaks of "the manifestations of an interruption of the [movement of the qi through the] three yang [vessels]," because
when [the movement of qi] is cut off from all yang vessels of the hands and
feet, the manifestations of such an interruption are identical [to those outlined
above]. Hence, they are not discussed here separately.

(8) *Zhang Shixian*: The "six yang" are the three yang [conduits] of hands and feet,
respectively. When the yang qi protect the external [sections of the body], the

8 Beginning with 太陽之脈, 其終也 *tai yang zhi mai, qi zhong ye* to the end of this chapter
the text is mostly identical with passages in SW 16. JYJ has 太陽脈絕, 其終也 *tai yang
mai jue, qi zhong ye*, „when the [movement in the] major yang vessel is interrupted, then
this is the end."

9 This is a modified quotation from *Su wen* treatise 16, "Zhen yao jing zhong lun" 診要經終
論.

pores are closed tightly. When the [flow of] yang [qi] is cut off, the pores are no longer closed firmly and the yin [qi] alone cannot remain [in their conduits. Hence,] the camp qi are drained off through the pores. The respective person is not yet dead but his qi have already died. Man is ruled by his qi. When the qi have died, man must die. [Hence, death] can be predicted for the [coming] morning or night.

THE TWENTY-FIFTH DIFFICULT ISSUE

二十五難曰：（一）有十二經，五藏六府十一耳，其一經者，何等經也？
（二）然：一經者，手少陰與心主別脈也。（三）心主與三焦為表裏，（四）俱
有名而無形，故言經有十二也。

The twenty-fifth difficult issue: (1) There are twelve conduits, but the [body's] five long-term depots and six short-term repositories [add up to only] eleven. Of what nature is the one [missing] conduit?

(2) It is like this. One of the conduits encompasses the hand minor yin [vessel] and the heart ruler [vessel] as separate vessels. (3) The heart ruler and the Triple Burner represent outside and inside. (4) Both have a name but no physical appearance. Hence, one speaks of twelve conduits.[1]

COMMENTARIES

(1) *Yang:* The hand minor yin [conduit] is the vessel [associated with] the true heart. The hand heart ruler [conduit] is the vessel [associated with] the heart enclosing network. Both vessels are heart vessels. Now, the [hand minor yin [conduit] is linked to the [vessel of the] small intestine, while the heart ruler [conduit] is linked to the vessel of the Triple Burner. The Triple Burner has a position but no physical appearance; the heart ruler [conduit] has a name but no long-term depot. Hence, the two conduits constitute "outside and inside." The five long-term depots and six short-term repositories have one vessel each; that equals eleven vessels. The heart has two vessels. That adds up to twelve vessels. Similarly, one

---

1 This difficult issue marks the beginning of a controversy that has not been settled even today. The heart ruler, also called heart-enclosing network, may originally have been a concept developed to meet the number six for the long-term depots, if they were to correspond to the three yin and three yang subcategories. The Triple Burner may have been conceptualized in correspondence to environmental symbolism. In the last centuries BCE, the entire physiological organism was seen as a mirror image of the state and its economy. The terms "long-term depot," "short-term repository," "conduits," the bureaucratic hierarchy of the organism, and so on reflect this understanding. In this context the assumption of some heating device in the organism – corresponding, for instance, to the most important economic functions of the saline and iron works – may have been a stringent consequence. See also *Medicine in China: A History of Ideas,* chapter 3.3. Obviously, it was apparent even during the Han era that no anatomical entity corresponded to the concepts of "heart ruler" / "heart-enclosing network" and "Triple Burner" in the same way that a morphologically present liver corresponds to the concept of the liver. Hence, the compromise approached here assigned a function to the heart ruler/heart-enclosing network and to the Triple Burner, but no anatomical substratum.

could state that of the six short-term repositories actually only five short-term repositories exist.[2]

Xu Dachun: The [treatise] "Jiu zhen lun" 九鍼論 of the *Ling* [*shu* states concerning] the five long-term depots: "The heart stores the spirit. The lung stores the *po* soul. The liver stores the *hun* soul. The spleen stores the intentions. The kidneys store the essence and the mind." The six short-term repositories include the small intestine, the large intestine, the stomach, the gall bladder, the urinary bladder, and the Triple Burner. They are responsible for emission and intake of water and grains, resembling a palace treasury that oversees expenditure and income. Hence, they are called *fu* 府, "short-term repository", "palace".

Liao Ping: Among the long-term depots and short-term repositories, the brain and the heart are designated with the same name. The inner and the outer kidneys are also designated with the same name. If five and six adds up to twelve, two [conduits] must be designated with the same name. Among the twelve conduits the brain constitutes an external ruler of the heart. This is similar to the inner kidney and the outer kidney (i.e., the testicles); if one differentiates among them, they, too, represent two [entities]. In old times one assumed that the yellow fat outside of the heart constituted a "heart enclosure." That was wrong.

(2)–(3) *Ding Deyong*: [The text] states: "[One of the conduits encompasses] the hand minor yin [vessel] and the heart ruler [vessel] as separate vessels." That is to say, the heart and the small intestine constitute outside and inside [of one unit,[3] and] the heart ruler and the Triple Burner constitute outside and inside [of one unit, too]. The minor yin [conduit] is the vessel of the true heart; [the latter] constitutes the ruler fire. The heart ruler constitutes, together with the Triple Burner, the minister fire. Hence, the [hand] minor yin and the heart ruler [conduits] are separate. The minister carries out the orders of the ruler. Hence, [the heart ruler] has the name of the heart but not its position.

Li Jiong: The heart ruler [conduit] is the hand ceasing yin [conduit]. The Triple Burner [conduit] is the hand minor yang [conduit]. The two conduits constitute "outside and inside."

Hua Shou: Someone asked: "The hand ceasing yin conduit is called 'heart ruler' and it is also called 'heart enclosing network'. Why is that?" [The answer is:] "It carries the name of the ruler fire, but it occupies the position of the minister fire. The hand ceasing yin [conduit] acts on behalf of the ruler fire. In terms of

---

2 The Triple Burner is a short-term repository.

3 Each long-term depot (yin, internal) is linked to a specific short-term repository (yang, external) – namely, lung to large intestine, spleen to stomach, heart to small intestine, kidneys to urinary bladder, heart ruler/heart-enclosing network to Triple Burner, and liver to gall bladder.

its function it is called 'hand heart ruler'; in terms of its [status as a separate] conduit it is called 'heart enclosing network'. It is one single conduit but carries two names and represents the minister fire."

(3) *Xu Dachun*: [According to the treatise] "Jiu zhen lun" 九鍼論 of the *Ling* [*shu*], the yang brilliance and the major yin [conduits] of the feet constitute outside and inside; the minor yang and the ceasing yin [conduits of the feet] constitute outside and inside; the major yang and the minor yin [conduits of the feet] constitute outside and inside; the yang brilliance and the major yin [conduits] of the hands constitute outside and inside; the minor yang and the heart ruler [conduits of the hands] constitute outside and inside; the major yang and the minor yin [conduits of the hands] constitute outside and inside. "Separate vessels" means that the heart ruler, encircling the heart, basically constitutes something like walls encircling a royal residence. One would expect that it forms outside and inside with the heart, but on the contrary, it is separate [from the heart], forms outside and inside with the Triple Burner, and has a separate conduit. Hence, there are twelve conduits.

(4) *Li Jiong*: The heart enclosing network constitutes a fine muscular membrane, located outside of the firm fat [of the heart]. It resembles silk threads and is linked to the heart and to the lung. For a detailed [discussion of the] Triple Burner, see the thirty-first difficult issue. Both have names but no physical appearance.

(2)–(4) *Zhang Shixian*: The hand minor yin [conduit] is the conduit of the true heart. The heart ruler is the heart enclosing network. The heart ruler [conduit] is a secondary vessel of the true heart. It does not coincide with the conduit of the true heart. The true heart constitutes the ruler fire; the heart ruler constitutes the minister fire. The Triple Burner is the father of the qi; the heart enclosing [network] is the mother of the blood. Together they form "outside and inside." The two have a real name but no substance. To the [eleven conduits of the] five long-term depots and six short-term repositories is added the one conduit of the heart enclosing [network]. Together that equals twelve conduits.

(4) *Xu Dachun*: [The text] states that the Triple Burner has no physical appearance. That cannot be. It states [further] that the hand heart ruler has no physical appearance, but such a doctrine definitely does not exist. The heart ruler is the network enclosing the heart; it consists of a fatty membrane protecting the heart. How could it have no physical appearance? It is not called a long-term depot because the heart ruler acts on behalf of the heart. In itself, it does not store anything. Hence, it is not called a depot.

(3)–(4) *Ding Jin*: This paragraph states that the heart ruler and the Triple Burner constitute outside and inside, and that both have a name but no physical appearance. Because of the two words "no physical appearance," people in later times who did not check the meaning of the [*Nei*] *jing* have engaged themselves in highly confused argumentations. They not only criticized the [alleged] mistakes of Yueren but also criticized [what they considered to be] erroneous interpretations forced [on this passage] by [Wang] Shuhe 王叔和. Over the past three thousand years, this has never been settled finally. I always think that the *Nan jing* was not yet distant from antiquity. Of all the authors who appeared [in later times to comment on the ancient scriptures, Yueren] was the very first. Also, one must base [his understanding of the *Nan jing*] word for word on the *Nei jing*. Why should misunderstandings and a deception of mankind be created just for the two key [concepts] of the [heart] enclosing network and the Triple Burner? There is no other way to elucidate [their meaning] except by comparing the meaning in the *Nei jing* with that in the *Nan jing*. Thus, the *Nei jing* states that all the five long-term depots have physical appearance and color, that the five short-term repositories, too, can be measured in *zhang* and feet, and that the water and the grains with which they are supplemented can be recorded in amounts of pints and pecks. If the [heart] enclosing network and the Triple Burner had a physical appearance, why would they be the only ones with colors, sizes, and capacities that are not clearly recorded? Well, one should look at what the *Nan jing* says about the [heart] enclosing network and pick its meaning from the term "enclosing," and [one should look] also at what [the *Nan jing*] says about the Triple Burner and pick its meaning from the term "triple." Thus, in the *Ling* [*shu*] and in the *Su* [*wen*], the treatise "Ben shu" 本輸 states: "The Triple Burner is the short-term repository functioning as central ditch. The [individual] water ways leave from it. It is linked to the urinary bladder. It is a solitary short-term repository." The treatise "Ben zang" 本藏 [states]: "When the [skin] structures are tight and when the skin is thick, the Triple Burner and the urinary bladder are thick [too]." The treatise "Jue qi" 決氣 states: "The Upper Burner [is responsible for] emissions; it disperses the flavor qi] of the five grains, [a process] resembling the gentle flow of mist. [What is distributed] is called 'the qi'. The Central Burner receives the qi. It extracts their juice and transforms it into something red. That is what is called ,blood'." In the treatise "Ying wei sheng hui" 營衛生會,[4] it is stated: "The camp [qi] emerge from the Central Burner; the guard [qi] emerge from the Lower Burner." It states further: "The Upper Burner is like fog. The Central Burner is like a humidifier. The Lower Burner is like a ditch." The discussion in the [treatise] "Wu long jin ye bie lun" 五癃津液別論 states: "The Triple Burner emits qi to warm the muscles and the

---

4   "Rong wei sheng hui" 榮衛生會 is a mistake for "Ying wei sheng hui" 營衛生會.

flesh, and to fill the skin." The treatise "Xie ke" 邪客 of the *Ling shu* states: "The minor yin [conduit] is the heart vessel. The heart is the big ruler among the five long-term depots and six short-term repositories. As long as this long-term depot is firm and stable, evil [qi] will not be accepted there. When they are accepted there, then the heart is damaged. [When the heart is damaged, then] the spirit will leave it. [When the spirit has left it, then that person] will die. The fact is: All evil [qi] that are present in the heart, they all are present in the heart enclosure." All the lines quoted above from the *Ling* [*shu*] and from the *Su* [*wen*][5] describe the Triple Burner as completely enclosing the five long-term depots and six short-term repositories. The [heart] enclosing network has the meaning of enclosing only the heart. The "short-term repository [acting as] central ditch" is the "solitary short-term repository." If it were not for the fact that the Triple Burner enclosed the [organism] externally, how could [this short-term repository] have this singularly honorable designation? It was said further that "when the pores are sealed tightly, and when the skin is thick, the Triple Burner is thick [too]." Now, if the inside of the skin and the flesh of the entire body were not supported by the Triple Burner, how could their thicknesses correspond to each other? It was said further that "the Upper Burner disperses the flavor [qi] of the grains; the Central Burner receives qi, absorbs the juices, transforms them, and turns them red." If the Triple Burner did not enclose all the body's long-term depots and short-term repositories, how could all the body's long-term depots and short-term repositories share in the qi of the Triple Burner in order to [further] diffuse and transform them? It was said further that "the camp [qi] emerge from the Central Burner; the guard [qi] emerge from the Lower Burner." The camp [qi] become the blood because they are [generated from] the essence of the flavor [qi] of the grains. The guard [qi] are qi [because they are] generated from the qi of the grains. All these [transformations occur] because of the [activities of the] stomach. But how could the stomach be stimulated to perform these transformations if it were not for the fact that the Triple Burner externally completely encloses [the stomach] and manages the movement of the qi? It was stated further: "[The Upper Burner] resembles fog; [the Central Burner] resembles a humidifier; [the Lower Burner] resembles a ditch." Above, [the Upper Burner] gives orders concerning emissions; below, [the Lower Burner] manages the passageways of water. How could this be if it were not for the fact that the Triple Burner externally encloses all the body's long-term depots and short-term repositories, exerting complete control over them? It was stated further: "[The Triple Burner] emits qi to warm the muscles and the flesh,

---

5   Actually, all the quotations are from the *Ling shu*.

and to fill the skin." That is a clear indication of the fact that the Triple Burner constitutes a layer supporting the skin and the flesh from inside. It was stated further: "Whenever evil [qi] are present in the heart, they are always in the network enclosing the heart." That is a clear indication of the fact that the enclosing network constitutes a layer holding the heart from outside. Later readers of these texts were to say, if the Triple Burner has no physical appearance, how can passageways of water emerge from it? How can it be thick or thin? How can it be like mist or fog or a humidifier or a ditch? How can it emit qi in order to supply warmth to the flesh? And if the enclosing network [of the heart] has no physical appearance, how can all the evil [qi] settle in this network enclosing the heart? Why is it the only [entity] that cannot be seen? Why does it lack color, width, and length? They obviously did not know that the [heart] enclosing network is a small bag providing a network internally and an enclosure externally. Thus, the name already states that it is an "enclosing network." Its physical appearance does not have to be described in terms of big or small, feet or inches. The Triple Burner is a large bag supporting [the organism] from outside and holding it inside. The uniqueness of its holding [function] is described fully by nothing but the term "triple." The term "burner" fully describes the provision of the entire [body] with qi. Hence, the name already states that it is a Triple Burner. Again, its physical appearance does not have to be described in terms of large or small, *zhang* or feet. Anybody who hitherto has harbored some doubts can have them resolved now if he follows this [argumentation]. Also, if one matches this small bag resembling a long-term depot and [therefore] constituting a separate long-term depot with that large bag resembling a short-term repository and [therefore] constituting a separate short-term repository, that is the principle of heavenly creation and earthly organization. Yueren stated the two words "no physical appearance" here, and again in the thirty-fourth difficult issue. An examination reveals that they are highly appropriate; an analysis shows that they are quite correct. How could the people of later times grasp but the hair on the skin of the *Nei jing* and then criticize exemplary men of former times? Often [enough, their statements] reveal only the dimensions of their ignorance.

Liao Ping: That is to say, the [Triple Burner] is spread out [to cover, internally,] the entire chest and back. It is unlike the other long-term depots and short-term repositories, which have a distinct location and a distinct form and which can be pointed out as concrete [entities]. If it is said [here] that if one assumes that "it has no physical appearance," that was not even followed by the authors of the apocryphal writings. It was a mistake of the one who said that.

二十六難曰：(一)經有十二，絡有十五，餘三絡者，是何等絡也？
(二)然：有陽絡，有陰絡，有脾之大絡。(三)陽絡者，陽蹻之絡也；陰絡
者，陰蹻之絡也。故絡有十五焉。

The twenty-sixth difficult issue: (1) There are twelve conduits and fifteen network [vessels]. Of what nature are the additional three network [vessels]?

(2) It is like this. They include the yang network [vessel], the yin network [vessel], and the great network [vessel] of the spleen. (3) The yang network [vessel] is the network [vessel] of the yang walker [conduit]; the yin network [vessel] is the network [vessel] of the yin walker. Hence, there are fifteen network [vessels].[1]

COMMENTARIES

(1)–(3) *Ding Deyong*: "[There are] twelve conduits and fifteen network [vessels]" is to say that each conduit has one network [vessel]. The conduits of liver, heart, and kidneys are located on the left; their network [vessels] are located on the right. The conduits of spleen, lung, and heart enclosing network are on the right; their network [vessels] are on the left. The yang walker conduit [starts from] the external ankle of the left foot; its network [vessel starts from] the external ankle of the right foot. The yin walker conduit [starts from] the internal ankle of the right foot; its network [vessel starts from] the internal ankle of the left foot. These are the network [vessels] of the yin walker and of the yang walker

---

1   This difficult issue briefly refers to the concept of the fifteen network vessels. A detailed discussion of their nature and courses had been presented by *Ling shu* treatise 10, "Jing mai." It was pointed out there that each of the twelve main conduits has a network – or "separate/diverging" (*bie* 別) – vessel, branching off from the respective main conduit at a specific point. These points are holes on the main conduits, and the network vessels are designated with the names of these holes. In addition, three further network vessels are named – those branching off from the controller and from the supervisor vessel, and one that is called the "great network[-vessel] of the spleen." The courses of the main conduits and of the network vessels differ, in that the former are said to proceed hidden in the body, invisible to the human eyes (except for the foot major yin conduit passing the outside of the outer ankle), while the latter proceed below the skin and can be seen. Hence, the accumulation of evil qi in the network vessels is treated mechanically; the *Ling shu* recommends opening them and letting the "entire blood" flow out. In contrast, diseases in the main conduits are, in general, treated functionally, in that the insertion of needles stimulates long-term depots, short-term repositories, or conduits to fulfill their respective physiological roles. This difficult issue differs from the account in *Ling shu* treatise 10 in referring to network vessels of the two walker conduits instead of to those of the supervisor and controller vessels. As usual, the early commentators accepted this replacement, while the conservatives of the second millennium either rejected it as a mistake or tried to reconcile it with the contents of the *Nei jing*.

[conduit vessels]. As for the great network [vessel] of the spleen, the spleen reflects the soil; it reigns in the central residence, and its rule extends through [all] four seasons. It provides nourishment to the four [remaining] long-term depots. Hence, the [*Ling shu* treatise "Jing mai"] states: "The big network [vessel] of the spleen is called *da bao* 大包. It appears in a distance of three inches below the *yuan ye* 淵腋[opening] and spreads in the chest and the flanks." It emerges between the ninth ribs.

Yang: The twelve conduits have one network [vessel] each; that accounts for twelve network [vessels]. Here now [the text] speaks of fifteen network [vessels, that is to say, in addition] there are two yin and yang network [vessels] and the great network [vessel] of the spleen. That adds up to fifteen network [vessels]. Man has the two yin and yang walker [conduit vessels]; they are located in both feet on the inner and outer sides, respectively. In males, those located at the outer side of the feet represent the conduits, while those located at the inner side of the feet represent the network [vessels]. In females, those located at the inner side of the feet represent the conduits, while those located at the outer side of the feet represent the network [vessels]. Hence, there are the two network [vessels] of the yin and yang walker [conduit vessels, respectively]. The [*Nei*] *jing* states: "In males the yang [vessels] are counted. In females the yin [vessels] are counted. Those counted, they are yin [vessels]. Those not counted, they are network [vessels]."[2] That is [what is] meant here. The great network [vessel] of the spleen is called *da bao* 大包 ("great enclosure"). The spleen, then, has two network [vessels]. All conduit vessels represent the inside; those that branch out and run crosswise are the network [vessels]. Those that depart from the network [vessels] are the tertiary [network vessels, *sun* 孫].[3]

Li Jiong: The yang walker conduit is located at the outer ankle of the left foot; [its] network [vessel] is located at the inner ankle of the right foot. The yin walker conduit is located at the inner ankle of the right foot; [its] network [vessel] is located at the outer ankle of the left foot. The great network [vessel] of the spleen starts from the spleen at a [hole] called *da bao* hole. It is located below the navel.[4]

Hua Shou: Those [vessels] proceeding straight [through the body] are called "conduits"; those that leave sideways are called "network [vessels]." The conduits resemble the real flow of the Han river; the network [vessels] are branches [resembling] streams diverging [from the main river]. Each conduit has a net-

---

2   *Ling shu* treatise 17, "Mai du" 脈度. See also difficult issue 23, X Dachun's commentary on sentence 6.

3   Literally, "grandchild."

4   *Qi* 臍 ("navel") may be a mistake here for *ye* 腋 ("armpits"). The *da bao* 大包 hole is located below the latter.

work [vessel]; the twelve conduits have twelve network [vessels]. For instance, the hand major yin [conduit] is associated with the lung; [its] network [vessel links it to] the large intestine. The hand yang brilliance [conduit] is associated with the large intestine; [its] network [vessel links it to] the lung. Here, [the text] states: "There are fifteen network [vessels]" because it includes the network [vessels] of the yang walker and of the yin walker [conduit vessels], as well as the great network [vessel] of the spleen. For the yang and yin walker [conduit vessels], see the twenty-eighth difficult issue. What are called "network [vessels]" here are the "single conduits" (*qi jing* 奇經) that are not included among the twelve conduits. It is quite possible to call them "network [vessels]."

Zhang Shixian: The yang walker [conduit] penetrates the five short-term repositories; it controls the external [affairs]. The yin walker [conduit] links and penetrates the five long-term depots; it controls the internal [affairs]. The network [vessel] of the spleen penetrates and links all conduits, including those in the yin or yang, in the external or internal, as well as in the upper or lower [sections of the body]. Hence, it is called the "great network [vessel]."

Xu Dachun: As far as the fifteen network [vessels] are concerned, the treatise "Jing mai" of the *Ling* [*shu*] clearly points out the [network vessels] leaving from the twelve [main] conduits as well as from the supervisor and controller [conduits]. Together with the great network [vessel] of the spleen, these are fifteen network [vessels]. They are all named after the hole [from which they branch off]. Diseases can be manifest in them, and methods exist to treat them. Here, [the text] takes recourse to the two walker [conduit vessels] to make up for the [number] fifteen. I do not know where that [doctrine] originated.

Katō Bankei: The *Ling shu* adds the [network vessels of the] controller and supervisor [conduits] to the network [vessels] of the twelve [main] conduits. [Together,] these are fifteen network [vessels]. This difficult issue replaces the [network vessels of the controller and supervisor conduits] by [those of] the yang walker and yin walker [conduit vessels]. Why is that? Well, if the single conduits (*qi jing* 奇經) are contrasted with the twelve [main] conduits, they all [count as] network [vessels]. Hence, one knows that – besides the controller and the supervisor [conduits] – the holes belonging to the two walkers are equivalent to the holes of all the other network [vessels]. The fifteen network [vessels] of the *Ling shu* include the two [network] vessels [associated with the] controller and the supervisor [conduits], but not the yin [walker] network [vessel] and yang [walker] network [vessel]. Now, the controller and the supervisor are part of the circulation system, and they have specific holes.⁵ Hence, they were replaced, in this difficult issue, by the [network vessels of the] yin and yang walkers.

Liao Ping: Including the [network vessels associated with the] supervisor and controller [conduits], there are fourteen network [vessels]. Altogether, the [main] conduits amount to fourteen, too. If each [main] conduit is matched with a great network [vessel], that amounts to twenty-eight .... The number of the network [vessels] should be fourteen. When [the text] states "fifteen," this may have resulted from a mistaken understanding and counting of the great network [vessel] of the spleen. A commentary to the [*Nei*] *jing* further adds a great network [vessel] of the stomach, thus reaching the number sixteen. These are all alike mistakes .... Yang walker vessel must refer here to the supervisor [conduit]. The names are identical but the substance is different. [Yin walker vessel] must refer to the controller [conduit].

---

5   In contrast to the network vessels, which are associated only with the one hole at the junction where they branch off from the main conduits. Katō Bankei's argumentation appears odd here. Usually, the walker, supervisor, and controller conduits are all considered "single conduits" (see also difficult issues 27 through 29). They all have a course and specific holes employed for functional needle treatment.

二十七難曰：（一）脈有奇經八脈者，不拘於十二經，何謂也？

（二）然：有陽維，有陰維，（三）有陽蹻，有陰蹻，（四）有衝，（五）有
督，（六）有任，（七）有帶之脈。（八）凡此八脈者，皆不拘於經，（九）故曰
奇經八脈也。

（十）經有十二，絡有十五，凡二十七，（十一）氣相隨上下，何獨不拘於經
也？

（十二）然：聖人圖設溝渠，通利水道，以備不然。（十三）天雨降下，溝渠
溢滿，當此之時，霧霈妄行，聖人不能復圖也。（十四）此絡脈滿溢，諸經
不能復拘也。

The twenty-seventh difficult issue: (1) Among the vessels are the eight single-conduit vessels which are not touched by the [movement of the qi circulating through
the] twelve [main] conduits. What does that mean?

(2) It is like this. [The eight single-conduit vessels] include the yang rope vessel
and the yin rope vessel, (3) the yang walker vessel and the yin walker vessel, (4) the
throughway vessel, (5) the supervisor vessel, (6) the controller vessel, (7) and the
belt vessel. (8) None of these eight vessels is touched by the [movement of the qi
circulating through the main] conduits. (9) Hence, they are called the eight "single-conduit" vessels.

(10) There are twelve [main] conduits and fifteen network [vessels], twenty-seven
altogether. (11) The qi move up and down [through these conduits and network
vessels], following their respective courses. What [does it mean when it is said that]
only [the eight single-conduit vessels] are not touched by the [movement of the qi
circulating through the main] conduits?

(12) It is like this. The sages [of antiquity] devised and constructed ditches and
reservoirs and they kept the waterways open in order to be prepared for any extraordinary [situation]. (13) When rains poured down from heaven, the ditches and
the reservoirs became filled. In times like that, when the rainfloods rushed wildly,
even the sages could not make plans again; [hence, they had to be prepared]. (14)
Here [in the organism], when the network vessels are filled to overflowing, none of
the [main] conduits could seize any [of their contents, and it is only then that the
surplus contents of these vessels flow into the single-conduit vessels].¹

---

1 The preceding difficult issue briefly referred to the network vessels. Their functions had
   already been elucidated, in detail, in the *Nei jing,* and obviously the *Nan jing* did not
   deem it necessary to add any new insights. In contrast, the functions of the eight single-conduit vessels are neither recognizable from their common designation, nor had
   they been outlined by the *Nei jing. Ling shu* treatise 65 ("Wu yin wu wei" 五音五味) and

Commentaries

(1) *Ding Deyong*: Earlier, [the text] talked about the twelve [main] conduits and fifteen network [vessels] – adding up to twenty-seven – through which the qi move up and down consecutively. [These twenty-seven conduit vessels] transmit the flow of the qi and the blood; they are tied to each other and there is no break [in the circulation proceeding in them]. Here, these eight vessels are passageways proceeding separately. Hence, they are called the eight "single-conduit" vessels. Their points of origin are discussed in a subsequent chapter.

Yang: Qi 奇 ("single") means *yi* 異 ("different"). These eight vessels are not part of [the system of] mutual seizure [of contents] among the twelve conduits; they constitute passageways proceeding separately. They are "different" from the main conduits. Hence, they are called "single-conduits." Their number is eight; hence, one speaks of eight [single-conduit] vessels.

Yu Shu: Qi 奇 is to be read like *ji* 基; it stands for *xie* 斜 ("diagonal") or *ling* 零 ("odd," "fraction"). The meaning implied here is "single." That is to say, these eight vessels are not linked to the yinyang classification of the proper conduits. They do not consist of matching [conduits, resembling the] outside and inside [classification of the main conduits]. They constitute separate passageways proceeding singly. That is why they are called "single-conduits." [The statement of the text that these vessels] are not touched by the [movement of the qi through the main] conduits is verified by these [arguments]. When Mr. Yang stated that "single" means "different," he was wrong.

Xu Dachun: Qi 奇 ("single") should be read like the *qi* in *qi ou* 奇偶 ("odd," "single"). That is to say, in contrast to the twelve [main] conduits, no pairs of foot and hand [conduits] exist in their case. For details, see the next treatise.

Liao Ping: The [*Nei*] *jing* has no clear textual passage on these eight vessels. If one were to say that those [vessels] with holes are the [main] conduits while those without holes are the single[-conduit vessels], then there should be only six single[-conduit vessels] because the supervisor and the controller [vessels] have holes. The latter add up [with the remaining twelve main conduits] to a total of

---

Su wen treatises 41 ("Ci yao tong lun" 刺腰痛論) and 60 ("Gu kong lun" 骨空論) refer to the names of these vessels, to their courses [with the exception of the yin rope], and to their diseases, but the term "eight single-conduit vessels" appears to be an innovation introduced by the *Nan jing*. Similarly, the idea that the single-conduit vessels act as "ditches and reservoirs," absorbing surplus contents of the main conduits, was expressed first in this book. The term *ju* 拘 appears in this paragraph with two different meanings. This discrepancy may have led Hua Shou to state that "single-conduit vessels" in the first sentence might stand for "network vessels." In that case, the meaning of *ju* in sentences 1 and 11 on the one hand, and in sentence 14 on the other hand would, of course, be identical.

fourteen conduits, as Mr. Hua [Shou] has pointed out correctly in his [book] *Shi si jing fa hui* 十四經發揮 ("Elucidations Concerning the Fourteen Conduits").

Li Jiong: *Wei* 維 ("tie") means *chi* 持 ("to support"). The [yang rope vessel] is tied to and supports all the yang [sections of the organism; the yin rope vessel] is tied to and supports all yin [sections of the organism].

(3) *Li Jiong*: *Qiao* 蹺 ("walker") stands for *jie ji* 捷疾 ("rapid") or *xie* 偞 ("to hasten"). That is to say, this vessel provides the mechanism for one's walking [ability]; it is the source of the movement of one's feet.

(4) *Li Jiong*: The throughway vessel is the sea [in which] the twelve conduit vessels [end]. *Chong* 衝 ("throughway") stands for *tong* 通 ("penetration"). That is to say, this vessel reaches down to the feet and up to the head. It receives qi and blood from [all] the twelve [main] conduits.

Ye Lin: *Chong* 衝 ("throughway") means *zhi shang* 直上 ("straight upward").

(5) *Li Jiong*: *Du* 督 ("supervisor") means *du* 都 ("administrative center"). It represents the central link of all the yang vessels.

Ye Lin: *Du* 督 ("supervisor") means "general supervision"(*zong du*) 總督 of all yang [sections].

(6) *Li Jiong*: *Ren* 任 ("controller") stands for *hui* 娃 ("commanding");[2] that is the origin of man's [coming to] life and nourishment.

Ye Lin: *Ren* 任 ("controller") means "controlling" (*tong ren*) 統任 all yin [sections].

(7) *Li Jiong*: *Dai* 帶 ("belt") stands for *shu* 束 ("to bind"). It binds all the other vessels, bringing [their contents] into balance.

(5)–(6) *Liao Ping*: They have special holes; they cannot be single-conduit vessels.

(8) *Liao Ping*: These should be six. The [*Nei*] *jing* does not have this designation [i.e., eight single-conduit vessels]. It was established by this book. Later people adopted it without checking [whether it already existed in the *Nei jing*].

(9) *Liao Ping*: Among the eight vessels [outlined in] this difficult issue are the supervisor and the controller [vessels]. Is this not a contradiction to [the statement in] the preceding difficult issue, [where it was said] that the yang network [vessel] is the network [vessel] of the yang walker, and that the yin network [vessel] is the network [vessel] of the yin walker?

(10) *Liao Ping*: If one counts the controller and the supervisor [vessels] among them, there should be fourteen [main conduits] .... There are [not fifteen but 1]4 [network vessels] .... It should be "[In all, 2]8 [of them]."

---

2 Although the meaning of the term *hui* 娃 ("commanding") corresponds to that of the term *ren* 任 ("controller"), from the statement that follows it one may assume that it is a mistake for *ren* 妊 ("pregnancy"). See also Yang's commentary on sentence 3 of difficult issue 28.

(12) *Li Jiong*: The earth has twenty-four waters, matching the twenty-four conduits and network [vessels]. In addition to these twenty-four waters, the sages devised and constructed ditches and reservoirs. This is used here as a metaphor for the eight single-conduit vessels. "Ditches and reservoirs" are passageways opening passages between all [the twenty-four] waters; they are [designed as] preventive measures against unforeseeable [conditions].

Xu Dachun: For *bu ran* 不然 ("extraordinary"), one could also say *bu yu* 不虞 ("unexpected").

(13) *Li Jiong*: In times when the rainfloods rushed wildly through the ditches and into the reservoirs, the sages just listened to their flow. They did not [have to] make any further plans [to prevent a catastrophe].

(14) *Li Jiong*: When the eight single-conduit vessels are full to overflowing, the twelve [main] conduits will not seize any [of their contents]. They let [the contents of] these passageways proceed separately.

Hua Shou: The movement [of the qi] through the [main] conduits and network [vessels] is marked by a continuing passage. The eight single-conduit vessels are not included in the sequence [of the main conduits and network vessels]. The planning and construction of ditches and reservoirs by the sages is used here as an analogy. It elucidates that when the network vessels are full to overflowing, none of the [main] conduits can seize any [of their surplus contents]; the single-conduit [vessels] serve this purpose. That means that the single-conduit [vessels] serve [as additional ditches and reservoirs] In the case of an overfilling of the network vessels.

Xu Dachun: The waterways are used here as a metaphor for the blood vessels of the human body. When the blood vessels are supplemented completely, the twelve [main] conduits do not suffice to accept the [surplus from the blood vessels]. Consequently, there is an overflow into the single-conduit [vessels]. Hence, the single-conduit [vessels] are separate vessels [branching off from] the twelve [main] conduits.

Katō Bankei: The network vessels are the fifteen network vessels mentioned earlier [in the preceding difficult issue]. Mr. Hua [Shou] believed [that the term "network vessel" could be interpreted here] as designating the single-conduit vessels. That was wrong.

二十八難曰：（一）其奇經八脈者，既不拘於十二經，皆何起何繼也？
（二）然：督脈者，起於下極之俞，並於脊裏，上至風府，入於腦。（三）任
脈者，起於中極之下，以上毛際，循腹裏，上關元，至喉咽。（四）衝脈
者，起於氣衝，並足陽明之經，夾齊上行，至胸中而散也。（五）帶脈者，
起於季脅，迴身一周。（六）陽蹻脈者，起於跟中，循外踝上行，入風
池。（七）陰蹻脈者，亦起於跟中，循內踝上行，至咽喉，交貫衝脈。（八）
陽維、陰維者，維絡于身，溢畜不能環流灌溉諸經者也。（九）故陽維起於
諸陽會也，陰維起於諸陰交也。（十）比于聖人圖設溝渠，（十一）溝渠滿
溢，流于深湖，故聖人不能拘通也。（十二）而人脈隆聖，入於八脈而不環
周，故十二經亦不能拘之。（十三）其受邪氣，畜則腫熱，（十四）砭射之也。

The twenty-eighth difficult issue: (1) If the eight single-conduit vessels are not touched by the [movement of the qi through the main] conduits, from where do they originate and where do their courses continue?

(2) It is like this. The supervisor vessel originates from the transportation [hole] at the [body's] lower end; it continues inside the backbone and moves upward toward the wind palace, where it enters the brain. (3) The controller vessel originates from below the *zhong ji* [hole] and moves upward toward the [pubic] hairline. It proceeds inside the abdomen, ascends to the *guan yuan* [hole], and reaches the throat. (4) The throughway vessel originates from the *qi chong* [hole], parallels the foot yang brilliance conduit, ascends near the navel, and reaches the chest, where it dissipates. (5) The belt vessel originates from the smallest rib and circles around the body. (6) The yang walker vessel originates in the heel; it proceeds along the outer ankle, ascends upward, and enters the *feng chi* [hole]. (7) The yin walker vessel also originates in the heel; it proceeds along the inner ankle, ascends upward, and reaches the throat, where it joins the throughway vessel. (8) The yang rope and the yin rope vessels are tied like a network to the body. When they are supplemented to overflowing, [their contents] stagnate; they cannot [return to the] circulating [qi] by drainage into the [main] conduits. (9) Hence, the yang rope [vessel] originates from a point where all yang [vessels] meet each other, and the yin rope [vessel] originates from a point where all yin [vessels] intersect. (10) This can be compared to the planning and construction of ditches and reservoirs by the sages of antiquity. (11) When the ditches and reservoirs are full, [their surplus contents] flow into deep lakes because [even] the sages were unable to [find other means to] seize [these contents and ensure the continuation of a circulatory] flow. (12) Similarly, when the [conduits and network vessels] of man are filled [to overflowing, their surplus contents] enter the eight [single-conduit] vessels – where they are no longer part of the circulation – because

the twelve [main] conduits cannot seize this [surplus]. (13) When the [single-conduit vessels] receive evil qi which stagnate in them, swelling and heat will result. (14) In this case one has to hit [the respective vessel] with a sharp stone to let [their contents] be discharged.[1]

COMMENTARIES

(1) *Xu Dachun*: For *ji* 繼 ("to continue"), the *Mai jing* 脈經 writes *xi* 繫 ("to be attached to").

    Liao Ping: The fourteen [main] conduits (*jing* 經) resemble the fixed stars (*jing xing* 經星) which do not move. The single[-conduit] vessels stop on their way [at the main conduits] in the same way that the planets utilize the fixed stars as their resting places. The movement and the stopping of the two [kinds of stars] are not identical. The [movement of the] fixed stars and that of the planets are opposite to each other. "Eight" should be "six."

(2) *Lü Guang*: The supervisor vessel is the sea [in which all] the yang vessels [end].

    Ding Deyong: [When the text states that] the supervisor vessel originates from the transportation [hole] at the [body's] lower end, it refers to the *chang qiang* 長強 hole at the lower end of the backbone.[2] That is where the supervisor and controller [vessels] meet and tie up with each other. The two ascend together inside the backbone to the *feng fu* 風府 hole, which is located one inch above the hair[-line]. There the supervisor vessel meets with the yang rope [vessel].

    Yu Shu: The [*Nan*] *jing* states: "The supervisor vessel originates from the [body's] lower end; it ascends and enters the brain." Mr. Lü has said: "It is the sea [in which] all yang [vessels end]." Mr. Yang has said: "It is the central link of all the yang vessels." The flow through the supervisor vessel starts from the *hui yin* 會陰 hole.[3] It follows the center of the backbone, ascending towards the *da chui* 大椎 hole,[4] where it meets in an intersection with the three yang [conduits] of the hands and feet. It ascends further to the *yin men* 瘂門 hole,[5] where it meets with the yang rope [vessel]. It ascends further to the *bai hui* 百會 hole,[6] where it meets in an intersection with the major yang [conduit]. Then it descends to the

---

1   Sentences 10 through 14 have been transferred, in Ding Jin's edition, to follow the text of difficult issue 27.

2   The *chang qiang* 長強 hole is situated three *fen* above the lower end of the spine. It is also the point where the foot minor yin and the foot minor yang vessels meet.

3   The *hui yin* 會陰 hole is situated on the perineum.

4   This hole is situated at the lower end of the neck.

5   This hole is situated at the hairline in the center of the back of the head.

6   This hole is situated on the top of the head.

nasal column, down to the *shui gou* 水溝 hole,[7] where it meets in an intersection with the hand yang brilliance [conduit]. From this course one may conclude that [the supervisor vessel] is indeed the "sea [in which] all yang [vessels end]" and the "central tie of all the yang vessels."

Xu Dachun: Yu 俞 ("transportation") stands for *xue* 穴 ("hole"). "Lower end" refers to the *chang duan* 長短 hole.[8] It belongs to the controller vessel and is located at the tip of the bone at the lower end of the spine.

Liao Ping: Of each conduit it is said: "It is tied to that-and-that [vessel] and constitutes [together with it] outside and inside, and it belongs to that-and-that, which represents its basic long-term depot." Here it is said that the [supervisor vessel] belongs to the brain. Well, if the supervisor vessel belongs to the brain, it must be the conduit vessel of the brain.

(3) *Ding Deyong*: Zhong ji 中極 ("central pole") is the name of a hole, located four inches below the navel. Below the "central pole" is the *qu gu* 曲骨 ("crooked bone") hole where the controller vessel originates. [When the text states that] it proceeds inside the abdomen, ascends to the *guan yuan* 關元 [hole], and reaches the throat, it refers to the *tian tu* 天突 hole.[9] This is the point where the controller vessel meets [with the yin rope vessel].

Yang: Ren 任 ("controller") stands for *ren* 妊 ("pregnancy"). This is the basis of man's [coming to] life and nourishment. Hence, [the text] states: "It is located below the *zhong ji* 中極 [hole] and above the *chang qiang* 長強 [hole]."

Yu Shu: According to the *Zhen jing* 鍼經,[10] the controller vessel originates from the *hui yin* 會陰 hole. [When the text of the *Nan jing* states that] it moves upward to the [pubic] hairline, it refers to the *qu gu* 曲骨 hole, which is located at the [pubic] hairline below the lower abdomen. There [the controller vessel] meets with the foot ceasing yin vessel. Then it ascends to the *guan yuan* 關元 [hole], which is located two inches below the navel. It reaches the throat where it meets with the yin rope vessel. The *Su wen* states: "With two times seven years, females reach sexual maturity. The controller vessel is passable and the throughway vessel is full. The monthly affair commences to descend and [the girl] is now able to bear children."[11] That is why Mr. Yang has said: "[The controller vessel] is the basis of man's [coming to] life and nourishment."

---

7 This hole is situated in the center between the nose and the upper lip.

8 *Chang duan* 長短 may be a mistake for *chang qiang* 長強.

9 The *tian tu* 天突 hole is situated in front of the trachea between the clavicles.

10 A "scripture on needling" mentioned in the *Nei jing* and in Sui and Tang bibliographies. It is no longer extant.

11 *Su wen* treatise 1, "Shang gu tian zhen lun" 上古天眞論.

(4) *Lü Guang*: The throughway vessel is the sea [in which all] the yin vessels [end].

Yang: The [*Nei*]*jing* states: "The throughway vessel is the sea [in which all] twelve conduits [end]." In this case it is not just the sea [in which] the yin vessels [end]. I fear Mr. Lü was wrong here. *Chong* 衝 ("throughway") stands for *tong* 通 ("penetration," "all"). That is to say, this vessel reaches down to the feet and up to the head. It receives qi and blood from all (*tong* 通) the twelve conduits. Hence, it is called *chong* 衝.

Yu Shu: The *Su wen* states: "The throughway vessel originates from the *qi jie* 氣街 [hole]." The *Nan jing* states: "It originates from the *qi chong* 氣衝 [hole]." Furthermore, the *Zhen jing* 鍼經 has both these names among its [designations of] holes. The meanings of both *chong* 衝 and *jie* 街 refer to "penetration." The *Su wen* states: "[The throughway vessel] parallels the foot minor yin conduit." The *Nan jing* states: "It parallels the foot yang- brilliance conduit." Moreover, the minor yin vessels pass the navel both to the left and right at a distance of five inches, respectively. The yang brilliance conduits pass the navel both to the left and right at a distance of two inches. The *qi chong* 氣衝 [hole] is the place where the qi of the yang brilliance vessel emerge. In conclusion, the throughway vessel originates from the *qi chong* 氣衝 [hole]. It ascends in between the yang brilliance and minor yin conduits, passing close by the navel. The reason for the [different statements in the *Su wen* and in the *Nan jing*] has become clear now. Principally, the supervisor vessel, the controller vessel, and the throughway vessel all three emerge from the *hui yin* 會陰 hole, where they are united. One vessel, then, branches out into three [vessels], which proceed separately through the yin and yang sections [of the organism]. Hence, they all have different names.

(5) *Ding Deyong*: One inch eight *fen* 分 below the smallest rib is the hole where the belt vessel [originates]. If forms one circle around the body.

(8) *Hua Shou*: The twelve characters *yi chu bu neng huan liu quan gai zhu jing zhe ye* 益畜不能環流灌溉諸經者也 ("when they are supplemented to overflowing ... into the main conduits") should follow the sentence, "similarly, the twelve [main] conduits cannot seize [the surplus contents of the eight single-conduit vessels]." They do not fit here, but there they would follow [the course of the argument]. Mr. Xie [Jinsun] has, therefore, reached the conclusion that some text must be missing in the beginning or at the end [of this difficult issue].

Xu Dachun: The [*Nei*]*jing* has no clear textual passage on the two rope vessels. Hence, one cannot check where they originate and where they end.

Liao Ping: Following [the words] *wei luo yu shen* 維絡于身 ("are tied like a network to the body"), some text must be missing. These two sentences may have been moved here mistakenly by later people. Hence, they are difficult to understand.

(9) *Nan jing 1962*: "Where all yang [vessels] meet each other" refers to the location of the *jin men* 金門 hole of the conduit [associated with the] urinary bladder; it is situated below the outer ankles of the feet to the front .... "Where all yin [vessels] intersect" refers to the location of the *zhu bin* 築賓 hole of the conduit [associated with] the kidneys; it is situated above the inner ankles of the feet.

(10)–(12) *Yang*: Within the nine geographical regions are twelve stream waters (*jing shui* 經水); their flow drains the qi of the earth. Man has twelve conduit/stream vessels (*jing mai* 經脈) reflecting these [stream waters]. They, too, by means of their flow, pour blood and qi through the body, supplying it with life. Hence, they are compared to ditches and reservoirs.

(12)–(14) *Yu Shu*: When the twelve conduits are filled [to overflowing, their surplus contents] enter the eight [single-conduit] vessels where they are no longer part of the circulation. When evil [qi] are present in the eight [single-conduit] vessels, they cause swelling, heat, and accumulations. Hence, one must hit and pierce them with a sharp stone. Hence, [the text] states: "Hit [the respective vessel] with a sharp stone."

(14) *Xu Dachun*: This refers to the method of treating [diseases in the single-conduit vessels]. The [contents of the] single-conduit vessels cannot join the circulation. Hence, evil qi [after having entered them] have no way of getting out. When one uses sharp stones to hit [these vessels], the evil qi follow the blood and will be drained. As a result, the disease will be cured.

THE TWENTY-NINTH DIFFICULT ISSUE

二十九難曰：（一）奇經之為病何如？

（二）然：陽維維於陽，陰維維於陰，（三）陰陽不能自相維，則悵然失志，溶溶不能自收持。（四）陽維為病苦寒熱（五）陰維為病苦心痛。（六）陰蹻為病，陽緩而陰急。（七）陽蹻為病，陰緩而陽急。（八）衝之為病，逆氣而裏急。（九）督之為病，脊強而厥。（十）任之為病，其內苦結，（十一）男子為七疝，（十二）女子為瘕聚。（十三）帶之為病，腹滿，腰溶溶若坐水中。（十四）此奇經八脈之為病也。

The twenty-ninth difficult issue: (1) What is it like when the single-conduit [vessels] have a disease?

(2) It is like this. The yang rope is tied to the yang [conduits]; the yin rope is tied to the yin [conduits]. (3) When the yin and yang [rope vessels] cannot maintain their respective ties, one feels uncomfortable and loses his mind, One is weak and cannot support his [stature]. (4) When the yang rope has a disease, one suffers from [fits of] cold and heat. (5) When the yin rope has a disease, one suffers from pain in the heart. (6) When the yin walker [vessel] has a disease, the yang [walker vessel] is relaxed while the yin [walker vessel] is tense. (7) When the yang walker [vessel] has a disease, the yin [walker vessel] is relaxed while the yang [walker vessel] is tense. (8) When the throughway [vessel] has a disease, the qi move contrary to their proper course and tensions occur inside [the abdomen]. (9) When the supervisor [vessel] has a disease, one's back is stiff and [it is bent] backward. (10) When the controller [vessel] has a disease, one suffers from internal knots. (11) Males will develop the seven elevation-illnesses; (12) females will develop conglomeration-illness-collections. (13) When the belt [vessel] has a disease, the abdomen will be full, and the loins will be bloated as if one were sitting in water. (14) That happens when the eight single-conduit vessels have a disease.

COMMENTARIES

(3) *Lü Guang: Chang ran* 悵然 ("uncomfortable") means that a person is afraid. When one is afraid, the rope vessels relax. Hence, the respective person will no longer be able to support his bodily [stature]. When one is afraid, he loses his mind; he has a tendency to forget, and he will be confused.

Ding Deyong: The [yin and] yang rope [vessels] are the ties linking the yin and the yang [vessels]; they are responsible for supporting the vessels of the yin and yang [sections of the organism]. Here, they cannot maintain their respective ties; that is, the yang [rope vessel] can no longer support all the yang [vessels], and the yin [rope vessel] can no longer support all the yin [vessels]. Hence, [the text] states: "One feels uncomfortable and loses his mind." *Rong rong* 溶溶 ("weak") means *nuan man* 緩慢 ("relaxed and slow"). Hence, one is unable to support his [bodily stature].

Xu Dachun: *Rong rong* 溶溶 ("weak") describes a drifting, unsettled state.

Liao Ping: That is a disease of one's muscles.

(4)–(5) *Lü Guang*: The yang [qi] are the guard [qi]; hence, [when the yang rope vessel has a disease one suffers from fits of] cold and heat. The yin [qi] are the camp [qi]; the camp [qi] are the blood. The blood is [associated with] the heart. Hence, [in the case of a disease in the yin rope vessel], one suffers from pain in the heart.

Ding Deyong: The yang rope vessel is attached[1] to all yang conduits; in the case of a disease [in the yang rope vessel], one suffers from [fits of] cold and heat. The yin rope [vessel] is attached to all yin conduits; in the case of a disease [in the yin rope vessel] one suffers from pain in the heart.

Xu Dachun: The yang [conduits] rule the external [sections of the organism]; in the case of an unbalanced [presence of] yang qi, [fits of] cold and heat will result. The yin [conduits] rule the internal [sections of the organism]. The heart is [associated with] the minor yin. In the case of an unbalanced [presence of] yin qi, pain in the heart [will result].

(6)–(7) *Lü Guang*: The yin walker [vessel] ascends at the inner ankle. In the case of a disease, this vessel will be tense from the inner ankle upward [while the yang walker vessel] will be relaxed from the outer ankle upward. The yang walker [vessel] ascends at the outer ankle. In the case of a disease, this vessel will be tense from the outer ankle upward [while the yin walker vessel] will be relaxed from the inner ankle upward.

Ding Deyong: The eight single-conduit vessels [reflect] the principle behind the planning and the construction of ditches and reservoirs by the sages in order to ensure the passability of the waterways [even under extraordinary circumstances]. The diseases [of these vessels] cannot emerge from within [these vessels] themselves; they are always caused by an influex [of surplus contents] from the [main] conduits when the latter are replete. These [surplus contents] are taken away [from the walker vessels] by piercing them with sharp stones. Whenever the yang vessels are replete, they distribute [their surplus contents] into the yang walker [vessel]; as a result, the yang walker [vessel] is ill. Whenever the yin vessels are replete, they distribute [their surplus contents] into the yin walker [vessel]; as a result, the yin walker [vessel] is ill. Hence, when the [text states that in case the] yin walker [vessel] or the yang walker [vessel] are ill, the [respective]

---

1   I interpret *zhu* 主 ("to rule") here as *zhu* 注 ("to be attached to").

yin or yang [walker vessels] are relaxed or tense, this means that they suffer from depletion or repletion. When the yin walker [vessel] is ill, the yang [walker vessel] is relaxed and the yin [walker vessel] is tense. That is, one suffers from a depletion of yin [qi]; one's feet are stiff and straight, and the fifteen[2] network [vessels] are blocked. When the yang walker [vessel] is ill, the yin [walker vessel] is relaxed and the yang [walker vessel] is tense. That is, one runs madly, does not lie down, and dies. *Qiao* 蹺 ("walker") stands for *jian* 健 ("active").

Zhang Shixian: All yin vessels distribute their excess contents into the yin walker. When the yin walker has received these evil [qi], the resulting disease will be manifest in the yin section, not in the yang section. Hence, the yang [walker vessel] will be relaxed while the yin [walker vessel] is tense. "Relaxed" and "tense" carry the meaning of "depletion" and "repletion," [respectively]. All yang vessels distribute their excess contents into the yang walker. When the yang walker has received these evil [qi], the resulting disease will be manifest in the yang section, not in the yin section. Hence, the yin [walker vessel] will be relaxed while the yang [walker vessel] is tense.

Ding Jin: When the yin walker receives evil [qi], the yang walker is relaxed while the yin walker is tense. The yin walker originates from the center of the heels and proceeds upward along the inner ankle. When the yang walker receives evil [qi] the yin walker is relaxed while the yang walker is tense. The yin walker originates from the center of the heels and proceeds upward along the outer ankle.

(8) *Lü Guang*: The throughway vessel proceeds from the *guan yuan* 關元 [hole] upward to the throat. Hence, when this vessel has a disease, [its] qi move contrary to their proper course and tensions occur inside [the body].

Ding Deyong: *Ni qi* 逆氣 ("qi moving contrary to their proper course") refers to [qi in the] abdomen moving contrary to their proper course; *li ji* 裏急 ("internal tensions") refers to pain in the abdomen.

Liao Ping: The throughway vessel is the sea [in which] the twelve conduits [end]; man's stem qi (*zong qi* 宗氣) emerge from it. In particular it rules the reproductive affairs. It is called "lymphatic vessel" (*lin ba guan* 淋巴管) by the Westerners. Its main [course proceeds] through the abdomen, but at the same time it proceeds along the back. Hence, Mr. Yang's *Tai su* considered the three vessels – the throughway, controller, and supervisor – to constitute one entity.

(9) *Lü Guang*: The supervisor vessel is in the spine. In the case of a disease, this vessel is tense. Hence, it causes the spine to be stiff.

Xu Dachun: *Jue* 厥 ("backward") has the same [meaning] as *ni* 逆 ("contrary to a proper direction").

---

2   The text says "five." That is probably a mistake for "fifteen."

(10)–(11) *Lü Guang*: The controller vessel starts from the cervical opening. Hence when this vessel is [blocked by] knots, it causes the seven elevation-illnesses [in males] and the conglomeration-illnesses [in females].

Yu Shu: The controller vessel ascends along the abdomen. Hence, [in the case of a disease] one suffers from internal knots; males will develop the seven elevation-illnesses[3] – namely, *jue* 厥 elevation, *pan* 盤 elevation, *han* 寒 elevation, *wei* 癀 elevation, *fu* 咐 elevation, *lang* 狼 elevation, and *qi* 氣 elevation. These seven diseases originate from [conditions of] depletion and weakness of the qi and the blood, and from imbalances of cold and warmth. Females will suffer from the conglomeration-illnesses. There are eight conglomeration-illnesses – namely, virid conglomeration, yellow conglomeration, dryness concentration, blood concentration, fox concentration, snake conglomeration, turtle conglomeration, and fat conglomeration. *Jia* 瘕 ("conglomeration-illness")[4] means [that one suffers from a disease] that "appears to assume" (*jia* 假) a [specific] material form.

Zhang Shixian: The controller vessel originates from below the *zhong ji* 中極 [hole] and moves upward toward the [pubic] hairline. It proceeds inside the abdomen, ascends to the *guan yuan* 關元 [hole] and reaches the throat. In the case of a disease [a condition emerges] inside the abdomen as if [the vessel][5]

---

3 *Shan* 疝 ("elevation-illness") is a term mentioned in the *Shi ji* 史記, biography of Chunyu Yi 淳于意, (ca. 100 BCE) and in the bibliography of the *Han shu* 漢書. It seems to refer to swellings due to various causes, and it has been associated mostly with diseases in the abdomen and, in particular, in the male reproductive organs. Chao Yuanfang 巢元方 (fl. 610 CE), in chapter 20 of his *Zhu bing yuan hou lun* 諸病源候論, named the "seven elevation-illnesses" as they are quoted here by Yu Shu. The origins of some of the seven designations are not clear, including *pan* ("bowl"), *fu* 咐, 附, 肘 (written variously in different texts), and *lang* ("wolf"). The others may be interpreted from their associated symptoms: *jue* ("backwards," i.e., vomiting resulting from accumulations), *wei* ("obstruction"), *han* ("cold"), and *qi* ("qi"). Zhang Zihe 張子和 (1156-1228), in chapter 2 of his *Ru men shi qin* 儒門事親 wrote perhaps the most detailed account of the seven elevation-illnesses, introducing, however, partly different designations – namely, *han* ("cold"), *shui* ("water"), *jin* ("muscles"), *xue* ("blood"), *qi* ("qi"), and *tui* (unclear here). Xu Dachun (see his commentary on sentence 11) referred to still another list when he quoted Chao Yuanfang's original sequence, exchanging, however, *lang* 狼 ("wolf") for *mai* 脈 ("vessel").

4 *Jia* 瘕 ("conglomeration-illness") is an ancient term; it appeared in the *Shan hai jing* 山海經 (eighth to second century BCE) and is also mentioned in the Chunyu Yi biography of the *Shi ji*. Commentators of the respective passages assumed that the term designated swellings caused by concentrations of worms/insects. In *Su wen* treatise 60, "Gu kong lun" 骨空論, *Ling shu* treatise 57, "Shui zhang" 水脹, and the bibliography of the *Sui shu* 隨書, which lists a title *Fu ren jia* 婦人瘕 ("Women's Conglomeration-illnesses"), *jia* is referred to solely in a gynecological sense. In this context, it came to be used to designate various swellings in the female reproductive tract, all specified by additional terms (as mentioned, for instance, in Zhang Shixian's commentary on sentences 10 and 11).

5 Or [the vessels].

were knotted and impassible. The disease manifests itself in males in the seven elevation-illnesses – namely, first, *jue* 厥; second, *pan* 盤; third, *han* 寒; fourth, *wei* 癀; fifth, *fu* 附; sixth, *mai* 脈; and seventh, *qi* 氣. In females this disease manifests itself as an abdominal conglomeration-illness. [Such a disease] often results from stagnating blood. One speaks of *jia* conglomeration-illness when they assume some specific material form. The *jia* 瘕 conglomeration-illnesses are known under eight different names, including snake conglomeration-illness; virid conglomeration-illness; fat conglomeration-illness; yellow conglomeration-illness; dryness conglomeration-illness; blood conglomeration-illness; fox conglomeration-illness; and turtle conglomeration-illness. The *ju* 聚 collections form lumps and do not remain at a specific location.

(10) *Xu Dachun*: *Jie* 結 ("knots") stands for *jin jie* 緊結 ("twisted tightly") or *ning zhi* 凝滯 ("congealed and obstructed"). The controller vessel originates from the cervical opening and proceeds along the abdomen. Hence, [in the case of a disease] internal knots will result.

(11) *Xu Dachun*: The seven elevation-illnesses include, first, the *jue* 厥; second, the *pan* 盤; third, the *han* 寒; fourth, the *wei* 癀; fifth, the *fu* 附; sixth, the *mai* 脈; and seventh, the *qi* 氣 [elevation-illnesses]. Some say [they include the] *han* 寒, *shui* 水, *jin* 筋, *xue* 血, *qi* 氣, *hu* 狐, and *tui* 穨, "breakdown[-illness]".

(12) *Xu Dachun*: *Jia* 瘕 means "to appear as some item and assume its material form." *Ju* 聚 refers to "concentrations that do not disperse." Because males are yang and are associated with the qi, while females are yin and are associated with the blood, their diseases differ. The *Su wen* [treatise] "Gu kong lun" 骨空論 [states]: "In case the controller vessel has a disease, males suffer from internal knots and from the seven accumulation illnesses; females suffer from concentrations below the belt-line. In case the throughway vessel has a disease, the qi move contrary to their proper course and internal tensions occur. In case the supervisor vessel has a disease, one's back is stiff and he is bent backward." That is truly identical with what is [said] here.

(13) *Lü Guang*: The belt vessel circles belt-like around the human body. In case it has a disease, the abdomen is relaxed. Hence, it causes the loins to be weak.

Xu Dachun: *Rong rong ru zuo shui zhong* 溶溶如坐在水中 ("[the loins will be] bloated as if one were sitting in water") refers to a state when one is at ease, relaxed, and shrinks back at cold.

(14) *Katō Bankei*: The [discussion of the] bodily [manifestations] of diseases in the eight [single-conduit] vessels is distributed in the *Nei jing* among many treatises as if they were unrelated to each other. Therefore Yueren has concentrated [all that scattered information], stating it as the present difficult issue.

THE THIRTIETH DIFFICULT ISSUE

三十難曰：（一）榮氣之行，常與衛氣相隨不？
（二）然：經言人受氣於穀。（三）穀入於胃，乃傳與五藏六府，（四）五藏
六府皆受於氣。（五）其清者為榮，濁者為衛，（六）榮行脈中，衛行脈
外，（七）榮周不息，五十而復大會。（八）陰陽相貫，如環之無端，（九）故
知榮衛相隨也。

The thirtieth difficult issue: (1) In general, the camp qi and the guard qi follow each other proceeding [through the organism]. Is it not so?

(2) It is like this. The scripture states: Man receives his qi from the grains. (3) The grains enter the stomach, from which they are transmitted further to the five long-term depots and six short-term repositories. (4) All the five long-term depots and six short-term repositories are supplied with qi [by the stomach]. (5) The clear [portion] turns into camp [qi]; the turbid [portion] turns into guard [qi]. (6) The camp [qi] proceed inside the vessels; the guard [qi] proceed outside of the vessels. (7) They circulate [through the organism] without a break; [after] every fifty [passages they have] another great meeting. (8) The yin and the yang [conduits] are tied to each other like a ring without end. (9) Hence, one knows that the camp and the guard [qi] follow each other.[1]

COMMENTARIES

(1)–(9) *Ding Deyong*: Once man is endowed with life through the true qi of heaven, the water he drinks and the grains he eats enter the stomach. From there they

---

1 The *Nan jing* quotes here, almost literally, a passage from *Ling shu* treatise 18, "Ying wei sheng hui" 營衛生會. The difference from the original wording of the *Nei jing* was pointed out by some of the commentators as insignificant; conservative authors considered it serious and unacceptable. Obviously, the *Nan jing* author(s) expressed here the innovative idea that the stomach supplied all the five long-term depots and the remaining short-term repositories directly with qi digested from food, while the *Nei jing* had offered, in its corresponding treatise, the insight that the qi emitted by the stomach reach the long-term depots and short-term repositories only via the lung.

are transmitted to the five long-term depots and six short-term repositories where they are transformed into essence and blood. Both essence and blood have clear and turbid [portions]. The clear [portion] of the essence turns to the lung where it supports the true qi of heaven. Its turbid [portion] strengthens the bones and the marrow. Hence, the clear [portion] in the blood turns to the heart where it nourishes the spirit. The turbid [portion] of the blood provides external splendor to the flesh. The clear [portion] proceeds inside the vessels; the turbid [portion] proceeds outside the vessels. *Wei* 衛 has the meaning of *wei hu* 衛護 ("to protect").

Yang: *Ying* 營 is written here as *rong* 榮 ("brightness"). *Rong* has the meaning of *rong hua* 榮華 ("splendor"), that is to say, man's hundred bones and the nine orifices receive their splendor from these blood qi. *Ying* 營 stands for *jing ying* 經營 ("operational"). That is to say, the movement in the conduit vessels continues without stop; it links the [entire] human body and provides it with long life. The two meanings [of *ying* and of *rong*] are identical here. *Wei* 衛 stands for *hu* 護 ("to guard"). That is, man has aggressive qi proceeding outside the conduit vessels. At day they proceed through the body, and at night they proceed through the long-term depots to protect the human body. Hence, they are called "guard" qi. Man's yin and yang qi meet in the head, in the hands, and in the feet. Their flow revolves [through the organism] without end. Hence, [the text] states: "Like a ring without end." The heart [is associated with] the operational [qi, i.e.,] the blood. The lung [is associated with] the guard qi. The flow of the blood relies on the [movement of the guard] qi. The movement of the [guard] qi follows the blood. They proceed [through the organism] depending on each other. Hence, one knows that "camp [qi] and guard [qi] follow each other."

Yu Shu: "The scripture states: 'Man receives his qi from the grains. The grains enter the stomach, from which they are transmitted to the five long-term depots and six short-term repositories'." That is to say, water and grains enter the mouth and move down into the stomach. The stomach transforms the grains into qi. [These qi] are transmitted upward into the lung. The lung controls the qi. [These] qi are the guard [qi]. The stomach transforms the water and transmits it upward into the heart. The heart generates the blood. The blood constitutes the camp [qi]. The [guard] qi represent the exterior; they proceed outside of the vessels. The blood represents the interior; it proceeds inside the vessels. Both depend on each other in their movement. Hence, in one day and one night they circulate fifty times through the body; then they meet again in the hand major yin [conduit. The conduits are tied to each other] like a ring without end; they pour [their contents] into each other, creating a revolving movement. The [*Nan*]*jing* states:

"The clear qi become the camp [qi]; the turbid qi become the guard [qi]." If one looks closely at the meaning of clear and turbid, exactly the opposite statement would have been correct. I fear that this is a mistake in writing that has occurred in the course of tradition. In the [treatise] "Yin yang ying xiang lun" 陰陽應象 論 [of the *Su wen*] it is stated: "The clear is yang; it supplements the four limbs. The turbid is yin; it turns to the six short-term repositories." That is the meaning.

Hua Shou: This chapter corresponds to what is said in the eighteenth chapter of the *Ling shu*. However, for [the sentence], "the grains enter the stomach, from which ... are supplied with qi [by the stomach]," the *Ling shu* states: "Man receives his qi from the grain. The grain enters the stomach, and from there [its qi] are transmitted to the lung. This way, all the five long-term depots and six short-term repositories receive qi." That is a minor difference.

Zhang Shixian: Rong 榮 stands for *hua* 華 ("splendor"). *Wei* 衛 ("guard") stands for *hu* 護 ("to protect"). Man's root and basis are his beverages and his food; they maintain his existence. Hence, man receives his qi from the grains. The grains enter the stomach,[2] from which their essence qi flow out to be transported upward to the spleen. The qi of the spleen distribute the essence [qi] further to the five long-term depots and to the six short-term repositories. They all [are supplied with] the qi of the grains in the stomach. The clear [portion] of these qi turns – as soon as the yin [phase of the day] emerges after the *wu* 午 [hour][3] – into camp [qi]. The turbid [portion] of these qi turns – as soon as the yang [phase of the day] emerges after the *zi* 子 [hour][4] – into guard [qi]. The camp [qi] are associated with the yin; they rule the interior. When they enter the conduits, they proceed inside the vessels. The guard [qi] are associated with the yang; they rule the exterior. When they enter the conduits they proceed outside of the vessels. Both circulate [through the organism] without[5] break; after fifty passages they have circulated through the [entire] body. The next morning, at the *yin* hour, they have another great meeting in the hand major yin [conduit]. The yin and the yang [qi proceed] in mutual succession through the twelve conduits like an annular movement revolving without end. Hence, one knows that the camp and the guard [qi] follow each other in their flow.

Xu Dachun: These are the words of the treatise "Ying wei sheng hui" 營衛生會 of the *Ling* [*shu*]. In the text of that scripture, though, following the sentence "the grains enter the stomach" are the four words *yi chuan yu fei* 以傳於肺 ("which

---

2   The text has *wei* 衛. That must be a mistake for *wei* 胃 ("stomach").
3   The *wu* 午 hour lasts over noon from 11 a.m. to 1 p.m.
4   The *zi* 子 hour lasts over midnight from 11 p.m. to 1 a.m.
5   The text has *gong* 工. That must be a mistake for *wu* 無 ("without").

transmits them to the lung"). Then the text continues: "This way, all the five long-term depots and six short-term repositories receive qi." The meaning of this [passage] is quite clear. Here now, [in the *Nan jing*], those four words are omitted. How could the stomach introduce [anything] directly into the five long-term depots and six short-term repositories? The consequences of this passage are very significant; how could it be shortened by that sentence? That amounts to a distortion of the pattern of the transmission [of the qi] through the long-term depots and short-term repositories.

Tamba Genkan: *Rong* 榮 is identical with *ying* 營; both have the meaning of *huan zhou* 環周 ("to encircle"). The *Ling shu* has a treatise entitled "Wu shi ying" 五十營; it elucidates the number of times the qi pass through the human [body each day]. Then there is a treatise entitled "Ying qi" 營氣. It states: "For the WAY of the camp qi, the intake of grain is its most precious function. The grain enter the stomach. The qi are forwarded to the lung. They flow into the center, and they disperse toward the outside. The pure essence, it passes through the conduit channels. It always circulates, without cease. When it has reached the end, it begins anew." Furthermore, the treatise "Ying wei sheng hui" 營衛生會 [also of the *Ling shu*] – it corresponds to the present paragraph – contains the words *ying zhou bu xi* 營周不息, ("they circulate without break"). The meaning is always the same. Now, if we check the *Shuo wen* [*jie zi*] 説文解字, it says: "*Ying* means *shi ju* 市居 ("to settle"). It derives from [the character] *gong* 宮 ("residence") and has the pronunciation of *ying* 榮." This does not correspond to the meaning of *huan zhou* 環周 ("to encircle"). However, *ying* 營 was read as *huan* 環 ("circle") in old times. In the chapter "Wu du" 五蠹 of the *Han fei zi* 韓非子, it is said: "[In ancient times] when Cang Jie 倉頡 created the system of writing, he used the character for 'private' to express the idea of self-centeredness (*zi huan* 子環), and combined the elements for 'private' and 'opposed' to form the character for 'public'."[6] The *Shuo wen* [*jie zi*] quoted the *Han Fei zi* but wrote: "He used the character for 'private' to express the idea of self-centeredness *(zi ying* 子營), and combined the elements for 'opposed' and 'private' to form the character for public." ... The *ying* in *ying wei* 營衛 carries the meaning of *huan* 環, too. The treatise "Mai-du" 脈度 of the *Ling shu* states: "The [yin] walker vessel links up with the major yang [conduit] and yang walker [vessel] and extends further upward. When the qi circulate (*huan* 環) through all [vessels] alike, they cause moistening. When the qi of the eyes fail to circulate (*rong* 榮), then the eyes cannot close." Here, then, *huan* 環 and *rong* 榮 are used interchangeably.

---

6   Cf. Burton Watson (transl.), *Han Fei Zi: Basic Writings* (New York, 1964, 106).

This is further evidence. When Yang commented that *rong* stands for *rong hua*, while *ying* stands for *jing ying*, he distorted the message of the [*Nei*] *jing*.

(1) *Xu Dachun*: *Xiang sui* 相隨 ("follow each other") is to say that they are united and proceed together.

   Liao Ping: This refers to the two paths, one of which is in accordance with the proper direction and one of which is contrary to it. That is also expressed in the saying, "husband and wife have the same way but they take different roads." [The present passage] by no means states that [the camp qi and the guard qi literally] follow each other in their movement. If they were [literally] following each other, [the text] could not say that they meet [each other]. Xu [Dachun] misinterpreted this metaphor. He believed that the camp and the guard [qi] proceed together through one vessel.

   Nan jing 1962: *Xiang sui* 相隨 has the meaning "united with each other and proceeding together."

三十一難曰：（一）三焦者，何稟何生？何始何終？其治常在何許？可曉以不？

（二）然：三焦者，水穀之道路，氣之所終始也。（三）上焦者，在心下，下膈，在胃上口，主內而不出。其治在膻中，玉堂下一寸六分，直兩乳間陷者是。（四）中焦者，在胃中脘，不上不下，主腐熟水穀。其治有齊傍。（五）下焦者，當膀胱上口，主分別清濁，主出而不內，以傳導也。其治在齊下一寸。（六）故名曰三焦，其府在氣街。一本曰衝。

The thirty-first difficult issue: (1) The Triple Burner: how is it supplied and what does it generate? Where does it start and where does it end? And where, in general, [are its disorders] regulated? Can that be known?

(2) It is like this. The Triple Burner encompasses the passageways of water and grain [in the organism]. It represents the conclusion and the start of [the course of] the qi. (3) The upper [section of the Triple] Burner extends from below the heart downward through the diaphragm [and ends] at the upper opening of the stomach. It is responsible for intake but not for discharge. [Disorders in this section are] regulated at the *dan zhong* [hole, located] one inch and six *fen* below the *yu tang* [hole], exactly in the fold between the two breasts. (4) The central [section of the Triple] Burner is located in the central duct of the stomach; it does not extend further upward or downward. It is responsible for the spoiling and processing of water and grains. [Disorders in this section are] regulated to the sides of the navel. (5) The lower [section of the Triple] Burner [begins] exactly at the upper opening of the urinary bladder [and extends downward]. It is responsible for separating the clear from the turbid [portions]. It controls discharge but not intake, and it serves as a transmitter. [Disorders in this section are] regulated one inch below the navel. (6) Hence, one speaks of it Triple Burner. Its [qi are] collected at the street of qi. Another copy [of this text] says "throughway" [of qi].[1]

---

1   The character of the so-called Triple Burner has remained a controversial issue for as long as we can trace this concept in medical literature. Not unlike their counterparts in ancient Greek medicine, ancient Chinese thinkers assumed the existence of some kind of a heat source in the organism. Hence, they conceptualized the ruler-fire and the minister-fire, as well as the Triple Burner. Obviously, the *Nei jing* documents the development of the Triple Burner from a designation of functions (see the various *Su wen* passages quoted by the commentators) to the designation of a tangible entity (see the *Ling shu* treatise quoted by Xu Dachun in his commentary on sentences 1 through 6). In the *Nan jing*, in contrast to both the *Su wen* and the *Ling shu*, the Triple Burner – with a name but no form itself (see difficult issue 38) – appears to be considered a functional description of the upper, central, and lower groups of organs in the body. Current textbooks in the People's Republic of China offer differing opinions as to whether one should interpret the

(1) *Xu Dachun*: *Bing* 稟 ("supplied") stands for *shou* 受 ("receives"). ["Where does it start and where does it end"] refers to origin and conclusion of its conduit. *Zhi* 治 ("disorders regulated") is identical with the *zhi* in *xian zhi* 縣治 ("county administration"); [it refers to] the place where [the three sections of the Triple Burner] are located.

Liao Ping: The text of the [*Nei*] *jing* is quite clear on this. Why should anybody make it the subject of a question?

(2-3) *Yang*: *Jiao* 焦 stands for *yuan* 元 ("origin"). Heaven has the qi of the three originals;[2] they serve to generate and form the ten thousand things. Man reflects heaven and earth. Hence, he too has the qi of the three originals to nourish the form of the human body. All three [sections of the Triple] Burner occupy a definite position and still they do not represent a proper long-term depot.

Li Jiong: The Triple Burner [has been compared in the *Su wen*] with the official responsible for maintaining the ditches; the passageways of water originate from there.[3] The passage of the water enters [the organism] through the upper [section of the Triple] Burner and leaves it through the lower [section of the Triple] Burner. The *dan zhong* 膻中 is the sea [in which all] qi [end]; it is located three inches below the navel.[4] Thus one knows that [the Triple Burner] represents conclusion and start of the [course of the] qi.

Triple Burner as an anatomical entity or simply as a functional description. The *Zhong yi xue gai lun* 中医学概论 of 1978 (Shanghai, 23) has found an interesting compromise. It distinguishes between the Triple Burner on the one hand and the three sections of the Triple Burner on the other. In the *Zhong yi xue gai lun*, the Triple Burner is considered to be a short-term repository responsible, first, for the passage of the original qi through the entire body – thus stimulating the remaining long-term depots and short-term repositories in their functions – and, second, for the passage of the liquids through the body. The upper, central, and lower sections of the Triple Burner are assumed to refer to the heart and lung, the spleen and stomach, and the liver, kidneys, and bladder, respectively. The wording of the present difficult issue is not as clear as one might wish. In sentence 3, I believe that *xin xia* 心下 ("below the heart") is a mistake for *xin shang* 心上 ("extends from above the heart"). My interpretation of sentence 5 is based on the description in sentence 4 of the central section of the Triple Burner, which is said here not to "extend further upward or downward." Hence, this should be the case with both the upper and the lower section.

2   This sentence is to be understood as "The universe consists of the three original principles – namely, heaven, earth, and water."

3   Cf. *Su wen* treatise 8, "Ling lan mi dian lun" 靈蘭祕典論.

4   The term *dan zhong* is mentioned in the *Nei jing* as an entity located in the chest. The *Ling shu*, in treatise 35, "Zhang lun" 脹論, calls it the "residential walls surrounding the heart ruler" (*xin zhu zhi gong cheng* 心主之宮城). The *Su wen*, in its treatise 8, "Ling lan mi dian lun," said of the *dan zhong*: "It is the emissary among the officials. Happiness

Hua Shou: The long-term depots and short-term repositories of the human body have physical appearance and shape; they are supplied [with qi] and they are generated. For instance, the liver receives qi from the [phase of] wood and is generated by the [phase of] water. The heart receives qi from the [phase of] fire and is generated by the [phase of] wood. There is no exception. Only the Triple Burner has no physical appearance and shape, and it is supplied and generated by nothing but the original qi and the qi [sent out] by the stomach. That is why [the text] states: "It encompasses the passageways of water and grain [in the organism]; it represents conclusion and start of [the course of] the qi."

(1)–(2) *Zhang Shixian*: *Bing* stands for *bing fu* (稟賦 "endowed"). *Sheng* 生 stands for *fa* 發 ("to emit"). *Shi* 始 stands for *qi* 起 ("to emerge"). *Zhong* 終 stands for *zhi* 止 ("to stop"). The Triple Burner is supplied with qi moving in the supervisor [vessel] as provision of its beginning; it relies on the qi of the grains in the stomach as provision for its [continuing] generation. It is the official responsible for the maintenance of the ditches; the waterways originate from it. Water and grains enter [the organism] through the upper [section of the Triple] Burner; they leave through the lower [section of the Triple] Burner. The *dan zhong* 膻中 is the sea [in which all] the qi [end]. A second "sea [in which all] the qi [end]," i.e., a *qi hai* 氣海 hole] is located one and a half inches below the navel. Hence, one knows that [the Triple Burner] represents the conclusion and the start of the [course of the] qi.

(2) *Xu Dachun*: This is a general summary of the meaning of the Triple Burner. It says that [the Triple Burner] is supplied and generated by water and grains, and that it constitutes the start and conclusion of the [course of the] qi.

(3) *Yang*: [The region] from the diaphragm upward is called the upper [section of the Triple] Burner. It controls the emission of yang qi, providing warmth to the space between the skin and the flesh. That resembles the gentle flow of fog. The "upper opening of the stomach" [is a] hole that lies two inches five *fen* 分 below the sternum.

Yu Shu: *Dan zhong* 膻中 is the name of a hole. It is a hole situated exactly in the center between the two breasts. The qi of the controller vessel are emitted from here. The *Su wen* states: "The *dan zhong* is the emissary among the officials." It controls the distribution of qi into the yin and yang [sections of the organism]. When the qi are balanced, and when one's mind reaches into the distance, happiness and joy originate. That is [what is] meant by "distribution of qi." Hence,

---

and joy emerge from there." *Ling shu* treatise 33, "Hai lun," calls it the "sea of the qi." Later commentators have identified the *dan zhong* with the heart ruler – that is, with the heart-enclosing network itself. Its allocation here to a place below the navel is rather unusual.

[disorders in the upper section of the Triple Burner] are regulated through [a hole located] in the center [between the breasts]. The upper [section of the Triple] Burner is responsible for the entry of water and grains [into the organism]. It takes in but it does not discharge. When [the upper section of the Triple Burner] has a disease, that is expressed only in terms of "cold" and "hot." In the case of a depletion one supplements its heart;[5] in the case of repletion one drains its lung. If one treats [disease] like this, not one failure will occur in ten thousand cases. The *Ling shu jing* states: "The upper [section of the Triple] Burner resembles fog." That is to say, when it passes the qi, that resembles mist gently flowing into all the conduits. In other words, the qi of the stomach and the qi distributed by the *dan zhong* are poured downward by the lung into all the long-term depots. The [*Nei*] *jing* states: "The lung passes the qi of heaven." That is the meaning implied here.

Hua Shou: *Zhi* 治 ("disorders regulated") is equal here to *si* 司 ("to oversee"); it corresponds to the *zhi* in *jun xian zhi* 郡縣治 ("commandary and county administration"). That is to say, [the *dan zhong* hole, the *tian shu* 天樞 hole, and the *yin jiao* 陰交 hole] are the locations where the three [sections of the Triple] Burner are located. According to other [commentators], *zhi* 治 should be read in the second tone as "when the three [sections of the Triple] Burner have a disease, treatment should be applied at these locations." That is a [reference to the] technique of needling. The Triple Burner represents the minister fire. Fire is capable of spoiling and processing the ten thousand things. [The character] *jiao* 焦 ("burner") is derived from "fire"; it, too, [refers to] qi which spoil things. The meaning is to be taken from the terms.

Xu Dachun: *Ge* 膈 stands for *ge* 隔 ("to screen off"). Below the heart is a membrane screening off the turbid qi. It is called *ge* 膈.

(4) *Yang*: [The region] from the navel upward is called the central [section of the Triple] Burner. It transforms the flavor [qi] of water and grain, and it generates the blood with which it nourishes the five long-term depots and six short-term repositories, as well as the [entire] body. The "central duct" [is a] hole that lies four inches below the sternum.

Yu Shu: The central [section of the Triple] Burner includes spleen and stomach. When the central [section of the Triple] Burner has a disease, that is expressed only in terms of "cold" or "hot." In the case of a depletion, one supplements its stomach; in the case of repletion, one drains its spleen. If one treats [disease] like that, not one failure will occur in ten thousand cases. The *Ling shu jing* states:

---

5   "Its heart" refers to the concept that the upper section of the Triple Burner encloses the heart (and the lung).

"The central [section of the Triple] Burner resembles a humidifier." That is to say, it spoils and processes the water and the grains. "Its [disorders are] regulated to the sides of the navel" – [that is to say], both to the left and to the right of the navel, at a distance of one inch each, emerge the stomach vessels of the foot yang brilliance [conduits]. To the sides of the navel are the *tian shu* 天樞 holes [of these conduits]. The central [section of the Triple] Burner controls spleen and stomach. Hence, its [disorders] are regulated at that conduit. Hence, [the text] states: "To the sides of the navel."

(5) *Yang*: [The region] below the navel is called lower [section of the Triple] Burner. One inch below the navel is the *yin jiao* 陰交 hole. [The lower section of the Triple Burner] controls the timely passage downward of the stools. Hence, [the text] states: "It [controls] discharge but does not take in."

Yu Shu: When the lower [section of the Triple] Burner has a disease, that is expressed only in terms of "cold" or "hot." In the case of a depletion one supplements its kidneys; in the case of repletion one drains its liver. If one treats [disease] like that, not one failure will occur in thousand cases. The *Ling shu jing* states: "The lower [section of the Triple] Burner resembles a ditch." That is to say, the urinary bladder controls the water. The *Su wen* states: "The Triple Burner represents the official responsible for maintaining the ditches. The waterways originate from there." One inch below the navel is the meeting point of the three yin [conduits] of the feet with the controller vessel. The [disorders of the lower section of the Triple Burner are] regulated here because the [entire] lower [region of the body] is linked [to this meeting point].

Li Jiong: [The lower section of the Triple Burner] separates the water and the grains which were taken in through the upper [section of the Triple] Burner. The clear [portions] become urine; the turbid [portions] become feces. They are then transmitted to the outside.

Xu Dachun: The clear [portions] enter the bladder and become the urine; the turbid [portions] enter the large intestine and become the dregs.

(6) *Yang*: The *qi jie* 氣街 ("street of qi") is a passageway of the qi. The Triple Burner controls the passage of the qi. Hence, [the text] states: "It collects [its qi] at the *qi jie*." *Jie* stands for *qu* 衢 ("crossing"). *Qu* is a place where four roads reach [into different directions]. Another copy [of this text] says *chong* 衝 ("throughway"). That is not the language of Bian Que. Hence, when Mr. Lü recorded this [term], he said that it appeared in "another copy" and that, because of its meaning, it should not be used.

Yu Shu: The *qi jie* 氣街 [holes] are located in a distance of two inches on both sides of the center in the hair of the lower abdomen. At these [two] holes, the qi of the foot yang brilliance vessel are emitted. It has been said that the Triple Burner controls the qi of the three originals, and that it collects [its qi] at the *qi jie*. This *qi jie* is called *qi chong* 氣衝 in the *Zhen jing* 鍼經. *Chong* means *tong* 通 ("to pass through"). That is not different from *si da* 四達 ("reaching into four directions"). It is quite possible to retain both [terms – namely, *qi jie* and *qi chong*]! Why is the *qi jie* regarded as the [place] where [the Triple Burner] collects [its qi]? Because the stomach [which is associated with] the foot yang brilliance [conduit] transforms the grains to qi. The Triple Burner controls the qi of the three originals. Hence, the *qi jie* is regarded as [the place] where [the Triple Burner] collects [its qi].

Hua Shou: In my opinion, the sentence "its short-term repository is situated at the street of qi" is either an erroneous abridgment [of a longer passage] or a [mistaken] amendment. The Triple Burner [itself] is one of the body's short-term repositories. Its conduits are the hand minor yang and the hand heart ruler [conduits]. It can be treated through both of them. Therefore, it does not need to have a short-term repository of its own.

Xu Dachun: *Fu* 府 ("short-term repository") is equal to *she* 舍 ("shelter"). It has the meaning of "storage and accumulation." That is to say, the qi [of the Triple Burner] are stored and accumulated here. Mr. Hua expressed the opinion that this sentence is an erroneous abridgment [of a longer passage]. That is incorrect.

(1)–(6) *Xu Dachun*: The [treatise] "Gu kong lun" 骨空論 of the *Su* [*wen* states]: "The throughway vessel emerges from the 'street of qi'." The commentary says: "That is a hole on the foot yang brilliance conduit; it is located at the hairline on both sides [of the center]." The treatise "Ying wei sheng hui" 營衛生會[6] of the *Ling* [*shu*] states: "The [qi of the] Upper Burner emerge from the upper opening of the stomach. they ascend parallel to the throat, penetrate the diaphragm and dissipate in the chest. They extend further into the armpit, follow a section of the major yin [conduit], turn around to the yang brilliance [conduit], ascend to the tongue and descend to the foot yang brilliance [conduit]. They usually move together with the camp [qi] in the yang [conduits] over 25 units, and in the yin [conduits] over 25 units. This constitutes one circulation. The fact is: After 50 units another grand meeting occurs in the hand major yin [conduit]. [The qi of] the Central Burner, they too [emerge] from the stomach opening; they emerge from behind the Upper Burner. The qi received there are discharged as dregs, steamed as *jin* 津 and *ye* 液 body liquids, and transformed to fine essence. [The latter] pours upward into the lung vessel where it is transformed to

6   This treatise is usually called "Ying wei sheng hui" 營衛生會. The following account suggests a conduit-like interpretation of the Triple Burner.

blood which in turn is supplied to the entire body. There is nothing more precious! Hence it may pass only through the conduit channels. It is called „camp qi". The Lower Burner discharges into the curved intestine and pours out into the urinary bladder where its liquids seep in. The fact is: Water and grain are regularly present together in the stomach. There they are transformed to dregs and together they descend into the large intestine. //where they constitute the Lower Burner, where its liquids seep in,// A separate juice is secreted along the Lower Burner and seeps into the urinary bladder." It is also said that the camp [qi] emerge from the central [section of the Triple] Burner, while the [qi of the stomach emerge from the lower [section of the Triple] Burner. The *Su* [*wen* treatise] "Ling lan mi dian lun" 靈蘭祕典論 states: "The Triple Burner is the official functioning as opener of channels. The paths of water originate in it." If one takes all these textual passages into consideration, the meaning [of the Triple Burner] becomes even more obvious.

Ye Lin: [It is stated that] the upper [section of the Triple] Burner is located below the diaphragm because its upper layer is attached to the lower layer of the diaphragm. Its qi move upward from below; they disperse in the chest and evaporate – like steam – into the skin and the pores. Hence, [the upper section of the Triple Burner ends] at the upper opening of the stomach; it is responsible for intake but not for discharge. Its [disorders are] regulated at the *dan zhong* 膻中 hole which belongs to the controller vessel. This [hole] is located – on the basis of the individually standardized inch – one inch and six *fen* below the *yu tang* 玉堂 [hole]. That is where the qi of the controller vessel are emitted. [The text states:] "The central [section of the Triple] Burner is located in the central duct of the stomach" because it includes the liver and encloses the stomach. Its [disorders are] regulated at the *tian shu* 天樞 [holes] to the sides of the navel. That is a hole of the stomach vessel. [The central section of the Triple Burner] functions in the central duct of the stomach. This central duct is a location where the twelve conduits originate and where they meet, and it is the place where yin and yang [portions] of the meat [consumed] are finished. Hence it is called *wan* 脘.[7] The lower [section of the Triple] Burner is located exactly at the upper opening of the urinary bladder. That is a separation line represented by the *lan* 闌 gate. From there the clear [portions] enter the bladder where they become qi and urine. The turbid [portions] enter the large intestine where they become dregs and waste. Hence, [the lower section of the Triple Burner] controls discharge

---

7   "Yin and yang [portions] of the meat [consumed]" may refer to liquid and solid portions in one's food. The term "finished" is used here for "processed" because the corresponding character *wan* 完 reappears, together with the radical *rou* 肉 ("meat"), in the character *wan* 脘 ("[stomach-]duct").

but not intake; it serves as a transmitter. Its [disorders] are regulated below the navel at the *yin jiao* 陰交 hole of the controller vessel. The [treatise] "Ling lan mi dian lun" of the *Su wen* states: "The Triple Burner is the official functioning as opener of channels. The paths of water originate in it." That is [what is] meant here. As to its location on the "street of qi," the *qi jie* 氣街 [holes] are located on both sides of the [center of the] hairline. They represent holes on the foot yang brilliance [conduits]. That is the root and the origin of the Triple Burner; it is the location of the qi. It is a fatty membrane emerging from the tie between the kidneys. The Triple Burner is associated with the residence of the minister fire. The nature of fire is to ascend from below. Hence, the [treatise] "Jing mai bie lun" 經脈別論 of the *Su wen* states: "Beverages enter [the organism] through the stomach. Overflowing essence qi are transported upward to the spleen." That is a reference to the central [section of the Triple] Burner. "The qi of the spleen spread the essence which ascends [further] and turns to the lung." That is a reference to the upper [section of the Triple] Burner. "From there they free and regulate the paths of water, moving downward to the urinary bladder." That is a reference to the lower [section of the Triple] Burner. But why are only beverages emphasized in this discussion of the qi of the upper, central, and lower [section of the Triple] Burner? [Anybody posing such a question] does not know that the qi are transformed from water. Through the inhalation of the heavenly yang, the water of the urinary bladder follows the fire of the heart downward to the lower [section of the Triple] Burner. There it evaporates like steam and is transformed into qi moving up again, where they become the jin 津 [liquids], the *ye* 液 [liquids], and the sweat. All of that rests on the principle that when fire meets water, a transformation into qi takes place.[8] The meaning is that heavenly yang [i.e., the qi of the sun] enters earthly yin [i.e., the water in the soil]. The [latter], following the movement of the yang qi, ascends and becomes clouds and rain.

Nan jing 1962: Throughout history, commentators have voiced all kinds of different opinions concerning the Triple Burner as one of the six short-term repositories. Most important was the argument over whether the [Triple Burner] represents an entity with a name and no physical appearance, or with both name and physical appearance. In addition there were [authors] proposing [that the Triple Burner] occupies three locations in the body's cavity, and others who referred to the lower [section of the Triple] Burner as simply a waterway penetrating the six short-term repositories. In the present paragraph, the discussion

---

8   The bodily liquids are occasionally distinguished, according to the yin and yang classification system, in *jin* 津 and *ye* 液 liquids. The former are said to be clear; the latter are defined as turbid. In the present enumeration, however, *jin* could also be used with its second meaning – namely, saliva – while *ye* might stand for internal liquids of the body.

of the Triple Burner refers to three locations in the body's cavity, and to the respective functions of the organs located in these sections.

Huang Weisan: The Triple Burner encloses all the long-term depots and short-term repositories externally. It is a fatty membrane covering the entire physical body from the inside. Although it has no definite physical appearance and shape, it represents a great short-term repository among the six short-term repositories. Hence, the final section [of difficult issue 31] states that it has three ruling centers and, in addition, that it has a specific location where it accumulates its qi.

三十二難曰：（一）五藏俱等，而心肺獨在膈上者，何也？

（二）然：心者血，肺者氣，（三）血為榮，氣為衛，相隨上下，（四）謂之榮衛，通行經絡，營周於外，（五）故令心肺在膈上也。

The thirty-second difficult issue: (1) All the body's five long-term depots are located on one level, with the exception of heart and lung, which are located above the diaphragm. How is that?

(2) It is like this. The heart [is associated with] the blood; the lung [is associated with] the qi. (3) The blood represents the camp [qi]; the qi represent the guard [qi]. They follow each other, moving up and down [in the organism]. (4) They are called camp and guard [qi, because the former] proceed through the conduits and network [vessels] and [the latter] circulate through [the body's] external regions. (5) Hence, heart and lung must occupy an [elevated] position above the diaphragm.

COMMENTARIES

(1) *Li Jiong*: All the five long-term depots are located in the abdomen. Only heart and lung are located in the chest above the diaphragm.

Liao Ping: The Five Phases are symbols. When they are matched with the long-term depots and short-term repositories, this is a doctrine fulfilling some specific purposes. However, when [the Five Phases] are brought together with the [higher or lower] positions [of the long-term depots and short-term repositories in the body], that is a false doctrine which serves only as an obstacle for the medical community.

(2) *Liao Ping*: ["Heart"] should be "liver." The guard [qi] are controlled by the lung; the camp [qi] are controlled by the liver.

(3) *Liao Ping*: If they move in opposite directions, they can have a great meeting. If they move together, they cannot meet [each other].

(1)–(5) *Ding Deyong*: Heart and lung control the passage of the qi of heaven. Hence, they are located above the diaphragm.

Yang: Everything above the navel is yang; everything below the navel is yin. Hence, the scripture states: "Above the hips is heaven; below the hips is earth." Heaven is yang; the earth is yin. That is the meaning. Here, heart and lung are located above the diaphragm, passing camp and guard [qi through the body]. Hence, [the text] states: "They circulate through the [body's] external regions."

Yu Shu: The heart is the supreme ruler. It resides on high and beholds what is far away. The lung is a canopy; it, too, is located [above] the diaphragm. The heart controls the blood; the blood represents the camp [qi]. The lung controls the qi;

the qi are the guard [qi]. The flow of the blood relies on the [movement of the] qi; the movement of the qi depends on the [flow of the] blood. Blood and qi proceed [through the organism] in mutual dependency. Hence, heart and lung are located in the upper [section of the Triple] Burner.

Hua Shou: Everybody has a diaphragm membrane below his heart. It is attached all the way round to the backbone and to the flanks. It provides a barrier screening off the turbid qi and preventing their steaming up to heart and lung. Mr. Chen from si-ming said: Heart and lung give life to and nourish the human body with blood and qi. Thus they constitute father and mother of the body. Given the high esteem in which father and mother are held, they must, of course, be located above.

Xu Dachun: The camp and the guard [qi] link the entire body; heart and lung are their controls. Hence, they are the only [long-term depots] located above the diaphragm so that they may carry out their rule [from there].

Ye Lin: Everybody has a layer of a diaphragm membrane below his heart and lung and above all the [remaining] long-term depots. It is thin like a fine net. It ascends and descends following exhalation and inhalation. It provides a barrier for the turbid qi, preventing their steaming up to heart and lung. The first paragraph[1] elucidated the functions of blood and qi; the present paragraph discusses the substance of blood and qi. [Both] demonstrate that the long-term depots and short-term repositories of the human body depend on the nourishment provided by the blood and by the qi.

Katō Bankei: This treatise explains why the five long-term depots are all located on one level, with the exception of heart and lung, which are located above the diaphragm. The three long-term depots – spleen, liver, and kidneys – are all located below the diaphragm. Above the [diaphragm] is the location of the clear yang; below the [diaphragm] is the place of the turbid yin. Thus, heart and lung appear to be the only [long-term depots] of value. The heart generates and transforms the camp [qi, i.e.,] the blood. The lung moves the guard qi through [the body]. Qi and blood in the entire body rely on the movements and transformations occurring in these two long-term depots. Hence, their duties are the most important. The fact that no other [depot] is as valuable as are heart and lung, rests solely with the blood and the qi.

Liao Ping: This answer differs from the meaning expressed in a subsequent difficult issue.

---

1 "The first paragraph" refers to difficult issue 30, which is the first in chapter 3 of Ye Lin's edition of the *Nan jing*.

三十三難曰：（一）肝青象木，肺白象金；肝得水而沉，木得水而浮；肺得
水而浮，金得水而沉。其意何也？

（二）然：肝者，非為純木也，乙角也，庚之柔。（三）大言陰與陽，小言
夫與婦。（四）釋其微陽，而吸其微陰之氣，（五）其意樂金，（六）又行陰
道多，（七）故令肝得水而沉也。（八）肺者，非為純金也，辛商也，丙之
柔。（九）大言陰與陽，小言夫與婦。（十）釋其微陰，婚而就火，（十一）其
意樂火，（十二）又行陽道多，（十三）故令肺得水而浮也。

（十四）肺熟而復沉，肝熟而復浮者，何也？

（十五）故知辛當歸庚，乙當歸甲也。

The thirty-third difficult issue: (1) The liver [is associated with] virid; it reflects
the [phase of] wood. The lung [is associated with] white; it reflects the [phase of]
metal. When the liver is brought into water it will sink; when wood is brought into
water it will float. When the lung is brought into water it will float; when metal
is brought into water it will sink. What are the respective sentiments [of liver and
lung]?

(2) It is like this. The liver is not pure wood; the *yi*, which is [associated with the
musical note] *yue*, constitutes the soft [partner] of *geng*.(3) In macro-terms, [*yi* and
geng] represent yin and yang; in micro-terms, they constitute husband and wife. (4)
[The liver] releases its feeble yang [qi] and absorbs feeble yin [qi]. (5) Its sentiment
is joy of metal. (6) Furthermore, it proceeds mostly through yin paths. (7) Hence,
when the liver is brought into water, it will sink. (8) The lung is not pure metal. The
xin, which is [associated with the musical note] *shang*, is the soft [partner] of *bing*.
(9)In macro-terms, [*xin* and *bing*] represent yin and yang; in micro-terms, they
constitute husband and wife. (10) [The lung] releases its feeble yin [qi]; through
marriage it approaches the fire. (11) Its sentiment is joy of fire. (12) Furthermore,
it proceeds mostly through yang paths. (13) Hence, when the lung is brought into
water, it will float.

(14) When the lung is mature it will take a turn and sink; when the liver is mature
it will take a turn and float. Why is that?

(15) It is because we know that *xin* must return to *geng*, and *yi* must return to *jia*.

COMMENTARIES

(1) *Liao Ping*: This is a special doctrine of the Five Phases school [of philosophy]. For details see the *Wu xing da yi* 五行大義.[1] The medical community has no such unreasonable [teachings] .... The lung is located above, the liver is located below. These are their natural positions. Why should it be necessary to distinguish them by bringing them into water? ... This question lacks any reason.

(2)–(7) *Ding Deyong*: Since the Five Phases have been determined, hard and soft [partners] have been matched as husband and wife. The soft [partner] takes in the hard [partner]. Here now, the [*Nan*] *jing* takes up the example of the liver, [which is associated with] virid and reflects the [phase of] wood. The basic nature of wood is to float. Here, [it is stated that] when the liver is brought into water it will sink. That is to say, it harbors the nature of metal. Furthermore, wood receives its qi in the seventh month; it assumes public duties in the first month. [Thus,] it proceeds mostly through the yin paths of the [year]. Hence, when the liver is brought into water it will sink.

Yang: Each of the four cardinal directions has a yin and a yang [aspect]. The East is [associated with the Celestial Stems] *jia* 甲 and *yi* 乙, and with wood. *Jia* is yang; *yi* is yin. The same applies to all the other [cardinal directions]. Also, *jia* represents wood, *yi* represents herbs; *bing* 丙 represents fire, *ding* 丁 represents ashes; *wu* 戊 represents soil, *ji* 己 represents refuse; *geng* 庚 represents metal, *xin* 辛 represents stone; *ren* 壬 represents water, *gui* 癸 represents ponds. Furthermore, *yi* carries qi of metal; *ding* carries qi of water; *ji* carries qi of wood; *xin* carries qi of fire; *gui* carries qi of soil.[2] In all these [instances] those [aspects of the] Five Phases ruling and [those aspects] serving are united to form a pair. Hence, [the text] states: "The liver is not pure wood." The reason is that yin and yang are interlocked. Wood is generated in the *hai* 亥 [period, i.e., in the tenth month] and dominates in the *mao* 卯 [period, i.e., in the second month]. Hence, [the text] states: "It proceeds mostly through yin paths." The East, [being associated with] *jia* and *yi*, and with wood, stands in awe of the West, [which is associated with] *geng* and *xin*, and with metal. Hence, it releases its younger sister *yi* and marries it to the *geng* as its wife. Hence, [the text] speaks [of *yi*] as the soft [part-

---

1 Title of a book ("The General Meaning of the Five Phases") written by Xiao Ji 蕭吉, probably in the first decades of the seventh century.

2 The combination *jia yi* corresponds to the phase of wood; metal is the phase that is able to destroy wood. The combination *bing ding* corresponds to the phase of fire; water is the phase that is able to destroy fire. The combination *wu ji* corresponds to the phase of soil; wood is the phase that is able to destroy soil. The combination *geng xin* corresponds to the phase of metal; fire is the phase that is able to destroy metal. The combination *ren gui* corresponds to the phase of water; soil is the phase that is able to overcome water.

ner] of *geng.* "Soft" stands for yin. The *yi* carries metal qi as its marriage present. Hence, when the liver is brought into water it will sink.

Yu Shu: When *yi* and *geng* are united, their nature [as a pair] will follow that of the husband. Hence, when [the liver] is brought into water it will sink.

Hua Shou: Mr. Chen from Siming has stated: The liver is associated with [the Celestial Stems] *jia* and *yi;* [it belongs to the phase of] wood and corresponds to the [musical] note *yue.* It is heavy and turbid. If one refers to [*jia* and *yi*] separately, *jia* represents the yang [aspect] of wood, *yi* represents the yin [aspect] of wood. If one refers to them together, they are yang. Because the [liver] is associated with the minor yang, and because it is located in the yin section of the human body, it represents the yang-in-yin. Now, yang must unite with yin. The yin and the yang represented in the [Celestial Stems] *jia* and *yi* originally constitute a [yin and yang] pair themselves. However, *yi* proceeds together with *geng* on the path of hardness and softness. *Yi,* then, is linked to the feeble yang of *jia* and, in contrast, has a liking for metal. Hence, it absorbs the metal of *geng,* [i.e., feeble qi], and the two become husband and wife. The original nature of wood is to float. Because it absorbs the qi of metal and resides at the yin paths, it will sink when it is brought into water. When it matures, the qi of metal, absorbed earlier, will leave. The *yi* will return to the *jia* and the original body of the wood will be restored and return to floating.

(2)–(3) *Zhang Shixian: Chun* 純 ("pure") stands for *bu za* 不雜 ("unmixed"). *Yue* is the [musical] note [associated with] wood. *Shang* is the [musical] note [associated with] metal. When wood is generated it is called "feeble yang." "Feeble yang" means that it contains lots of yin. When metal is generated it is called "feeble yin." "Feeble yin" means that it contains lots of yang. [Liver and lung] do not represent pure wood or pure metal, respectively, because of the interactions of yin and yang [aspects. The combination of] *yi* and *geng,* as well as of *bing* and *xin* [corresponds], in macro-terms, to [the combination of] yin and yang, and, in micro-terms, [the union of] husband and wife. Husband and wife represent yin and yang.

(2) *Liao Ping:* The doctrines of the [Celestial] Stems and of the [Earth] Branches have emerged from the [doctrine of the] [Five] Periods [and Six] Qi.[3] They rep-

---

3   The Chinese term is *wu yun liu qi* 五運六氣. The statement that follows – "they represent a pattern of imperial rule over the empire" – refers to the political application of the *wu yun* concept alone (here, "five dynastic phases") as an explanatory model for the cyclical succession of dynastic eras. In this model each dynasty was associated with one of the Five Phases, permitting the legitimization of their mutual destruction or generation. In a medical context the *wu yun liu qi* concept usually refers to the normal and abnormal occurrences of "five phases and six [climatic] qi" in the course of one year. For a detailed account, see Lu and Needham, *Celestial Lancets* (Cambridge, 1980, 137-153).

resent a pattern of [imperial] rule over the empire, and they are special teachings of the ancient yinyang school [of philosophy]. Here, they have been combined with the sayings of the [*Nei*] *jing*. Nobody who studies medicine needs to take pains to make them his own.

(3) *Xu Dachun*: "In macro-terms" means to discuss this in terms of yin and yang of heaven and earth. "In micro-terms" means to discuss this in terms of husband and wife as human relations. The principle is identical.

(4)–(5) *Xu Dachun*: To be a wife means to follow a husband. *Yi* is yin and wood. Hence, it is called feeble yang. "Joy of metal" means that it finds joy in following the metal.

(4)–(6) *Zhang Shixian*: *Shi* 釋 stands for *qu* 去 ("to send away"). *Xi* 吸 stands for *shou* 受 ("to receive"). The wood receives qi in the *shen* 申 [period]; the *shen* [period] is the seventh month. It grows in the *hai* 亥 [period]; the *hai* [period] is the tenth month. These are all yin paths. It assumes public duties in the *yin* 寅 [period]; the *yin* [period] is the first month. It dominates in the *mao* 卯 [period]; the *mao* [period] is the second month. These are yang paths. Hence, [the text] states: "It proceeds mostly through yin paths."

(6) *Xu Dachun*: The liver is associated with the foot ceasing yin conduit. Its position is below the diaphragm. Hence, [the text] states: "It proceeds mostly through yin paths."

(8)–(13) *Ding Deyong*: The lung [is associated with] white; it reflects the [phase of] metal. The basic nature of metal is to sink down. Here now, in contrast, the lung [is said to] float. That is to say, *xin* has adopted the nature of fire. Furthermore, [metal] receives its qi in the first month; it assumes public duties in the seventh month. [Thus,] it proceeds mostly through the yang paths of the [year]. Hence, when the lung is brought into water it will float.

Yang: Metal is generated in the *si* 巳 [period, i.e., in the fourth month] and dominates in the *you* 酉 [period, i.e., in the eighth month]. Hence, [the text] states: "It proceeds mostly through yang paths." The West, [being associated with] *bing* and *ding*, and with metal, stands in awe of the South, [which is associated with] *bing* and *ding* and with fire. Hence, it releases its younger sister *xin* and marries her to the *bing* as the latter's wife. Hence, [the text] states: "[The *xin*] is the soft [partner] of *bing*." The *xin* carries qi of fire as its wedding present. Hence, when the lung is brought into water it will float.

Yu Shu: When *bing* and *xin* are untied, their nature [as a pair] will follow that of the husband. Flames ascend and float. Hence [the text contains] that statement.

(9) *Liao Ping*: Beginning with the *Nan* [*jing*], the [contents of the] *Nei jing* were erroneously combined with the teachings of [the correspondences between]

man and heaven. Thereupon the Five Phases [doctrine] was added to medical literature. [Those who did this] were unaware that the Five Phases and yinyang school represented one of the nine currents [in ancient philosophy]. Originally, [these ideas] constituted a pattern of imperial rule over the empire. Yet medical literature was counted in the bibliographical section of the *Han shu* 漢書 among the technical arts, and it was listed only following the [literature of the] nine [philosophical] currents. [Medicine and philosophy] must not be mixed up! Such a tradition started with the *Nan jing*.

(12) *Zhang Shixian*: The metal receives qi in the *yin* [period]; it grows in the *si* [period]. The *si* [period] is the fourth month. These are all yang paths. [Metal] assumes public duties in the *shen* [period], and it dominates in the *you* [period]. The *you* [period] is the eighth month. These are yin paths. Hence, [the text] states: "It proceeds mostly through yang paths."

 Xu Dachun: The lung is associated with the hand major yin conduit. Its position is above the diaphragm. Hence, [the text] states: "It proceeds mostly through yang paths."

(13) *Liao Ping*: This is surplus from the ball of threads of the [doctrine of the] [Five] Periods [and Six] Qi. Medical people should not weave this together into a deceptive net.

(14)–(15) *Yang*: In a fresh state the liver sinks; in a mature state it floats. In a fresh state the lung floats; in a mature state it sinks. The meaning implied here is that at death everything returns to its origin. "Mature" illustrates death here, as among humans, when a husband and his wife die without offspring, each of them returns to his or her original [family]. Extreme yin changes to yang; cold in abundance generates heat; long-time obstruction produces passage; accumulations must disperse. For this same reason [a mature liver or lung act differently than fresh ones].

 Zhang Shixian: "Mature" stands for dead. Dead [partners] can no longer unite with each other. When wood is dead it changes to pure yang; when metal is dead it changes to pure yin. Hence, what has floated [when alive] will sink when it is mature; what has sunk [when alive] will float when mature. *Xin* returns to *geng;* its sentiment is no [longer] joy of fire; rather it will be pure metal. *Yi* returns to *jia;* its sentiment is no [longer] joy of metal; rather it will be pure wood. Pure metal is pure yin; pure wood is pure yang.

三十四難曰：（一）五藏各有聲、色、臭、味、，可曉知以不？
（二）然：《十變》言，（三）肝色青，其臭臊，其味酸，其聲呼，其液
泣；（四）心色赤，其臭焦，其味苦，其聲言，其液汗；（五）脾色黃，其臭
香，其味甘，其聲歌，其液涎；（六）肺色白，其臭腥，其味辛，其聲哭，
其液涕；（七）腎色黑，其臭腐，其味鹹，其聲呻，其液唾。（八）是五藏
聲、色、臭、味、也。
（九）五藏有七神，各何所藏耶？
（十）然：藏者，人之神氣所舍藏也。（十一）故肝藏魂，肺藏魄，心藏神，
脾藏意與智，腎藏精與志也。

The thirty-fourth difficult issue: (1) Each of the five long-term depots has a [specific] sound, complexion, odor, and flavor. Can they be known?

(2) It is like this. The "Ten Transformations" states: (3) The color of the liver is virid; its odor is fetid; its flavor is sour; its sound is the shout; its liquid is the tears. (4) The color of the heart is red; its smell is burned; its flavor is bitter; its sound is talk; its liquid is sweat. (5) The color of the spleen is yellow; its odor is aromatic; its flavor is sweet; its sound is singing; its liquid is saliva. (6) The color of the lung is white; its odor is frowzy; its flavor is acrid; its sound is wailing; its liquid is snivel. (7) The color of the kidneys is black; their odor is foul; their flavor is salty; their sound is groaning; their liquid is spittle. (8) These are the sounds, colors, odors, flavors, [and liquids] of the five long-term depots.

(9) The five long-term depots have seven spirits. Which [spirit] lodges in each of them, respectively?

(10) It is like this. The long-term depots are storage depots containing man's spirit qi. (11) Hence, the liver stores the *hun;* the lung stores the *po;* the heart stores the spirit; the spleen stores sentiment and wisdom; the kidneys store the essence and the mind.[1]

---

1 The *Nan jing* may be called *the* classic of systematic correspondence. The restriction of vessel diagnosis to but two locations at the hands necessitated a consistent adherence to the concepts of systematic correspondence. Otherwise it would have been impossible to examine the condition of each long-term depot and of each conduit vessel at just the two inch sections. This consistent application of the Five Phases and yinyang doctrines of systematic correspondence reappears here where the functional structure of the organism is elucidated. In difficult issue 33, an attempt was made at demonstrating that even apparent contradictions between sensorial perception and the claims of theory should not jeopardize the all-encompassing validity of the concepts of systematic correspondence. Here, in difficult issue 34, two additional spirits are named, thus exceeding the number five. Obviously, earlier authors had already recognized that not all existential phenomena

(1) *Hua Shou*: These are the functions of the five long-term depots. Below "sound, color, odor, and flavor," the character for "liquid" is missing.

Liao Ping: That has been made clear in the *Nei jing* already. There was no need to ask further questions.

(2) *Li Jiong*: That is to say, in the five long-term depots only five transformations [of the sounds, colors, odors, flavors, and liquids] take place. If the long-term depots and the short-term repositories are counted together [one may speak of] "Ten Transformations."

Hua Shou: Mr. Chen from Siming states: The lung controls the sounds; the liver controls the colors; the heart controls the odors; the spleen controls the flavors; the kidneys control the liquids. The five long-term depots are mutually interconnected and provide each other [with the respective sounds, colors, odors, flavors, and liquids]. Hence, [the text] speaks of "Ten Transformations."

Zhang Shixian: The liver controls the colors: the transformation of the five colors takes place in the wood. The heart controls the odors; the transformation of the five odors takes place in the fire. The spleen controls the flavors; the transformation of the five flavors takes place in the soil. The lung controls the sounds; the transformation of the five sounds takes place in the metal. The kidneys control the liquids; the transformation of the liquids takes place in the water.

Xu Dachun: [The meaning of] "Ten Transformations" is not clear.

Katō Bankei: *Shi Bian* 十變 ("Ten Transformations") is the title of an ancient book; it does not appear in the extant versions of the *Nei jing*.

Liao Ping: [The meaning of] *shi bian* is not known. One possibility is that *shi* 十 ("ten") should be *wu* 五 ("five"). *Wu* was written, in ancient times, as X, closely resembling *shi*. The *Nei jing* has many treatises with *wu* ("five") in their titles.

(3) *Yu Shu*: The transformations of the five colors occur in the wood. The five colors are poured into the respective five long-term depots by the qi of the liver, which represents [the phase of] wood. Hence, in each long-term depot a specific color may appear that corresponds to the [Five Phases'] categorization of that [depot]. The *Huang ting jing* 黃庭經.[2] states: "The liver is [associated with] the

---

can be put into five categories. The *Su wen*, for instance, records a dialogue on the actual numbers of long-term depots and short-term repositories. This was a truly serious problem, since it could have cracked the rigid categorizations of the Five Phases doctrine. The present difficult issue and various subsequent ones demonstrate the compromises that appeared acceptable.

2 This title refers to at least four books of Daoist orientation.

essence of water and with the qi of *zhen* 震.³ Its color is virid; its position is the East. [Wood] may be transformed by fire; hence, its odor is then fetid. When the soil receives the flavor [= qi] of the wood, they will be sour." The "Hong fan" 洪範⁴ states: "That which is crooked and straight becomes sour." When metal and wood are brought together the sound emitted is a shout. *Hu* 呼 ("to shout") can also be *xiao* 嘯 ("to scream"). *Qi* 泣 ("tears") stands for *lei* 淚 ("tears"). These are qi proceeding [through the organism] with water. Here they are poured into the child [depot];⁵ hence, tears are generated.

Hua Shou: Its liquid is tears; it passes through the eyes.

Xu Dachun: The orifices of the liver are the eyes; hence, [its liquid] is the tears.

(4) *Yu Shu*: The color spread out by wood [turns] red when it is brought into fire. The transformation of the five odors takes place in the fire. The five long-term depots [are associated with] five odors. When the fire blazes, a burned [odor and a] bitter [flavor] emerge from it. Hence, [the text] states: "Its odor is burned." The nature of fire is to flame upward. Hence, it generates a burned [odor and a] bitter [flavor]. When metal and fire come into contact, or when a husband and his wife see each other, the sound emitted is talk. The *Su wen* says "laughter." When water and fire have close contact, steam will rise and sweat is generated.

Hua Shou: Its liquid is sweat. The heart controls the blood. Sweat belongs to the blood.

Xu Dachun: Sweat is an external sign of blood. The heart controls the blood. Hence, [its liquid] is sweat.

(5) *Yu Shu*: The spleen [is associated with] the soil; it is located in the center. The respective color is yellow. That is, the color spread out by wood [turns] yellow when it is in the soil. When fire transforms soil, the latter's odor will be aromatic. The spleen is [associated with] the soil; its flavor is sweet. Sweet is a flavor that can be consumed in order to make use of its [ability to] soothe. [The spleen] moves the five flavors [through the organism] in order to nourish the five long-term depots. In each case [a depot] is matched with a specific flavor that corresponds to [the respective depot's Five Phases'] classification. But in its basic nature [the flavors transmitted] remain sweet. When metal is generated by the soil, or when a mother and a child see each other, the sound emitted

---

3 *Zhen* is the designation of a trigram in the *Yi jing* 易經. It is associated with the phase of wood and with the East.

4 Title of Book IV of the Books of Zhou of the *Shu Jing* 書經.

5 The liver (wood) is the child long-term depot of the kidneys (water); the latter master the liquids.

is singing. The liquids proceeding with water [through the organism] become saliva in the spleen.

Hua Shou: Its liquid is saliva; it passes through the mouth.

Xu Dachun: The orifice of the spleen is the mouth; hence, [its liquid] is saliva.

(6) *Yu Shu*: The color spread out by wood [turns] white in the lung. When it is transformed by fire, metal develops a frowzy odor. When the flavor [that originates from the spleen, i.e.,] from the soil, is received by the lung, it becomes acrid. With [the consumption of] acrid [flavor] one makes use of [its ability to] disperse and moisten. All the five [musical] notes are emitted from the metal. The metal emits the five [musical] notes in order to send them out to the five long-term depots. Each [depot] has its specific note emitted corresponding to its [Five Phases'] classification. The basic nature of metal makes it wail. That is to say, the lung belongs to the [phase of] metal. Metal is [associated with the musical] note *shang* 商. *Shang* stands for *shang* 傷 ("injured"). (The phase of metal) dominates in autumn. *Qiu* 秋 stands for *chou* 愁 ("grief"). Hence, its mental state is wailing because of sadness. That is [what is] meant here. The liquids proceeding with water [through the organism] become snivel in the lung.

Hua Shou: Its liquid is snivel; it passes through the nose.

Xu Dachun: The orifice of the lung is the nose; hence, [its liquid] is snivel.

(7) *Yu Shu*: The color spread out by wood [turns] black in the kidneys. Fire controls the odors. In water it develops a foul odor. When the flavor of the soil is received [by the kidneys, i.e.,] by water, it becomes salty. With [the consumption of] salty [flavor], one can make use of its [ability to] soften. When a child sees its mother, the sound emitted is a happy groaning. All five liquids originate from water. The water moves the five liquids [through the organism] and passes them into the respective long-term depots. Hence, each long-term depot has its specific liquid. In its original residence [the liquid] is spittle.

Hua Shou: Their liquid is spittle which belongs to the water.

Zhang Shixian: Spittle is the liquid next to the teeth.

Xu Dachun: The orifice of the kidneys is below the tongue; hence, [their liquid] is spittle.

(3)–(8) *Xu Dachun*: The *Ling* [*shu*] treatise "Jiu zhen" 九鍼 and the *Su* [*wen* treatise] "Xuan ming wu qi lun" 宣明五氣論 both state concerning the sounds [associated with the] five long-term depots: "The heart controls sighing. The lung controls coughing. The liver controls speaking. The spleen controls swallowing. The kidneys control yawning." Here, though, shouting, speaking; singing, wailing, and groaning are listed based on the *Su* [*wen* treatise] "Yin yang ying xiang da lun" 陰陽應象大論. Well, the former refer to the sounds emitted in the case of a disease; here, the sounds [are listed that are] emitted with respect to specific emotions. The principle is the same. When one reads the classics one must always fathom their meaning. This way not a single [passage] will remain incomprehensible.

(9)-(11) *Ding Deyong*: The commentary to the [treatise] "Xuan ming wu qi" 宣明五氣 [of the *Su wen*] states [the following] on the five long-term depots and their seven spirits. On "the heart stores the spirit," [it says: "The spirit] is a transformation product of the essence qi." On "the lung stores the *po*," [it says: „The *po*] is an aide to the essence qi. The *Ling shu jing* states: 'That which leaves and enters together with the essence is called the *po*'." On "the liver stores the *hun*," [it says: „The *hun*] is an assistant to the spirit qi. The *Ling shu* states: 'That which comes with the spirit qi is called the *hun*'." On "the spleen stores sentiment and wisdom," [it says:] "The sentiment controls the thoughts; wisdom controls the memory." On "the kidneys store the essence and the mind," [it says]:⁶ "They harbor a specific sentiment which does not undergo any change. The *Ling shu jing* states: 'The location where the intentions are that is called the mind.' It states further: 'That which guards the essence is called the mind'."

Yang: The liver, the heart, and the lung have one spirit each. The spleen and the kidneys have two spirits each. The five long-term depots together have seven spirits.

Hua Shou: *Zang* 臟 stands for *cang* 藏 ("to store"). Man's spirit qi are stored in the internal [sections of the organism]. The *hun* is an assistant to the spirit brilliance. What comes together with the spirit is called *hun*. The *po* is an aide to the essence qi. That which leaves and enters together with the essence is called *po*. The spirit is a transformation product of the essence qi. When the two essences [of yin and yang] interact, [the product] is called spirit. The spleen controls the thoughts; hence, it stores sentiment and wisdom. The kidneys serve as the official of strength; techniques and skills originate from them. Hence, they store the essence and the mind. This listing of the spirits in the body's five long-term depots is based on the functions of these long-term depots. Hence, the five

---

6 Actually, the commentary to the *Su wen* treatise "Xuan ming wu qi lun" refers only to five long-term depots and five spirits. The Su wen says: "The spleen stores the *yi* 意 ("sentiment"; here, possibly 'memory')." The commentary states: "[*Yi*] means to remember and not to forget. The *Ling shu jing* states: 'When the heart reflects on something that is called *yi*'." The *Su wen* continues with: "The kidneys store the mind." The commentary states: "They harbor a specific sentiment which does not change. The *Ling shu jing* states: 'That which preserves the sentiment is called the mind'." The passage "the sentiment controls the thoughts" may have been added by Ding Deyong; I could not find it in the *Su wen* editions available to me.

functions appear outside [of the long-term depots]; the seven spirits are kept inside [of the five long-term depots].

Zhang Shixian: She 舍 stands for *zhai she* 宅舍 ("dwelling"). Each of man's spirit qi is stored in one of the body's long-term depots. The *Ling shu* states:[7] "When the two essences [of yin and yang] interact, [the product] is called spirit. That which comes with the spirit is called *hun*.[8] That which enters and leaves with the essence is called *po*. That which controls all things is called the heart. When the heart reflects on something, that is called sentiment. If one considers something and [is able] to locate it, that is called wisdom. That which preserves the sentiment is called the essence. It is the basis of generation and of one's physical appearance."

Xu Dachun: In the *Ling [shu]*, treatise "Jiu zhen" 九鍼 [it is stated]: "The heart stores the spirit. The lung stores the *po* soul. The liver stores the *hun* soul. The spleen stores the intentions. The kidneys store the essence and the mind." The *Su [wen* treatise] "Tiao jing lun" 調經論 states: "The heart stores the spirit; the lung stores the qi; the liver stores the blood; the spleen stores the flesh; the kidneys store the will. [Together] this completes the [body's] physical appearance." That is quite different from [the statement in the *Nan jing*] here. The [*Nan*] *jing* contains no answer to the two words "seven spirits." There is no explanation [as to what that might mean]. Even the "essence" of the kidneys is called a spirit. Maybe this listing is incomplete.

(9) *Liao Ping:* There are five spirits and five long-term depots. The text of the [*Nei*] *jing* is clear about that. The character *qi* 七 ("seven") makes absolutely no sense. Is not this a good example proving that [the *Nan jing*] introduced deviant teachings and did not care about the meaning of the [corresponding *Nei jing*] passages? ... The sentence ["Which spirit lodges in each of them respectively?"] does not fit in with the preceding sentence. If [the preceding sentence] had stated "five long-term depots and five spirits," they would have matched each other.

(10) *Liao Ping:* The character *qi* 氣 ("qi") is an amendment. "Spirit" reflects something abstract. "Essence" and "qi" reflect something tangible; they cannot be spiritual.

(11) *Katō Bankei:* Spleen and kidneys both have two spirits because the spleen is the basis for the generation and transformation of the camp and guard [qi] and because the kidneys harbor, in the yin [region], the true and original qi.

Liao Ping: The two characters *yu zhi* 與智 ("and wisdom") are false additions .... The two characters *yu zhi* 與志 ("and the mind") are false additions.

---

7   In its treatise 8, "Ben shen."

8   All *Tu zhu Nan jing* 圖諸難經 editions available to me have *po* here instead of *hun*. That is a mistake.

THE THIRTY-FIFTH DIFFICULT ISSUE

三十五難曰：（一）五藏各有所，府皆相近，而心肺獨去大腸、小腸遠者，何謂也？

（二）經言心榮肺衛，（三）通行陽氣，故居有上；（四）大腸、小腸傳陰氣而下，故居在下。（五）所以相去而遠也。

（六）又諸府者，皆陽也，清淨之處。今大腸、小腸、胃與膀胱，皆受不淨，其意何也？

（七）然：諸府者，謂是非也。（八）經言：小腸者，受盛之府也；（九）大腸者，傳瀉行道之府也；（十）膽者，清淨之府也；（十一）胃者，水穀之府也；（十二）膀胱者，津液之府也。（十三）一府猶無兩名，故知非也。（十四）小腸者，心之府；大腸者，肺之府；胃者，脾之府；膽者，肝之府；膀胱者，腎之府。（十五）小腸謂赤腸，大腸謂白腸，膽者謂青腸，胃者謂黃腸，膀胱者謂黑腸。（十六）下焦所治也。

The thirty-fifth difficult issue: (1) All the five long-term depots occupy a specific location, and the short-term repositories are all in the vicinity [of the individual long-term depots with which they are associated], except for the heart and the lung, which are located far away from the large and small intestines, respectively. What does that mean?

(2) It is like this. The scripture states: The heart [is responsible for the] camp [qi]; the lung [is responsible for the] guard [qi]. (3) Both [the heart and the lung] send yang qi through [the organism]. (4) The large and the small intestines transmit yin qi in a downward direction. Hence, they are located in the lower parts [of the body]. (5) That is the reason why [the heart and the lung on the one side, and the large and the small intestines on the other side] are situated so far away from each other.

(6) Also, all short-term repositories are [categorized as] yang; they are places of clarity and purity. Now, the large intestine, the small intestine, the stomach, and the urinary bladder all receive that which is not clean. What does that mean?

(7) It is like this. It is not correct to say that all short-term repositories are [places of clarity and purity]. (8) The scripture states: The small intestine is the short-term repository of receiving in abundance. (9) The large intestine is a short-term repository that constitutes a pathway for transmission and drainage. (10) The gall bladder is the short-term repository of clarity and purity. (11) The stomach is the short-term repository of water and grains. (12) The urinary bladder is the short-term repository of *jin* and *ye* liquids. (13) One single short-term repository cannot have two designations; thus one knows that [the point stated in the question] is wrong. (14) The small intestine is the short-term repository of the heart; the large intestine is

the short-term repository of the lung; the gall bladder is the short-term repository of the liver; the stomach is the short-term repository of the spleen; the urinary bladder is the short-term repository of the kidneys. (15) The small intestine is called red intestine; the large intestine is called white intestine; the gall bladder is called virid intestine; the stomach is called yellow intestine; the urinary bladder is called black intestine. (16) They belong to the governing district of the lower [section of the Triple] Burner.¹

COMMENTARIES

(1) *Li Jiong*: Suo 所 stands for *suo zhi zhi di* 所止之地 ("a place where they remain") .... The stomach is located near the spleen. The gall bladder is near the liver. The urinary bladder is near the kidneys. Heart and lung are located above the diaphragm. Large intestine and small intestine are located below. [The latter two long-term depots and short-term repositories] are all distant from each other; they are not near to each other.

Liao Ping: Not all of them are located close to each other. That applies only to liver and gall bladder. ... This statement is based on [the mutual proximity of] liver and gall bladder. [The author(s)] did not know that it is incorrect [with respect to all the other long-term depots and short-term repositories] .... The outer kidney – [that is, the] gall bladder – is the short-term repository of the liver. The urinary bladder is the short-term repository of the [inner] kidney. The [latter] are not close to each other either.

(2)–(3) *Li Jiong*: The upper section reflects heaven. Heaven is yang. Heart and lung are located above the diaphragm. The heart controls the blood. The blood represents the camp [qi]. The lung controls the qi. These qi are the guard [qi]. Yang [qi] float upward. Both heart and lung pass yang qi [through the organism]. Hence, they are located above.

(2) *Liao Ping*: Xin 心 ("heart") should be *gan* 肝 ("liver").

(3) *Xu Dachun*: "Yang qi" refers to the camp and to the guard qi. In the treatise "Ying wei sheng hui" 營衛生會 of the *Ling* [*shu*], it is stated: "They pass through twenty-five passages during the yang [section of one day] and they pass through

---

1 The last sentence is worded, in some editions, *xia jiao zhi suo zhi ye* 下焦之所治也. The present difficult issue provides two further examples for attempts to reconcile apparent contradictions between certain realities that can be perceived with one's senses and the claims of systematic correspondence. It is interesting to note that Liao Ping – the commentator who has, thus far, followed most closely the lines of the *Nei jing* – here gives priority to the consistency of theory over the text of the *Nei jing*. Since, in his eyes, the outer kidney resembles a short-term repository in its functions, while the gall bladder resembles a long-term depot, he suggests exchanging their names (i.e., calling the outer kidney the gall bladder, and vice versa).

twenty-five passages during the yin [section of one day]." [These qi are what is] meant here.

Liao Ping: This book [propagates] examining the [conditions of] heart and lung at the inch [sections] of the two [hands] only, because both [the heart and the lung] are located above [in the body]. Such doctrines are unreasonable additions [to the teachings of the *Nei jing*].

(4) *Li Jiong*: The lower section reflects the earth. [The earth] is yin. The large intestine and the small intestine are both located below the diaphragm. They transmit yin qi downward. Hence, they are situated in the lower section [of the body]. Because heart and lung pass yang qi while the large intestine and the small intestine pass yin qi, they are distant from each other.

Xu Dachun: "Yin qi" refers to the turbid qi. That is to say, [these short-term repositories are the places] to which the impure dregs turn.

Liao Ping: This strange doctrine has been developed simply because [the *Nan jing*] claims that the condition of these two short-term repositories can be examined at the] foot section.

(5) *Xu Dachun*: Their respective governing districts differ. Thus, although they are linked by a conduit, their locations are distant from each other.

(6)–(7) *Ding Deyong*: The statement of the [*Nan*] *jing*, "all short-term repositories are [categorized as] yang; they are places of clarity and purity," refers to [the understanding that] the short-term repositories [associated with the] three yang [conduits] of the hands and of the feet [serve to] pass qi [through the organism]. Hence, they are called "places of clarity and purity." Here, [it is pointed out that] the large intestine, the small intestine, the stomach, and the bladder are short-term repositories which transmit and transform. Hence, [the text] says [that the statement in the question] is incorrect.

(6) *Li Jiong*: The six short-term repositories are all [categorized as] yang. The yang [appears as] the qi. The three yang [conduits] of the hands and of the feet are [associated with] short-term repositories passing the qi [through the organism]. The yang is the clearest and the purest. Hence, [these short-term repositories] are called "places of clarity and purity." The large intestine transmits the impure [portions] of water and grain. The small intestine is supplemented with the impure [portions] of water and grains. The stomach takes in and contains the impure [portions] of water and grains. The bladder stores the impure [portions] of the *jin* 津 and *ye* 液 liquids. Only the gall bladder is clear and pure.

Xu Dachun: That is to say, [the short-term repositories are] yang and they should be [associated with] clarity and purity. But, on the contrary, they receive impure and turbid [refuse]. Only the gall bladder is not reached [by refuse] because it is not a function of the gall bladder to receive.

Liao Ping: This question refers to the difference between the four short-term repositories [mentioned on the one hand,] and the Triple Burner and the gall bladder [on the other hand].

(7) *Yang*: The statement "it is not correct to say that [all short-term repositories are places of clarity and purity]" means [the following]. All the short-term repositories are individual entities [the function of which is] to transmit. That is correct. The small intestine is a short-term repository. That is incorrect. How can that be? It is like this. Although the small intestine is matched with the heart as its external [correspondence], its governing district is different. Their qi are the same. Although their qi are the same, that which they each control is different again. Thus, although it is said [that the small intestine partakes of] the qi[2] of the heart, it does not constitute [a short-term repository associated with] the heart but is located separately from it. Hence, [the text] states: "It is not correct."

Xu Dachun: This means that although all short-term repositories belong to the yang, they are not all places of clarity and purity.

Ding Jin: It is correct to say that all the short-term repositories are yang, but it is not correct to say that all the short-term repositories could be named [places of] clarity and purity. The *Nei jing* refers only to the gall bladder as the "short-term repository of clarity and purity." Each of the remaining four short-term repositories is named with a specific designation too. Thus, two names cannot be mixed up. Therefore, it is obvious that "clarity and purity" refers only to the gall bladder. Furthermore, all the four remaining short-term repositories belong to the lower [section of the Triple] Burner. They all are responsible for receiving and transmission. How could they be called "[places of] clarity and purity?"

(8) *Li Jiong*: [The small intestine] receives orders from the stomach. It is filled with refuse. When the receiving is completed, it transforms [that refuse] again and transmits it to the large intestine.

Xu Dachun: [The *Su wen* treatise] "Ling lan mi dian lun" 靈蘭祕典論 [states]: "The small intestine is the official functioning as recipient of what has been perfected. The transformation of things originates from here." That is to say, it receives items from the stomach and transforms them into refuse.

(9) *Li Jiong*: The large intestine is capable of transmitting and draining impure things because it constitutes a passageway through which anything can flow.

---

2   The *Nan jing ji zhu* edition has *xin bing* 心病 ("illnesses of the heart"). Here I have followed Li Jiong's edition in the *Dao zang* 道藏, which has *xin qi* 心氣.

Xu Dachun: The *Su* [*wen* states]: "The large intestine is the official functioning as transmitter along the way. Changes and transformations originate from here."

(10) *Li Jiong*: The gall bladder is located between the short lobes of the liver. The qi of the liver pass through the eyes. When the [qi passing through the] eyes are in harmonious [balance], one can perceive black and white. The gall bladder is the short-term repository of the liver. It is most happy about clarity and purity.

Xu Dachun: The *Su* [*wen* states]: "The gall bladder is the official functioning as rectifier. Decisions and judgments originate from here." The gall bladder does not receive and it does not serve to drain; it supports the liver in its decision-making and in its considerations, and that is it. Therefore, it is called a "place of clarity and purity."

(11) *Li Jiong*: The stomach is the official responsible for storage of grain. Also, [the stomach] is the ruler of the lung. All the water and the grains are accumulated in it.

Xu Dachun: The *Su* [*wen* states]: "The spleen and the stomach are officials responsible for grain storage. The five foods[3] originate from here."

(12) *Li Jiong*: As to the *jin* and *ye* liquids, that which is emitted as sweat and leaves through the pores is the *jin* liquid. Those of the liquids that flow into hollow cavities where they stagnate and do not move are the *ye* liquids. *Jin* and *ye* liquids are contained in the bladder.

Xu Dachun: The *Su* [*wen* states]: "The bladder is the official functioning as regional rectifier. It stores the *jin* and *ye* liquids."

(6)-(13) *Hua Shou*: When [the question] states, "all short-term repositories are places of clarity and purity," that is incorrect. Now, the large intestine, the small intestine, the stomach, and ·the bladder are all responsible for receiving. Therefore, they cannot be yang [places of] clarity and purity.[4] They all constitute short-term repositories of the five long-term depots. It is definitely impossible that they could have two designations [at the same time]. The substance of all the short-term repositories is yang, but their function is yin. [The question in the text] states: "All the short-term repositories are [categorized as] yang; they are short-term repositories of clarity and purity." Only the gall bladder corresponds to that [description].

Zhang Shixian: Each short-term repository has only one designation. When here all [short-term repositories] are called "places of clarity and purity," then

3   It is difficult to reflect the dual meaning of the term *wu wei* 五味 with an English word. In the literal (and medical) sense, it should be rendered as "five flavors." In the present metaphor, though, the term refers to the foods of all flavors that are handed out by the officials responsible for storage and granaries.

4   "Receiving" is categorized as female, as yin.

each short-term repository has two designations. Hence, one knows that not all short-term repositories are places of clarity and purity; that [designation] applies only to the one long-term depot of the gall bladder.

Xu Dachun: [The answer given] here does not exactly correspond to the meaning of the question. The question states that yang should go along with clarity and purity. Why then, in contrast, do [some short-term repositories] receive impure [things]? [The answer] states that ["place of clarity and purity"] is not the [proper] designation [for all the short-term repositories. But we may ask] why they are not called ["places of] clarity and purity"? Here the [*Nan jing*] quotes only from the text of the [*Nei*] *jing* in order to elucidate the fact that these [short-term repositories] are not clear and pure. But that [kind of an answer] fails to elucidate the meaning of the association of all short-term repositories with yang [in comparison to the categorization of all long-term depots as yin]. It should have said: "When the long-term depots and the short-term repositories are distinguished as yin and yang, that does not refer to [categorizations such as] clear and turbid, but to those of movement and rest, of internal and external [location in the body]. Hence, [what is categorized as] yin [can be] clear – in contrast [to the claims of systematic correspondence,] [while that which is categorized as] yang [can be] turbid – also in contrast [to the claims of systematic correspondence]." If [the explanation in the *Nan jing* had been formulated] like that, the meaning would have been understandable.

Liao Ping: The inner kidney and the outer kidney are both named kidneys. The heart, the brain, and the [heart] enclosing network are all called heart. Some long-term depots and short-term repositories are different entities in reality but have identical names. Thus, "gall bladder" should be "kidney." The "inner kidney" should be named "[heart] enclosing network." The "outer kidney" should be named "gall bladder." The outer kidney drains the essence. It is called traditionally "small intestine short-term repository." ... ["Thus one knows that the point stated in the question is wrong"] means that all the short-term repositories are receptacles for some [liquid] leaking into them. The gall bladder is a long-term depot; [its name] should be changed to "outer kidney." All the short-term repositories serve to drain [liquids]. ... The gall bladder should be a long-term depot. It can be replete but it cannot be full. The outer kidney serves to pass liquids; it equals the short-term repositories. Hence, statements in the [*Nei*] *jing* such as "when the five long-term depots have a surplus they can be drained" are all incorrect. Xu [Dachun's] statement is incorrect too. All these [statements have been made] because [their authors] did not know that the gall bladder is not a short-term repository. If it were one of the short-term repositories, the meaning [of "long-term depot" and "short-term repository"] would not be consistent in all respects.

(15)–(16) *Li Jiong*: The color of the heart is red; hence, the small intestine is the red intestine, reflecting [the color of the heart]. The color of the lung is white; hence, the large intestine is the white intestine. The color of the liver is virid; hence, the gall is the virid intestine. The color of the spleen is yellow; hence, the stomach is the yellow intestine. The color of the kidneys is black; hence, the bladder is the black intestine. All these intestines are located in the [region of the] lower [section of the Triple] Burner.

  Liao Ping: The gall bladder has an upper opening but has no lower opening. It cannot be termed "virid intestine." The outer kidney controls the passing of liquids. Thus, it can be called "intestine."

(16) *Hua Shou*: The sentence *xia jiao suo zhi ye* 下焦所治也 refers to the urinary bladder. That is to say, the urinary bladder separates the clear from the turbid in accordance with instructions from the lower [section of the Triple] Burner.

  Zhang Shixian: [All the short-term repositories] receive water and grains from the stomach, which they transform and transmit down to the lower [section of the Triple] Burner. In this process of drainage, clear and turbid [portions] are not separated before they are emitted.[5] Hence, [the text] states: "They belong to the governing district of the lower [section of the Triple] Burner."

  Xu Dachun: The *Ling* [*shu*] treatise "Ying wei sheng hui" 營衛生會 states: "Water and grains should be present in the stomach simultaneously. They become dregs and move down together. When they reach the large intestine, they enter the [realm of the] lower [section of the Triple] Burner. [The liquids and the solid dregs] leak downward together. The liquid [portions] are then strained off; they follow the lower [section of the Triple] Burner and leak into the bladder." Hence, all the five short-term repositories are governed by the qi from the lower [section of the Triple] Burner.

  Katō Bankei: Hua Shou has commented that the sentence *xia jiao zhi suo zhi ye* 下焦之所治也 refers to the gall bladder. That is incorrect because everything from the stomach downward represents the governing district of the lower [section of the Triple] Burner. Hence, all short-term repositories could be termed as belonging [to the lower section of the Triple Burner].

---

5   This sentence contradicts some of the commentaries on the lower section of the Triple Burner following difficult issue 31. Perhaps its wording is corrupt.

三十六難曰：（一）藏各有一耳，腎獨有兩者，何也？
（二）然：腎兩者，非皆腎也。其左者為腎，右者為命門。（三）命門者，諸
神精之所舍，原氣之所繫也。（四）故男子以藏精，女子以繫胞，（五）故知
腎有一也。

The thirty-sixth difficult issue: (1) Each of the long-term depots is a single [entity], except for the kidneys which represent a twin [entity]. Why is that so?

(2) It is like this. The two kidneys are not both kidneys. The one on the left is the kidney; the one on the right is the gate of life. (3) The gate of life is the place where the spirit-essence lodges; it is the place to which the original qi are tied. (4) Hence, in males it stores the essence; in females it holds the womb. (5) Hence, one knows that there is only one kidney.[1]

COMMENTARIES

(1) *Li Jiong*: Liver, spleen, lung, and heart have one lobe each. The kidney has two lobes. Why is that so?

Liao Ping: The following is the erroneous explanation of this book [of the false doctrine that there are two kidneys].

(2) *Ding Deyong*: "The gate of life is the place where the spirit essence lodges; it is the place to which the original qi are tied. Hence, in males it stores the essence; in females it holds the womb. Hence, one knows that there is only one kidney." The so-called gate of life is not [the right kidney, the vessel of which can be felt] at the foot [section] of the right [hand]. It is a gate controlling man's existence. The kidneys belong to the (phase of) water. Hence, one knows that what [can be felt] at the foot [section] of the right [hand] is the minister fire carrying out the orders (*ming* 命) of the ruler fire. It is also called *ming men* 命門 (here, "gate of orders") today; that is not the *ming men* of the kidneys. The name is identical but the meaning differs.

Yang: Although there are two kidneys, not each of them is a kidney. Hence the *Mai jing* 脈經 states: "The kidney [movement in the] vessels [appears] in the foot [section] of the left hand. The spirit gate [movement in the] vessels [appears] in the foot [section] of the right hand." That is the meaning. The kidney is the root and the basis of human life; the "spirit gate" is the source of the original

---

1   The *Nan jing* editions compiled by Ding Jin, Ye Lin, and Liao Ping have, as the last sentence of the present difficult issue, *gu zhi shen you er ye* 故知腎有二也 ("hence, one knows that there are two kidneys"). This should be kept in mind when reading their commentaries.

qi. Hence, [the text] states: "It is the place where the spirit essence lodges." The "spirit gate" (*shen men* 神門) is also called the "gate of life."

Yu Shu: The [*Nan*] *jing* states: "The one on the right is the gate of life; it is the place to which the original qi are tied." The *Mai jing* 脈經 says that the [gate of life] is related to the Triple Burner like outside and inside. The Triple Burner, furthermore, controls the qi of the three originals. From this one may infer that the Triple Burner originates from the gate of life. It is associated with the fire of the hand minor yang [conduit], and it matches the fire of the heart enclosing [network, which is associated with the] hand ceasing yin[conduit], like outside and inside. The principle is clear now.

Xu Dachun: Neither in the *Ling* [*shu*] nor in the *Su* [*wen*] are there statements that [one] kidney constitutes the gate of life. The only reference [to the gate of life appears in a different context, in that] the treatise "Gen jie" 根結 of the *Ling* [*shu*] states: "The major yang [conduit]: Its root lies in the *zhi yin* [opening]; it is connected to the gates of life. The ,gates of life' are the eyes." The treatise "Wei qi" 衛氣 of the *Ling* [*shu*] states also that the eyes are the gate of life. The [treatise] "Yin yang li he lun" 陰陽離合倫 of the *Su* [*wen*] states: "The major yang [vessel] originates from the *zhi yin* 至陰 [hole], and ends in the gate of life. It is called yang-in-yin." The [*Nei*] *jing* texts say nothing else [on the gate of life]. Also, in the [treatise] "Da huo lun" 大惑論 of the *Ling* [*shu*] it is stated: "All the essence qi of the five long-term depots and six short-term repositories pour upwards into the eyes and let them be clear." That is the meaning underlying the designation of the eyes as the gate of life. If the kidney has two [lobes], then both must be called kidney. [One of them] cannot be called the gate of life. Now, the kidneys are a female depot. Their number [i.e., two] is even. Hence, it is [associated with the] North [and with the stellar division] *xuan wu* 玄武. Also, it is related to the two beings, the tortoise and the snake. The tortoise is [categorized as] yin-in-yin; the snake is [categorized as] yang-in-yin. It is that principle. But the one on the right controls the fire in the kidneys; the one on the left controls the water in the kidneys. Each has its specific responsibilities. As for the doctrine concerning the gate of life, the *Huang ting jing* 黃庭經 states: "Behind is the dark gate; in front is the gate of life." The meanings come close to each other. Some of the [previous] commentators have considered the gate of life to be the navel. But such statements are not sufficiently [grounded in fact] to be mentioned [here]. In my own opinion there is enough [evidence for the assumption] that it corresponds to the starting point of the throughway vessel. In the [treatise] "Ju tong lun" 舉痛論 of the *Su* [*wen*] it is said: "The throughway vessel emerges from the *guan yuan* 關元." The *guan yuan* hole is located three inches below the navel. In the [treatise] "Ni shun fei shou lun" 逆順肥瘦論 of the *Ling* [*shu*] it is said: "The throughway vessel is the sea of the five long-term depots and six short-term repositories. Its extension downward pours [its contents] into the big network [vessels] of the minor yin [conduit], it appears at the *qi jie* 氣街 [opening]." Furthermore, the [treatise] "Hai lun" 海論 considers the throughway vessel to be the sea of blood. Thus, its position is exactly between the two kidneys. It can truly be called the "gate of life." Although its qi communicate with the kidneys, [the gate of life] cannot be identified as the right kidney.

　Liao Ping: That is to say, one is the outer kidney, one is the [heart] enclosing network. It is not a kidney. ["Left"] should be read as "inner." That is the [heart] enclosing network. ["Right"] should be read as "outer." ["Gate of life"] is another name for the outer kidney.... [The gate of life] corresponds to the "outer kidney." It is also called "gall bladder."

(3) *Li Jiong*: There is a hole in the fourteenth vertebra [called] *ming men* 命門 ("gate of life"). Furthermore, there are two *zhi shi* 志室 holes on both sides below the fourteenth vertebra, at a distance of three inches each. A spirit holds guard at the gate of life; it does not allow any evil to enter. *Zhi shi* 志室 ("dwelling of the mind") stands for *she zhai* 舍宅 ("dwelling"). That is where the spirit-essence resides .... *Yuan* 原 ("original") stands for *yuan* 元 ("original"). The original qi originate from the [branch] *zi* 子.[2] *Zi* refers to the cardinal direction [associated with the trigram] *kan* 坎.[3] *Kan* represents the original qi of both father and mother. [The trigram] *qian* 乾 represents heaven and father. [The trigram] *kun* 坤 represents earth and mother. Now, [the trigram] *kan* has six on first place and six on third place. That is [identical with] the six on first place and the six on third place of [the trigram] *kun*. The nine on second place of *kan* is [identical] with the nine on second place of [the trigram] *qian*. That is to say, *qian* and *kun* interact with six on third place and with nine on second place and form the trigram *kan*. Therefore, the original qi are tied to the kidneys.

(4) *Li Jiong*: The essence qi flow from the five long-term depots and six short-term repositories and leak into the kidneys. The long-term depot of the kidneys receives and stores them. Each of the five long-term depots contains essence.

2　*Zi* is the first of the Twelve Earth Branches (*di zhi* 地枝). It is associated with the North.

3　The trigram *kan* 坎 is associated with the North and with water. Its upper and lower lines are yin lines, they are broken. Its central line is a yang line, it is unbroken. The following sentences refer to the trigram *qian* 乾, consisting of three yang lines, and the trigram *kun* 坤, consisting of three yin lines. The number "six" refers, in the commentaries to the *Yi jing*, to the yin lines; "nine" refers to the yang lines. *Kan* unites elements of *qian* (father) and *kun* (mother).

Whenever necessary, the [long-term depots] pour it into the kidneys. The kidneys are the location from which the city gates are controlled. The essence of the body is stored here.

Hua Shou: There are two kidneys. The one on the left is the kidney; the one on the right is the gate of life. In males, the essence is stored here. The essence [transmitted] from the five long-term depots and six short-term repositories is received and stored here. In females, the womb is tied here. It receives the essence [from the males] and transforms it. The womb is the location where the embryo is conceived.

(1)–(5) *Ye Lin*: The kidney has two lobes; one on the left and one on the right side. One controls the water; one controls the fire. They correspond to the mechanics of rise and fall. The gate of life is the root of the Triple Burner and the sea of the original qi of the 12 conduits; it is the utensil that stores and transforms the essence, and it is the place to which the womb, which conceives the embryo, is tied. Thus, it is the origin of man's life. Hence, it is called gate of life. According to the treatise "Gen jie" 根結 of the *Ling shu*, and according to the treatise "Yin yang li he lun" 陰陽離合論 of the *Su wen*, the major yang [conduit] is rooted at the *zhi yin* 至陰 [hole], and it ties up with the gate of life. [In that context] the gate of life refers to the eyes. These [treatises] point out that the final hole of the major yang conduit is the *qing ming* 晴明 [hole].[4] The *qing ming* [hole is passed by qi that] come from the brain and from the heart. [The eyes] are therefore the holes where one's life arrives. Hence, they are called gate of life. That, however, differs from the meaning implied here. If [the present difficult issue] did in fact state that the right kidney is the gate of life, I fear that such [a statement] is not entirely correct. If one discusses this subject in terms of the [movement of the] qi in the vessels, water rises on the left, fire descends on the right. The left and the right are the passageways of yin and yang, respectively. They are the pivotal mechanisms of rise and fall. When Yueren examined the [movement in the] vessels, he relied only on the inch openings. He diagnosed the water at the foot [section] of the left hand; and he diagnosed the fire at the foot [section] of the right hand. Hence, he called the [kidney] on the left "kidney," and the one on the right "gate of life." Maybe he based the meaning [of his terminology] on such [considerations].

---

4 The *qing ming* hole is located at the inner corner of the eye. It is usually listed as the first hole of the foot major yang conduit.

三十七難曰：（一）五藏之氣，於何發起，通於何許，可曉以不？
（二）然：五藏者，當上關於九竅也。（三）故肺氣通於鼻，鼻和則知香臭
矣；肝氣通於目，目和則知白黑矣；脾氣通於口，口和則知穀味矣；心
氣通於舌，舌和則知五味矣；腎氣通於耳，耳和則知五音矣。（四）五藏不
和，則九竅不通；（五）六府不和，則留結為癰。
（六）邪在六府，則陽脈不和；陽脈不和，則氣留之；氣留之，則陽脈盛
矣。（七）邪在五藏，則陰脈不和；陰脈不和，則血留之；血留之，則陰脈
盛矣。（八）陰氣太盛，則陽氣不得相營也，故曰格。（九）陽氣太盛，則陰
氣不得相營也，故曰關。（十）陰陽俱盛，不得相營也，故曰關格。關格
者，不得盡其命而死矣。
（十一）經言氣獨行於五藏，不營於六府者，何也？
（十二）然：氣之所行也，如水之流，不得息也。故陰脈營於五藏，陽脈營
於六府，如環之無端，莫知其紀，終而復始，（十三）其不覆溢，人氣內溫
於藏府，外濡於腠理。

The thirty-seventh difficult issue: (1) The qi of the five long-term depots, where do they originate, where do they pass through. Can that be known?

(2) It is like this. The nine orifices are the upper gates of the five long-term depots. (3) Hence, the qi of the lung pass through the nose; as long as the nose is at ease, one knows [the differences between] aroma and stench. The qi of the liver pass through the eyes; as long as the eyes are at ease, one knows [the differences between] black and white. The qi of the spleen pass through the mouth; as long as the mouth is at ease, one knows [the differences between] the grains. The qi of the heart pass through the tongue; as long as the tongue is at ease, one knows [the differences between] the five flavors. The qi of the kidneys pass through the ears; as long as the ears are at ease, one knows [the differences between] the five [musical] notes. (4) When the five long-term depots are not at ease, the nine orifices are not passable. (5) When the six short-term repositories are not at ease, the [qi] will stagnate and accumulate, causing obstruction-illness. (6) When evil [qi] are present in [any of] the six short-term repositories, the yang vessels will not be at ease. When the yang vessels are not at ease, the qi will stagnate in them. When the qi stagnate in them, the yang vessels will be overfilled. (7) When evil [qi] are present in the five long-term depots, the yin vessels will not be at ease. When the yin vessels are not at ease, the blood will stagnate in them. When the blood stagnates in them, the yin vessels will be overfilled. (8) In the case of a great surplus of qi in the yin [vessels], qi from the yang [vessels] cannot circulate [into the yin vessels]. Therefore, one speaks of "barrier." (9) In the case of a great surplus of qi in the yang [vessels], the qi from

the yin [vessels] cannot circulate [into the yang vessels]. Therefore, one speaks of "closure." (10) When there is a surplus of [qi in] both yin and yang [vessels], no circulation will be possible between them. Hence, one speaks of "closure and barrier." When closure and barrier are present, one may not complete his life-span and shall die [a premature death].

(11) The scripture states: The qi proceed only through the five long-term depots; they do not circulate through the six short-term repositories. Why is that so?

(12) It is like this. The passage of the qi is like the flow of water; it never comes to rest. Hence, [when the qi are in the] yin vessels, they circulate through the five long-term depots, and [when the qi are in] the yang vessels, they circulate through the six short-term repositories. It is like a ring without end. Nobody knows its break; it ends and begins anew. (13) In case there is no turnover or overflow, man's qi provide [all] the long-term depots and short-term repositories with warmth internally, and they moisten the pores externally.[5]

COMMENTARIES

(2) *Yang*: The seven orifices are the door gates of the five long-term depots. As long as the qi in the long-term depots are well balanced, the door gates will be at ease and passable.

Zhang Shixian: The five long-term depots are below; the nine orifices are above. Hence, [the text] states: "The nine orifices are the upper gates." "Upper" means "upper part of the body." The nine orifices have been explained by [previous] commentators as seven yang orifices and two yin orifices; the latter being located at the lower, the former being located at the upper [end of the body]. Only [Zhang] Jiegu 張潔古[6] speaks of "nine orifices as upper gates" – namely, two ears, two eyes, two nose-holes, one mouth, one tongue, and one throat, adding up to nine orifices. However, no other author has considered the tongue to be an orifice, and that was quite reasonable. But they have probably missed the meaning intended by Yueren. From "the qi of the liver pass through the eyes" to "the qi of the kidneys pass through the ears," the nine orifices are properly outlined as upper gates of the five long-term depots. If one considers it right to speak of seven yang orifices and two yin orifices, then the two sentences in the original text – "the qi of the heart pass through the tongue. As long as the

---

5   For the concepts of "barrier" and "closure," "turnover" and "overflow," see also difficult issue 3.

6   Jiegu is the *zi* name of Zhang Yuansu 張元素, a Jin author who lived around 1180. Among his works is the *Bing ji qi yi bao ming ji* 病機氣宜保命集.

tongue is at ease, one knows [the differences between] the fives flavors" – are superfluous. But if one counts the tongue as an orifice one gets a sum of ten orifices. [To speak of] ten, eight, or seven[7] orifices is not as good as [Zhang] Jiegu's statement, which makes very good sense – especially because it does not neglect the original text [of the *Nan jing*, which speaks] of the nine orifices as the upper gates. The word "upper" is quite apposite. Hence, I follow the discourse of [Zhang] Jiegu and point out the errors of all the [previous] authors here.

Xu Dachun: This paragraph [corresponds to] the treatise "Mai du" 脈度 of the *Ling* [*shu*]. Of the entire text only a few words have been altered, but many problems have resulted from this. The [*Nei*] *jing* states: "The five long-term depots internally always communicate with the seven orifices." That is to say, the nose represents two, the eyes represent two, and the ears represent two [orifices], while mouth and tongue – although distinguished [as two entities] – represent, in fact, only one orifice. That adds up to seven orifices. If one speaks of nine orifices, one should include the two yin orifices [for urine and stools] because the [qi of the] kidneys pass through the two yin [orifices]. Here, the two yin [orifices] are excluded, and still [the text] speaks of "nine orifices." Now, if one distinguishes between mouth and tongue as two orifices, there are still only eight orifices. One cannot speak of nine orifices. Also, instead of the five phrases "when the nose is at ease; when the eyes are at ease," and so on, the [*Nei*] *jing* states: "When the [qi of the] lung are in harmony; when the [qi of the] liver are in harmony; ...." When the qi of the long-term depots are in harmony, the seven orifices reflect this as [external locations where the conditions of the long-term depots] become visible. If one says "the nose is at ease; ... the eyes are at ease; ...." then [one should ask] how can the seven orifices be at ease out of themselves? This [answer], once again, does not correspond to the meaning of the question asked.

(3) *Yang*: When the five long-term depots lose their ease internally, the nine orifices will be blocked externally. Now, there are seven orifices in the upper [part of the body], but [the text] speaks of nine. Two orifices are dark and hidden; hence, they are not mentioned. Above, the qi of the kidneys pass through the ears; below, they pass through the two yin [openings]. Hence, [the text] speaks of nine orifices.

Zhang Shixian: "Not at ease" means evil [qi] reside in them.

Liao Ping: The foot minor yin conduit and [its] network [vessel] do not reach the ears. What reaches the ears is the minor yang conduit [associated with the] gall bladder. This "kidneys" must refer to the outer kidney.

---

7   The text has "nine." That must be an error in writing.

(5) *Yang*: "Six short-term repositories" stands for "yang qi." When the yang qi cannot move at ease, they accumulate to obstruction-illnesses and swelling. Hence, [the text] speaks of "causing obstruction-illness." When evil [qi] arrive to seize the [place originally supplemented by proper] qi, they travel into the short-term repositories first.

(6) *Li Jiong*: The six short-term repositories belong to the yang; the yang vessels are above the flesh. When evil qi move into the six short-term repositories, then the vessels above the flesh are not at ease. The yang constitutes the qi which rule the exterior. When the vessels above the flesh are not at ease, then evil qi stagnate in the skin and do not disperse. When evil qi stagnate [there], the yang vessels will be unilaterally overfilled.

(7) *Li Jiong*: The five long-term depots belong to the yin; below the flesh are the yin vessels. When evil qi are present in the five long-term depots, then the vessels below the flesh are not at ease. The yin constitutes the blood which rules the interior. When the vessels below the flesh are not at ease, then blood evil will stagnate in the flesh. When blood evil stagnates [there], the yin vessels will be unilaterally overfilled.

(8) *Zhang Shixian*: Ge 格 ("barrier") stands for *ju* 拒 ("to ward off"). "Internal barrier" [means that the qi of the] external vessels cannot enter [the internal vessels] because the [qi in the] yin [vessels] stagnate unilaterally and the qi of the yang [vessels] cannot circulate [either]. Hence, [this condition] is called "barrier against [qi from the] yang [vessels]."

(9) *Zhang Shixian*: Guan 関 ("closure") stands for *bi* 閉 ("closed"). "External closure" [means that the qi of] the internal vessels cannot exit [into the external vessels] because the yang [vessels] are unilaterally overfilled and, as a consequence, the qi of the yin [vessels] cannot circulate. Hence, [this condition] is called "closure against [qi from the] yin [vessels]."

(6)–(10) *Xu Dachun*: This section, from beginning to end, is original text from the treatise "Mai du" 脈度 of the *Ling* [*shu*]. Only a few words have been changed. Nothing is explained. In addition, by inverting the yin and yang [categorizations] of the two words "closure" and "barrier," an age-old controversy has been set up. [I] do not know whether it originated from an error in writing or whether Yueren himself did indeed change the text of the [*Nei*] *jing* on his own. The treatise "Mai du" states: "When the yin qi abound excessively, then the yang qi are unable to circulate. Hence that is called "closure". When the yang qi abound excessively, then the yin qi are unable to circulate. Hence that is called "barrier". In the treatise "Liu jie zang xiang" 六節藏象 of the *Su* [*wen*] it is stated: "A fourfold or stronger overfilling [perceived] at the *ren ying* 人迎 [holes] indicates barrier in the yang [section against the influx of qi from the yin section]. A fourfold or stronger overfilling [perceived] at the inch opening indicates closure of the yin [section against the influx of qi from the yang section]." Also, the treatise "Zhong shi" 終始 of the *Ling* [*shu*] states: "If they abound at the *ren ying* [opening an additional] four times [more than normal] and [if their movement is] both massive and increased in speed, that is called 'overflowing yang'." Overflowing yang generates an external barrier. If they abound at the vessel opening [an additional] four times [more than normal], and [if their movement is] both massive and increased in speed, that is called 'overflowing yin'. Overflowing yin generates an internal closure." Indisputably, the texts of the [*Nei*] *jing* nowhere regard yin overfilling as "barrier" and yang overfilling as "closure." Why did Yueren turn away from that?

(10) *Zhang Shixian*: If the yin [vessels] in the internal and the yang [vessels] in the external [sections of the organism] are both overfilled, the camp and the guard [qi] are blocked, [that is,] the qi and the blood cannot reach each other easily. That is [a condition called] "closure and barrier." Now, human life depends on the circulatory movement of qi and blood. When the qi and the blood fail to continue their circulatory movement, one cannot complete his life-span and will die.

(11) *Hua Shou*: [The text] states: "The qi proceed only through the five long-term depots; they do not circulate through the six short-term repositories," That does not mean that they do not circulate through the six short-term repositories. It means that when they proceed through the yin conduits [which are associated with the long-term depots], they circulate through the five long-term depots, When they proceed through the yang conduits [which are associated with the short-term repositories], they circulate through the six short-term repositories.

(12) *Yang*: "Turnover or overflow" means that [a movement of the foot sections] ascends to the fish [line, or that a movement that should be limited to the inch section] enters the foot [section]. If that is not the case, [the qi] should proceed without break, Hence, [the text] states: "It ends and begins anew."

Hua Shou: When the qi in the vessels continue their circulatory flow as if they were [moving in] a ring without end, then no suffering from closure or barrier, from turnover or overflow is present and man's qi are able to provide the long-term depots and short-term repositories with warmth internally and to moisten the pores externally, Mr. Chen from Siming states: When evil [qi] are present in the short-term repositories, then the yang vessels are overfilled, When evil [qi] are present in the long-term depots, then the yin vessels are overfilled, When the yin vessels are overfilled, the yin qi close the lower [section of the body against the influx of yang qi]. When the yang vessels are replete, the yang qi resist [against the influx of yin qi] in the upper [section of the body]. But such a situation does not yet lead to death. When both the yin and yang [vessels] are overfilled, then closure and barrier occur at the same time. Barrier means that one vomits and cannot get his food down, closure means that the two yin [orifices] are blocked and that urine and stools cannot pass. Hence, death follows. When the qi of the long-term depots and short-term repositories are at ease and circulate from one [section] into the other, when yin [qi] do not turn over, and when yang [qi] do not overflow, why should there be any closure or barrier?

(11)–(12) *Ding Deyong*: Whenever there are not enough yin [qi], yang [qi] will enter [their space] and seize it. That is a "turnover." Whenever there are not enough yang [qi], yin [qi] will come out to seize [their space]. That is an "overflow." That is meant by "the qi proceed only through [the five long-term depots]."

Xu Dachun: Camp and guard [qi] proceed through [all] long-term depots and short-term repositories. There is absolutely no such doctrine that they proceed through the long-term depots but do not proceed through the short-term repositories. Question and answer in this paragraph quote the treatise "Mai du" 脈度 of the *Ling* [*shu*], but the meaning is once again interpreted erroneously. The original text of the [*Nei*] *jing* states: "The qi pass only through the five long-term depots, they do not circulate through the six short-term repositories. How is that? Qi Bo replied: It is simply impossible that there is a place not passed through by the qi. This is like the flow of water, like the movement of sun and moon – they will never stop. The fact is: The [qi of the] yin vessels circulate through the long-term depots. The [qi of the] yang vessels circulate through the short-term repositories. This is like a ring without end. And nobody knows the underlying set-up. Where it ends there is a new begin. The qi that spill over, they moisten the long-term depots and the short-term repositories internally. Externally they moisten the skin structures." That is the text of the [*Nei*] *jing*. The qi mentioned here are those of the walker vessel. The phrase "They pass only through the five long-term depots, they do not circulate through the six short-term repositories" refers, as the answer of Qi Bo points out quite clearly, to the course of the yin walker; it does not refer to the yang walker. There were some doubts as to whether only yin passageways had been discussed [in the previous paragraph of the respective *Nei jing* treatise], hence, [the Yellow Thearch] posed his second question. Here, [in the present difficult issue], the section on the walker vessel is omitted. Thus, what qi are the qi mentioned? To what does the statement "they proceed through the five long-term depots, they do not circulate through the six short-term repositories" refer? Answer and question quote the text of the [*Nei*] *jing*, but virtually nothing is explained. That is completely useless. Also, erroneous omissions occur to such an extent! How could Yueren be so careless?

(12) *Liao Ping*: The camp [qi] circulate through the twelve conduits; they do not distinguish between long-term depots and short-term repositories. The guard [qi] also circulate through the twelve conduits and do not distinguish between long-term depots and short-term repositories.

(13) *Li Jiong*: *Cou li* 腠理 ("skin structures", "pores") refers to *mao kong* 毛孔 ("the openings through which the hairs grow") and to *wen li* 文理 ("the line structures on the skin").

三十八難曰：（一）藏唯有五，府獨有六者，何也？
（二）然：所以府有六者，謂三焦也。（三）有原氣之別焉，主持諸氣，（四）有名而無形，（五）其經屬手少陽，（六）此外府也，（七）故言府有六焉。

The thirty-eighth difficult issue: (1) The long-term depots are but five; only the short-term repositories are six. Why is that so?

(2) It is like this. The [existence of the] Triple Burner is to be named as the reason for the fact that there are six short-term repositories. (3) The Triple Burner represents an additional [source] of original qi; it governs all the qi [circulating in the body]. (4) It has a name but no physical appearance. (5) It is associated with the hand minor yang conduit. (6) This is an external short-term repository. (7) Hence, one speaks of the existence of six short-term repositories.

COMMENTARIES

(1) *Liao Ping*: If there were only five long-term depots, how could they [and the six short-term repositories] be matched with the twelve conduits? Basically, [the twelve conduits] are associated with six short-term repositories and six long-term depots. The [*Nei*] *jing* has resorted to the designations "five" and "six" because "five" corresponds to the earth while "six" reflects heaven. The short-term repositories are yang; they match heaven. The long-term depots are yin; they match the earth. The [*Nei*] *jing* says: "Heaven has six as its ordering [principle]; the earth has five [seasonal] terms." Also, there are five [circulatory] phases and six [climatic] qi. But when they are to be matched with the Twelve [Earth] Branches, then there are six long-term depots.

(3) *Li Jiong*: The kidneys are the proper [source] of the original qi; the Triple Burner represents an additional [source] of original qi. The *dan zhong* 膻中 is a sea of qi; it is located in the upper [section of the Triple] Burner. Also, a sea-of-qi hole exists two inches below the navel; it is located in the lower [section of the Triple] Burner. [Hence, the Triple Burner] controls the qi of the entire body.

Hua Shou: The Triple Burner governs all the qi; it is an additional transmitter of original qi. [That is to say], the original qi depend on the guidance of the [Triple Burner] in their ceaseless hidden movement and secret circulation through the entire body.

Xu Dachun: That is the "additional transmitter of the original qi," [as mentioned] in the sixty-sixth difficult issue.

(4) *Li Jiong*: The Triple Burner represents nothing but membranes attached to the upper, central, and lower opening of the stomach. The Triple Burner has a name, but no real form.

　Xu Dachun: The *Ling* [*shu*] and the *Su* [*wen*] discuss the Triple Burner more than once. These are individual statements the grammatical styles of which are more or less transparent. [The Triple Burner] is called a short-term repository because it emits and takes in, because it links and because it spreads. That makes it obvious that [the Triple Burner] has the function of storing and draining. How could one say that it has no physical appearance! It is spread out all around the upper and the lower [parts of the body], enclosing [all the other] long-term depots and short-term repositories. Its form differs from that of the [remaining] five short-term repositories, each of which has its distinct body. Hence, its appearance cannot be defined [in the same way]. But to say "it has no physical appearance" – that is impossible.

　Ding Jin: "It has a name but no physical appearance" because it encloses [everything else like a cover] on the outside. Hence, [the text] speaks of an "external short-term repository." In the twenty-fifth difficult issue, my commentary stated that the Triple Burner holds all the long-term depots and short-term repositories like a large bag. If one compares that [difficult issue] with the meaning of the present paragraph, one could become confused. People of later times have said that the Triple Burner has a physical appearance and that the *Nan jing* is wrong. Well, they failed to penetrate the entire corpus of the *Nan jing*.

　Ye Lin: The Triple Burner has a physical appearance! That has already been discussed in sufficient detail in the commentaries on difficult issue 25 .... It can be proven that the Triple Burner has a physical appearance. But the transformation of qi through the Triple Burner is difficult to perceive. Hence, [the text] says: "It has a name but no physical appearance."

(4) *Liao Ping*: This question is superfluous. [The author] issued this question – inquiring about the meaning [of five long-term depots versus six short-term repositories] – because he had not studied the [*Nei*] *jing* in its entirety. The Triple Burner has been discussed in detail in the thirty-first difficult issue. "No physical appearance" means that it does not occupy a fixed position. The [*Ling shu*] treatise "Jing mai" 經脈 elucidates [the course of] the Triple Burner from its origin to its end, with all its holes. It names, altogether, twenty-three holes. If [the present passage] is to say that [the Triple Burner] has, in fact, no physical appearance, the author[s] of this book could hardly have been foolish enough themselves to arrive at such [a statement]. Later people must have altered the original version, adding to the seriousness [of its mistakes].

(6) *Yang*: The Triple Burner has no [corresponding] depot[1] in the internal [section of the body]; it has only a conduit vessel named hand minor yang. Hence, [the text] speaks of an "external short-term repository."

Hua Shou: "External short-term repository" refers to its conduit, which is the hand minor yang [conduit]. Thus, the Triple Burner has a conduit externally, but it has no physical appearance internally. Hence, the [respective] statement [of the text].

Xu Dachun: That is to say, it is located outside of all the [remaining] short-term repositories. Hence, it is called an "external short-term repository." According to the treatise "Ben shu" 本輸 of the *Ling* [*shu*], "the Triple Burner is the short-term repository of the central ditch. The waterways originate from there. It is associated with the bladder. It is a solitary short-term repository." It is called "solitary short-term repository" because it is not attached to a depot. That is the meaning of "external short-term repository."

Liao Ping: That is to say, its territory is much broader than that of the remaining long-term depots, it does not really mean that it has no physical appearance.

(7) *Ding Deyong*: [The text] speaks of "five long-term depots" and "six short-term repositories." That is to say, the five long-term depots correspond to the Five Phases on earth, while the six short-term repositories correspond to the six qi of heaven. In reference to the six qi of heaven, the Triple Burner represents the minister fire. It is associated with the hand minor yang [conduit]. Hence, [the text] states: "Only the short-term repositories are six."

Liao Ping: This kind of answer is fool's talk.

(1)–(7) *Katō Bankei*: If [one speaks of] but five short-term repositories and long-term depots, this is so because of the principle of the Five Phases. Two times five is ten. That completes the number [associated with] generation and maturing. An extension [of the number of long-term depots and short-term repositories] to six corresponds to the six qi. Adding [six and six] makes twelve. That parallels [the number of the Twelve] Branches and pitch pipes. All [the numbers five, six, ten, and twelve] are symbols matching the nature of heaven and earth. Now, the Triple Burner is not a proper short-term repository. However, without its qi all the other short-term repositories could not fulfill their functions of emitting, intake, revolution, and transformation. It is not a proper short-term repository; hence, it steams inside of the membrane;[2] it moves in between the short-term

---

1 The text has *fu* 府 ("short-term repository"). That must be a mistake in writing.

2 The phrase repeats, almost literally, a passage from *Su wen* treatise 43, "Pi lun" 痺論, where it is stated that because of their aggressive nature, the guard qi cannot find entrance into the vessels but "proceed through the skin and in the flesh, steaming against the membrane, and dispersing in the chest." The meaning here is different. "It steams inside of the

repositories and long-term depots. It resembles an external wall. Hence, it is called "external short-term repository." The *Ling shu* calls it "solitary short-term repository." That is the same meaning. The commentary by Hua [Shou] stated: "The Triple Burner has a conduit externally, but it has no physical appearance internally. Hence, it is called 'external short-term repository'." That is incorrect. The twenty-fifth treatise of the old version [of the *Nan jing*][3] speaks of the Triple Burner and of the heart enclosing [network] as outside and inside. The present paragraph calls it an "additional [source] of original qi." There, [in difficult issue 25,] the Triple Burner and the heart enclosing [network] were discussed together as long-term depot and short-term repository, and [the Triple Burner was associated with] the minister fire because [the heart enclosing network was associated with it, too]. Here, the gate of life and the Triple Burner are referred to as beginning and end. The meaning implied is different.

---

membrane" refers to the functions of the Triple Burner below the diaphragm by alluding to the literal meaning of the term "Burner."

3   Katō Bankei, in his *Nan jing* edition, extensively rearranged the order of the difficult issues and distinguished his "present version" from what he called the "old version." However, difficult issue 25 is numbered identically in both versions.

三十九難曰：（一）經言府有五，藏有六者，何也？

（二）然：六府者，正有五府也。（三）然五藏亦有六藏者，謂腎有兩藏也。（四）其左為腎，右為命門。（五）命門者，謂精神之所舍也；（六）男子以藏精，女子以繫胞，（七）其氣與腎通，故言藏有六也。

（八）府有五者，何也？

（九）然：五藏各一府，三焦亦是一府，然不屬於五藏，故言府有五焉。

The thirty-ninth difficult issue: (1) The scripture states: There are five short-term repositories and six long-term depots. What [does that mean]?

(2) It is like this. [Usually one speaks of] six short-term repositories, but actually there are five short-term repositories. (3) Although [one commonly speaks of] five long-term depots, there are also [arguments pointing out an existence of] six long-term depots. They state that the kidneys consist of two long-term depots. (4) The one on the left is the kidney; the one on the right is the gate of life. (5) The gate of life is the place where the essence spirit is harbored.[1] (6) In males it stores the essence; in females it holds the womb. (7) The qi of the gate of life are identical with [those of] the kidney. That is why [some] speak of an existence of six long-term depots.

(8) There are five short-term repositories. What does that mean?

(9) It is like this. Each of the body's five long-term depots has one short-term repository associated with it. The Triple Burner is a short-term repository, too, but even so it is not related to any of the five long-term depots. Hence [some] speak of an existence of [only] five short-term repositories.

COMMENTARIES

(1) *Li Jiong*: Gall bladder, stomach, large intestine, small intestine, and urinary bladder [are the five short-term repositories]; liver, heart, spleen, lung, kidney, and gate of life [are the six long-term depots]. Why is that so?

Xu Dachun: The text of the [*Nei*] *jing* has no [corresponding passage] that could be examined [for comparison].

Liao Ping: Since it quotes the *jing* 經 (here, "classic"), this book itself should not be called a "classic." ... The three characters [*fu you wu* 府有五 ("there are five short-term repositories")] are a mistaken amendment [by later editors]. If they represented the original text [of the *Nan jing*], then this would be yet another [example for the fact that its authors] did not understand [the *Nei jing*]. ....

---

1   Compare difficult issue 36, sentence 3.

Those without learning dare to wage false accusations against the [*Nei*] *jing*, using boastful words. Xu [Dachun] maintained that the [*Nei jing*] has no [corresponding passage] that could be examined [for comparison]. His words are but an excuse.

(2) *Li Jiong*: The Triple Burner is [sometimes] added as a sixth short-term repository. But in reality it would be appropriate [to speak of] five long-term depots.

Xu Dachun: That is to say, the Triple Burner is not attached to any [specific] depot. Hence it is not designated "short-term repository."

Liao Ping: All the [six] long-term depots and [six] short-term repositories [associated with] the twelve conduits are related to each other like outside and inside. The term "five long-term depots and six short-term repositories" was created for a special purpose. Here, this [expression] is reversed to "six long-term depots and five short-term repositories." Such daydreams are dangerous beyond conception.

(3) *Liao Ping*: It is difficult to count it but it may be a hundred times that the [*Nei*] *jing* calls the heart ruler, [i.e., the heart] enclosing network, the sixth short-term repository. Here, that is set aside and the term "gate of life" is introduced instead. This is really acting in defiance of what is right!

(1)–(9) *Ding Deyong*: In principle, the five long-term depots have five short-term repositories. Here [the text] states that the Triple Burner is a short-term repository, too. It is matched with the heart enclosing network as its depot. Thus, there are six long-term depots and six short-term repositories. The two conduits [associated with the heart enclosing network and the Triple Burner] both represent the minister fire. The minister carries out the orders (*ming* 命) of the ruler. Hence one speaks of a *ming men* 命門 (here, "gate of orders").

Yang: [Although one commonly speaks of] five long-term depots and six short-term repositories, [the number] five [applies to] both of them. [In fact,] they can be numbered five and six. One may speak of both five [long-term depots and short-term repositories] and of both six [long-term depots and short-term repositories], or of five on the one side and six on the other side. Each [constellation] likewise corresponds to numbers found in heaven and on earth. If one talks about proper long-term depots and short-term repositories, then both the long-term depots and the short-term repositories number five. The five long-term depots correspond to the five sacred mountains on earth while the five short-term repositories correspond to the five stars in heaven. If one talks in terms of six [long-term depots and short-term repositories], then the six long-term depots correspond to the six [yang notes of the twelve] pitch pipes, while the six short-term repositories correspond to the number of the [diagram] *qian*

乾 [i.e., of heaven]. If one talks about five long-term depots and six short-term repositories, then the five long-term depots correspond to the Five Phases while the six short-term repositories correspond to the six qi. If one talks about five short-term repositories and six long-term depots, then the six long-term depots reflect the six yin[2] while the five short-term repositories reflect the five constant virtues. Thus, if long-term depots and short-term repositories are both considered to be five, the hand heart ruler is not [considered to be] a depot, and the Triple Burner is not [considered to be] a short-term repository. If long-term depots and short-term repositories are both considered to be six, the hand heart ruler and the Triple Burner are added.

Yu Shu: Heaven manages [the world] below with the six qi; the earth presents the Five Phases [to the world] above. Heaven and earth exchange [their qi] liberally. [That which reflects their] numbers "five" and "six" is perfect. Man reflects the three powers.[3] Therefore, the long-term depots and the short-term repositories reflect the numbers five and six, respectively. That is to say, the human head is round; it reflects heaven. The feet are rectangular; they reflect the earth. The long-term depots and the short-term repositories, numbering five and six respectively, reflect man. Thus, the three powers are [reflected] completely.

Hua Shou: The preceding treatise spoke of five long-term depots and six short-term repositories. The present [difficult issue] speaks of five short-term repositories and six long-term depots because there are two kidneys. Although there are two kidneys, and although one distinguishes between one on the left and one on the right, [with the latter being called] the "gate of life," their qi are identical and both are kidneys. [One could speak of] five short-term repositories because the Triple Burner is matched with the hand heart ruler. Taking all treatises [of the *Nan jing*] into consideration, it is quite possible to speak of five long-term depots and six short-term repositories. It is also possible to speak of five long-term depots and five short-term repositories. And it is also possible to speak of six long-term depots and six short-term repositories.

Xu Dachun: The difficult issues raised in this and in the preceding paragraph are very important, but the respective answers do not exactly correspond to the questions. Now, the Triple Burner and the heart ruler constitute outside and inside [like other short-term repository - long-term depot pairs]. But the heart ruler is the residential wall encircling the heart. Although it is associated with the hand ceasing yin conduit it does, in fact, represent the external membrane of the heart, thus constituting one body together with the heart. Hence it cannot

2   I am not sure what is meant by "six yin", *liu yin* 六陰.

3   These are the *san cai* 三才 – that is, heaven, earth, and man.

be distinguished as a separate long-term depot. The Triple Burner is [the official who is] responsible for ditches and waterways. It forms a short-term repository by itself. It would be inappropriate to say that it is not a short-term repository simply because it cannot be matched with a [specific] long-term depot. Hence, the names of the long-term depots and short-term repositories cannot be increased or decreased. If one wished to continue this discussion, the [heart] enclosing network could be separated from the heart as a long-term depot of its own. Together with the gate of life, that would give a total of seven long-term depots. If one were to point out the [heart] enclosing network as a short-term repository, then one could speak of seven short-term repositories.

Ding Jin: The preceding chapter explained the meaning of six short-term repositories; the present chapter, in turn, explains the meaning of six long-term depots. In the preceding [chapter] the external short-term repository was included; here the [*Nan*] *jing* states that there are six long-term depots because the kidneys consist of two lobes. The left [lobe] is the kidney; the right [lobe] is the gate of life. It states further: "The gate of life is the place where the essence spirit is harbored. In males it stores the essence; in females it holds the womb. Its qi are identical with [those of] the kidney." Obviously, Yueren linked the designation gate of life to the right kidney. But the location of the gate of life is, in fact, in between the two kidneys. If that were not so, how could one say that it stores the essence and holds the womb? How could one say that its qi are identical with [those of] the kidney? I suspect the designation "gate of life" has been confused with the long-term depot of the hand heart ruler, [i.e., the heart] enclosing network. Hence, the text further down says: "The short-term repository of the Triple Burner does not belong to the five long-term depots." That makes it quite clear that it is associated with the long-term depot of the [heart] enclosing network. "Its qi are identical with [those of] the kidney" points out that the qi of the gate of life and of the right kidney are identical. All this becomes obvious by itself if one but carefully reads [the text].

四十難曰：（一）經言肝主色，（二）心主臭，（三）脾主味，（四）肺主聲，（五）腎主液。（六）鼻者，肺之候，而反知香臭；耳者，腎之候，而反聞聲，其意何也？

（七）然：肺者，西方金也，金生於巳，巳者南方火也，火者心，心主臭，故令鼻知香臭；（八）腎者，北方水也，水生於申，申者西方金，金者肺，肺主聲，故令耳聞聲。

The fortieth difficult issue: (1) The scripture states: The liver is responsible for the colors. (2) The heart is responsible for the odors. (3) The spleen is responsible for the flavors. (4) The lung is responsible for the sounds. (5) The kidneys are responsible for the liquids. (6) However, the nose indicates the [condition of the] lung and, contrary [to what one might expect, it does not differentiate the sounds but] knows [how to distinguish] aroma and stench. The ears indicate the [condition of the] kidneys and, contrary [to what one might expect, they have nothing to do with liquids but] hear the sounds. What does that mean?

(7) It is like this. The lung [corresponds to the] Western regions and [to the phase of] metal. Metal comes to life during [the time of the year associated with the branch] *si*, and [the branch] *si* [corresponds to the] Southern regions and to fire. Fire [corresponds to the] heart, and the heart is responsible for the odors. Hence it lets the nose know [how to distinguish] aroma and stench. (8) The kidneys are [associated with the] Northern regions and with water. Water comes to life during [the time of the year associated with the branch] *shen,* and [the branch] *shen* [corresponds to the] Western regions and to metal. Metal [corresponds to the] lung, and the lung is responsible for the sounds. Hence it lets the ears hear the sounds.[1]

---

1 This is another example of attempts to dissolve apparent contradictions in the system of correspondences. In this case they result from the association of the body's five long-term depots with specific orifices and their respective functions. The explanation given in the answer has been interpreted by some authors as referring, for the first time in this book, to a relationship among the Five Phases that is more sophisticated than the sequences of mutual generation and destruction quoted earlier. This third relationship among the Five Phases is known as *wu xing zhang sheng* 五行長生. In general, the term *chang sheng* carries the meaning of "long life." In the present context, it seems to have two meanings. On the one hand, it could be read as "life cycle"; on the other hand, it could be rendered as "coming to life" because the character *chang* is often omitted and the remaining term *sheng* is used as part of the sequence "birth, maturity, and death." In Zhang Shixian's list of the twelve stages of the "life cycle of the Five Phases" (*wu xing zhang sheng*), stage four – designated *zhang sheng* – should therefore be read as "coming to life." The *wu xing zhang sheng* concept is based on the assumption that each of the four phases associated with one of the four annual seasons (i.e., wood, fire, metal, and water) pass through a life

cycle of twelve stages. According to the *Tu zhu Nan jing* 圖註難經 by Zhang Shixian, these stages are the following:

1. *shou qi* 受氣   "conception"
2. *pei tai* 培胎   "nourishment of the fetus"
3. *yang* 養   "birth"
4. *zhang sheng* 長生   "coming to life"
5. *mu yu* 沐浴   "bathing"
6. *guan dai* 冠帶   "cap and sash"
7. *lin guan* 臨官   "taking over an official rank"
8. *di wang* 帝旺   "flourishing as ruler"
9. *shuai* 衰   "decline"
10. *bing* 病   "illness"
11. *si* 死   "death"
12. *gui mu* 歸墓   "burial"

Each of the four cycles is associated differently with the Twelve Earth Branches, but the underlying structure is always the same. Stages (7), (8), and (9) are associated with the three branches that are, in turn, associated with the season during which the respective phase occupies the dominating position. For example, stages (7), (8), and (9) of the life cycle of wood are associated with spring (because the phase of wood dominates during the three months of spring), and hence with the branches *yin* 寅, *mao* 卯, and *chen* 辰. The entire schema can be illustrated graphically as follows.

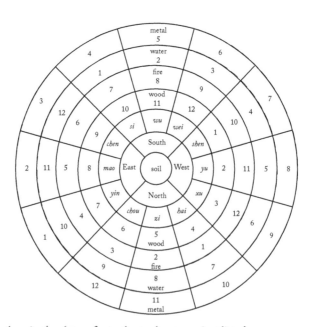

The numbers in the slots refer to the twelve stages just listed.

COMMENTARIES

(1) *Yu Shu*: The liver is [associated with] wood. The flowers of wood² display the five colors. Hence, [the liver] is responsible for the colors.

(2) *Yu Shu*: The heart is [associated with] fire. When fire transforms things, the five odors emerge. Hence, only the heart is responsible for the five odors.

(3) *Yu Shu*: The spleen is [associated with] soil. The soil is sweet. Sweetness absorbs [all other] flavors. Hence, [the spleen] is responsible for the flavors. The *Li* [*ji*] 禮記³ states: "Sweetness absorbs and harmonizes the flavors." That is [what is] meant here.

Zhang Shixian: The spleen is [associated with] soil. The flavors are generated by the soil. Hence, the spleen is responsible for the flavors.

(4) *Yu Shu*: The lung is [associated with] metal. A hit against metal produces a sound. Hence, all the five tones emerge from the lung.

(5) *Yu Shu*: The kidneys are [associated with] water. Water flows and is moist. [Hence, the kidneys] are responsible for the liquids.

Li Jiong: All the five liquids originate from water. The kidneys control the water [in the body]. Hence, they are responsible for the [bodily] liquids.

(1)–(5) *Xu Dachun*: [I] do not know on what original [text] the question voiced in this paragraph is based. The forty-ninth difficult issue provides a very detailed elucidation [of the topic touched on here], allowing for a good understanding. The explanations given in the present [difficult issue] are completely irrelevant.

As Zhang Shixian elucidated, both the contradiction between the association of the nose with the lung (which is responsible for the sounds) on the one hand and with the function of distinguishing odors on the other hand, and the contradiction between the association of the ears with the kidneys (which are responsible for the bodily liquids) on the one hand and with the function of hearing the sounds on the other hand can be dissolved on the basis of the life cycle relationship among the Five Phases. However, Zhang's argument is not pervasive. If we extend it to tongue and eyes, the former should not be able to distinguish the flavors but should be able to distinguish the colors, and the latter should not be able to distinguish the colors but should be associated with the bodily liquids. We do not know whether the author(s) of the *Nan jing* had the life cycle relationship among the Five Phases in mind when they raised and answered difficult issue 40. The incongruity of the schema should not argue against such an assumption because incongruity appears to be an unavoidable – and, to some authors, acceptable – characteristic of the paradigm of systematic correspondence, which, despite its sophistication, could never make all ends meet. While people such as Zhang Shixian and, possibly, the *Nan jing* authors themselves seem to have been able to live with these incongruities, others (such as Xu Dachun, who mocked at the logical consequences of the life cycle concept) searched for more coherent explanations.

2 "Wood" stands here for "plants."

3 A work of the Confucian canon attributed to Dai Sheng 戴聖 (first and second century BCE), but probably compiled by Cao Bao 曹褒 of the first century CE.

Liver and heart are both [categorized as] yang. Hence, when one can see and speak, [the qi of liver and heart] leave from inside toward outside. The lung and the kidneys belong both to the yin. Hence, when one can smell and hear, [qi] enter from outside toward inside. All that is very meaningful; no forced interpretations are necessary. Furthermore, one could explain all that with the meaning of the mutual generation [sequence of the Five Phases. If] the wood of the liver comes to life during [the period of the year associated with the branch] *hai,* why does one not spit with one's eyes?[4] [If] the fire of the heart comes to life during [the period of the year associated with the branch] *yin,* why does one not distinguish the colors with one's tongue?[5] [If] the soil of the spleen comes to life during [the period of the year associated with the branch] *shen,* why can one not hear sounds with one's mouth?[6]

(6)–(8) *Yang:* Among the Five Phases, there are those that accomplish things in relation with others and there are those that accomplish things individually. For instance, the two long-term depots lung and kidneys accomplish [their tasks] in mutual relation [with another depot]. The remaining three long-term depots accomplish their [tasks] by themselves.[7]

(6) *Li Jiong:* The lung is responsible for the sounds. The nose is associated with the lung but it cannot hear sounds and tones; instead, it knows [how to distinguish] aroma and stench. The kidneys are responsible for the liquids. The ears are associated with the kidneys but they have nothing to do with the bodily liquids; instead, they are able to hear the sounds.

(7) *Li Jiong:* The nose is associated with the lung. The metal of the lung comes to life while the fire of the heart occupies the [dominating] position. Hence, it is able to distinguish the odors, which are controlled by the fire of the heart.

  Hua Shou: Mr. Chen from Siming states: "The odors are controlled by the heart; the nose is the orifice of the lung. The vessel [associated with] the heart ascends to the lung. Hence, it enables the nose to know [how to distinguish] aroma and stench."

(8) *Li Jiong:* The ears are associated with the kidneys. The water of the kidneys comes to life while the metal of the lung occupies the [dominating] position. Hence, [the latter] enables the ears to hear the sounds.

---

4   The branch *hai* 亥 is associated with the North and with water, and hence with the kidneys, which control the liquids.

5   The branch *yin* 寅 is associated with the East and with wood, and hence with the liver, which controls the colors.

6   The branch *shen* 申 is associated with the West and with metal, and hence with the lung, which controls the sounds.

7   A noteworthy explanation, since it assumed qualitative differences among the Five Phases.

Hua Shou: Mr. Chen from Siming states: "The ears are the orifices of the kidneys. The sounds are controlled by the lung. The vessel [associated with the] kidneys ascends to the lung. Hence, it enables the ears to hear the sounds.

(6)–(8) *Zhang Shixian*: The lung belongs to the Western regions and to [the phase] metal. Metal comes to life during [the time of the year associated with the branch] *si*. The Southern regions [are associated with the branches] *si* 巳, *wu* 午 and *wei* 未. During [the time of the year associated with the branch] *si*, the fire happens to occupy the position where it "takes over an official rank." Among the long-term depots, the fire is [associated with] the heart. The heart controls the odors. The nose belongs to the lung, but the metal of the lung comes to life when the fire of the heart occupies the [dominating] position. Hence, [the fire] lets the nose know [how to distinguish] aroma and stench. The kidneys belong[8] to the Northern regions and to [the phase] water. Water comes to life during [the time of the year associated with the branch] *shen*. The Western regions [are associated with the branches] *shen* 申, *you* 酉, and *xu* 戌. During [the time of the year associated with the branch] *shen*, the metal happens to occupy a position where it "takes over an official rank." Among the long-term depots, the metal is [associated with] the lung. The lung controls the sounds. The ears belong to the kidneys, but the water of the kidneys comes to life when the metal of the lung occupies a [dominating] position. Hence, [the metal] lets the ears be able to hear the sounds.

Ding Jin: This [difficult issue] explains the meaning of the "coming to life" of the Five Phases. The [term *sheng* ("life") in the phrase *zhang sheng* 長生 ("coming to life")] is different from the [term] *sheng* in [the phrase] *sheng ke* 生剋 ("[mutual] generation and destruction [of the Five Phases]"). For instance, when [the text states] *Jin sheng yu si* 金生於巳 that means *jin zhang sheng zai si* 金長生在巳 ("metal comes to life during [the period of the year associated with the branch] *si*"). And when [the text states] *shui sheng yu shen* 水生於申 that means *shui zhang sheng zai shen* 水長生在申("water comes to life during [the period of the year associated with the branch] *shen*").

Katō Bankei: This [difficult issue] takes up the text of the treatise "Mai du" 脈度 that was quoted in the preceding difficult issue, [in which] it was pointed out that the qi of the long-term depots pass through [specific] orifices and [in which] a question [provoking an explanation] was asked. When it was said [in the answer] that the orifices kept open by the [qi of the liver] are the eyes and, further, that the liver is responsible for the five colors, these [two statements] corresponded to each other. [Similarly, when it was said that] the orifice kept

---

8   The text has *zhu* 主 ("to rule").

open by the [qi of the] spleen is the mouth and, further, that the spleen is responsible for the flavors, [the former statement] followed from the latter. Only the kidneys, the heart, and the lung are responsible for something that does not correspond to the orifices kept open by their [qi]. Hence, the present difficult issue was raised. In general, the way of the Five Phases is differentiated as to [whether it proceeds in accordance with the sequences of mutual] generation or destruction. But in addition there is also the principle of "fetal transformation" (*tai hua* 胎化). The present treatise is a discourse on the changes associated with fetal transformation. What does that mean? When the nose knows [how to distinguish] the odors, that is [evidence of a relationship among the Five Phases of] mutual destruction.[9] When the ears hear the sounds, that is [evidence of a relationship among the Five Phases of] mutual generation.[10] Hence one knows that the usual order of the Five Phases cannot be implied here. Now, metal has its fetal stage in the East, [which is associated with] wood; it is transformed in the South, [which is associated with] fire. Its qi flourish in the West. From the [period of the year associated with the branch] *mao* 卯 to [the period associated with] *you* 酉 the metal retains its qi. Water has its fetal stage in the South, which is yang. It is transformed in the West, [which is associated with] metal. Its qi flourish in the North. From [the period associated with] *wu* 午 to the [period associated with] *zi* 子 the water retains its qi. The same applies to the fetal [stage and subsequent] transformation of fire and wood. The intention of Yueren here is to let the student know that, in addition to the [principle of mutual] generation and destruction [of the Five Phases], the human body contains the principle of fetal [stage and subsequent] transformation [of each of the Five Phases]. The same is implied in the statement in the [*Su wen* treatise] "Liu yuan zheng ji da lun" 六元正紀大論. "The qi of spring move to the West; the qi of summer move to the South; the qi of autumn move to the East; the qi of winter move to the North." The [chapter] "Tian men xun" 天門訓[11] of the *Huai nan zi* 淮南子 states: "Metal comes to life during *si* 巳; it is vigorous during *you* 酉; it dies during *chou* 丑. These three periods are all metal. Water comes to life during *shen* 申; it is vigorous during *zi* 子; it dies during *chen* 辰. These three periods are all water." That corresponds to the meaning of the present treatise.

---

9   The nose is associated with the phase of metal; the odors are controlled by the heart, which is associated with fire. Fire destroys metal.

10 The ears are associated with the phase of water; the sounds are controlled by the lung, which is associated with metal. Metal generates water.

11 This should be "Tian wen xun" 天聞訊.

四十一難曰：（一）肝獨有兩葉，以何應也？

（二）然：肝者，東方木也。木者，春也。（三）萬物始生，其尚幼小，（四）意無所親，（五）去太陰尚近，（六）離太陽不遠，（七）猶有兩心，（八）故有兩葉，亦應木葉也。

The forty-first difficult issue: (1) Only the liver has two lobes. What does that correspond to?

(2) It is like this. The liver is [associated with the] East and [with the phase of] wood. Wood [corresponds to] spring. (3) [During the time of spring] all things begin to come to life; they are still young and small. (4) In their sentiments they are not [yet] close to anything. (5) [The period of spring] moves away from the major yin [of winter] and is still near to it. (6) It is separated from the major yang [of summer] but is not far away from it. (7) It appears to have two hearts. (8) Hence, [the liver] has two lobes. This is also in correspondence to the leaves of the woods.

_{COMMENTARIES}

(2) *Yu Shu*: Among the five regular [categories of correspondence], wood reflects spring; it corresponds to benevolence. Hence [the text] states: "Wood [corresponds to] spring." That is [the season] when human benevolence is put into practice.

Li Jiong: The liver belongs to the East, to [the constellation] *jia yi* 甲乙, [of the Celestial Stems], and to wood. Spring is the time when wood comes to life.

Ding Deyong: The [*Nan*] *jing* says: "The liver is [associated with the] East and [with the phase of] wood; it corresponds to spring, [which is the season] when all things come to life and are still young and small." That is as follows. What comes to life has not yet had a long life. That is to say, when the wood receives its first qi, that [condition] is called "young and small."

(3) *Yu Shu*: The liver [corresponds to the phase of] wood [and is associated with] the foot ceasing yin [conduit]; it is matched with the gall bladder [which also corresponds to the phase of] wood [and is associated with] the foot minor yang [conduit]. The arrival of a minor yang [movement in the vessels] is at times strong and at times weak, at times short and at times extensive. Hence, [the text] calls it "young and small."

Li Jiong: When the roots and the buds begin to shoot forth, they are still young and small and have not yet penetrated [their protective covers entirely].

(4) *Ding Deyong*: "In their sentiments they are not close to anything" means that one has lost his father and does not know his mother. Hence, [the text] states: "In their sentiments they are not close to anything."

Yu Shu: The wood corresponds to spring and reflects benevolence; [spring is the period when one] bestows favors without asking for recompensation. [It is the period when] transforming and sustaining [qi] are applied [even] to those who are not close. Hence, [the text] states: "In their sentiments they are not close to anything."

Li Jiong: All things, when they come to life, move forward and stand up by themselves. They have nothing [any longer] to be close to.

(5) *Ding Deyong*: "Moves away from the major yin and is still near to it." The major yin [month] is the seventh month. [That is the time when] the wood receives its first qi.[12]

Yu Shu: The twelve conduits pour [their contents] into each other. [The contents of] the foot ceasing yin [conduit] return and flow back into the hand major yin [conduit]. Hence, [the text] states: "Moves towards the major yin and is close to it."[13]

(6) *Ding Deyong*: "Separated from the major yang but not far away from it." The major yang [month] is the sixth month. Hence, [the text] states: "It is separated from the major yang but is not far away from it."

Yu Shu: The [*Nan*] *jing* itself states: "The foot ceasing yin and the [foot] minor yang [conduits] are [associated with the phase of] wood; it generates the [phase of] fire, [which is associated with the] hand major yang and the [hand] minor yin [conduits]."[14] Hence [the text here] states: "It is separated from the major yang but is not far away from it." That is the meaning implied here.

(4)–(6) *Xu Dachun*: In the [treatise] "Jin kui zhen yan lun" 金匱眞言論 of the *Su* [*wen*] it is stated: "The yang in the yang is the heart; the yin in the yin are the kidneys. The yang in the yin is the liver." The kidneys [are associated with the] water [and with the] major yin; they constitute the mother [depot] of the liver. The heart [is associated with] fire [and with the] major yang; it constitutes the child [depot] of the liver. The liver is the yang in the yin; it is located above the kidneys and below the heart. Hence, [the text] states: "is still near to it" and "is not

---

12　See difficult issue 40, note 1. "Receives its first qi" corresponds to "conception" – that is, to the first stage in the life cycle of the phases.

13　*Qu* 去 is read here by most commentators as "to move away"; Yu Shu, possibly following Ding Deyong (see his commentary on sentence 7), interpreted it in the opposite sense – namely, as "moving toward."

14　See difficult issue 18, sentence 3.

far away from it." "Not close to anything" means that [the liver] belongs to neither [the heart nor to the kidneys] in particular.

(6) *Liao Ping*: The matching of the five long-term depots with the Five Phases represents an application of the inductive doctrines of the Five Phases school [of philosophy] by a Chinese person. For instance, in the *Wu xing da yi* 五行大義 all the facts and beings below heaven are matched with the Five Phases. That is the doctrine of the matching [of all phenomena with] the Five Phases. Hence the ancient texts on the matching of the five long-term depots differ from current texts. The Five Phases school [of philosophy] originally referred with the Five Phases to the people of the five cardinal directions. Forced interpretations, as applied here, are a great mistake.

(7) *Ding Deyong*: "It appears to have two hearts" means it moves toward the major yin and hankers after the major yang. Because of this "moving toward" and "hankering after," [the text] speaks of "two hearts." Hence, the liver has two lobes corresponding to the leaves of the woods.

Yu Shu: *You* 猶 stands for *ru* 如 ("as if"). "As if it had two hearts" means [the following]. When [the qi of the liver] flow into the major yin [conduit, the liver] has a heart that fears the metal.[15] When it gives life to the major yang [conduit], it has a heart that produces fire. Hence, [the text] states: "It appears to have two hearts."

Xu Dachun: "Two hearts" – that is, one follows the yang and one follows the yin.

(8) *Yang*: If one speaks of the liver in terms of large lobes, then it consists of two lobes. If one speaks of it in terms of small lobes, then it has many lobes. This will be explained in a later chapter.

Xu Dachun: All woods have two leaves when their buds break open. This, then, is the original body [structure] of wood. Hence, the [wood] and the liver correspond to each other.

Liao Ping: Not even the demons could come up with such talk!

(1)–(8) *Hua Shou*: Mr. Chen from Siming states: "The mutual generation of the body's five long-term depots is [based on] the mother-child principle. Hence, the kidneys are the mother of the liver; they belong to the [subcategory] major yin within the [main category] yin. The heart is the child of the liver; it belongs to the major yang within the yang. The position of the liver is close to the kidneys and it is not far removed from the heart." I myself venture to say that the liver has two lobes; it corresponds to the Eastern regions and to wood. Wood is spring. [Spring is the season when] all things come to life, when herbs and woods begin to spring open. This is where Yueren happened to visualize the meaning of the two lobes. Hence,

---

15 The concept "heart" corresponds here to the Western concept of the heart as the seat of love and fear.

he set up this discussion. It must not necessarily be as he stated it, but it could be like that. When he spoke of "major yin" and "major yang," he did not necessarily refer to the qi in the body's long-term depots, but may have referred to the seasons of the year. The peak of winter is the apex of yin; the begin of summer marks the flourishing of yang. To call these [seasons] "major yin" and "major yang" is quite possible. Whenever one reads a book one must be flexible; one should not always strictly adhere [to the written word]. In a later paragraph it is stated that the liver has three lobes on the left and four lobes on the right. Here [the text] speaks of "two lobes." That is but a general remark on [its two] main [sections].

Zhang Shixian: The water is the father of wood; the soil is the mother of wood.[16] [Wood] comes to life in spring. In spring the roots and the buds start shooting forth; their appearance is still young and small and has not yet become large. When [things] come to life and stand up by themselves, their sentiments have nothing else to which they are close. Water and soil support the generation [of wood] and are, therefore, close to it. But only these two [are close to it] and nothing else. To come here from somewhere else, is called *li* 離 ("to separate oneself from"); to proceed from here to somewhere else is called *qu* 去 ("to move away"). "Major yin" refers to the spleen, [which is associated with] soil; "major yang" refers to the urinary bladder, [which is associated with] water. The position of the liver is on the right, below the spleen and above the urinary bladder. The spleen is very near to the liver. Hence, [the text] says: "It is still near to it." Water and soil occupy different locations, thus "it appears to have two hearts." Because of its two hearts it has two lobes. That, too, corresponds to the life of wood. The liver has a total of seven lobes. Here [the text] speaks of two lobes. That is because the three lobes on the left constitute one lobe and the four lobes on the right constitute one lobe.

Ding Jin: This [paragraph] elucidates the emotions between the five long-term depots and the Five Phases, and it takes the liver as an example. The liver is located to the left of the spleen, [which is categorized as] major yin [and which is associated with] wood. Hence [the text] states: "Still near." It is located above the urinary bladder, [which is categorized as] major yang [and which is associated with] water. Hence [the text] states: "Not far away." Wood without soil is worthless; without water it cannot live. [The wood] is tied emotionally to water and soil because nature has it that it depends on them in its transformation. Hence [the text] states: "It appears to have two hearts." "Two lobes" means that the liver basically consists of two lobes.

---

16 While the mutual generation order of the Five Phases defines the soil as the child of wood (possibly because the burning or rotting of wood produces "soil"), a more immediate environmental symbolism is quoted here to demonstrate the opposite – namely, that the soil can be regarded as the mother of wood.

四十二難曰：（一）人腸胃長短，受水穀多少，各幾何？

（二）然：胃大一尺五寸，徑五寸，長二尺六寸，橫屈受水穀三斗五升，其中常留穀二斗，水一斗五升。（三）小腸大二寸半，徑八分分之少半，長三丈二尺，受穀二斗四升，水六升合合之太半。（四）迴腸大四寸，徑一寸半，長二丈一尺，受穀一斗，水七升半。（五）廣腸大八寸，徑二寸半，長二尺八寸，受穀九升三合八分合之一。（六）故腸胃凡長五丈八尺四寸，合受水穀八斗七升六合八分合之一，此腸胃長短，受水穀之數也。

（七）肝重四斤四兩，左三葉，右四葉，凡七葉，（八）主藏魂。（九）心重十二兩，中有七孔三毛，盛精汁三合，主藏神。（十）脾重二斤三兩，扁廣三寸，長五寸，有散膏半斤，主裹血，溫五藏，主藏意。（十一）肺重三兩三兩，六葉兩耳，凡八葉，（十二）主藏魂。（十三）腎有兩枚，重一斤一兩，主藏志。（十四）膽在肝之短葉間，重三兩三銖，盛精汁三合。（十五）胃重二斤二兩，紆曲屈伸，長二尺六寸，大一尺五寸，徑五寸，盛穀二斗，水一斗五升。（十六）小腸重二斤十四兩，長三丈二尺，廣二寸半，徑八分分之少半，左迴疊積十六曲，盛穀二斗四升，水六升三合合之太半。（十七）大腸重二斤十二兩，長二丈一尺，廣四寸，徑一寸，當齊右迴十六曲，盛穀一斗，水七升半。（十八）膀胱重九兩二銖，縱廣九寸，盛溺九升九合。

（十九）口廣二寸半，唇至齒長九分，齒以後至會厭，深三寸半，大容五合。（二十）舌重十兩，長七寸，廣二寸半。（二十一）咽門重十兩，廣二寸半，至胃長一尺六寸。（二十二）喉嚨重十二兩，廣二寸，長一尺二寸，九節。（二十三）肛門重十二兩，大八寸，徑二寸大半，長二尺八寸，受穀九升二合八分合之一。

The forty-second difficult issue: (1) What are the dimensions of each of the intestines and of the stomach, and what are the respective amounts of water and grains they can hold?

(2) It is like this. The size[1] of the stomach is one foot and five inches. Its diameter is five inches. Its length is two feet and six inches. It is coiled transversally and holds three pecks and five pints of water and grains. Of these, [the stomach] normally contains two pecks of grains and one peck and five pints of water. (3) The size of the small intestine is two and one half inches. Its diameter is eight and one third *fen*.[2] Its length is three *zhang* and two feet. It holds two pecks and four pints of grains,

---

1   *Da* 大 ("size") refers to the circumference of the stomach and, later, of the intestines. Similarly, sentence 10 speaks of *Bian guang* 扁廣 ("flat width"), which may refer to the width that is measured if one cuts the stomach or the intestines open and spreads them flat on a board. The term *bian* refers to a flat board.

2   The Chinese expressions *xiao ban* 小半 and *da ban* 大半 are rendered here as "one third" and "two thirds," respectively, following Yang's commentary on this sentence.

and six pints and three and two thirds *ge* of water. (4) The size of the returning intestine is four inches. Its diameter is one and a half inches. Its length is two *zhang* and
one foot. It holds one peck of grains, and seven and one half pints of water.(5) The
size of the wide intestine is eight inches. Its diameter is two and a half inches; its
length is two feet and eight inches. It holds nine pints and three and one eighth *ge*
of grains. (6) Hence the length of the intestines and of the stomach adds up to five
zhang, eight feet and four inches. Together they hold eight pecks, seven pints and
six and one eighth *ge* of water and grains. These are the figures of the dimensions
of the intestines and of the stomach, and of the amounts of water and grains they
hold. (7) The liver weighs two catties and four ounces. It has three lobes on its left
and four lobes on its right side, adding up to seven lobes.(8) [The liver] is responsible for harboring the *hun*. (9) The heart weighs twelve ounces. It has seven holes
and three hairs.[3] It is supplemented with three *ge* of essence sap. It is responsible for
harboring of the spirit. (10) The spleen weighs two catties and three ounces. Its flat
width is three inches. Its length is five inches. It has a half catty of dispersed fat. It
controls the containment of the blood and supplies the five long-term depots with
warmth. It is responsible for the harboring of the sentiments. (11) The lung weighs
three catties and three ounces. It has six lobes and two ears, adding up to eight lobes.
(12) It is responsible for harboring the *po*. (13) The kidneys consist of two [separate]
entities; they weigh one catty and one ounce. They are responsible for harboring the
mind. (14) The gall bladder is located between the short lobes of the liver. It weighs
three ounces and three *zhu*. It is filled with three *ge* of essential sap. (15) The stomach
weighs two catties and two ounces. Its shape is twisted. It bends and stretches. Its
length is two feet and six inches. Its size is one foot and five inches. Its diameter is
five inches. It is filled with two pecks of grains and with one peck and five pints of
water. (16) The small intestine weighs two catties and fourteen ounces. Its length is
three *zhang* and two feet. Its width is two and a half inches. Its diameter is eight and
one third *fen*. It lies folded, turning to the left, with sixteen bends. It is filled with
two pecks and four pints of grains, and with six pints and three and two thirds *ge* of
water. (17) The large intestine weighs two catties and twelve ounces. Its length is two
zhang and one foot. Its width is four inches. Its diameter is one inch. It is located
exactly at the navel, turning to the right with sixteen bends. It is filled with one peck
of grains and seven and a half pints of water. (18) The urinary bladder weighs nine
ounces and two *zhu*. Its longitudinal width is nine inches. It is filled with nine pints
and nine *ge* of urine. (19) The mouth is two and a half inches wide. The distance from
the lips to the teeth is nine *fen*. The depth from the teeth backward to the epiglottis
is three and a half inches. [The oral cavity] holds, at most, five *ge*. (20) The tongue

---

3   The origin and meaning of this concept of hairs on the heart are unknown.

weighs ten ounces; its length is seven inches. Its width is two and a half inches. (21) The throat-gate weighs twelve ounces. Its width is two and a half inches. It extends to the stomach over one foot and six inches. (22) The windpipe weighs twelve ounces; its width is two inches. Its length is one foot two inches. It has nine sections. (23) The rectum weighs twelve ounces. Its size is eight inches. Its diameter is two and two thirds inches. Its length is two feet and eight inches. It holds nine pints and two and one eighth *ge* of grains.⁴

COMMENTARIES

(2) *Yang*: All the food man consumes enters through the mouth and is collected in the stomach. Hence the [*Nei*] *jing* states: "The stomach is the sea of water and grains." Once the grains have been processed in the stomach, they are transferred into the small intestine.

　　Zhang Shixian: *Wei* 胃 ("stomach") stands for *hui* 會 ("to meet"). *Wei* means that all the items from the market meet here.

(3) *Yang*: The small intestine receives the grains from the stomach and transmits them further into the large intestine. When the grains are divided into three parts, two parts constitute the larger half, one part constitutes the smaller half.

(4) *Yang*: The "returning intestine" is the large intestine. It receives the grains from the small intestine and transmits them into the wide intestine.

　　Yu Shu: The amount of water and grains [held by] the stomach is three pecks and five pints. From [the stomach, water and grains] are transmitted into the small intestine, which [is capable of holding] an additional [amount of] four pints of grains, while the [capacity for holding] water is decreased by eight pints and six

---

4　The text of this difficult issue may be partially corrupt. It corresponds largely to the two *Ling shu* treatises, "Chang wei" 腸胃 and "Ping ren jue gu" 平人絕穀, which are, however, structured much more systematically than the present text. The account given here of the weight, capacity, and sizes of all the organs passed by food on its way through the body – from the lips to the rectum – is difficult to define with respect to its age. It could be knowledge accumulated in centuries BCE and adopted by the *Nan jing* from the *Nei jing*. Until the appearance of better evidence, however, we cannot discard the possibility that these measurements were introduced into Chinese medicine by the *Nan jing* itself – possibly as a result of the interest in anatomy, which is documented from the time of Wang Mang 王莽 in the first century CE – whence they found their way into the *Tai su* and *Ling shu* editions of the *Nei jing*. Although only a handful of dissections are recorded in Chinese historical sources prior to the nineteenth century, an interest in the concrete structure of the organism – and discussions on many related topics – had long preceded the arrival of Western medicine. For reasons not yet understood, the questions raised in this regard were approached almost exclusively by means of speculation and logic (rather than by concrete examination of the body itself) until Wang Qingren 王清任 (1768-1831), the author of the *Yi lin gai cuo* 醫林改錯, propagated the maxim that an understanding of functions is impossible without a knowledge of tangible structures.

and one third *ge*. [Water and grains] are then transmitted further into the large intestine. If one compares the amount of water and grains [held by the large intestine] with that [held by] the stomach, it has decreased by one half for both [water and grains]. When they have reached the [large intestine], the aqueous portion enters into the urinary bladder while the grains are transmitted to the rectum gate:

Hua Shou: "Returning intestine" is a designation encompassing the large intestine, the wide intestine, and the rectum.

Zhang Shixian: The "returning intestine" is the large intestine.

(5) *Yang*: The "wide intestine" is the "greasy intestine" (*zhi chang* 膱腸). Another name is "rectum gate"(*gang men* 肛門). It receives the grains from the large intestine and transmits them toward outside [of the body].

Katō Bankei: The *Ling shu* has "two thirds of one *ge*."

Nan jing 1962: The "wide intestine" is the final end of the large intestine.

(6) *Yang*: According to the *Jia yi jing* 甲乙經, the total length of the intestines, including the stomach, is six *zhang*, four inches and four *fen*. That [figure] differs from the one given here because the *Jia yi jing* calculates it from the mouth to the rectum. Hence [the distance] is long. The [*Nan*] *jing* calculates it from the stomach to the intestines. Hence [the distance] is short. Both [figures] explain each other; no error is involved here.

Xu Dachun: The total amount of water and grains held [by the short-term repositories] listed above is given in the treatise "Ping ren jue gu" 平人絕穀 of the *Ling shu* as nine pecks, two pints, and one and two thirds *ge*. That is the correct amount. But it differs from the amount given in the text above. [I] do not know the reason. Maybe it is an error in writing.

Qian Xizuo: This figure is wrong. According to the preceding text it should be nine pecks, two pints and one *ge*.

(1)–(6) *Katō Bankei*: The amounts of water and grains held by each short-term repository are identical with those given in the *Ling shu*, but the present treatise sums them up as eight pecks, seven pints, and six and one eighth *ge*, which is four pints and five *ge* less [than the sum given in the *Ling shu*]. Personally, I suspect that the "two pecks four pints" of the small intestine should be one peck nine pints. How is that? The stomach processes the water and the grains. It transforms them and generates the dregs. These are then diminished, further transmitted, and moved here and there – why should they increase [on their way to the small intestine]? It was probably such that Bian Que saw the amount of grains stored by the small intestine as written down in the *Ling shu*. He compared this [amount] with the amount given for the stomach and [realized that the contents of the small intestine surpassed those of the stomach by] four pints. Hence he must have changed [the amount held by the small intestine] in such a way that he arrived at the sum total [of eight pecks, seven pints and six and one eighth *ge* for all the short-term repositories]. Later on, [Bian Que's] correction disappeared; later people [who edited the *Nan jing*] followed the text of the *Ling shu* and filled in [its figures]. For the time being, I write it down as is until someone knows better.

(7) *Yu Shu*: The liver [is associated with the] foot ceasing yin [conduit], which is matched with the foot minor yang [conduit].[5] The minor yang occupies rank seven.[6] Hence [the liver] has seven lobes.

   Qian Xizuo: All the other sources speak of two catties and four ounces. Only the *Shi ji zheng yi* 史記正義[7] speaks of four catties and four ounces, agreeing with [the data given] here.

(8) *Yu Shu*: The *hun* 魂 is an assistant to the spirit qi.

(9) *Li Jiong*: The heart of people with superior knowledge has seven holes – some say nine holes – and three hairs. The heart of people with mediocre knowledge has five holes and two hairs. The heart of people with inferior knowledge has three holes and one hair. The heart of the ordinary people has two holes and no hair. The heart of stupid people has one hole. The heart of extremely stupid people has one very small hole. Those people who act foolishly throughout their lives have a heart but no hole in it. Hence it has no gate through which the spirit could leave or enter. Nothing can be expected [from such a heart].

   Liao Ping: That is to say, the essential fluid stored by the heart is identical with [the amount stored by] the gall bladder. That is correct.

(10) *Liao Ping*: The three characters *zhu guo xue* 主裹血 ("it controls the containment of the blood") should be deleted.

(11) *Yu Shu*: The lung is the [depot] manifesting [the phase of] metal; it [represents] the qi of [trigram] *dui* 兌. During the [month associated with the branch] *you* 酉 [the metal] occupies the [ruling] position. The [month] *you* represents the eighth gate [in the life cycle of metal]. The eight lobes [of the lung] reflect that pattern.

---

5   The foot minor yang conduit is associated with the gall bladder, which is the short-term repository matched with the liver.

6   In general, seven is associated with heaven, with the South and with full yang, not with minor yang. In a personal communication, Dr. Yamada Keiji suggested regarding the character *ci* 次 ("rank") as a mistake for *su* 宿 ("to stop"). In this case, the sentence would read: "The minor yang [conduit] stops [in the liver] seven times. Hence [the liver] has seven lobes."

7   A Tang commentary on the *Shi ji* 史記, written by Zhang Shoujie 張守節.

(12) *Yu Shu*: The *po* 魄 is an assistant of the essence qi.

(13) *Zhang Shixian*: The kidneys consist of two lobes, situated opposite to each other in the waist. The one to the left of the navel is the kidney; the one to the right is the gate of life. The mind is the residence of one's sentiments.

 Xu Dachun: In a former paragraph, the right [kidney] was considered to be the gate of life. Here [the text] says: "The kidneys consist of two lobes." That is different from what was said earlier.

 Liao Ping: The gall bladder is attached [as a short-term repository] to the [long-term depot of the] liver; it is located opposite to the heart. Together with [the heart], it is [associated with] the minor yin [conduit]. It constitutes the real kidney.[8] It has no lower opening. It stores but does not drain. The outer kidney is also called gall bladder. Sometimes it fulfills draining functions, sometimes it does not. Thus, it differs from the [remaining] five short-term repositories, which have the special function of draining. Hence it is called the "short-term repository of clarity and purity."

(14) *Zhang Shixian*: The gall bladder is the short-term repository of clarity and purity; it does not accept anything dirty. It contains only three *ge* of essence sap.

 Liao Ping: The essence sap of the liver is stored in the gall bladder. [Both liver and gall bladder] control the blood. The two long-term depots [liver and gall] are tied to each other; they constitute one entity. In this they resemble heart and lung.

(17) *Katō Bankei*: The *Ling shu* has *zuo huan* 左環 ("winding to the left"). That is correct.

(19) *Li Jiong*: The epiglottis suppresses exhalation and inhalation whenever water and grains move down the throat.

(22) *Xu Dachun*: The windpipe is the place through which the sounds leave [the body].

(1)–(23) *Ding Deyong*: The measurements of the diameter [on the one side] and of the circumference of the intestines and of the stomach [on the other side] do not [in all cases] correspond to each other. When [the text] states: "The size of the stomach is one foot and five inches; its diameter is five inches," then the circumference is three times the diameter. The diameter of the small intestine is eight *fen*. Its correct size, then, should be two inches and four *fen*. Here [the text] speaks of [a circumference of] two and one half inches. That is [for the diameter a difference of] one third of a *fen*. The diameter of the returning intestine is one and one half inches. Its size, then, should be four inches five *fen*.

---

8 Liao Ping suggested exchanging the names for gall bladder and outer kidney. See his comments on difficult issues 35 and 36.

Here [the text] speaks of [a circumference of] four inches. That is five *fen* too small. The wide intestine has a diameter of two and one half inches. Its size, then, should be seven inches five *fen*. Here [the text] speaks of [a circumference of] eight inches. That is five *fen* too many. [If one works with] pecks, pints, inches and feet, one must first establish [the standard length of] a foot with respect to [the specific person to be measured]. Only then [can] one construct the respective pints, pecks, and weights. They all must be defined on the basis of the respective person's individually standardized inch. With the foot [defined], one constructs a peck. A peck is one foot wide at its face and seven inches wide at its bottom; its height is four inches and [the walls are] all three *fen* thick. It can hold ten pints. A piece of wood the size of one finger weighs one *liang* if its length is exactly one inch. Sixteen *liang* constitute one catty. This is how to construct inch, foot, pint, and peck, all standardized according to the individual body, as measurements reflecting the patterns of weight and extension of man's intestines and stomach.

Hua Shou: The entire contents of this paragraph can [also] be found in paragraphs 31 and 32 of the *Ling shu*. Yueren has brought them together into one paragraph. He has added a section on the weight, the capacity, and the contents of the five long-term depots. I believe that the repetitions in [what is said] earlier and later [in this paragraph] are of no harm – they are [like] repeated injunctions. But the figures given on the receptive capacity [of the individual short-term repositories given here in the *Nan jing* and given in the *Ling shu*] do not all agree with each other. Because they do not touch the general meaning, I have kept them [as is] for the time being until someone who knows better [can correct them].

Xu Dachun: The paragraphs "Chang wei" 腸胃 and "Ping ren jue gu" 平人絕穀 of the *Ling* [*shu*] discuss the size and the extension of the intestines and of the stomach in the same terms as the text here. But as far as the weight of the long-term depots and short-term repositories is concerned, the "Chang wei" paragraph of the *Ling* [*shu*] has only [the data] that the tongue weighs ten *liang* and that the throat gate weighs ten *liang*. [I] do not know the source for all the other [data]. Also, the text of the [*Ling shu*] *jing* does not contain any [information] on the amounts of essence sap contained in the long-term depots and short-term repositories. [I] do not know whether there was another [source] that could have provided [these data]. It may well be that two scriptures existed originally, of which only fragments are extant.

Katō Bankei: This [difficult issue] corresponds to the text of the *Ling shu* treatise "Jue gu" 絕穀. Its major message is that the three pecks and five pints of water and grains held by the stomach, if consumed by a person on a normal day as his amount of food, are sufficient to nourish the long-term depots and short-term repositories. If [one consumes] more or less, that will not only be harmful to the harmonious balance of his qi but can also lead to disease. The large and the small intestines as well as the wide intestine all receive unclean refuse. Their function is to transmit and quickly excrete. This treatise has been compiled as the basis for [the argument of the following difficult issue – namely,] that one must die if his [consumption of] grains is interrupted for seven days. The 109 characters from "the liver weighs ..." on cannot be found in the *Ling shu*. [Although] they appear in this treatise, I suspect they are not the words of Bian Que. Why do I say so? In the preceding [difficult issue], it was said that the liver has two lobes. Here [the text] speaks of seven lobes. According to the *Ling shu*, the large and the small intestines wind in left turns; here [the text] says: "The large intestine turns to the right." Furthermore, the amounts given for the intestines and the stomach in this treatise are repeated in its earlier and later sections. The 99 characters from "The mouth is ... wide" on are quoted from the treatise "Chang wei" [of the *Ling shu*] to follow [the data provided on] the urinary bladder. That is a gross misinterpretation of the meaning implied in the *Ling shu*. Hence I have developed some doubts. However, throughout the ages, famous physicians, in discussing the appearance of the long-term depots, have relied on [the data offered] here. Also, the origin [of these data] is already quite old. Hence for the time being I write [the text of this difficult issue as is] until someone knows better.

四十三難曰：（一）人不食飲，七日而死者，何也？

（二）然：人胃中常有留穀二斗，水一斗五升。故平人日再至圊，一行二升半，日中五升，七日五七三斗五升，而水穀盡矣。故平人不食飲七日而死者，水穀津液俱盡，即死矣。

The forty-third difficult issue: (1) When someone does not eat or drink, that person will die after seven days. Why is that so?

(2) It is like this. In the stomach and in the intestines there usually remain 2 pecks of grain and 1 peck, 5 pints of water. The fact is: A healthy person has two discharges per day; each discharge amounts to 2 ½ pecks. These are 5 pecks per day. Within seven days these are 5 times 7, amounting to 3 pints 5 pecks, and all those waters and grains present will be used up. The fact is: When a health person fails to eat and drink for seven days and dies, it is because all his water and grain, essence and qi, *jin* and *ye* liquids are all used up.

<small>COMMENTARIES</small>

(1)–(2) *Ding Deyong*: The qi that man receives from the grains nourish his spirit. When water and grains are exhausted, his spirit departs. Hence, enough grains maintain one's life; an interruption of [the supply of] grains leads to death.

Yang: *Qing* 圊 stands for *ce* 廁 ("privy").

Li Jiong: Man has no root or trunk; food and beverages provide his existence. The stomach is the sea of water and grains; it serves as the receptacle for water and grains. Under regular circumstances it contains two pecks and five pints.

Hua Shou: This paragraph corresponds largely to the thirtieth treatise of the *Ling shu*. When, in a normal person, the stomach is filled, the intestines are empty. When the intestines are filled, the stomach is empty. Because of these alternating states of being filled and being empty, the qi can move up and down, the [functions of the] body's five long-term depots are arranged perfectly, the blood vessels are passable, and the essence spirit is settled down. Hence the essence qi of water and grains constitute the spirit. [The fact] that a normal person dies if he does not eat or drink for seven days results from a complete exhaustion of water, grains, and internal liquids. Hence the saying: "When the water departs, the camp [qi] will disperse; when the grains diminish, the guard [qi] will vanish. With the camp [qi] dispersed and with the guard [qi] vanished, the spirit has nothing to lean on." That is [what is] meant here.

Zhang Shixian: "A normal person" is a person without disease. Man needs water and grains to support his internal liquids, his [guard] qi, and his blood.

When water and grains are exhausted, his internal liquids, his qi, and his blood will also become exhausted. Hence his existence will fade away. Mr. Ding has said: "The qi that man receives from the grains nourish his spirit. When water and grains are exhausted, his spirit departs." The [*Nei*] *jing* states: "If one gets enough grains, he will prosper; if the [supply of] grains is cut off, he will perish." [Zhang] Zhongjing 張仲景 says: "When water enters the conduits, blood will be generated. When grains enter the stomach, the vessel [transportation] paths will be passable." Hence one must nourish the blood and one must provide warmth to the guard [qi]. When they are provided with warmth, the guard and the camp [qi] will proceed [through the body] and the heavenly mandate [of life] will persist continuously.

Xu Dachun: This section [corresponds exactly] to the questions and answers in the treatise "Ping ren jue gu" 平人絕穀 of the *Ling shu;* not a single word has been changed. No explanation whatsoever is provided. Also, the text of the [*Nei*] *jing* has, in addition [to what is quoted here], a number of words discussing depletion and repletion in the intestines and in the stomach. Preceding this section they are highly meaningful. Here they have been left out; that is a sign of great ignorance.

Katō Bankei: [The statement] that one will die if [his consumption of] grains is interrupted for seven days is based on two visits to the latrine per day, with two and a half pints passed each time. Hence, [seven days] are set as limit. However, human hearts are as [different as are human] faces. Similarly, the transmission and transformation [of food] in the intestines and in the stomach differ [from person to person]. Thus, when people go to the latrine, some may do so once a day, others twice or three times. Or in two days, some may go once, others may go twice or three times. No fixed standards can be determined here. Hence [the text] makes the general statement: "Death has come because water, grains, and internal liquids have been exhausted completely." Thus, one should not just pay attention to one sentence only of this difficult issue. When [the text] speaks of "seven days," this is also based on two visits to the latrine per day. There is no reason to adhere to this number of days too closely. The reader must think it all over. The wording here is slightly different from that of the *Ling shu* treatise "[Ping ren] jue gu," 平人絕穀 but the meaning is entirely the same.

Liao Ping: Why would [the authors of the *Nan jing*] waste their writing materials on issues such as the present one? Because they wished to come up with eighty-one treatises. Even under hard bargaining, more than half [of the eighty-one treatises of the *Nan jing*] are of this character.

四十四難曰：（一）七衝門何在？

（二）然：唇為飛門，（三）齒為戶門，（四）會厭為吸門，（五）胃為賁
門，（六）太倉下口為幽門，（七）太腸小腸會為闌門，（八）下極為魄
門，（九）故曰七衝門也。

The forty-fourth difficult issue: (1) The seven through-gates, where are they located?

(2) It is like this. The lips constitute the flying gate. (3) The teeth constitute the door gate. (4) The epiglottis constitutes the inhalation gate. (5) The stomach constitutes the strong gate. (6) The lower opening of the great granary constitutes the dark gate. (7) Where the large and small intestines meet is the screen gate. (8) The lower end is the *po* gate. (9) Hence one speaks of seven through-gates.

COMMENTARIES

(1)–(9) *Ding Deyong*: The [*Nan*] *jing* states: "The lips constitute the flying gate"; it does so in order to illustrate the meaning of movement. [It states] "the teeth constitute the door gate" because [the teeth] represent the bolt with which one opens and closes [a door]. The five kinds of grain enter here to become crushed, and then leave again. "The epiglottis constitutes the inhalation gate" because it suppresses exhalation and inhalation whenever the throat moves water and grains down. "The stomach constitutes the strong gate" because the stomach is also called a "hero of tiger-like strength" in order to convey the image of enclosure and penetration. Hence it is called "strong gate." Furthermore, *wei* 胃 ("stomach") stands for *wei* 圍 ("enclosure"). It controls the storage of grains. Hence it is also called "great granary." The lower opening of the great granary is the opening [leading into the] intestines. [The *Nan jing* states further:] "Where the large and small intestines meet is the screen gate." *Hui* 會 ("to meet") stands for *he* 合 ("to join"). The place where the large and the small intestines join is [the location] where water and grains are separated [to be transformed into] essence and blood; each has its destination to move toward. Hence [the *Nan jing*] speaks of a "screen gate." [Finally, the text states:] "The lower end is the *po* gate." The large intestine is the short-term repository of the lung. It stores the *po*. The lower [section] of the large intestine is called "rectum gate"; another name is "*po* gate."

Yang: Man has seven orifices. These are the gates of the five long-term depots. They all leave through the face. The seven through-gates referred to here are also exits of the long-term depots and short-term repositories. They appear both internally and externally. The flying gate is the exit of the qi of the spleen. The spleen controls the lips as its flying gate. *Fei* 飛 ("to fly") stands for *dong* 動 ("to move"). That is to say, the lips receive the water and the grains. They move and transmit them into the interior [of the body. The statement] "the teeth constitute the door gate" [implies the following]: Mouth and teeth are the exit of the qi of the heart. In the heart [these qi] constitute the mind; when they leave through the mouth they constitute one's language. Hence the teeth constitute the door gate of the heart. The designation [door gate] refers also to their function of crushing the five grains and transmitting them into the mouth. [The statement] "the epiglottis constitutes the inhalation gate" [refers to the following]: The epiglottis is the gate of the sounds emitted by the five long-term depots. Hence [the text] states: "The epiglottis is the inhalation gate." [The statement] "the stomach constitutes the strong gate" [refers to the following]: *Ben* 賁 ("strong") stands for *ge* 膈 ("diaphragm"). [The strong gate] is the exit of the qi of the stomach. The stomach emits the qi of the grains and transmits them to the lung. The lung is located above the diaphragm. Hence the stomach is considered to be the strong gate. [The statement] "the lower opening of the great granary constitutes the dark gate" [refers to the following: The dark gate] is the exit of the qi of the kidneys. The "great granary" is the stomach. The lower opening of the stomach is located three inches above[1] the navel. That is a dark and hidden location. Hence it is called "dark gate." [The statement] "where the large and small intestines meet is the screen gate," [refers to the following]: "Screen gate" carries the meaning of *yi* 遺 ("to hand down") and *shi* 失 ("to lose"). That is to say, the [contents of the] large and small intestines are drained into the wide intestine. The wide intestine receives, transmits, and emits what [is sent to it]. That is the idea of "to hand down" and "to lose." Hence [the text] speaks of a "screen gate." [The statement] "the lower end is the *po* gate" [refers to the following]: The *po* gate is the rectum gate at the lowest end [of the body]. The qi of the lung move upward and pass through the windpipe; when they move downward they pass through the rectum gate, which is the exit of the qi of the lung. The lung stores the *po*. *Chong* 衝 ("through") stands for *tong* 通 ("to pass through") and for *chu* 出 ("to exit"). That is to say, these [gates] are locations through which the qi of the long-term depots and short-term repositories exit.

(1) *Hua Shou*: *Chong* 衝 stands for *chong yao* 衝要 ("important intersection").

Zhang Shixian: *Chong* 衝 stands for *tong* 通 ("to pass through"). These [gates] are important locations. Things enter the [body] from above and leave it from below; [the body] opens and closes at specific times. Hence one calls these [openings] "gates."

Liao Ping: If we examine [this book] closely, all the difficult issues that are not based directly on quotations from the text of the [*Nei*]*jing* commit hundreds of

---

1   Some editions have "below."

errors, trumping up false doctrines. They have absolutely no meaning. In general, this book has been compiled with the special intention of [introducing the doctrine of] the two inch [sections]. Whenever it deals with the diagnostic patterns reflected at the two inch [sections], one should pay attention. All the remaining strange talk was supposed to demonstrate [that the author of the *Nan jing*] was a learned and accomplished [scholar].

(2) *Zhang Shixian*: Fei 飛 ("flying") stands for *dong* 動 ("to move"). The movement of the lips resembles the flying of some being.

Ye Lin: Fei 飛 ("flying") was used in antiquity for *fei* 扉 ("door leaf"). *Fei* 扉 stands for *hu shan* 戶扇 ("door leaf"). [The term is used here] because the teeth constitute the door gate and the lips are the door leaves. Hence they are called *fei men* 飛門. In the treatise "You wei wu yan"² 憂恚無言 of the *Ling shu*, it is stated: "The lips are the door leaves (*shan* 扇) of the sounds." That is [what is] meant here.

(3) *Zhang Shixian*: A "door" is a gate with but one wing. Large items cannot enter [the body] directly; they must be crushed by the teeth. Only then can they enter.

(4) *Hua Shou*: Hui yan 會厭 ("epiglottis") refers to [the location] where the *yan* 咽 and the *yi* 嗌 throats join (*hui* 會) each other. *Yan* 厭 stands for *yan* 偃 ("to conceal"). That is to say, whenever some item is swallowed, [the epiglottis] covers the windpipe lest food is mistakenly sent into it, blocking the moving in and out of the breathing qi.

Zhang Shixian: The epiglottis is the place where the *yan* 咽 and the *yi* 嗌 throats join each other.³

(5) *Ye Lin*: The stomach can collect things like a granary. Hence it is called "great granary." *Ben* 賁 ("strong") is equivalent to *ben* 奔 ("hasty"). The *ben* gate is located at the upper opening of the stomach. That is to say, when things enter the stomach, they hastily move downward into the great granary.

(6) *Ye Lin*: The lower opening of the stomach is the place where [the stomach] is linked to the small intestine. It is called "dark gate" because that is a deep and hidden location. It is very far away from the upper and lower points of exit and entry [of the body].

(7) *Zhang Shixian*: Lan 闌 ("screen") stands for *zhe lan* 遮攔 ("to fence off"). Where the large and the small intestines meet, the clear is separated from the turbid. The dregs and the unclean [portions] enter the large intestine. The water and the clear liquids flow into the urinary bladder. Hence [the designation "screen gate"] draws on the meaning "to fence off" [of the word *lan*].

---

2 The text has "You huan 患 wu yan." That must be an error in writing.

3 *Yan* 咽 may refer here to the esophagus; *yi* 嗌 may refer here to the windpipe. Both terms are usually used interchangeably.

(8) *Xu Dachun*: When beverages and food reach here, their essence and splendor have already left them. All that remains is their material appearance. Hence when [the rectum gate] is called *po* gate, this is to express [the meaning of] *gui men* 鬼門 ("demons' gate"). Also, the lung harbors the *po*. The rectum is tied to the large intestine which, in turn, is associated with the lung as an outside [short-term repository] to an inside [long-term depot]. Hence [the rectum] is called "*po* gate."

Ye Lin: [The term] *po* 魄 was used in ancient times for *po* 粕 ("dregs"). In the treatise "Tian dao" 天道 of Zhuangzi it is said: "This is nothing but refuse and dregs of the people in antiquity" (*gu ren zhi zao po yi fu* 古人之糟粕已父). That is to say, when food and beverages have reached here, their essence and splendor have already left them. All that remains are the refuse and dregs of their material appearance.

(9) *Zhang Shixian*: These seven gates are the short-term repositories which are opened or closed [to control] – as important intersections – the passage of water and grains. Hence they are called the "seven through-gates."

(1)–(9) *Xu Dachun*: I do not know the source of this paragraph.

Katō Bankei: The strong, the dark, the screen, and the *po* gates, these four are mentioned in various treatises of the *Nei jing*. But they are not brought together [in a single discourse] there. The flying , the door, and the inhalation gates – these three cannot be found in the ancient texts and are named only in the present treatise for reasons we do not know. The so-called seven through[-gates] are gates through which the water and the grains are taken in and emitted. From the flying gate to the strong gate they control intake; from the dark gate to the *po* gate they control emission. If the four gates of the upper section of the path [of food through the body] lose their functions, choking, turned over stomach,[4] vomiting, and heartburn are all diseases resulting from the individual sections [that should be closed by said gates]. When the lower three gates discontinue their services, this results in diarrhea, constipation, loss or retention of urine, hemorrhoids, and wasting away.[5]

(9) *Liao Ping*: It would be correct to speak of "seven gates." The character *chong* 衝 ("through") is quite incomprehensible.

---

4   The term "turned over stomach" indicates that the stomach turns back the food without digesting it. The Chinese expression is written here with the character, *fan* 翻 ("to turn over"). Another character used more commonly is *fan* 反.

5   The term *tuo* 脫 conveys several meanings. It could refer, as in my rendering, to a wasting away as a result, for instance, of continuing diarrhea. It is also used to indicate a prolapse of the rectum. The term *tuo gang zhi* 脫肛痔 refers to hemorrhoids combined with a prolapse of the rectum.

THE FORTY-FIFTH DIFFICULT ISSUE

四十五難曰：（一）經言八會者，何也？

（二）然：府會大倉，（三）藏會季脅，（四）筋會陽陵泉，（五）髓會絕骨，（六）血會鬲俞，（七）骨會大抒，（八）脈太淵，（九）氣會三焦外一筋直兩乳內也。（十）熱病在內者，取其會之氣穴也。

The forty-fifth difficult issue: (1) The scripture speaks of eight gathering points; what are they?

(2) It is like this. The [qi of the] short-term repositories gather at the *tai cang* [hole]. (3) The [qi of the] long-term depots gather at the *ji xie* [hole]. (4) The [qi of the] muscles gather at the *yang ling quan* [hole]. (5) The [qi of the] bone marrow gather at the *jue gu* [hole]. (6) The [qi of the] blood gather at the *ge shu* [hole]. (7) The [qi of the] bones gather at the *da shu* [hole]. (8) The [qi of the] vessels gather at the *tai yuan* [hole]. (9) The qi gather in the Triple Burner, that is, in one muscle exactly between the two breasts at the outside [of the body].[1] (10) Whenever a disease resulting from heat is present inside [the body, one should] select [for treatment] the respective holes where the qi [of the affected entity] gather.[2]

---

1 My rendering here corresponds to the interpretation of this sentence by a number of commentators who read it as ... *san jiao, wai* .... Others, including Xu Dachun (see his comments below), have interpreted *san jiao wai* as "outside of the Triple Burner." Xu Dachun appears to have preferred such an interpretation since, as a conservative commentator who gave priority to the sayings of the *Nei jing*, he believed in a tangible quality of the Triple Burner (see also his comments on difficult issue 31, where he quotes the respective passage from the *Ling shu*). The *Nan jing* itself, in contrast, did not consider the Triple Burner to be a tangible entity; in difficult issue 38, it states: "It has a name but no form." Therefore, when the author(s) of the *Nan jing* wrote here that "the qi gather in the Triple Burner," they must have seen the need to add an explanation to the effect that this statement refers to a specific location on the surface of the body. One may of course ask why, in sentence 9, in contrast to the preceding sentences, no specific hole was named in the first place.

2 In this difficult issue, a new concept is introduced that has, apparently, no parallel in the *Nei jing*. The author presents the idea that each of the organism's functional systems (all the long-term depots are seen here as constituting one functional system, and so are the short-term repositories, the muscles, etc.) has one point where its qi accumulate and where, consequently, evil qi that have entered a particular system can be removed. The pattern of the "eight gathering-points" mentioned here constitutes one of two brief references by the *Nan jing* to possibilities of needling the trunk without resorting to a needling of the circulating qi in the conduits (the second reference appears in difficult issue 67). In general, however, the *Nan jing* stressed the needling of individual streams in the four limbs as an alternative to circuit-needling (see difficult issue 62 ff).

(1) *Zhang Shixian*: *Hui* 會 stands for *ju hui* 聚會 ("to gather together").

Xu Dachun: *Hui* 會 stands for *ju* 聚 ("to come together"). This refers to the eight holes where the qi gather together.

Liao Ping: This difficult issue is probably based on the one sentence [in the *Nei jing*] that the vessels meet at the *tai yuan* 太淵 [hole]. But it is unclear how the present sentence could be formulated. The following [sentences] are even less founded [in any *Nei jing* statement].

(2) *Ding Deyong*: "The [qi of the] short-term repositories gather at the *tai cang* ("great granary")" refers to the stomach. The hole [to be used for treatment] is the *zhong wan* 中脘 [hole].

Yu Shu: The *tai cang* [hole] is located in front of the heart, four inches below the *jiu wei* 鳩尾 [hole]. It is the gathering point of the foot yang brilliance vessel of the stomach, of the hand major yang vessel of the small intestine, of the hand minor yang vessel of the Triple Burner, and of the controller vessel. Its original name is *zhong wan* 中脘. Here it is called *tai cang*, It is the place where [the qi of] the stomach are accumulated. The stomach transforms [food and beverages into] qi and nourishes the six short-term repositories. Hence [the text] speaks of a "gathering point."

Hua Shou: Another name for *tai cang* is *zhong wan*. It is located four inches above the navel. The six short-term repositories receive their provisions from the stomach. Hence [the stomach] constitutes the gathering point of the short-term repositories.

Xu Dachun: The *tai cang* [hole] belongs to the controller vessel.

Liao Ping: The [term "gathering"] corresponds to the [term] "to gather" (*hui*) in the [expression] "to gather for an alliance" (*meng hui* 盟會) that was in use during the Spring-and-Autumn period. One speaks of a "gathering" only if two or more people are involved. Also, each of them should come his own way. For instance, one does not speak of a gathering in the case of two related [phenomena], such as male and female spirits, or camp and guard qi. Also, if no movement is involved, one also does not speak of a gathering. Hence, in the present context the meaning of the term "gather" is obscure.

(3) *Ding Deyong*: "The [qi of the] long-term depots gather at the *ji xie*. *Ji xie* is another name for the soft ribs. At their end is a hole called *zhang men* 章門. It is located on one level with the navel. This is the place where the [qi of the] spleen are accumulated. It is the gathering point of the foot ceasing yin and [foot] minor yang [conduits]. Hence [the text] states: "The [qi of the] long-term depots gather at the youngest ribs."

Yu Shu: This is the *zhang men* hole. It is the place where the [qi of the] spleen are accumulated. It is located exactly at the end of the youngest ribs, on one level with the navel. [To locate this hole, have the patient] lie on his side, [ask him] to pull up [his] upper leg and to extend [his] lower leg. Then you will find it next to his arm [as it is stretched down along his side]. It is the gathering point of the foot ceasing yin and [foot minor yang [conduits].

Hua Shou: The five long-term depots receive their provisions from the spleen. Hence [the spleen] constitutes the gathering point of the long-term depots.

Xu Dachun: The *ji xie* [hole] belongs to the foot ceasing yin [vessel].

(4) *Ding Deyong*: *Yang ling quan* is the name of a hole. It is located one inch below[3] the knee at the outer angle.

Yu Shu: The *yang ling quan* hole is located in the center of the bend below the knee. It is the place where the qi of the foot minor yang vessel [which is associated with] the gall bladder are emitted.

Hua Shou: The muscles [associated with the] foot minor yang [vessel] are tied to the outer angle of the knee. That is the *yang ling quan*. It is located in the bend at the outer angle one inch below the knee. Also, the gall and the liver constitute one pair. The liver is associated with the muscles. Hence [the *yang ling quan*] is the gathering point of the muscles.

Zhang Shixian: *Yang ling quan* is the name of a hole of the foot minor yang [conduit]. It is located one inch below the knee in the bend at the outer angle. It is the place where all the muscles come together. Also, the lung is responsible for the muscles. The minor yang [short-term repository] is the short-term repository of the liver. Hence all the muscles gather at the *yang ling quan*.

Xu Dachun: The *yang ling quan* [hole] belongs to the foot minor yang [vessel].

(5) *Ding Deyong*: "The [qi of the] bone marrow gather at the *jue gu*." [*Jue gu*] is the name of a bone. This hole is located four inches above[4] the outer ankle. It is the *yang fu* hole.

Yu Shu: The *jue gu* is the *yang fu* 陽輔 hole. It too is a location where qi of the foot minor yang vessel leave [the organism].

Hua Shou: All marrow is associated with the bones. Hence this is the gathering point of the marrow .... Mr. Chen from Siming states: The marrow is associated with the kidneys; the kidneys are responsible for the bones. They have nothing to do with the foot minor yang [conduit]. The brain is the "sea of marrow." The brain has the *zhen gu* 枕骨 hole. [The marrow], hence, should meet at the *zhen gu* [hole. The reference here to] the *jue gu* [hole] is a mistake.

---

3   Li Jiong's edition has *shang* 上 ("above"). That must be a mistake.
4   Li Jiong's edition has *xia* 下 ("below"). That, too, must be a mistake.

Xu Dachun: The *jue gu* [hole] belongs to the foot minor yang [vessel]. It is the *xuan zhong* 懸鍾 hole, which is located four inches above the outer ankle. In the treatise "Jing mai" 經脈 of the *Ling* [*shu*], it is stated in a discussion of the foot minor yang vessel: "It controls the bones. Now, because all marrow is associated with the bones, this is the gathering point of the marrow."

Ye Lin: The *jue gu* [bone] is the *zhen gu* [bone – i.e., the back of the skull]. The name [of the hole] is the *yu zhen* 玉枕 hole. It is located behind the *luo que* 絡卻 [hole] at a distance of one inch five *fen*, based on an individually standardized inch. It is located one inch three *fen* to the side of the *nao hu* 腦戶 [hole]. The character *jue* 絕 may be an error resulting from careless [copying].

(6) *Ding Deyong*: "The [qi of the] blood gather at the *ge shu*." [*Ge shu*] is the name for holes located on both sides below the seventh vertebra. The distance [from the spinal column] is on both [sides] one inch and five *fen* on the basis of an individually standardized inch.

Yu Shu: The two *ge shu* holes are located on both sides of the spinal bone, one inch and five *fen* below the seventh vertebra. They are the locations where the qi of the foot major yang vessel [which is associated with] the urinary bladder are emitted.

Hua Shou: Mr. Chen from Siming states: The blood is ruled by the heart and it is stored by the liver. The *ge shu* [holes] are located on both sides of the seventh vertebra. Above they constitute the transportation [point] associated with the heart; below it is the transportation [point] associated with the liver. Hence it constitutes the gathering point of the blood.

Zhang Shixian: "The gathering point of the blood" refers to the blood of the entire body. *Ge shu* is the name of holes which are located at a distance of one inch and five *fen* on both sides of the spine below the seventh vertebra. The blood of all the conduits moves from the diaphragm (*ge mo* 膈膜) upward and downward. The heart generates the blood and the liver stores the blood. The heart is located above the diaphragm; the liver is located below the diaphragm. [The blood] travels through the diaphragm. Hence the "diaphragm transportation" [hole, i.e., the *ge shu*] is the gathering point of the blood.

Xu Dachun: The *ge shu* [holes] belong to the foot major yang [vessel] .... They are locations in the central section of the [Triple] Burner where the essence is transformed into blood. Hence they are the gathering points of the blood.

(7) *Ding Deyong*: "The [qi of the] bones meet at the *da shu*." [*Da shu*] is the name of holes located behind the neck on both sides of the first vertebra at a distance of one inch five *fen* each, on the basis of an individually standardized inch.

Yu Shu: The *da shu* too is a location where qi of the foot major yang vessel are emitted.

Hua Shou: Mr. Chen from Siming states: The bones are nourished by the marrow. The marrow flows downward from the brain into the *da shu* [hole]. From the *da shu* [hole] it leaks into the backbone below the heart down to the tail [bone, whence] it leaks into all the bones and joints. Hence all the qi of the bones gather here.

Zhang Shixian: "Bones" refers to the bones of the entire body. *Da shu* is the name of holes located behind the neck on both sides of the first vertebra at a distance of one inch five *fen*. The framework of all bones has its origin here; branches develop downward. Hence the *da shu* is the gathering point of the bones.

Xu Dachun: The *da shu* [holes] belong to the foot major yang [vessel]. In the treatise "Hai lun" 海論 of the *Ling* [*shu*] it is stated: "The throughway vessel is the sea of the twelve conduits. Its transport [openings] are the *da zhu* [holes]." In the treatise "Yun shu" 運輸 it is stated: "The throughway vessel and the big network [vessel] of the minor yin [conduit] emerge from the kidneys and descend." Now, the kidneys control the bones, and the bladder is linked to the kidneys. Hence [the *da shu* holes] are the gathering points of the bones.

Ding Jin: The *da shu* is a hole of the supervisor vessel. The bones of shoulder and spine meet here. Hence [the text] calls it the gathering-point of the bones.

(8) *Ding Deyong*: "The [qi of the] vessels meet at the *tai yuan* [hole." This hole] is located at the right [hand] in the inch-interior [section] below the fish-line.

Yu Shu: The *tai yuan* [hole] is located at the hand in the fish-line where a movement in the vessel can be felt by one's hand. It is a location where the qi of the hand major yin conduit are emitted.

Xu Dachun: The *tai yuan* [hole] belongs to the hand major yin [vessel]; it is located in the bend behind the palm. It is the inch opening. The lung [resembles] a court that is visited by all vessels. Hence [the *tai yuan* hole] is the gathering point of all vessels. The meaning of this [statement] is discussed in detail as the first difficult issue.

Liao Ping: The vessels cannot gather at the *tai yuan* [hole] because the vessels cannot move from one place to another. The camp and the guard [qi] circulate [through the organism]; in their case one may speak of a "gathering."

(9) *Ding Deyong*: "The qi gather in the Triple Burner, that is, in one muscle exactly between the two breasts at the outside of the body" refers to the *dan zhong* hole.

Li Jiong: The upper [section of the Triple] Burner is located below the heart; it extends to the upper opening of the stomach. It is treated at the *dan zhong*, which is located one inch six *fen* below the *yu tang* 玉堂, exactly in the hollow where the two breasts meet. "The muscles outside [of the Triple Burner] right between the two breasts" refers to the *dan zhong* hole.

Hua Shou: Xie Jinsun states: "*San jiao* 三焦 ("Triple Burner") should be *shang jiao* 上焦 ("upper section of the Triple Burner")."

Zhang Shixian: "Triple Burner" stands for the upper, central, and lower [sections of the Triple] Burner. Between the two breasts is the *dan zhong* hole. The *dan zhong* is the upper [section of the Triple] Burner; the *zhong wan* 中脘 is the central [section of the Triple] Burner; the *qi hai* 氣海 ("sea of qi") is the lower [section of the Triple] Burner. "Outside" refers to the entire conduit from below the *qi hai* directly upward to in between the two breasts.

Xu Dachun: "Outside of the Triple Burner" means "outside of the Burner's membrane (*jiao mo* 焦膜)". "Between the two breasts" refers to the location in the middle between the two breasts where the controller vessel passes through. This is the *dan zhong* hole. In the treatise "Jing mai" 經脈 of the *Ling* [*shu* it is stated:] "The hand minor yang vessel controls the qi." Furthermore, in the [treatise] "Hai lun" 海論 it is stated: "The *dan zhong* is the sea of the qi." Hence it is the gathering point of the qi.

Liao Ping: In the text of the [*Nei*] *jing* it is stated clearly that the Triple Burner is the place where the original and true [qi] pass through and gather. The present book changes this and states: "The qi gather in the Triple Burner." I do not know what that means.

(10) *Yang*: Man's long-term depots, short-term repositories, muscles, bones, marrow, blood, vessels and qi, all these eight [entities] are associated with a specific hole that is the gathering point [of their respective qi]. When a disease due to heat is present inside [the body], one selects outside the appropriate hole where [the evil qi] gather in order to eliminate the disease.

Xu Dachun: When a disease due to heat is present in the interior [of the body], evil qi have already deeply penetrated [the organism] and a superficial treatment is of no avail. One must take the location where these qi have gathered together as a starting point to attack and seize the evil. Only then can one eliminate the disease. "Where respective [qi] gather" means that in each case one should see [first] where the disease is located and [then] select the appropriate place for treatment.

Ding Jin: Whenever a disease [due to] heat is present inside [of the body, one should] take hold of the qi and of the blood where [the heat] has gathered and treat this location with needles. This is a reference to the *qi men* 期門 hole. When Zhang Zhongjing treated the minor yang [conduits] because of the intrusion of heat into the blood chamber, he pierced the *qi men* [hole. His approach] was based on the [statement made] here.

(1)–(10) *Xu Dachun*: The "eight gathering points" do not appear in the [*Nei*] *jing*. But the meaning [of this difficult issue] has undoubtedly been derived from somewhere. These must be the words of an ancient scripture. Today no [such scripture] is extant to check [the origin of statements here].[5]

---

5 Liao Ping could not agree with this opinion. He commented on this statement: "Xu was wrong!"

四十六難曰：（一）老人臥而不寐，少壯寐而不寤者，何也？
（二）然：經言少壯者，血氣盛，肌肉滑，氣道通，榮衛之行不失於常，故
晝日精，夜不寤。（三）老人血氣衰，氣肉不滑，榮衛之道澀，故晝日不能
精，夜不得寐也，故知老人不得寐也。

The forty-sixth difficult issue: (1) Old people lie down but do not sleep; young and vigorous [people] sleep and do not wake up. Why is that so?

(2) It is like this. The scripture states: Those who are young and vigorous have plenty of blood and qi. Their flesh is smooth. Their passageways for the qi are passable. Their camp and guard [qi] proceed regularly without fail. Hence they are alert during the daytime and do not wake up during the nighttime. (3) In old people blood and qi diminish. The flesh is no longer smooth. The passageways of the camp and guard [qi] are rough. Hence they cannot be alert during the daytime, and they cannot find sleep at night. Hence one knows [the reason why] old people cannot find sleep.[1]

COMMENTARIES

(1)–(3) *Ding Deyong*: Heaven and earth communicate as opposites; sun and moon [go through periods of] brightness and darkness. Man's sleeping and being awake is closely tied to [these macrocosmic processes]. In those who are young and vigorous, the camp and the guard [qi] are not yet damaged; hence [their states of] being awake and being asleep follow the course of heaven and earth, of yin and yang. Thus, they are alert and vigorous during the daytime, and they sleep during the nighttime. Those who are old are damaged and distressed. Hence they cannot be alert and vigorous during the daytime; [the flow of their]

---

1 At first glance, this difficult issue appears to convey a rather straight-forward message. Yet some of the commentators felt the need for a theoretical underpinning of the insights offered, while the conservatives blamed the author(s) of the *Nan jing* for having grossly misrepresented the corresponding text of the *Ling shu*. Xu Dachun's critique seems to be overdrawn. For comparison, the short *Nei jing* passage is quoted here in full: "The Yellow Thearch said: 'Which qi cause old people not to sleep at night; which qi cause young and vigorous people not to sleep during the daytime?' Qi Bo replied: 'The qi and the blood of vigorous [people) are plentiful; their flesh is smooth; their passageways of the qi are passable; their camp and guard [qi) proceed regularly without fail. Hence they are alert during the daytime and they sleep at night. In old people, qi and blood diminish. Their flesh dries out. The passageways of the qi are rough; the qi of the five long-term depots clash against each other. Their camp qi are diminished and the guard qi attack the interior. Hence they are not alert during the daytime and they do not sleep at night'."

camp and guard [qi] is rough and obstructed. Therefore, at night they cannot find sleep.

Yang: During the daytime, the guard qi proceed through the yang [sections]; the yang [sections] are the body.[2] During the nighttime, they proceed through the yin [sections]. The yin [sections] constitute the interior of the abdomen. When man opens his eyes, the guard qi come out [of the abdomen] and he will be awake. When they enter [the abdomen] he will sleep. In those who are young, the guard qi proceed without fail. Hence during the daytime these [people] are settled and calm, and at night they find sound sleep. In old people, the guard qi – in leaving and entering [the abdomen] – do not correspond to the time [of the day]. Hence during the daytime [these old people] are not settled and calm, and during the nighttime they cannot find sleep. *Jing* 精 ("alert") stands for *jing* 靜 ("calm"); *jing* ("calm") means *an* 安 ("settled").

Hua Shou: [The fact that] old people are awake and cannot find sleep, and that young and strong people [can] sleep and do not wake up is related to repletion and depletion of the camp and guard qi, [i.e.,] of blood and qi. [This paragraph] corresponds to the eighteenth treatise of the *Ling shu.*

Zhang Shixian: The *Ling shu* states: "Those above fifty are old; those above twenty are strong; those below eighteen are young." *Sheng* 盛 ("plenty") stands for *wang* 旺 ("flourishing"). *Chang* ("regularly") stands for *chang du* 常度 "regular degree". The yang rules the day; the yin rules the night. When the yang [qi] move, the yin [qi] rest. The movement [of the yang qi] is responsible for alertness; the resting [of the yang qi] is responsible for sleep. The [movement in the] vessels of man circulates – during one day and one night – fifty times through the body. During the daytime, the camp and the guard [qi] proceed twenty-five times through the yang [sections of the organism]; during the nighttime they proceed twenty-five times through the yin [sections of the organism]. Young and vigorous people have plenty of camp and guard [qi]; their flesh is smooth, their passageways for the blood and for the qi are passable; [their blood and their qi proceed] regularly without fail. In the morning, the yin [qi] withdraw and the yang qi come out. [Hence] during the daytime [these people] are alert and strong. When the sun goes down, the yang [qi] withdraw and the yin [sections] receive their qi. As a consequence [these people] fall asleep and do not wake up. In old people, this is reversed.

Xu Dachun: The treatise "Ying wei sheng hui" 營衛生會 of the *Ling [shu]* states: "The camp and the guard [qi] proceed twenty-five times through the yang and twenty-five times through the yin [sections of the body]." At dawn, the yang

---

2   See difficult issue 1.

[sections] receive the qi; at dusk, the yin [sections] receive the qi. This continues without end. That is [what is] meant here. *Jing* 精 ("alert") stands for *jing min bu juan* 精敏不倦 ("alert and not tired").

(1)–(3) *Xu Dachun*: This paragraph contains even more mistakes [than others]. The *Nan jing* was basically [compiled in order to] explain the [meaning of the *Nei*] *jing*. However, in the present [dialogue of] question and answer it merely transcribes the words of the treatise "Ying wei sheng hui" 營衛生會 of the *Ling* [*shu*], and in changing a number of characters it creates many errors. The [*Nei*] *jing* states: "The Yellow Thearch asked: 'When old people cannot close their eyes during the night, which qi cause this to be so? When young[3], strong people are unable to close their eyes during daytime, which qi cause this to be so?' " The wording of these questions is both simple and encompassing. When it says "unable to close their eyes during daytime" it implies that [young people] are alert during the daytime and sleep soundly during the nighttime. That is changed here [in the *Nan jing*] to "sleep and do not awake." Apparently, day and night are not differentiated, and the language is muddled. Furthermore, the sentence "the passageways of the camp and guard [qi] are rough" reads in the text of the [*Nei*] *jing*: "the paths of their qi are rough. The camp qi are weak and diminished, and the guard qi attack their own interior." Now, if there are only few camp qi, the blood is diminished and the spirit, too, cannot be contained. When the guard qi attack the interior, one's qi are not plentiful and one's strength is easily exhausted. "Hence they are not of a clear [mind] during daytime, and they do not close their eyes at night." [All of this] is changed here to "the passageways of the camp and guard [qi] are rough." That is quite unclear and does not elucidate anything. Also, [this wording] does not enable one to thoroughly investigate the meaning of the [*Nei*] *jing*. Even the changing of a single character must lead to many errors. Therefore I do not explain this [paragraph].

Katō Bankei: This [difficult issue] appears to discuss the differences between old and young people concerning their being awake and finding sleep during day and night. In fact, however, [this paragraph] elucidates that, as far as the amount of circulation of the camp and guard [qi through the body] is concerned, old people have fewer [qi] and no longer reflect the [correct] amount [of circulation]. This meaning agrees with that of the treatise "[Ying wei] sheng hui" 營衛生會 of the *Ling shu*; the question is raised here once more because in strong [people], the blood and the qi are normally plentiful, but when one reaches

---

3 Further down the text speaks of 壯者 *zhuang zhe*, "strong ones", and 老者 *lao zhe*, "old ones". The character 少 *shao*, "young", breaks the rhyme structure and may be a later addition.

old age, the amount of blood and qi constantly present [in the body] is diminished. This is all the more true when [an old person] suffers from a disease. Consequently, in considering the [application of] drugs, one must differentiate [between old and young people]. Hence, if one compares the diseases of old [people] with those of young and strong [people], although they may appear as repletion, they are still based on a depletion. An ordinary internal or external disease [of old people] may appear just like the disease of young and strong [people], but when it comes down to attack them and to supplement [a depletion], one must be very careful. One cannot always apply the same treatment just because the diseases appear to be the same. It is for this special reason that Bian Que has raised this present issue.

Liao Ping: That is a transcription of the old book; it is not an explanation of the meaning of the text. Mr. Huang Kunzai[4] 黃崑載 reveres [Yueren] as one of the four sages. How can one avoid a sigh!

---

4   *Zi* name of Huang Yuanyu 黃元御, an author of numerous medical works dated between 1755 and 1760.

四十七難曰：（一）人面獨能耐寒者，何也？

（二）然：人頭者，諸陽之會也。（三）諸陰脈皆至頸胸中而還，（四）獨諸陽脈皆上至頭耳，故令面耐寒也。

The forty-seventh difficult issue: (1) Only man's face can stand cold. Why is that so?

(2) It is like this. Man's head is the meeting point of all yang [vessels]. (3) All the yin vessels reach into neck and chest, from which they return. (4) Only all the yang vessels reach upward into the head. Hence they let the face endure cold.

COMMENTARIES

(1)–(4) *Ding Deyong:* The ascending and descending of yin and yang [qi] between heaven and earth has a beginning and an end. The [ascending and descending of the] yang qi begins at [the solar term] "spring begins"; it ends with [the solar term] "winter begins." The [ascending and descending of the] yin qi begins at [the solar term] "autumn begins" and ends with [the solar term] "summer begins." The five [solar] terms "grain fills," "grain-in-ear," "summer solstice," "slight heat," and "great heat," [during which no yin qi are present,] correspond to the head. Hence only the face can stand cold. The five [solar] terms "little snow," "heavy snow," "winter solstice," "minor cold," and "massive cold," [during which no yang qi are present,] correspond to man's feet. They cannot stand cold. That is [what is] meant here.

Yang: The statement "all the yin vessels reach into neck and chest, from which they return" may be based on [the assumption] that while all yang [vessels] meet in head and face, only a few yin [vessels] reach head and face. The [*Nei*] *jing* states: "All 365 vessels meet in the eyes." If this is so, all the yin and yang vessels reach the face, and one cannot say that only the yang vessels reach head and face.

Hua Shou: The fourth treatise of the *Ling shu* states: "Huang Di asked Qi Bo:
'The head, the face and the entire physical body are tied to bones and connected through sinews. They all have identical blood forming a union with the qi. When the heaven is cold, then the earth will crack and the waters freeze. If the cold arrives unexpectedly, it may well be that hands and feet remain relaxed [because they are covered], while the face may remain uncovered. Why is that?' Qi Bo replied: '[Humans have] twelve conduit vessels and 365 network [vessels]. Their blood and qi all rise into the face and move into the empty orifices. The essence yang qi rise and move into the eyes where they enable the eyesight. The remaining qi move into the ears where they enable hearing. The stem qi rise and leave [the face] through the nose. They enable smelling. The turbid qi leave

the stomach and move into the lips and the tongue where they generate taste. The body liquids of the qi, they all evaporate into the face. As a result, the skin thickens, and the flesh becomes firm. The fact is: The qi of heaven may be very cold, and yet they are unable to subdue [the face]'." In my own opinion, the three yang [conduits] of the hands proceed from the hands upward to the head; the three yang [conduits] of the feet proceed from the head downward to the feet. The three yin [conduits] of the hands run from the abdomen to the hands; and the three yin [conduits] of the feet run from the feet into the abdomen. For this reason [the *Nan jing* states] that all yin vessels reach into neck and chest, from which they return, while only all the yang vessels reach upward into the head.

Zhang Shixian: "All yang [vessels]" refers to the three yang [vessels] of the hands and feet. "All yin [vessels]" refers to the three yin [vessels] of the hands and feet. The three yin vessels of the hands reach from the chest to the hands; the three yin vessels of the feet [include, first,] the [foot] major yin [vessel], which starts from the end of the big toe, ascends to the diaphragm, continues on both sides of the throat, and links up with the base of the tongue. It dissipates below the tongue. [Second, there is] the [foot] minor yin [vessel], which starts from the end of the small toe, ascends from the kidneys, passes the liver and the diaphragm, enters the lung, and proceeds on both sides of the base of the tongue. [Third, there is] the [foot] ceasing yin [vessel], which starts from the thicket of hairs on the big toe, ascends through the ribs, and meets with the top of the head. The [*Nan*] *jing* states: "All the vessels of the yin conduits reach into neck and chest, from which they return." Is that not in stark conflict with the [real courses of the] vessels of the yin conduits? The face constitutes the yang in yang. It is for this reason that it can stand cold! If the face, however, has an antipathy against cold, this is so because the major yin [qi] do not gather in the head. Such [a condition] is called "yin abundance, yang depletion."

Xu Dachun: In the treatise "Ni shun fei shou lun" 逆順肥瘦論 of the *Ling* [*shu*], it is stated: "The three yin [conduits] of the hands proceed from the long-term depots to the hands; the three yang [conduits] of the hands proceed from the hands to the head. The three yang [conduits] of the feet proceed from the head to the feet. The three yin [conduits] of the feet proceed from the feet to the abdomen." That is [what is] meant here .... This [dialogue of] question and answer is also based on the *Ling* [*shu*] treatise "Xie qi zang fu bing xing lun" 邪氣藏府病形論. The text of the *Nei jing* states: "All the blood and all the qi of the twelve conduits and 365 network [vessels] ascend to the face and proceed through the orifices." It states further: "The skin is thick, and the flesh is firm. Hence neither extreme heat nor massive cold can do harm to it." That has been changed here [in the *Nan jing*] to "the qi of all the yang conduits ascend to the head." This is, of course, based on the meaning of the treatise "Ni shun fei shou lun," [the words of which] have been moved here as an explanation. The underlying principle is very clear and to the point. In such instances, the [*Nan jing*] and the text of the *Nei jing* may follow different paths but their destinations are identical.

Liao Ping: The [corresponding] text of the [*Nei*] *jing* is clear and by no means obscure. Why should it be necessary to bring [this topic] up again? If difficult issues are formulated this way, it is not at all difficult to immediately understand hundreds or thousands of such paragraphs. This is all the more true if only eighty-one difficult issues are concerned!

Chapter Four
On Diseases

THE FORTY-EIGHTH DIFFICULT ISSUE

四十八難曰：（一）人有三虛三實，何謂也？

（二）然：有脈之虛實，有病之虛實，有診之虛實也。（三）脈之虛實者，濡者為虛，緊牢者為實。（四）病之虛實者，出者為虛，入者為實；（五）言者為虛，不言者為實；（六）緩者為虛，急者為實。（七）診之虛實者，濡者為虛，牢者為實；（八）癢者為虛，痛者為實；（九）外痛內快，為外實內虛；內痛外快，為內實外虛。（十）故曰虛實也。

The forty-eighth difficult issue: (1) A person may have three [kinds of] depletion and three [kinds of] repletion. What does that mean?

(2) It is like this. The, [movement in the] vessels may display depletion or repletion; the [course and the nature of a] disease may reveal depletion or repletion; and the examination [of the patient] may reveal depletion or repletion. (3) As for [the display of] depletion or repletion by the [movement in the] vessels, a soft [movement] indicates depletion, a tight and firm [movement] indicates repletion. (4) [There are three possibilities for a display of] depletion and repletion by the [course and nature of a] disease, [including the following]. If [the disease] moves toward the outside, that indicates a depletion; if it moves toward the interior, that marks a repletion. (5) If [the patient] speaks, that indicates a depletion; if he does not speak, that indicates a repletion. (6) If [the patient is] relaxed, that marks a depletion; if he is tense, that marks a repletion. (7) [There are four possibilities for a display of] depletion and repletion through an examination [of the patient]. If [by touching the patient one perceives] softness, that marks a depletion; if [one perceives] firmness, that marks a repletion. (8) Itching marks a depletion; pain indicates repletion. (9) [If the patient feels] pain externally but is comfortable internally, that indicates repletion in the exterior [sections of the body and] a depletion in the interior; if he feels pain internally and is comfortable in the exterior [sections of the organism], that marks

an internal repletion and an external depletion. (10) Hence one speaks of depletion and repletion.[1]

COMMENTARIES

(1) *Zhang Shixian*: *Xu* 虛 ("depletion") stands for *kong xu* 空虛 ("empty"); that is, the proper qi are lost. *Shi* 實 ("repletion") stands for *qiang shi* 強實 ("vigorous and full"); that is, evil qi are present in abundance.

---

1 The terms "three depletions" and "three repletions" first appear in the *Tai su* treatise "San xu san shi" (see Unschuld, *Medicine in China: A History of Ideas*, 69-70 and 267-269). But the concept of an "abundance" that must be drained and of an "insufficiency" that must be supplemented is already recorded in the Ma wang dui 馬王堆 fragment of the *Mai fa* 脈法, which may have been compiled around 200 BCE or earlier. The concepts of "abundance" or "repletion" and of "insufficiency" or "depletion" may have originated from agricultural experiences. A good harvest ensured well-being; a harvest creating a surplus had to be shared lest it provoke envy. A bad harvest led to famine and, as a result, disease. The linkage of repletion and depletion with different degrees of susceptibility to disease is quite evident in the *Tai su* treatise "San xu san shi" 三虛三實 and in the *Ling shu* treatise "Sui lu lun" 歲露論, which repeats the contents of the former. In these treatises it is stated that each person is characterized at all times by a combination of three variables accounting for his susceptibility to disease. These variables include the so-called decline of the years, the state of the moon, and one's harmony with the time (of the year?). The "decline of the years" may refer to critical years, cyclically returning in man's life – at least that is how Yang Shangshan 楊上善, the *Tai su* compiler/commentator of the seventh century, explained this concept. According to him, the seventh, sixteenth, twenty-fifth, thirty-fourth, and forty-third years of life and so on are critical years in which one is particularly susceptible to disease. The second variable causing depletion or repletion in the organism is the rhythm of the changing phases of the moon. The full moon produces repletion, while a new or waning moon entails weakness and susceptibility to injury. The third variable appears to be a person's ability to live in harmony with time. This may refer to man's ability to adapt to the climate of the individual seasons. Hence, a person may have "three repletions" if he is not in his critical years, if the moon is full, and if he lives in harmony with the time (of the year). In such a state of "three repletions," one is not susceptible to disease even if he is attacked by evil qi. Three depletions indicate the opposite state, with an extreme susceptibility to disease. There are numerous other states in between, such as "two repletions" and "one depletion," which account for gradations in one's susceptibility to disease. Basically, the concept of the "three depletions" and "three repletions" in the *Tai su* should be seen as a paradigm explaining why some people fall ill and others do not, although they appear to have been subjected to identical pathological qi. As the commentaries of the present difficult issue demonstrate, the concepts of depletion and repletion underwent many changes in later centuries; for the most part, they seem to have referred to a lack of proper qi (depletion) or to the presence of evil qi (repletion) that may have originated from outside the body (as, for instance, wind, moisture, heat) or from another long-term depot (when, for instance, qi from the liver seize the region of the spleen). The *Nan jing* interpretation of "repletion" and "depletion" appears in the fiftieth difficult issue; here, only various diagnostic patterns permitting one to distinguish whether a person suffers from a depletion or from a repletion are introduced.

Katō Bankei: In discussing the three depletions and the three repletions, the *Ling shu* distinguishes between "abundance" and "weakness" of the year, "depletion" and "fullness" of the moon, and "to be in harmony" and "not to be in harmony" with time. In that way, the meaning of "three depletions" and "three repletions" was broad and far-reaching; it did not come close to the current pattern [of the *Nan jing*]. Hence, this treatise has continued the terms but has revolutionized the pattern [for which they stand. Here,] the so-called three depletions and three repletions refer to the [movement in the] vessels, to [the course of a] disease, and to examination.

(2) *Liao Ping*: Such a list is inappropriate. The [movement in the] vessels and the [course of a] disease can be perceived only through examination. It is impossible to designate the former two and the latter one with different names [as if they constituted a series of three].

(3) *Ding Deyong*: [A movement in the] vessels that is slow and tender is [called] "soft." If one presses [the vessel] and if [its movement then] displays strength, it is [called] "firm" and "replete."

Yang: If one presses [the vessel] and [has a feeling] like touching a rope, that is called "tight."

Li Jiong: "Soft" indicates a yin [movement in the] vessels. Hence [the text] speaks of "depletion." "Tight" and "firm" indicate a yang [movement in the] vessels. Hence [the text] speaks of "repletion."

Zhang Shixian: "[Movement in the] vessels" refers to the [movement in the] vessels at the inch, gate, and foot [sections] of both hands. If [that movement] is soft, the arrival of qi is insufficient. That marks a depletion. If [the movement] is tight and firm, the arrival of qi exceeds [its normal level]. That marks a repletion.

Xu Dachun: Ru 濡 ("soft") stands for *rou ruo* 柔弱 ("soft"), *ruan zhi* 軟滯 ("yielding"). The *Shang han lun* 傷寒論 states: "A soft (*ru*) [movement in the vessels indicates] loss of blood." It states further: "A soft [movement in the vessels] indicates diminished guard qi." From these [quotations] one can see that a "soft" [movement in the vessels] is a sign for a depletion of both blood and qi. A string-like and stiff [movement in the vessels] is called "tight"; a hard and replete [movement] is called "firm."

(4) *Ding Deyong*: Yin and yang [qi] control the [body's] internal and external [sections], respectively. Here, in the case of an insufficiency of yang [qi], the yin [qi] leave [the interior sections of the body] and seize the [exterior section, which should be occupied by yang qi]. In the interior [section] only yin [qi] are present. Hence one knows that "if [the qi] move toward the outside, that marks a depletion [of yang qi]." In the case of an insufficiency of yin [qi], the yang [qi]

move in and seize the [interior section, which should be occupied by *yin* qi]. In the external [sections] only yang [qi] are present. Hence one knows that "if [the qi] move toward the interior [section of the organism], that indicates a repletion [of yang qi]."

Yang: ["A movement toward the outside indicates a depletion" refers to] many exhalations and few inhalations; ["a movement toward the interior indicates a repletion" refers to] many inhalations and few exhalations.

Hua Shou: "A movement toward the outside indicates a depletion" means that the body's five long-term depots have developed a disease by themselves which proceeds outward from the interior. [Li] Dongyuan calls such [a situation] "internal damages." "A movement toward the interior indicates a repletion" refers to a damage caused by the five evil [qi] from outside that moves toward the interior [sections of the organism. Li] Dongyuan calls such [a situation] "external damages."

Zhang Shixian: Chu 出 ("move toward the outside") means that [something] comes from the interior and proceeds toward the exterior. *Ru* 入 ("move toward the interior") means that [something] comes from the exterior and proceeds toward the interior. "Moves toward the outside" means that the five [long-term depots] in the interior [sections of the organism] have fallen ill by themselves and are depleted. "Moves toward the interior" means that the exterior [sections of the organism] have been harmed by evil qi and [suffer from] repletion.

Xu Dachun: *Chu* 出 ("move toward the outside") means that the essence qi are drained toward the outside as, for instance, through sweating, vomiting, or diarrhea. All instances when something moves from inside toward outside are meant here. *Ru* 入 ("move toward the interior") means that external qi accumulate inside [the body]. These are, for instance, wind and cold which – after having been accepted [by the body] – are able to block [the passageways of] food and stools. All instances when something enters from outside are meant here.

Liao Ping: The [terms] *chu* 出 ("move toward the outside") and *ru* 入 ("move toward the interior") refer, in the [*Nei*] *jing*, to the courses of the conduits and network [vessels] from the interior to the exterior [sections of the organism], and vice versa. There are many passages in the [*Nei*] *jing* clearly elucidating the diseases that belong [to each of these vessels proceeding toward the outside or toward the interior]. Why should one use these two characters [in the present context]? Xu [Dachun's] words are equally far-fetched.

(5) *Yang Xuancao*: The lung controls the sounds. When [its qi] enter the heart, they cause [a person] to speak. Hence one knows that "if [the patient] speaks, that indicates a depletion." The liver controls planning and considering; thus, when

[its qi] enter the heart, one does not speak. That is a manifestation of a repletion evil.² Hence one knows that "if [the patient] does not speak, that indicates a repletion."

Yang Kanghou: When the qi of the long-term depots are depleted, the essence qi are lost; as a result, the respective person will speak a lot. When the qi of the long-term depots are replete, evil qi are present in abundance. Hence one is not willing to speak.

Hua Shou: "If he speaks, that indicates a depletion" means that the body's five long-term depots have fallen ill by themselves, not because of an external evil [qi]. Hence one remains alert and there is nothing that hinders one to speak. "If he does not speak, that indicates a repletion" means that evil qi depress a person internally. Hence he is confused and does not speak.

(6) *Ding Deyong*: Yang [qi] are responsible for haste; yin [qi] are responsible for calmness. [Thus,] if yin [qi are present in abundance, the patient] is relaxed; if yang [qi are present in abundance, the patient] is tense. Hence one knows that a relaxed [state of the patient] indicates a depletion; a tense [state of the patient] indicates a repletion.

Yang: ["Relaxed"] refers to relaxed skin and flesh; ["tense" refers to] a full and tense skin.

Hua Shou: "Relaxation indicates a depletion." *Huan* 緩 ("relaxed") stands for *bu ji* 不急 ("not speedy").³ That is to say, what leaves from the interior outward proceeds slowly, step by step. These are not diseases which complete their course in one morning and in one night. "Speed indicates a repletion" means that in the case of a disease caused by being struck by wind, cold, warmth, or heat, one will die or recover within five or six days.

Xu Dachun: *Huan* 緩 ("relaxed") means that the disease proceeds slowly. When the proper qi are lost and when the presence of evil qi is minimal, the disease penetrates deeper at a slow pace. *Ji* 急 ("speedy") means that the disease comes all of a sudden. When the proper qi have not yet leaked out [completely], and when evil qi are present in abundance, the disease will be fast.

(7) *Yang*: [In the case of depletion] the skin is soft and relaxed. [In the case of repletion] the skin is firm and vigorous.

Hua Shou: *Zhen* 診 ("examination") includes *an* 按 ("pressing") and *hou* 候 ("checking for symptoms"). To press someone externally and recognize his [condition]

---

2   This interpretation does not correspond to the definition of "repletion evil" in the fiftieth difficult issue.

3   *Ji* 急 carries the meanings of "tense" and "speedy."

is not the "examination" [implied by] the [term] *zhen mai* 診脈 ("examination of the [movement in the] vessels").

Zhang Shixian: *Zhen* 診 ("examination") stands for *shi yan* 睞眼 ("inspection"). That is an all-encompassing designation for the examination of a disease by means of observation, listening/smelling, asking the patient questions, and feeling [the movement in his vessels].

Xu Dachun: The *Mai jing* 脈經 quotes this [passage] but has omitted these two sentences. I suspect [the *Mai jing* author assumed] that they constitute a repetition of the text above and therefore discarded them.

(8) *Yang*: When the body [suffers from] depletion, that [causes] itching; painful locations on the body indicate repletion.

Xu Dachun: If blood and qi are depleted and cannot supplement skin and flesh, itching results. If evil qi gather together and if, [as a result,] camp and guard [qi] cannot [proceed] in harmony, pain results.

(9) *Yang*: If light pressure with one's hand causes pain, that indicates an external repletion; the reason is that the disease is near the surface. If heavy pressure with one's hand makes the patient feel comfortable, that indicates internal depletion; the reason is that the disease is located in the depth.

Xu Dachun: In the case of a depletion, pressure will cause joy; in the case of a repletion, one cannot stand being touched by a hand.

(10) *Yang*: if heavy pressure with one's hand causes pain, that indicates an internal repletion; the reason is that the disease is located in the depth. If light pressure with one's hand makes the patient feel comfortable, that indicates external depletion; the reason is that the disease is located near the surface. Whenever a person has a disease and feels pain if pressed, that is always due to a repletion. If [the patient] feels comfortable despite the pressure, that is always a sign of depletion.

Ding Deyong: For an examination one presses the skin [of the patient] at the heart and on the abdomen, at the inner and at the outer side [of the body].[4] If the pain stops under pressure, that marks a depletion. If the pain becomes even stronger under pressure, that marks a repletion. The same pattern applies to the internal and external [sections of the organism].

4　"Inner and outer" may refer to front and back of the body, respectively.

THE FORTY-NINTH DIFFICULT ISSUE

四十九難曰：(一)有正經自病，有五邪所傷，何以別之？

(二)然：經言憂愁思慮則傷心；(三)形寒飲冷則傷肺；(四)恚怒氣逆，上而不下則傷肝；(五)飲食勞倦則傷脾；(六)久坐濕地，強力入水則傷腎。(七)是正經之自病也。

(八)何謂五邪？

(九)然：有中風，(十)有傷暑，(十一)有飲食勞倦，(十二)有傷寒，(十三)有中濕，(十四)此之謂五邪。

(十五)假令心病，何以知中風得之？

(十六)然：其色當赤。何以言之？(十七)肝主色，(十八)自入為青，(十九)入心為赤，(二十)入脾為黃，(二十一)入肺為白，(二十二)入腎為黑。(二十三)肝為心邪，故知當赤色也。(二十四)其病身熱，脅下滿痛，(二十五)其脈浮大而弦。

(二十六)何以知傷暑得之？

(二十七)然：當惡臭。何以言之？(二十八)心主臭，(二十九)自入為焦臭，(三十)入脾為香臭，(三十一)入肝為臊臭，(三十二)入腎為腐臭，(三十三)入肺為腥臭。(三十四)故知心病傷暑得之也，當惡臭。其病身熱而煩，心痛，其脈浮大而散。

(三十五)何以知飲食勞倦得之？

(三十六)然：當喜苦味也。(三十七)虛為不欲食，實為欲食。何以言之？(三十八)脾主味，(三十九)入肝為酸，(四十)入心為苦，(四十一)入肺為辛，(四十二)入腎為鹹，(四十三)自入為甘。(四十四)故知脾邪入心，為喜苦味也。(四十五)其病身熱而體重嗜臥，四肢不收，(四十六)其脈浮大而緩。

(四十七)何以知傷寒得之？

(四十八)然：當譫言妄語。何以言之？(四十九)肺主聲，(五十)入肝為呼，(五十一)入心為言，(五十二)入脾為歌，(五十三)入腎為呻，(五十四)自入為哭，(五十五)故知肺邪入心為譫言妄語也。(五十六)其病身熱，灑灑惡寒，甚則喘咳，(五十七)其脈浮大而濇。

(五十八)何以知中濕得之？

(五十九)然：當喜汗出不可止。何以言之？(六十)腎主濕，(六十一)入肝為泣，(六十二)入心為汗，(六十三)入脾為液，(六十四)入肺為涕，(六十五)自入為唾。(六十六)故知腎邪入心，為汗出不可止也。(六十七)其病身熱而小腹痛，足脛寒而逆，(六十八)其脈沉濡而大。(六十九)此五邪之法也。

The forty-ninth difficult issue: (1) It happens that the regular conduits fall ill by themselves, or that one is harmed by any of the five evils. How can these [situations] be distinguished?

(2) It is like this. The scripture states: Grief and anxiety, thoughts and considerations harm the heart; (3) a cold body and chilled beverages harm the lung; (4) hate and anger let the qi flow contrary to their proper direction; they move upward but not downward. This harms the liver. (5) Drinking and eating [without restraint], as well as weariness and exhaustion, harm the spleen. (6) If one sits at a humid place for an extended period, or if one exerts his strength and goes into water, that harms the kidneys. (7) These are [examples of situations where] the regular conduits fall ill by themselves.

(8) What is meant by "the five evils"?

(9) It is like this. To be struck by wind, (10) to be harmed by heat, (11) to drink and eat [without restraint], as well as weariness and exhaustion, (12) to be harmed by cold, (13) to be struck by moisture, (14) these [conditions] are called the five evils.

(15) Let us take a disease in the heart as an example. How does one know that [the patient] has contracted it because he was struck by wind?

(16) It is like this. His complexion should be red. Why do I say so? (17) The liver rules the colors. (18) [The color it keeps] itself is virid. (19) [The color that is generated when its qi] enter the heart is red. (20) [The color that is generated when its qi] enter the spleen is yellow. (21) [The color that is generated when its qi] enter the lung is white. (22) [The color that is generated when its qi] enter the kidneys is black. (23) Hence one knows from the red complexion [of a patient] that the liver has [sent its qi into] the heart, causing the presence of evil [qi there]. (24) [The patient] will suffer from a hot body, and [he will perceive] fullness and pain below the ribs. (25) [The movement of the qi in] his vessels is at the surface, strong, and like a string.

(26) How does one know that [the patient has] contracted [his disease in the heart] because he was harmed by heat?

(27) It is like this. He should have a bad odor. Why do I say so? (28) The heart rules the odors. (29) [The odor that is generated by] itself is burnt. (30) [The odor that is generated when the heart sends its qi] into the spleen is aromatic. (31) [The odor that is generated when the heart sends its qi] into the liver is fetid. (32) [The odor that is generated when it sends its qi] into the kidneys is foul. (33) [The odor that is generated when it sends its qi] into the lung is frowzy. (34) Hence one knows if a disease in the heart has been contracted because of harm caused by heat, there should be a detestable[1] odor. The patient will suffer from a hot body and will feel uneasy. He has pain in the heart, and [the movement in] his vessels is at the surface, strong, and dispersed.

---

1 *E* 惡 ("detestable") may be a mistake for *jiao* 焦 ("burnt").

(35) How does one know that [the patient has] contracted [his disease in the heart] because of [unrestrained] drinking and eating, or because of weariness and exhaustion?

(36) It is like this. He should prefer [to consume food with a] bitter flavor. (37) [When one's spleen is] depleted, he will not wish to eat; [when one's spleen] is replete, he will wish to eat. Why do I say so? (38) The spleen rules [one's preferences for a specific] flavor. (39) [The flavor one prefers when the spleen sends its qi] into the liver is sour. (40) [The flavor one prefers when the spleen sends its qi] into the heart is bitter. (41) [The flavor one prefers when the spleen sends its qi] into the lung is acrid. (42) [The flavor one prefers when the spleen sends its qi] into the kidneys is salty. (43) [The flavor one prefers when the spleen keeps its qi] within itself is sweet. (44) Hence one knows that if evil [qi] from the spleen enter the heart, that causes a preference for bitter flavor. (45) The patient will suffer from a hot body; [he will perceive] his body to be heavy and will have a desire to lie down. He cannot contract his four limbs. (46) [The movement in] his vessels is at the surface, strong and relaxed.

(47) How does one know that [the patient has] contracted [his disease in the heart] because of harm caused by cold?

(48) It is like this. He should talk incoherently and utter nonsense. Why do I say so? (49) The lung rules the sounds. (50) [The qi it sends] into the liver [cause one] to call. (51) [The qi it sends] into the heart [cause one] to speak. (52) [The qi it sends] into the spleen [cause one] to sing. (53) [The qi it sends] into the kidneys [cause one] to groan. (54) [The qi it keeps] within itself [cause one] to wail. (55) Hence one knows that if evil [qi] from the lung have entered the heart, they cause [the patient] to talk incoherently and to utter nonsense. (56) The patient will suffer from a hot body, he will shiver, and he will dislike cold. In extreme cases, that leads to panting and coughing. (57) [The movement in] his vessels is at the surface, strong, and rough.

(58) How does one know that [the patient has] contracted [his disease in the heart] because he was struck by moisture?

(59) It is like this. He should have a tendency to sweat without end. Why do I say so? (60) The kidneys rule the liquids. (61) [The liquid that is generated when they send their qi] into the liver is tears. (62) [The liquid that is generated when they send their qi] into the heart is sweat. (63) [The liquid that is generated when they send their qi] into the spleen is saliva. (64) [The liquid that is generated when they send their qi] into the lung is snivel. (65) [The liquid that is generated when they keep their qi] within themselves is spittle. (66) Hence one knows that if evil [qi] from the kidneys have entered the heart, that causes [the patient] to sweat without end. (67) He will suffer from a hot body and from pain in the lower abdomen; his feet and shinbones will be cold, and [the qi will] move contrary to their proper course. (68)

[The movement in] his vessels is deep, soft, and strong. (69) These are the patterns of the five evils.[2]

---

2   This difficult issue presents two different concepts of disease causation. Some commentators have approved of them, others have rejected them as inappropriate. In my own understanding, the first – which is called here "the regular conduits fall ill by themselves" – refers to five different illness causing agents which, if the organism is subjected to them, harm the specific long-term depot associated with them through the system of correspondences. The second concept is much more sophisticated and may not be as old as the first; it could be an innovation introduced by the *Nan jing*. While the first of the two concepts appears to be rather rigid – in that it implies that, for instance, lung diseases are always caused by a cold body or by chilled drinks, while a disease in the spleen cannot result from these causes – the second concept explains that five major pathological agents may affect each long-term depot, either as a primary or as a secondary affection, and that there are specific symptoms allowing one to recognize whether a primary or a secondary affection is involved and which long-term depots are affected. The general idea is that (1) each long-term depot may be subject to a primary affection by an agent associated with it through systematic correspondence, and (2) each long-term depot that has been subject to a primary affection may then send its qi into any other depot, causing a secondary affection there with specific symptoms. The entire scheme, of which only one example is presented in the text, is based on the Five Phases doctrine. The underlying pattern can be tabularized as follows.

Illness causing agent	Primary affection	Secondary affection	Symptoms of secondary affection	Type of symptoms
wind	liver	liver	virid	complexion
		heart	red	
		spleen	yellow	
		lung	white	
		kidneys	black	
heat	heart	liver	fetid	odor
		heart	burnt	
		spleen	aromatic	
		lung	frowzy	
		kidneys	foul	
drinking eating weariness exhaustion	spleen	liver	sour	(preference for) flavor
		heart	bitter	
		spleen	sweet	
		lung	acrid	
		kidneys	salty	
cold	lung	liver	to call	sound
		heart	to speak	
		spleen	to sing	
		lung	to wail	
		kidneys	to groan	
humidity	kidneys	liver	tears	liquid
		heart	sweat	
		spleen	saliva	
		lung	snivel	
		kidneys	spittel	

COMMENTARIES

(1) *Li Jiong*: When the regular conduits are depleted, the pores open. When the pores open, [evil qi] enter [from outside. Such diseases] originate from the [regular conduits] themselves; they are not initiated from the outside. ["To be harmed by any of the five evils" refers to] the mutual destruction among the [long-term depots on the basis of their association with the] Five Phases, [as a result of] harm caused by evil [qi] from outside.

(2) *Ding Deyong*: The heart rules [the movement in the] vessels. In the case of grief and anxiety, thoughts and considerations, the [qi in the] vessels of the heart cannot be spread [through the entire body]; hence the heart will be harmed.

   Lü Guang: The heart is the spirit; it constitutes the lord among the five long-term depots. Intelligence, skills, and wisdom all originate from the heart. If one is severely taxed by grief, that will harm his heart. When the heart is harmed, the spirit is weak.

   Yu Shu: [That which is] responsible for governing everything, [that which is] calm and dispassionate is called "heart." Here, grief and anxiety, thoughts and considerations are present, with no rest. Hence the heart will be harmed.

   Hua Shou: The heart rules the thoughts and the considerations. It represents the lord-ruler among the officials. Hence grief and anxiety, thoughts and considerations cause harm to the heart.

   Zhang Shixian: The heart harbors the spirit; to nourish the heart, nothing is better than to restrain one's desires and grief. Excessive thoughts and considerations will exhaust the spirit and harm the heart.

   Xu Dachun: Thoughts and considerations come from the heart. Hence if one uses them excessively, [the heart] will be harmed.

   Liao Ping: "Heart" stands for "brain"; it rules the thoughts.

(3) *Ding Deyong*: The lung rules the skin [and its] hair; it dislikes to see them being cold. Therefore, when the body is cold and when one's beverages are cold, too, that causes harm to the lung.

   Lü Guang: The lung rules the skin [and its] hair. When the body is cold, the skin [and its] hair are cold, too. Cold drinks harm the lung. The lung rules the intake of water and soups. Water and soups cannot be consumed cold. Also, the lung dislikes cold. Hence [the text] speaks of "harm."

For the movements in the vessels – providing essential supplementary diagnostic information – see also difficult issue 10. The pattern outlined there does not entirely correspond to the pattern outlined in the present difficult issue.

Hua Shou: The lung rules the skin [and its] hair; it is located in the upper [section of the body]. It constitutes a tender depot. Hence, if the body is cold and if one's beverages are chilled, one's lung will be harmed.

Zhang Shixian: The lung rules the qi and it should be warm. "A cold body" [refers to] cold skin [and] hair. When the body is cold outside and when chilled beverages are present inside, the qi do not pass and the lung receives harm.

Xu Dachun: The long-term depot of the lung is basically cold. Hence, if it receives [additional] wind cold from outside and [is affected by] chilled beverages from inside, that will harm the lung.

(4) *Ding Deyong*: The liver rules one's planning and considerations. The gall bladder rules one's courage and decision-making. Hence extreme anger will harm the liver.

Lü Guang: Liver and gall bladder constitute long-term depot and short-term repository. Their qi [constitute] one's courage. Hence, they rule one's anger. If one's anger [is out of control, the liver will be] harmed.

Yu Shu: The *Su wen* states: "In the case of anger, the blood will accumulate in great amounts in the upper [section of the Triple] Burner. That is called a 'flow contrary to the proper direction'." It states further: "In the case of severe anger, one vomits blood. That is caused by qi flowing contrary to their proper direction." Harm is the result.

Hua Shou: The liver rules the anger. In the case of anger, the liver will be harmed.

(5) *Ding Deyong*: The spleen rules [one's preference for a specific] flavor. One drinks and eats fine flavors [to support one's organism]. But if one consumes too much of them without restraint, if one exhausts his strength, and if one is tired to a point that he drags his feet, that will cause harm to his spleen.

Lü Guang: If one drinks and eats to repletion, the stomach is filled with qi. The network [vessel leading to the] spleen will be constantly tense. Or the vessels and the network [vessels] may crack as a result of horse riding, leaping, or because of sexual exhaustion. Hence the spleen will be harmed.

Yu Shu: The spleen is the official responsible for the granaries. The [preferences for any of the] five flavors originate from there. That is to say, [the spleen] receives the five flavors[3] and transforms them, generating the five qi in order to nourish the human body. Here, drinking and eating [without restraint], as well as weariness and exhaustion, have led to harm that is caused by oneself. It is for this reason that the sages paid great attention to a balanced [intake of the] five flavors in order to keep their bones straight and their muscles tender. They

---

3　When reading these statements, it should be kept in mind that the term *wei* 味 ("flavor") also refers to food items as carriers of flavor.

paid great attention to conducting their lives in accordance with the rules. Their [existence on earth through] heavenly mandate was long; how could they ever have done harm to themselves? And how could anybody not be careful on his way of nourishing his life?

Hua Shou: The spleen rules food and beverages and the four limbs. Hence, drinking and eating [without restraint], as well as weariness and exhaustion, harm the spleen.

(6) *Ding Deyong*: The kidneys rule the loins. The loins constitute the repository⁴ of the kidneys. If one sits for an extended period [at a humid location], the qi of the kidneys cannot be spread [through the body]. Hence damage will result. The hole [associated with] the kidneys is located in the center of the sole of the foot; it is called *yong quan* 湧泉. If one resides at a humid location or enters water, [the kidneys] will be harmed as a result. *Qiang li* 強力 ("to exert one's strength") means that one devotes [all his strength] to please his heart and to force the union of yin and yang. As a result, he will harm his kidneys.

Lü Guang: "To sit at a humid place for an extended period" means to meet with grief and mourning. "To exert one's strength" means to lift something heavy or to pull a crossbow. "To go into water" means to repeatedly sink down into water, or to force the union of yin and yang before the menstruation period is over.

Yu Shu: The soil rules the moisture; that is a natural principle. Now, if one sits at a humid place for an extended period, external moisture will enter and affect the kidneys. If it comes together with wind and cold, it will develop into a *zhang* 瘴 disease.⁵ "To exert one's strength" – that is, to overtax oneself – must result in harm which is caused by oneself.⁶ The "Jing mai bie lun" 經脈別論 states that to bear a heavy load and walk over a long distance will harm the kidneys. The [treatise] "Sheng qi tong tian lun" 生氣通天論 states: "Due to exertion of strength, the qi of the kidneys are damaged and the lumbar vertebrae are harmed." The [treatise] "Jing mai bie lun" 經脈別論 states: "When one crosses through water

---

4 Here, the term *fu* 府 ("short-term repository") may have been used not with its usual technical meaning, as in "long-term depots" and "short-term repositories," but simply as a reference to the location of the kidneys.

5 *Zhang* 瘴 diseases are supposed to be caused by the intrusion of so-called *zhang* 瘴 qi into the organism. These are humid qi of mountains and rivers, especially in the southern parts of China. The resulting disease is frequently categorized as a kind of *yao/nue* 瘧 ("malaria"), since the patient suffers from alternating fits of cold and heat. Whether such a disease was implied here cannot be ascertained.

6 The text has *yin* 飲 ("to drink") instead of *shang* 傷 ("harm"). That must be a mistake because the expression *zhi zi shang* 致自傷 appears twice in Yu Shu's comment on sentence 5, and was obviously repeated here.

and when one stumbles and falls to the ground, the [resulting] panting will originate from the kidneys and from the bones."

Hua Shou: The kidneys rule the bones and are associated with water. Hence if one exerts his strength and forces himself to do [certain things], if one sits at a humid place and goes into water, he will harm his kidneys.

(2)–(6) *Hua Shou*: In conclusion, grief, thoughts, rage, anger, drinking and eating, movement and exertion cause these [harms] if they are developed excessively. Of course, man cannot get along without grief, thoughts, rage, anger, food and beverages, movement and exertion. If the development [of these states] remains in a medium range, how could they result in injuries?! However, in the case of excess, harm to man is inevitable. Hence those who are well versed in nourishing their life eliminate extremes and exaggerations. They adapt themselves to the mean, and that is sufficient!

(7) *Ding Deyong*: These five [diseases] result from the regular conduits falling ill by themselves. This means that no outside evils are involved here.

Lü Guang: These are all diseases which develop in the long-term depots themselves; they do not come from outside.

Yu Shu: Mr. Lü has said that these are diseases which develop in the long-term depots themselves; they do not come from outside. That is not the meaning implied [by the *Nan jing*]. If one only takes the example of "a cold body and chilled beverages harm the lung," it means that an external cold affects the skin [and its] hair. Internally, [this cold] comes together with the lung. The [resulting disease, then,] has come from outside. Furthermore, chilled beverages enter the mouth and cause harm to the lung internally. This [disease] has also come from outside. All the other [examples] are based on the same [principle]. The important meaning [implied here] by the sages is that if the regular conduits are depleted, the pores open. When the pores are open, external [qi] affect the interior [of the body]. This is why [the text] states: "The regular conduits fall ill by themselves."

(9) *Ding Deyong*: *Zhong* 中 ("to be hit") stands for *shang* 傷 ("to be harmed"). When [the *Nan jing*] states "to be struck by wind," it means that the liver corresponds to wind. [The liver] rules the color evil. It distributes [its qi] to the five long-term depots, where they become the five colors.

Lü Guang: The liver rules the winds.

Yu Shun: The Eastern regions generate the winds. The winds generate the wood. [Wood] dislikes the winds. Also, [the trigram] *sun* 巽 stands for wood and represents wind.

Hua Shou: Wind is wood; it tends to harm the liver.

(10) *Ding Deyong*: "To be harmed by heat" is to say that the heart corresponds to
heat; it rules the odor evil. It distributes [its qi] to the five long-term depots,
where they become the five odors.

Lü Guang: The heart rules the heat.

Yu Shun: The heart fire rules the heat; it dominates during summer. *Shu* 署 ("heat")
stands for *re* 熱 ("hot"). The *Su wen* states: "If one is harmed by heat in summer,
he will develop cough and fever in autumn."

Hua Shou: Heat is fire; it tends to harm the heart.

(11) *Ding Deyong*: The spleen corresponds to moisture; it rules the flavor evil. It distributes [its qi] to the five long-term depots, where they cause [one's preferences
for any of] the five flavors.

Lü Guang: The spleen rules weariness and exhaustion.

Yu Shu: "The regular conduits fall ill by themselves," [as outlined above], includes
[situations] where drinking and eating [without restraint], as well as weariness
and exhaustion, harm the spleen. Here, drinking and eating, weariness and exhaustion are included among the five evils. "The regular conduits fall ill" means
that the regular conduits are depleted. Also, "to be harmed by drinking and
eating" as a disease caused by the five evils means that eating and drinking cause
harm to the spleen, thus causing a disease.

Hua Shou: The soil is subject to farming; the spleen rules the four limbs. Hence
eating and drinking [without restraint], as well as weariness and exhaustions,
tend to harm the spleen.

Liao Ping: The four characters *yin shi lao juan* 飲食勞倦 ("to drink and to eat
[without restraint], as well as weariness and exhaustion") must be an error of
writing that has occurred in the transmission [of this text]. According to the
fifth [evil mentioned] below – that is, harm due to cold – this here should be
"[harm caused by] warmth."

(12) *Ding Deyong*: The lung rules dryness; its season is extremely clear. It dislikes
cold. It controls the sound evil. It distributes [its qi] to the five long-term depots,
where they become the five sounds.

Lü Guang: The lung controls cold.

Yu Shu: That is to say, the cold affects the skin [and its] hair. Hence, [the text]
speaks of "harmed by cold."

Hua Shou: Cold constitutes the qi of metal; it tends to harm the lung.

(13) *Ding Deyong*: The kidneys correspond to cold; they rule the water evil. They
distribute [their qi] to the five long-term depots where they become the liquids.

Lü Guang: The kidneys rule moisture.

Yu Shu: The moisture of flowing water is [what is] meant here.

Hua Shou: Moisture is water; it tends to harm the kidneys. Dew, rain, and steam are examples [of moisture].

(14) *Lü Guang*: These five diseases come from outside.

(2)–(14) *Xu Dachun*: The two sections above deal separately with diseases [resulting from the conduits falling ill] by themselves and with [those caused by] the five evils. But the distinction is not at all clear. Drinking and eating as well as weariness and exhaustion, harm caused by cold, and to be struck by moisture – these three complexes are discussed in the first section [as well as in the second section]. This means that those diseases [resulting from the conduits falling ill] by themselves are [also those caused by] the five evils, and that [those caused by] the five evils are exactly the diseases [resulting from the conduits falling ill] by themselves. How could one avoid confusion?! The first section [of this difficult issue] consists of the original text of the treatise "Xie qi zang fu bing xing" 邪氣藏府病形 of the *Ling* [*shu*] and of the [treatise] "Ben bing lun" 本病論 of the *Su wen;* only a few characters have been changed. But neither the *Ling* [*shu*] nor the *Su* [*wen*] distinguish between diseases [resulting from the conduits falling ill] by themselves and [those caused by] the five evils. Thus, as far as the two long-term depots heart and liver are concerned, they are discussed in terms of grief and sadness, rage and anger. All the remaining [long-term depots] are discussed in terms of the six evils of excess. For each [long-term depot, the evil] that is important is pointed out. Here another meaning is presented. If one wishes to differentiate, the *Nei jing* itself has a sophisticated meaning that can be considered [for this purpose]. In the [treatise] "Yin yang ying xiang da lun" 陰陽應象大論 of the *Su* [*wen*], it is stated: "Anger harms the liver; joy harms the heart; pensiveness harms the spleen; anxiety harms the lung; fear harms the kidneys." These are truly symptoms of the basic conduits falling ill by themselves. As to effects from outside, the treatise "Jiu zhen" 九鍼 of the *Ling* [*shu*] states: "The liver has an aversion to wind. The heart has an aversion to heat. The lung has an aversion to cold. The kidneys have an aversion to dryness. The spleen has an aversion to dampness." That is a reference to symptoms of harm caused by external evils. Is not this clear and reliable? [The author of the *Nan jing* may have] intended to differentiate [between these two principles of disease causation], but he offered only one and the same principle. Not only does the scope of his argument remain unclear but also the wording is inappropriate. How could it be that an author of those days did not think about this? Or could it be that he searched for but did not get the meaning of the [respective passages in the *Nei jing*]?

(15) *Liao Ping:* This refers to pain in one's brain.[7]

(17) *Yu Shu:* The [trigram] *sun* 巽 represents the wind; it belongs to [the phase of] wood. Hence it rules [whether one is] struck by the wind. [The liver corresponds to] the flower calyx of the woods; it distributes the five colors. It produces the five evil [qi leading to the generation of the five colors], as is outlined below.

(18) *Yu Shu:* That is case when the conduit [associated with] wood has fallen ill by itself.

(19) *Yu Shu:* If evil [qi sent out by the] liver enter the heart, the [patient's] complexion will be red.

(20) *Yu Shu:* If evil [qi sent out by the] liver enter the spleen, the [patient's] complexion will be yellow.

(21) *Yu Shu:* If evil [qi sent out by the] liver enter the lung, the [patient's] complexion will be white.

(22) *Yu Shu:* If evil [qi sent out by the] liver enter the kidneys, the [patient's] complexion will be black.

(23) *Lü Guang:* The liver rules [whether one is] struck by wind. The heart rules harm due to heat. Here, the heart suffers from being struck by wind. Hence one knows that evil [qi] from the liver have moved to the heart, causing harm there.

(24) *Lü Guang:* A hot body [points to] the heart; fullness and pain [point to] the liver. The symptoms [described here] are those of a disease affecting these two long-term depots.

  Yu Shu: The heart rules harm due to heat. If one suffers from such a disease, the body will be hot. The liver spreads through both flanks. Hence, if one perceives fullness in his flanks, that is [a sign that the qi of] the liver have seized the heart.

(25) *Lü Guang:* [A movement that is] at the surface and strong [points to] the heart; a string-like [movement points to] the liver. The [movements associated with the] vessels of both long-term depots can be seen because they correspond [to the respective disease that has affected these two long-term depots].

(15)–(25) *Zhang Shixian:* This [section] discusses diseases in the heart which result from one's being struck by wind. A disease resulting from being struck by wind is first contracted by the liver. The colors are ruled by the liver. When evil [qi sent out by the] liver enter the heart, the complexion of the [patient] will be red.

(26) *Yu Shu:* The heart is the fire. When fire transforms things, the five odors emerge.

(29) *Yu Shu:* The nature of fire is to flame upward. When it generates a burnt odor, that is called "the regular conduit has fallen ill by itself."

(30) *Yu Shu:* When fire transforms soil, the respective odor is aromatic.

---

7 Liao Ping's *Nan jing* edition has *xin tong* 心痛 ("pain in the heart") in sentence 15 instead of *xin bing* 心病 ("illness in the heart").

(31) *Yu Shu*: When fire transforms wood, the respective odor is fetid.

(32) *Yu Shu*: When fire transforms water, the respective odor is foul.

(33) *Yu Shu*: When fire transforms metal, the respective odor is frowzy.

(34) *Yu Shu*: The heart rules the heat. Here, harm was caused by heat. That is [a case in which] the regular conduit has fallen ill by itself; it was not struck by an evil from somewhere else.

(26)–(34) *Zhang Shixian*: This [section] discusses diseases in the heart which result from harm due to heat. A disease resulting from harm caused by heat is first contracted by the heart. The heart is the fire. When fire transforms the five items, the five odors originate. Hence the odors are ruled by the fire. When the fire of the heart flames excessively, it generates a burnt [odor] and a bitter [flavor]. A bitter [flavor] is associated with the heart; a burnt [odor] is also associated with the heart. The evil in the heart has originated from the heart itself, hence [the odor] is burnt.

(39) *Yu Shu*: The spleen rules the flavors. In case one is ill because evil [qi from the spleen] have seized the liver, he will prefer [to consume] sour flavor.

(40) *Yu Shu*: The spleen rules the flavors. In case one is ill because evil [qi from the spleen] have attacked the heart, he will prefer [to consume] bitter flavor.

(41) *Yu Shu*: The spleen rules the flavors. In case one is ill because evil [qi from the spleen] have attacked the lung, he will prefer [to consume] acrid flavor.

(42) *Yu Shu*: The spleen rules the flavors. In case one is ill because evil [qi from the spleen] have attacked the kidneys, he will prefer [to consume] salty flavor.

(43) *Yu Shu*: Soil means sowing and reaping. If the basic conduit has fallen ill by itself, he will prefer [to consume] sweet flavor.

(44) *Lü Guang*: The heart rules harm due to heat. The spleen rules weariness and exhaustion. Here, a disease in the heart has been contracted as a result of [unrestrained] drinking and eating, as well as weariness and exhaustion. Hence one knows that evil [qi] from the spleen have entered the heart.

(45) *Lü Guang*: A hot body [points to] the heart. A heavy body [points to] the spleen. The symptoms [described here] are those of a disease affecting these two long-term depots.

(46) *Lü Guang*: [A movement in the] vessels that is at the surface and strong [points to] the heart. A relaxed [movement in the] vessels [points to the] spleen.

(35)–(46) *Zhang Shixian*: This [section] discusses diseases in the heart which result from [unrestrained] drinking and eating, from weariness and exhaustion. Diseases [due to unrestrained] drinking and eating, as well [as those due to] weariness and exhaustion, are first contracted by the spleen. When the spleen is depleted, there is no desire to eat; when the spleen is replete, there will be a desire to eat. Hence the flavors are ruled by the spleen. When evil [qi from the] spleen enter the heart, one prefers [to consume] bitter drinks and food. The flavors are associated with the spleen; a bitter [flavor] is associated with the heart.

Ye Lin: When the spleen is depleted, it has no qi that could transform the grains; [when the spleen is] replete, it can transform the grains. Hence there is the difference between [situations where] one can eat and others where one cannot eat.

(49) *Yu Shu*: If one hits against any of the five metals, that will [create] a sound. Hence the five sounds originate from the lung.

(50) *Yu Shu*: Wood fears metal, hence it "calls" out. *Qixuan zi* 啓玄子 states: "*Hu* 呼 ('to call') can also be *xiao* 嘯 ('to scream')."

(51) *Yu Shu*: Here [the text] says *yan* 言 ("to speak"). The *Su wen* says *xiao* 笑 ("to laugh"). That is to say, metal and fire fit each other. That is like husband and wife seeing each other. Hence they will speak [to each other or] laugh.

(52) *Yu Shu*: The soil is the mother; the metal is the child. [Here] mother and child see each other. Hence the meaning of "singing."

(53) *Yu Shu*: The metal is the mother, the water is the child. When the child sees the mother, it will produce sounds of happy groaning.

(54) *Yu Shu*: The lung rules during autumn. *Qiu* 秋 ("autumn") stands for *chou* 愁 ("grief"). The respective [musical] note is *shang* 商 [The note] *shang* 商 stands for *shang* 傷 ("injury"). Hence the [sound it produces] itself is wailing.

(55) *Lü Guang*: The heart rules the heat. The lung rules the cold. [In this case a disease in the heart] has been contracted due to harm caused by cold. Hence one knows that evil [qi] from the lung have entered the heart, causing a disease there.

(56) *Lü Guang*: A hot body [points to] the heart. A dislike of cold [points to] the lung. The symptoms [described here] are those of a disease affecting these two long-term depots.

(57) *Lü Guang*: [A movement in the] vessels that is at the surface and strong [points to the] heart; [a movement in the] vessels that is rough [points to the] lung.

(47)–(57) *Zhang Shixian*: This section discusses diseases in the heart which result from harm caused by cold. A disease of being harmed by cold is first contracted by the lung. The sounds are ruled by the lung. When evil [qi from the] lung enter the heart, the respective sound is [that it causes one to] speak. The sounds are associated with the lung; speaking is associated with the heart.

(60) *Ding Deyong*: The kidneys rule the water. Water is transformed into the five liquids.

Yu Shu: The kidneys rule the water. Water constitutes flowing moisture. Hence all the five kinds of moisture originate from the kidneys.

(61) *Yu Shu*: When mourning and sympathy move one's center, his *hun* 魂 will be harmed. When the *hun* is harmed, one will be moved and tears will flow. That is to say, the lung rules the mourning. If one mourns, there will be a surplus of metal. The wood fears this. The water is the mother of wood. The mother feels sorry for her child. Hence [when the evil qi of the kidneys have entered] the liver, they will cause tears.

(62) *Yu Shu*: When water and fire come into close contact, the resulting steam will produce sweating.

(63) *Yu Shu*: The soil is the husband; the water is the wife. When a wife follows her husband, saliva will be produced.[8]

(64) *Yu Shu*: The northern regions produce the cold. The cold produces the kidneys. Here, cold has affected skin and hair; internally, it has come into contact with the lung. When the lung is affected by cold, snivel results. From this one knows that [evil qi from the kidneys] entering the lung cause snivel.

(65) *Yu Shu*: The vessel of the kidneys moves upward and is tied to the tongue. Hence it produces spittle. That is six on second place in the center of the [trigram] *li* 離. This then [is a case in which] the regular conduit has fallen ill by itself.

(66) *Lü Guang*: The heart rules the heat. The kidneys rule the moisture. Here, the heart has contracted a disease due to harm caused by moisture. Hence one knows that evil [qi] from the kidneys have entered the heart.

(67) *Lü Guang*: A hot body [points to] the heart. Pain in the lower abdomen [points to] the kidneys. [In this case] evil [qi] from the kidneys have attacked the heart. The symptoms [described here] are those of a disease affecting these two long-term depots.

(68) *Lü Guang*: A strong [movement in the] vessels points to the heart. A deep and soft [movement] in the vessels [points to] the kidneys.

(58)–(68) *Zhang Shixian*: This [section] discusses diseases in the heart which result from being struck by moisture. A disease of being struck by moisture is first contracted by the kidneys. Moisture is ruled by the kidneys. When evil [qi from the] kidneys enter the heart, sweat will come out without end. Nothing can stop it. Moisture is associated with the kidneys; sweat is associated with the heart.

(69) *Xu Dachun*: The general message conveyed here is that diseases in the liver are indicated by one's complexion, diseases in the heart are indicated by one's odors, diseases in the spleen are indicated by one's [preference for a specific] flavor, diseases in the lung are indicated by one's sounds, and diseases in the kidneys are

---

8   This is a metaphorical etymology of the character *xian* 涎 ("saliva"), which can be considered as consisting of the elements "soil" (*tu* 土), "to move on" (*yin* 廴), and "water" (*shui* 水).

indicated by [the kind of] liquid [the body produces]. As far as the [movement in the] vessels is concerned, the [movement in the] vessels associated with the basic long-term depot [that has fallen ill] dominates; a vessel [movement associated with the long-term depot] that has accepted the evil [in the first place] accompanies [the dominant movement).

Liao Ping: It is quite possible to set up a doctrine to the effect that each of the five long-term depots represents a distinct department [with its specific symptoms in the case of disease], and to present one example [as is done here]. However, it is most difficult to distinguish the sounds, the complexions, the odors, and the [preferences for a specific] flavor [characterizing a particular person]. There are always contradictions. Sometimes these [symptoms] are obvious, sometimes they are not. Since Jin and Song times, the [diagnostic] patterns of medicine have become increasingly complex day by day, and they have become increasingly chaotic day by day. On the whole, the Five Phases [doctrine] serves to legitimate all this.

五十難曰：（一）病有虛邪，有實邪，有賊邪，有微邪，有正邪，何以別之？（二）然：從後來者為虛邪，（三）從前來者為實邪，（四）從所不勝來者為賊邪，（五）從所勝來者為微邪，（六）自病者為正邪。（七）何以言之？（八）假令心病，中風得之為虛邪，（九）傷暑得之為正邪，（十）飲食勞倦得之為實邪，（十一）傷寒得之為微邪，（十二）中濕得之為賊邪。

The fiftieth difficult issue: (1) Among the diseases are the depletion evil, the repletion evil, the robber evil, the weakness evil, and the regular evil. How can they be distinguished?

(2) It is like this. Those [diseases] coming from behind represent a depletion evil; (3) those coming from ahead represent a repletion evil; (4) those coming from what cannot be overcome represent a robber evil; (5) those coming from what can be overcome represent a weakness evil. (6) If the [respective depot] is afflicted from within itself, that represents a regular evil. (7) Why do I say so? (8) Take a disease in the heart as an example. If it was contracted because [the patient] was struck by wind, that represents a depletion evil. (9) If it was contracted because [the patient] was harmed by heat, that represents a regular evil. (10) If it was contracted because of [unrestrained] drinking and eating, or because of weariness and exhaustion, that represents a repletion evil. (11) If it was contracted because [the patient] was harmed by cold, that represents a weakness evil. (12) If it was contracted because [the patient] was struck by moisture, that represents a robber evil.[1]

COMMENTARIES

(2) *Ding Deyong*: Take a disease in the heart as an example: If it has been contracted because [evil qi] have come from the vessel of the liver to seize [the heart], that constitutes a "depletion evil." The liver represents the mother; the heart represents the child. A child is capable of causing a depletion in its mother. Hence [the text] states: "Those coming from behind represent a depletion evil."

Lü Guang: At a time when the heart dominates, the [movement in the] vessels should be vast, strong, and extended. If, in contrast, one perceives a string-like, weak, and tense [movement], that indicates that the wood of the liver extends its domination to the heart and strips the heart of its dominating [position]. That is

1 The fiftieth difficult issue further develops the concepts of the preceding two treatises. Supplementing the diagnostic and pathological data provided in difficult issues 48 and 49, the present treatise introduces (again on the basis of the Five Phases doctrine) new terms denoting the five possible origins of evil qi in case a specific long-term depot has fallen ill. This is, once again, the concept of primary and secondary affliction. The theoretical pattern underlying the present discourse is depicted graphically as follows:

to say, the liver [qi] proceed toward and seize the heart. Hence [the text] speaks of a "coming from behind." The liver represents the mother of the heart. When a mother seizes a child, that constitutes a "depletion evil."

Zhang Shixian: The origins of [these] diseases are all different; thus, the names of the evils [causing them] are different too. Let us take the long-term depot of the heart as an example to discuss this. A disease in the heart [which is associated with the phase of] fire [may have] resulted from the arrival of evil [qi] from the liver, [which is associated with the phase of] wood. Fire is generated by wood. This represents [a disease] that has come from behind. In fire is wood; wood is capable of checking soil. If no soil is present, the water will arrive.[2] Hence [this disease] represents a "depletion evil."

Liao Ping: The [*Nei*] *jing* refers to a robber wind. Hence it [can] say that it "comes." In the case of cold, heat, moisture, and so forth, one cannot say that they "come."

(3) *Ding Deyong*: [If the disease in the heart has been contracted because evil qi] have come from the vessel of the spleen to seize [the heart], that constitutes a "repletion evil." The heart represents the mother; the spleen represents the child. A mother is capable of causing repletion in her child. Hence [the text] states: "Those coming from ahead represent a repletion evil."

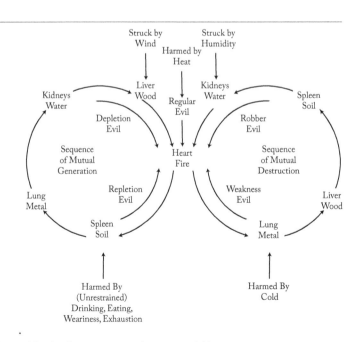

2   This could refer, for instance, to the image of dikes.

Lü Guang: That is to say, at a time when the heart dominates, one perceives a [movement in the] vessels [that is associated with the] spleen. Once the [period of] domination of the heart is concluded, its [dominating position] should be transferred to the spleen. Here – before the domination [period] of the heart was concluded – the [qi from the] spleen arrive, flowing contrary to their proper direction, to seize this domination. Hence [the text] speaks of a "coming from ahead." The spleen represents the child of the heart. When a child seizes its mother, that constitutes a "repletion evil."

Zhang Shixian: [A disease in the heart may have] resulted from the arrival of evil [qi] from the spleen [which is associated with the phase of] soil. Soil is generated by fire. This represents [an evil] that has come from ahead. In fire is soil;[3] the water cannot arrive and, as a consequence, it cannot subdue the evil.[4] Hence [this disease] represents a "repletion evil"

(4) *Ding Deyong*: Fire cannot overcome water. Hence, when a disease in the heart results from [the fact that evil qi from the] vessel of the kidneys have come to seize [the heart], that constitutes a "robber evil."

Lü Guang: One perceives a [movement in the] vessels [that is associated with the] kidneys during the domination [period] of the heart. Water overcomes fire. Hence this constitutes a "robber evil."

Zhang Shixian: [A disease in the heart may have] resulted from the arrival of evil [qi] from the kidneys, [which are associated with the phase of] water. Water is capable of overpowering fire. This represents [a disease] that has come from what cannot be overcome. Hence it constitutes a "robber evil."

(5) *Ding Deyong*: Fire can overcome metal. Hence, when a disease in the heart results from [the fact that evil qi from the] vessel of the lung have come to seize [the heart], that is called a "weakness evil."

Lü Guang: One perceives – contrary [to what would be proper] – a [movement in the] vessels [that is associated with the] lung during the domination [period] of the heart. Fire overcomes metal. Hence this constitutes a "weakness evil"

Zhang Shixian: [A disease in the heart may have] resulted from the arrival of evil [qi] from the lung, [which is associated with the phase of] metal. Fire can overcome metal. This represents [a disease] that has come from what can be overcome. What can be overcome cannot cause harm. Hence [this disease] represents a "weakness evil."

---

3   This could refer to the image that fire creates ashes (i.e., soil).

4   The text states *mu neng zhi gui* 木能制鬼 ("the wood can keep the demons in check"). This could be understood as a reference to peach wood, which is associated with apotropaic powers against demons. However, in the present context, *mu neng zhi gui* is probably a mistake for *bu neng zhi xie* 不能制邪 ("cannot subdue the evil").

(6) *Ding Deyong*: If no evil [qi] from another [source] are present which have seized [the afflicted depot], that indicates a "regular evil."

Lü Guang: As long as the heart dominates, the [movement in the] vessels is replete, vigorous, and greatly excessive. If, in contrast, one perceives a depleted and slight [movement in the vessels], that indicates a "regular evil."

Zhang Shixian: If one has contracted a disease that is limited to the heart, that is [a situation where] the regular conduit has fallen ill itself; no evil [qi] from another [source have come] to attack. Hence [this disease] represents a regular evil. The same applies to all the other long-term depots.

(8) *Zhang Shixian*: This [section] uses a disease in the heart as an example to once again explain the meaning of the text above. In the case of [harm caused by] being struck by wind, the liver, [which is associated with the phase of] wood, has contracted the disease first.

(9) *Lü Guang*: The heart rules the heat. Here the heart itself suffers from harm caused by heat. Hence this represents a "regular evil."

Zhang Shixian: In the case of harm caused by heat, the heart, [which is associated with the phase of] fire, has contracted the disease first.

(10) *Lü Guang*: "Those coming from ahead" means that [qi of] the spleen have seized the heart. The spleen rules weariness and exhaustion. Hence this represents a "repletion evil."

Zhang Shixian: In the case of [harm caused by unrestrained] drinking and eating, weariness and exhaustion, the spleen, [which is associated with the phase of] soil, has contracted the disease first.

(11) *Lü Guang*: "Those coming from what can be overcome" means that [qi of] the lung have seized the heart. The lung rules the cold; furthermore, it fears the heart. Hence this represents a "weakness evil."

Zhang Shixian: In the case of harm caused by cold, the lung, [which is associated with the phase of] metal, has contracted the disease first.

(12) *Lü Guang*: "Those coming from what cannot be overcome" means that [qi of] the kidneys have seized the heart. The kidneys rule the moisture. Water overpowers fire. Hence this represents a "robber evil."

Zhang Shixian: In the case of [harm caused by] being struck by moisture, the kidneys, [which are associated with the phase of] water, have contracted the disease first.

(7)–(12) *Ding Deyong*: The cold in heaven becomes the water on earth, and it constitutes the kidneys in man. The kidneys rule water and cold. The wind in heaven becomes the wood on earth, and it constitutes the liver in man. The liver rules the wind. The warmth and heat in heaven become the fire on earth, and they constitute the heart in man. The heart rules the heat. The dryness in heaven becomes the metal on earth, and it constitutes the lung in man. The lung rules the dryness. The moisture in heaven becomes the soil on earth, and it constitutes the spleen in man. The spleen rules the moisture. This constitutes the mutual penetration of the three powers heaven, earth, and man. Here, the [*Nan*] *jing* links cold with the lung, moisture with the kidneys, and drinking and eating, weariness and exhaustion with the spleen. The meaning of these three [statements] is somewhat deficient; their message is not outlined in detail.

Xu Dachun: The [treatise] "Ba zheng shen ming lun" 八正神明論 of the *Su* [*wen*] states: "The depletion evil, this is the depletion evil of the eight cardinal [turning points]. As for the 'evil of the [eight] cardinal [turning points],' [this is to say] when the body is exerted and sweat flows and when the interstice structures open, [and meet with depletion wind, …]" Hence, the so-called depletion evil constitutes [in the *Su wen*] the "depletion wind." Those [winds] rushing against the short-term repository where *Tai yi⁵* 太乙 resides represent "depletion winds." A "regular wind" is a wind which is received when the pores open because sweat flows out. The details can be seen in the treatise "Jiu gong ba feng" 九宮八風 of the *Ling shu.* The [explanation given there] does not correspond to what is said here about depletion evil and regular evil. But there is no reason why one should not adopt the [old] terms and provide them with a different meaning.⁶

---

5   Book 28 of the *Tai su* refers to a spirit called Tai yi which resides successively in eight different palaces in the eight cardinal directions for almost equal lengths of time each year, concluding one full cycle. This spirit moves from one palace to the next on the eight seasonal dates dividing a year. A wind that comes, on these dates, from the direction of the palace where Tai yi is supposed to take his residence, promises repletion; a wind that comes from the opposite direction indicates depletion. These concepts may mirror ancient agricultural experiences and divination practices that found their way into medicine. See also *Ling shu* treatise 58, "Zei feng 賊風"; *Ling shu* treatise 79, "Sui lu lun" 崴路論; and Unschuld, *Medicine in China: A History of Ideas,* 68-73 and 263-267.

6   Liao Ping commented on this statement: "It seems as if Mr. Xu has tolerated these mistaken doctrines!"

五十一難曰：（一）病有欲得溫者，有欲得寒者，（二）有欲得見人者，有不欲得見人者，而各不同，病在何藏府也？

（三）然：病欲得寒，而欲見人者，病在府也；（四）病欲得溫，而不欲得見人者，病在藏也。（五）何以言之？府者陽也，陽病欲得寒，又欲見人；（六）藏者陰也，陰病欲得溫，又欲閉戶獨處，惡聞人聲，（七）故以別知藏府之病也。

The fifty-first difficult issue: (1) In the case of a disease one may desire warmth or one may desire cold; (2) there are those who desire to see other people, and there are others who [in the case of a disease] do not desire to see anybody. With all these different [desires], in which long-term depots or short-term repositories are the [respective] diseases?

(3) It is like this. If, in the case of a disease, one desires cold, or if one desires to see people, the disease is in the [body's] short-term repositories. (4) If, in the case of a disease, one desires warmth, or if one does not desire to see anybody, the disease is in the [body's] long-term depots. (5) Why do I say so? The short-term repositories are yang; in the case of a yang disease one desires cold and, further, one desires to see people. (6) The long-term depots are yin; in the case of a yin disease one desires warmth and, further, one desires to close the doors and live by himself. One dislikes to hear other people's voices. (7) Hence, with [these different desires in mind] one knows how to distinguish whether a disease has affected the long-term depots or the short-term repositories.[1]

COMMENTARIES

(1) *Li Jiong*: In the case of a disease, one may have a desire to be at a warm place, or one may have a desire to be at a cold place.

   Liao Ping: This is elucidated in the [*Nei*] *jing* with great clarity. Why should one pose this question?

(4) *Li Jiong*: The long-term depots are associated with yin. Hence, if the disease is in the long-term depots, one desires warmth and does not wish to see anybody.

(5) *Ding Deyong*: The three yin and the three yang [conduits] of the hands correspond to heaven; they rule warmth, heat, and dryness. In the case of a disease

---

1 For comparison, see difficult issue 9. The allegation of conservative commentators like Liao Ping that the *Nan jing* focuses exclusively on a diagnosis of the movement in the vessels appears unfounded. The first twenty-two difficult issues emphasize a diagnosis of the movement in the vessels, but there are also references in the *Nan jing* as to how to take into account a person's complexion, feelings, odors, pitch of voice, and so forth, in one's assessment of his disease.

[in these conduits], one has a desire for cold. Now, yang means brilliance. For this reason one wishes to see other people [in the case of yang diseases. In the body] the yang constitutes the short-term repositories; hence [the text] states: "The disease is in the short-term repositories."

Ji Tianxi: The short-term repositories represent the yang. In the case of a yang disease, heat is present in surplus, while one's cold is insufficient. Hence, in drinking and eating, in one's clothing and in one's place of residence one always looks for cold. The yang rules the movement and corresponds to the outside. Hence one desires to see people.

(6) *Ding Deyong:* The three yin and the three yang [conduits] of the feet correspond to the earth; they rule winds, cold, and moisture. Hence, in the case of a disease [in these conduits], one has a desire for warmth. The yin rules the long-term depots. Hence one does not wish to see other people.

Li Jiong: The yin rules the interior. Hence one desires to close the doors and to live by himself inside.[2] The yin rules quietude. Hence one dislikes to hear the voices of other people.

Ji Tianxi: The long-term depots represent the yin. In the case of a yin disease, cold is present in surplus, while one's heat is insufficient. Hence, in drinking and eating, in one's clothing and in one's place of residence one always looks for warmth. The yin rules quietude and corresponds to the inside. Hence one desires to close the doors, to live by himself, and he dislikes to hear the voices of other people.

(1)–(7) *Xu Dachun:* In the [treatise] "Yang ming mai jie lun" 陽明脈解論 of the *Su [wen]* it is stated: "In the case of a disease in] the yang brilliance vessels, one dislikes other people and fire." Here [the *Nan jing*] states: "[In the case of a yang disease] one desires to see other people." Why do the meanings [of these two statements] directly contradict each other? Well, [in the *Su wen*] it is pointed out that if just the one conduit of yang brilliance [is affected by a disease], extreme heat and disturbance [develop]. Here, [the *Nan jing*] discusses the diseases of the short-term repositories and long-term depots in general terms. That is to say, of the proper meaning of yin and yang, the [*Nei*] *jing* has emphasized only one aspect, while [the *Nan jing*] here discusses the general outline. The meaning itself is, indeed, not affected.

Katō Bankei: The discourse recorded in this treatise focuses on the feelings that [become apparent in] one's desires, and on the utilization [of these feelings] in order to distinguish whether a disease has affected the long-term depots or the short-term repositories. In winter one drinks hot beverages, in summer one

---

2　The text has *wai* 外 ("outside"). That must be a mistake.

drinks water. One's normal feelings cause him to [have desires] like this. In the case of a disease one's feelings should similarly [guide his desires on the basis of his needs]. Now, in winter the yang [qi] lie hidden and the yin [qi] flourish. Hence there are few qi in the external [yang sections] of the body, while a surplus [of yin qi] is present in the interior [sections. A situation of] so-called yang depletion entails being cold in the external [sections of the body; in case of] yin abundance, one is cold in the internal [sections of the organism]. When both the internal and the external [sections] are cold, one wishes to drink hot beverages because he seeks warmth. In summer the yin lies [hidden] in the depth, while the yang is at the surface. Hence there is fullness in the external [sections of the organism] and emptiness in the internal [sections. In a situation of] so-called yang abundance, one is hot in the external [sections of the organism; in case of] yin depletion, one is hot in the internal [sections]. When both the internal and the external [sections of the organism] are hot, one wishes to drink water in order to take in some cold. These are one's feelings under regular circumstances. The same applies all the more to one's feelings in the case of a disease!

Liao Ping: This book is quite self-contradictory in its discussions of how to examine the long-term depots and short-term repositories, and in the way it sets up patterns to be taught [to physicians. Its concepts] cannot be applied in practice. All its doctrines, [such as the one indicating that] one can examine – at the inch opening – only the long-term depots but not the short-term repositories, are wrong.

五十二難曰：（一）府藏發病，根本等不？

（二）然：不等也。

（三）其不等奈何？

（四）然：藏病者，止而不移，其病不離其處；（五）府病者，彷彿賁嚮，上下行流，居處無常。（六）故以此知藏府根本不同也。

The fifty-second difficult issue: (1) When diseases develop in the [body's] short-term repositories and long-term depots, are they basically the same?

(2) It is like this. They are not [always] the same.

(3) Why is it that they are not [always] the same?

(4) It is like this. A disease [that develops] in a long-term depot is static and does not move; such a disease does not leave its place. (5) A disease [that develops] in a short-term repository runs around; it flows up and down and does not stay at any place permanently. (6) From this one knows that [diseases that develop in the] long-term depots and short-term repositories are basically different.

COMMENTARIES

(1) *Xu Dachun*: This refers to material diseases, like constipation. Hence [the text] speaks of a "basis."

Liao Ping: The meaning [of the present difficult issue] is identical with that of the fifty-fifth difficult issue below. Mr. Xu [Dachun] was right when he suggested that the two be brought together into one paragraph.

(4) *Ding Deyong*: Diseases in the long-term depots represent the yin. The yin rules quietude. Hence [such diseases] are static and do not move.

Lü Guang: The long-term depots represent the yin; they reflect[1] the earth. Hence they do not move.

Xu Dachun: In the case of a disease in a long-term depot, either the [material] body of that long-term depot is damaged or the qi of that long-term depot have received a disease. Basically, the five long-term depots do not emit and do not take in. Hence their diseases occupy their positions permanently and do not move.

(5) *Ding Deyong*: Diseases in the short-term repositories represent the yang. [The yang] rules movement. Hence [such diseases] flow up and down and do not stay at any place permanently.

1　The text has *jue* 決 ("to decide"). That must be a mistake for *fa* 法 ("to reflect").

Lü Guang: The short-term repositories represent the yang. The yang reflects heaven. The heaven revolves without break. Hence the diseases [of the short-term repositories] flow around; they do not stay at any place permanently.

Xu Dachun: "A disease in the short-term repositories" [means that one of the] six short-term repositories has received a disease. [Such diseases] move here and there and are immaterial. *Ben xiang* 賁嚮 means "to move vigorously and noisily." Suddenly they move up, suddenly they move down; they do not occupy any fixed position. The [function of the] six short-term repositories is to drain and not to store. Their qi are never fixed permanently [at one place]. Hence the same applies to their diseases.[2]

(1)–(6) *Ding Jin:* The question raised here is whether diseases that develop in the short-term repositories and in the long-term depots have the same basis. That is a discourse on the sources of the development of "accumulations" and "concentrations." It is designed to introduce the meaning of the following paragraph.[3] *Gen ben* 根本 ("basis") means that accumulations [of qi in the body] have a basis. *Bu deng* 不等 ("not the same") means that collections [of qi in the body] do not have a basis.[4] "Is static and does not move; [such a disease] does not leave its place" – that is to say, accumulations have a basis. Hence they do not leave [their place of origin]; they do not move. [A disease] "runs around; it flows up and down" – that is to say, concentrations have no basis. Hence they run around and flow [from one place to another].

---

2   The text says *bing ti* 病體 (literally, "the body of the illness"). Xu may have chosen this term because he assumed a material character for the diseases discussed here.

3   Ding Jin, and also Katō Bankei, listed the present difficult issue as difficult issue 54.

4   The concepts of "accumulation" and "collection" are introduced in difficult issue 55.

五十三難曰：（一）經言七傳者死，間藏者生，何謂也？

（二）然：七傳者，傳其所勝也。間藏者，傳其子也。（三）何以言之？假令心病傳肺，肺傳肝，肝傳脾，脾傳腎，腎傳心，一藏不再傷，故言七傳者死也。（四）間藏者，傳其所生也。假令心病傳脾，脾傳肺，肺傳腎，腎傳肝，肝傳心，是母子相傳，竟而復始，如環之無端，故言生也。

The fifty-third difficult issue: (1) The scripture states: [Diseases that are] transmitted through seven [long-term depots will result in] death; [diseases] that skip a long-term depot [in their transmission through the organism will not take the patient's] life. What does that mean?

(2) It is like this. [Diseases that are] transmitted through seven [long-term depots] are those that are transmitted to the [depot] that can be overcome, while [diseases] that skip a long-term depot [in their transmission through the organism] are those that are transmitted to the child [long-term depot of the transmitting depot]. (3) Why do I say so? Consider, for example, a disease in the heart. It is transmitted to the lung. The lung transmits it to the liver. The liver transmits it to the spleen. The spleen transmits it to the kidneys. The kidneys transmit it to the heart. One long-term depot cannot be harmed twice. Hence it is stated: [Diseases that are] transmitted through seven [long-term depots will result in] death. (4) [Diseases] that skip a long-term depot [in their transmission through the organism] are transmitted to those [long-term depots] which are generated [by the transmitting depot]. Consider, for example, a disease in the heart. It is transmitted to the spleen. The spleen transmits it to the lung. The lung transmits it to the kidneys. The kidneys transmit it to the liver. The liver transmits it to the heart. In that case, transmission takes place between child and mother [long-term depots]; when it reaches the end [of the cycle] it will begin anew, as in a ring without beginning or end. Hence it is stated [that such diseases will not take the patient's] life.[1]

---

1 The *Nan jing* may be called *the* classic of systematic correspondence; the intention of its author(s) to expand the paradigm of systematic correspondence to all aspects of diagnostics, physiology, pathology, and (in the final chapters) treatment is obvious. The consistent application of the Five Phases doctrine in the *Nan jing*, as in the present difficult issue, irritated conservative commentators because it greatly exceeds the limits set by the *Nei jing*. It is difficult to decide whether the character *qi* 七 ("seven") in sentences 1 through 3 is indeed a mistake for *ci* 次 ("consecutively") as some commentators have claimed. Both alternatives can be interpreted on the basis of the Five Phases doctrine. The pattern of the sequences of mutual generation and destruction of the Five Phases which is alluded to in the text and in the commentaries is the following:

(3) *Ding Deyong*: The [*Nan*] *jing* speaks first of "[diseases] transmitted through seven [long-term depots that will end in] death" and then of "[diseases] that skip a long-term depot [in their transmission through the organism and will not take the patient's] life." When it speaks of a transmission through seven [long-term depots], it refers to the five long-term depots that represent the yin. They transmit [the disease] to the [depot] which they can overcome. [The statement on diseases] that skip one long-term depot [in their transmission through the organism] refers to the six short-term repositories that represent the yang. Hence [in their case] transmission [of a disease] occurs toward those that are generated [by the transmitting entity]. Both the five long-term depots and the six short-term repositories correspond to the Five Phases. When transmission occurs toward those which are generated, there will be life; when transmission occurs toward those that can be overcome, there will be death. That is to say, when [the heart transmits the disease] to the lung [for the second time], the lung will die and will not transmit [the disease] further. Hence "one long-term depot cannot be harmed twice."

Lü Guang: Qi 七 ("seven") must be a mistake for *ci* 次 ("consecutively"). Further down is the character *jian* 閒 ("to skip"). Hence one knows that the one above should read *ci* 次. Also, there are five long-term depots with only the heart being harmed twice. That adds up to a transmission through six [long-term depots. The meaning implied here is] such that transmission occurs consecutively be-

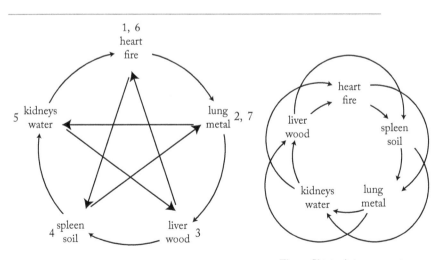

Zhang Shixian's interpretation

tween those long-term depots that overcome each other. Hence such diseases [will end in] death.

Yu Shu: The character *qi* 七 ("seven") in "[diseases that are] transmitted through seven [long-term depots will result in] death" is perfectly clear. Mr. Lü [Guang] reads it as *ci* 次. That is a grave mistake. Also, the pronunciations [of these two characters] do not even come close to each other. Here I shall clarify [the meaning implied] to demonstrate it to students of later times. That is to say, if one counts the [steps in the cycle of the] mutual generation of the Five Phases, one will reach the total number of five. Then one counts twice again, reaching [the number] two, which adds up [with five] to seven. The Five [Phases mentioned] above transmit [the disease] up to the seventh [position in their cycle]. The seventh is the one that becomes overpowered [by the original transmitter]. Hence [the text] speaks of "death." [I] shall provide an example now to elucidate this. Let us enumerate the mutual generation [sequence]. We enumerate wood, fire, soil, metal, water, wood, and fire. The fifth was the character for water. It is separated by the sixth character – that is, wood – from coming to overpower the seventh – that is, fire. Fire is overpowered by water. Hence [the text] speaks of a transmission [of the disease] through seven [long-term depots]. Further down, the text speaks of *jian zang* 間藏 ("skipping a long-term depot"). That is, the fifth character, which is water, transmits [the disease] to the sixth character, which is wood. Obviously, [water and wood are linked to each other through] the mutual generation [sequence of the Five Phases]. Hence [the text] states: "[Diseases] that skip a long-term depot [in their transmission through the organism will not take the patient's] life."

Hua Shou: Mr. Ji [Tianxi] states: "The fire of the heart transmits [the disease] to the metal of the lung; the metal of the lung transmits [the disease] to the wood of the liver; the wood of the liver transmits [the disease] to the soil of the spleen; the soil of the spleen transmits [the disease] to the water of the kidneys; the water of the kidneys transmits [the disease] to the fire of the heart. When the fire of the heart receives the transmission from the water [of the kidneys], that is the first [complete cycle of transmission]. When the metal of the lung once again receives the transmission from the fire [of the heart], that means a "second" [cycle of transmission is started]. The transmission [of the disease] proceeds consecutively, beginning from the heart, until it reaches the lung for the second time. That is a transmission through seven [long-term depots]. Hence, "[diseases that are] transmitted through seven [long-term depots will result in] death" means that one long-term depot cannot be harmed twice.

(4) *Ding Deyong*: When the [text] says "the heart transmits [the disease] to the spleen," [that is to say] the spleen receives vital qi [from the heart]. Then, transmission continues towards the lung. That is a transmission between mother and child. Hence [the text] speaks of "life."

Lü Guang: *Jian zang* 間藏 ("to skip a long-term depot") means that transmission occurs towards those long-term depots (*zang* 藏) which are located between (*jian* 間) those overcoming each other. The heart overcomes the lung; the spleen is located in between them. The liver overcomes the spleen; the heart is located in between them. The spleen overcomes the kidneys; the lung is located in between them. The lung overcomes the liver; the kidneys lie in between them. The kidneys overcome the heart; the liver lies in between them. That is the so-called transmission toward the [depot] which is generated [by the transmitting depot].

(1)–(4) *Zhang Shixian*: "Transmission through seven [long-term depots]" means that [a disease is] transmitted to the seventh [depot. The course of this] transmission through seven [long-term depots is comparable to] a transmission from husband to wife or children. Hence [the text] speaks of a "transmission to [the long-term depot] that can be overcome." Let us take a disease in the heart as an example. Beginning with the heart section, [this disease] will be transmitted consecutively among [the long-term depots]. After having been transmitted to the sixth [long-term depot in the cycle], it reaches the heart [again]. The heart should transmit it once again to the lung. But the lung is not willing to accept it. That is [what is] meant by "one long-term depot cannot be harmed twice." Transmission toward [a depot] that can be overcome is called "robber evil." Hence it ends in death. *Jian* 間 ("to skip") stands for *ge* 隔 ("to separate"). *Jian zang* 間藏 (here in the sense of "[transmission to] the separating long-term depot") refers to a transmission from mother to child. Hence it is called "transmission to what is generated." Let us take a disease in the heart as an example. The heart overcomes the lung. In this case [the heart] does not transmit [the disease] directly toward the lung, but transmits it to the spleen. The spleen separates [the heart] from the [depot] that [the heart] can overcome. The spleen overcomes the kidneys. In this case [the spleen] does not transmit [the disease] directly to the kidneys but transmits it to the lung. The lung separates [the spleen] from the [depot] that it can overcome. The lung overcomes the liver. In this case [the lung] does not transmit [the disease] directly to the liver but transmits it to the kidneys. The kidneys separate [the lung] from the [depot] that it can overcome.[2] The kidneys overcome the heart. In this case [the kidneys] do not transmit [the disease] directly to the heart but transmit it to the liver. The liver separates [the

---

2 The text has *sheng* 生 ("generate"). That must be a mistake.

kidneys] from the [depot] that they can overcome. *Sheng* 生 ("life") means "life without end; conclusion and new beginning." [Such a] transmission will never exhaust itself. It is called "depletion evil." No damage resulting from the mutual destruction [of the Five Phases] is involved here. Hence life is maintained.

Xu Dachun: The [*Nei*] *jing* contains no text passage that could be checked for comparison on the [meaning of] "transmission through seven [long-term depots]" and "[transmission] skipping [a depot]." The [treatise] "Yu ji zhen zang lun" 玉機真藏論 of the *Su* [*wen*] states: "[Each of] the five depots receives qi from the [depot] which it generates; it transmits it to the one which it dominates. The qi rests in [that depot] by which [the transmitting depot] is generated. Death results [when it is] in that [depot] which [the transmitting depot] cannot dominate. If a disease will result in death, it must[3] first be transmitted and pass [from one depot to another]. When it has reached [a depot] which [the transmitting depot] cannot dominate, the patient will die." That is a discourse concerning [a situation in which] qi proceed contrary to their proper course. Hence [such diseases will end in] death. The [*Nei jing*] text following [the passage quoted above] explains it by stating: "The liver receives qi from the heart, and transmits them to the spleen. The qi rest in the kidneys; death occurs when they reach the lung." "Death at the [long-term depot] that cannot be dominated" refers to a transmission from the long-term depot which was ill in the first place to the kidneys, which it cannot overcome, with the result of death. But that has nothing to do with the statements [in the *Nan jing*] on transmissions through seven [long-term depots] and on transmissions skipping [a depot]. When the [*Nei jing*] talks about "receiving qi from the [depot] which they generate," that refers to what was said in the fiftieth difficult issue – namely "those that come from ahead constitute a repletion evil." Also, the [treatises] "Biao ben bing chuan" 標本病傳 of the *Su* [*wen*] and "Bing chuan" 病傳 of the *Ling* [*shu*] both mention "transmissions to the long-term depots that can be overcome," as in "the heart transmits it to the lung, the lung transmits it to the liver; these are symptoms indicating death." Again, this is not a statement which refers to a transmission through all the five long-term depots up to the seventh position, with death as a consequence. As to the statements on transmissions skipping [a depot], the [treatise] "Biao ben bing chuan" of the *Su* [*wen*] states: "If in the course [of the transmission, the disease] skips one long-term depot and comes to a halt, and if it [eventually continues and] reaches the third or fourth long-term depot, then one can pierce." The meaning of the expression *jian zang* 間藏 ("to skip a depot") is approached here rather closely by the text

---

3   The *Nei jing* has *si bi* 死必 but the text here says *bi si* 必死.

of the [*Nei*] *jing*. If transmission occurs toward the second [possible stop of a] transmission, it skips the long-term depot separating [the transmitting long-term depot from the long-term depot that can be overcome by the transmitter]. After three [skipping] transmissions, [the disease] reaches the long-term depot which is generated by the original [depot]. After four [skipping] transmissions, [the disease] reaches the long-term depot which overcomes the original [depot]. If the disease skips one long-term depot [in each transmission] and comes to a stop [after having reached the third or fourth] depot, with no further transmissions, one can needle it. That is also somewhat different from the transmissions skipping [a long-term depot as outlined in the *Nan jing*].

Liao Ping: The medical classics focus on the long-term depots and short-term repositories, on the conduits and network vessels; they seek truth through facts. If one speculates on the basis of the Five Phases, it is as if one drew a picture of demons and spirits. [The medical classics are concerned with the] concrete; [the theories of the Five Phases are but] empty [talk. The medical classics are] difficult, [the theories of the Five Phases are] easy [to comprehend]. Because [the physicians have] set aside the long-term depots and the short-term repositories, the conduits and the network [vessels], and because they have focused on the Five Phases, medicine has deteriorated day by day. [In its discourses on] general laws, the *Nei jing* frequently refers to the Five Phases. But in those treatises that deal with diseases, it does not refer to the Five Phases. In the medical literature of later generations – just as [in the writings of the] astrologers – one finds detailed discussions of the Five Phases as they generate and overcome, control and transform each other. The *Nan jing* has originated this.

五十四難曰：（一）藏病難治，府病易治，何謂也？

（二）然：藏病所以難治者，傳其所勝也；（三）府病易治者，傳其子也。（四）與七傳間藏同法也。

The fifty-fourth difficult issue: (1) diseases in the long-term depots are difficult to cure; diseases in the short-term repositories are easy to cure. What does that mean?

(2) It is like this. Diseases in the long-term depots are difficult to cure because they are transmitted to [long-term depots that can be] overcome. (3) Diseases in the short-term repositories are easy to cure because they are transmitted to the respective child. (4) This pattern coincides with that of the "transmission through seven [long-term depots]" and with that of the "[transmission] skipping one depot" [outlined in the preceding difficult issue].

COMMENTARIES

(1)–(4) *Ding Deyong*: The long-term depots are yin. "Diseases [in the long-term depots] are difficult to cure" means that these [diseases] are transmitted to [the respective long-term depot that can be overcome]. "Those that can be overcome" means that the liver overcomes the spleen, the spleen overcomes the kidneys, the kidneys overcome the heart, the heart overcomes the lung, the lung overcomes the liver. Hence [diseases transmitted this way] are difficult to cure. The short-term repositories are yang. When [the text] says yang diseases "are transmitted to the respective child," that means a disease in the [short-term repository associated with the phase of] wood is transmitted to the [short-term repository associated with the phase of] fire. A disease in the [short-term repository associated with the phase of] fire is transmitted to the short-term repository associated with the phase of] soil. A disease in the [short-term repository associated with the phase of] soil is transmitted to the [short-term repository associated with the phase of] metal. A disease in the [short-term repository associated with the phase of] metal is transmitted to the [short-term repository associated with the phase of] water. The transmission [of the diseases] from the [short-term repository associated with the phase of] water to the [short-term repository associated with the phase of] wood [follows the] mutual generation [sequence of the Five Phases]. Hence diseases in the short-term repositories are easy to cure. Therefore [the text states]: "This pattern coincides with that of the 'transmission through seven [long-term depots]' and with that of the '[transmission] skipping one depot'."

Hua Shou: Mr. Chen from Siming states: As long as the five long-term depots are guarded internally by the seven spirits, evil [qi] of minor significance will not be transmitted easily. However, if major [evil] qi enter [the long-term depots], the spirits will lose their guarding [function] and the disease will penetrate deeply [into the body]. Hence diseases [in the long-term depots] are difficult to cure; they may even result in death. The [function of the] six short-term repositories is to revolve and transport, to transmit and transform [their contents]. It is quite normal that qi pass through them. Also, the gall bladder is the place of clarity and purity. Even if evil [qi] were to enter it, it would be difficult for them to penetrate deeply and to stay. Hence diseases in the short-term repositories are easy to cure.

Zhang Shixian: When a disease is located deeply, it will be transmitted to [the long-term depot that can be] overcome. When a disease is located below the surface, it will be transmitted to [the short-term repository that is] generated [by the transmitting short-term repository]. Diseases in the long-term depots are those that already have penetrated deeply; hence they are transmitted to [the long-term depot that can be] overcome. Diseases in the short-term repositories are still below the surface; hence they are transmitted to [the short-term repository that is] generated. The *Su wen* states "Those who are well versed in treatment will treat [a disease as long as it is located in] the skin [and its] hair. Next come those who treat [a disease when it is located in] the flesh [below the] skin. Next come those who treat [a disease when it is located in] the muscles and vessels. Next come those who treat [a disease when it is located in] the six short-term repositories. Next come those who treat [a disease when it is located in] the five long-term depots. One half of [those cases treated while the disease is located in] the five short-term repositories will die, one half will survive." According to this statement, as diseases gradually penetrate deeper [into the body], physicians have increasing difficulties in achieving a cure. Diseases are distinguished [according to their location in] either the long-term depots or the short-term repositories. In therapy, one distinguishes between those [cures] that are difficult to achieve and others that are easy to achieve. That is quite obvious.

Xu Dachun: This paragraph certainly does not agree with the [text of the *Nei*] *jing;* also, it contradicts the preceding paragraph. The treatise "Bing chuan" 病 傳 of the [*Ling*] *shu* states that the liver transmits [a disease] to the spleen, the spleen transmits it to the stomach, the stomach transmits it to the kidneys, the kidneys transmit it to the urinary bladder, and so on. That is to say, the long-term depots and the short-term repositories do transmit [diseases] among each other. The preceding treatise states: "The spleen transmits [the disease] to the lung; the lung transmits it to the kidneys." That is [to say], the transmission among the long-term depots can also proceed [from the mother] to the child. Here it is stated: "Diseases in the long-term depots are transmitted to [the long-term depot that can be] overcome" and "diseases in the short-term repositories are transmitted to the child." How could that make any sense? Now, diseases in the long-term depots are located in the depth; diseases in the short-term repositories are located below the surface. It would make perfect sense if one distinguished, on this basis, between [diseases that are] difficult and others that are easy to cure. Everything else is irrelevant.

Ding Jin: This [difficult issue] elucidates once again that the pattern of the transmission [of diseases] through seven [long-term depots] and that of the [transmission of diseases] skipping one long-term depot apply to both long-term depots and short-term repositories. That is to say, [diseases in] the long-term depots are difficult to cure when they are transmitted [to the long-term depot] that can be overcome [by the transmitting depot]; when they are transmitted to the respective child [depot], they are easy to cure. [Diseases in] the short-term repositories are easy to cure when they are transmitted to the respective child [short-term repository]; they are difficult to cure when they are transmitted to the [short-term repository] that can be overcome. Hence [the text] states: "This pattern coincides with that of [diseases that are transmitted] through seven [long-term depots] and with that [of diseases that are transmitted] skipping one depot."

(1) *Liao Ping*: The text of the [*Nei*] *jing* is very clear on this. Why should one raise such a question?

(2) *Liao Ping*: That is a false statement.

(3) *Liao Ping*: How could anybody distinguish between long-term depots and short-term repositories on the basis of such criteria?

(4) *Liao Ping*: To read this is sufficient to make it clear that the authors [of the *Nan jing*] have not penetrated the meaning of the text [of the *Nei jing*]. For details, see Xu [Dachun's] critique.

五十五難曰：（一）病有積、有聚，何以別之？

（二）然：積者，陰氣也；聚者，陽氣也，（三）故陰沉而伏，陽浮而動。（四）氣之所積名曰積，氣之所聚名曰聚。（五）故積者，五藏所生；聚者，六府所成也。（六）積者，陰氣也，其始發有常處，其痛不離其部，上下有所終始，左右有所窮處；（七）聚者，陽氣也，其始發無根本，上下無所留止，其痛無常處，謂之聚。（八）故以是別知積聚也。

The fifty-fifth difficult issue: (1) Among the diseases are "accumulations" and "collections." How can they be distinguished?

(2) Accumulations [consist of] yin qi; collections [consist of] yang qi. (3) Yin [qi stay] in the depth and are hidden; yang [qi remain] at the surface and move. (4) Accumulations of qi are called "accumulations"; collections of qi are called "collections." (5) Hence accumulations emerge in the five long-term depots; collections are formed in the six short-term repositories. (6) Accumulations [consist of] yin qi. They stay where they developed in the first place. The pain [they cause] does not leave its section. Their upper and lower [extensions are clearly marked by] end and beginning; to the left and to the right are [clearly defined] locations where they subside. (7) Collections [consist of] yang qi. They develop without roots. They move upward and downward and do not remain at a specific place; the pain [they cause] has no permanent location. Such [syndromes] are called "collections." (8) With these [criteria in mind], one knows how to distinguish accumulations and collections.

COMMENTARIES

(1)–(8) *Ding Deyong*: "Accumulations" are accumulations of yin qi. That is, when a long-term depot transmits [qi] to a [depot] by which it can be overcome and which – at this moment – is in its ruling period, the latter will not accept the evil. Hence [the evil qi] remain where they are and lump into accumulations. That is why [the text says]: "They stop and do not move." "Collections" are diseases in the six short-term repositories; they represent the yang. [The short-term repositories] transmit [evil qi] to the respective child [short-term repository; such diseases] revolve [in the organism] without fixed location. Also, the yang [qi] rule movement. Hence [such diseases] do not occupy a permanent location.

Lü Guang: All diseases with yin symptoms are located at a permanent place. They are firm and vigorous; they have head and foot. They stand and do not move. They are formed by the qi in the long-term depots. [The patient will] die and cannot be cured. Hence [the text] has stated [earlier]: "Diseases in the long-term depots are difficult to cure." Those symptoms of a disease that move up and down, to the right and to the left without permanent location are the so-called yang symptoms. Although this is difficult, they can be cured. Basically, [the patient should] not die. Hence [his life] will continue for years and months. Hence the [*Nan jing*] states: "Diseases in the short-term repositories are easy to cure."

Hua Shou: Mr. Yang states: "*Ji* 積 ("accumulation") stands for *xu* 蓄 ("to store"). That is to say, when the blood vessels are impassable, [their contents] accumulate and form a disease."

Zhang Shixian: "Accumulations" are generated by yin qi. They reflect the earth and do not move. "Collections" are generated by yang qi. They reflect heaven and revolve. Diseases due to an accumulation [of qi are such that if they occur in] the liver, [they are located] in the left flank;[1] [if they occur in] the lung, [they are located] in the right flank; [if they occur in] the heart, [they are located] above the navel; [if they occur in] the kidneys, [they are located] below the navel; [if they occur in] the spleen, they occupy the center. That is to say, they occupy a permanent location. "The pain [they cause] does not leave its section" means that it does not exceed its original location.[2] "Their upper and lower [extensions]" refers to the upper and lower [extensions] of the accumulations. "End and beginning" refers to where [these accumulations] rise and where they stop. "Left and right" refers to the two sides – namely, the left and the right – of accumulations. "Locations where they subside" are the locations where the concrete appearance of the accumulations ends and where the pain stops too. Diseases due to a collection [of qi] seem to be present [at a specific location and then] it is as if they were not. Hence [the text states]: "They develop without roots." They come and go; they move upward and downward without a specific [borderline where they might] stop. The pain [caused by these diseases] is not tied to a specific location either. Because one of these diseases moves around while the other rests at one place, one understands why they are called "accumulations" and "collections."

(4) *Xu Dachun*: This is an explanation of the origin of the names "accumulation" and "collection." Accumulations are formed through a gradual accumulation [of qi]; collections are conglomerations [of qi] that do not disperse again. Accumulations, then, are [material] entities; collections have no shape.

(5) *Xu Dachun*: This is another explanation of the origin of accumulations and collections. The long-term depots belong to the yin; hence yin qi accumulate in the interior [sections of the body] and form accumulations. The short-term reposi-

---

1   The text has *xi* 膝 ("knee"). That must be a mistake.
2   The text has *qi* 奇 ("strange"). That may be an error in writing for *ji* 寄 ("location").

tories belong to the yang. Hence yang qi concentrate in the exterior [sections of the body] and form collections. Each follows its category.

(1)–(8) *Xu Dachun*: In this paragraph, the two characters "accumulation" and "collection" are distinguished most clearly. However, it should be united with the fifty-second difficult issue into one paragraph. It is not necessary to make two separate chapters [out of the topic treated].

Tamba Genkan: The treatise "Bai bing shi sheng" 百病始生 of the *Ling shu* states: "The early generation of an accumulation results from getting cold. [The qi] recede and accumulations form." It states further: "When a depletion evil[3] hits a person, it will be transmitted further and settled outside of the intestines and the stomach, in the membrane plain.[4] There they attach themselves to the vessels.[5] When they have stayed there for some time without being removed, they rest and accumulate."

(1) *Liao Ping*: The text below discusses accumulations but does not discuss collections. Why? The present [paragraph] contradicts everything preceding and following it; it is random talk; it is the greatest nonsense!

(5) *Liao Ping*: The [*Nei*] *jing* speaks of "accumulations" in the case of both long-term depots and short-term repositories.

(8) *Liao Ping*: Tamba Genkan quoted the treatise "Bai bing shi sheng" of the *Ling shu*, which says that [in case of] accumulations [evil qi] rest outside of intestines and stomach and within the membrane field; that they remain in the abdomen [*sic!*],[6] that they stop and form accumulations. Long-term depots and short-term repositories are not distinguished [in the *Ling shu*]. The meaning [outlined here] is the same as that of the fifty-second difficult issue. This is sufficient evidence for the absurdity of seeking a division into eighty-one chapters.

---

3   The concept of "depletion evil" in the *Ling shu* is different from that in the *Nan jing*. The *Ling shu* uses the term "depletion evil" in reference to external evil qi that take advantage of a depletion in the organism to enter the body and seize the space depleted.

4   The membrane plain (*mu yuan* 募原) cannot be defined in exact anatomical terms. It seems to have been considered to be a region between heart and diaphragm.

5   MS: „募原之間 *mu yuan zhi jian* is to say: inside the skin, outside of the membrane."

6   Liao Ping, who repeated this quotation (see below), has exchanged *mai* 脈 ("vessel") for *fu* 腹 ("abdomen"), which makes better sense.

五十六難曰：（一）五藏之積，各有名乎？（二）以何月何日得之？
（三）然：肝之積名曰肥氣，（四）在左脅下，如覆杯，（五）有頭足。（六）久
不愈，令人發咳逆，瘡瘧，（七）連歲不已。（八）以季夏戊己日得之。（九）
何以言之？肺病傳於肝，肝當傳脾，脾季夏適王，王者不受邪，肝復欲還
肺，肺不肯受，故留結為積。故知肥氣以季夏戊己日得之。（十）心之積
名曰伏梁，（十一）起齊上，大如臂，（十二）上至心下。（十三）久不愈，
令人病煩心，（十四）以秋庚辛日得之。（十五）何以言之？腎病傳心，心
當傳肺，肺以秋適王，王者不受邪，心復欲還腎，腎不肯受，故留結為
積。故知伏梁以秋庚辛日得之。（十六）脾之積名曰痞氣，（十七）在胃脘，
覆大如盤。（十八）久不愈，令人四肢不收，發黃疸，（十九）飲食不為肌
膚。（二十）以冬壬癸日得之。（二十一）何以言之？肝病傳脾，脾當傳腎，
腎以冬適王，王者不受邪，脾復欲還肝，肝不肯受，故留結為積。故知痞
氣以冬壬癸日得之。（二十二）肺之積名曰息賁，（二十三）在右脅下，覆大
如杯。（二十四）久不已，令人洒淅寒熱，喘咳，發肺壅。（二十五）以春
甲乙日得之。（二十六）何以言之？心病傳肺，肺當傳肝，肝以春適王，
王者不受邪，肺復欲還心，心不肯受，故留結為積。故知息賁以春甲乙日
得之。（二十七）腎之積名曰賁豚，（二十八）發於少腹，上至心下，（二十
九）若豚狀，或上或下無時，（三十）久不已，令人喘逆，（三十一）骨痿少
氣，（三十二）以夏丙丁日得之。（三十三）何以言之？脾病傳腎，腎當傳
心，心以夏適王，王者不受邪，腎復欲還脾，脾不肯受，故留結為積。故
知賁豚以夏丙丁日得之。（三十四）此是五積之要法也。

The fifty-sixth difficult issue: (1) What are the names of all the accumulations in the
five long-term depots? (2) In what month and on what day does one contract them?

(3) It is like this. Accumulations in the liver are called "fat qi." (4) They are located
below the ribs on the left side and resemble a cup turned upside down. (5) They have
head and foot. (6) When they last a long time without healing, they let the [afflict-
ed] person develop a cough [with qi] moving contrary to their proper direction, and
they [cause] *jie* and *yao* [fevers]. (7) Even after a year, [such accumulations] do not
yet come to an end. (8) [Such diseases] are contracted in late summer on a *wu ji* day.
(9) Why do I say so? When the lung is ill, it will transmit [evil qi] to the liver, and
the liver should transmit them to the spleen. In the last month of summer, however,
the spleen acts as king. A king does not accept evil. Therefore, the liver wishes to
return [the evil qi] to the lung, but the lung is unwilling to accept them. Hence
[the evil qi] stay [in the liver] and conglomerate, causing accumulations. Hence one
knows that "fat qi" are acquired in late summer on a *wu ji* day. (10) Accumulations
in the heart are called "hidden beams." (11) They rise above the navel and are as large

as a lower arm. (12) They extend upward to below the heart. (13) When they last a long time without being healed, they let the [afflicted] person suffer from a feeling of uneasiness in his heart. (14) [Such diseases] are contracted in autumn on a *geng xin* day. (15) Why do I say so? When the kidneys are ill, they will transmit [evil qi] to the heart, and the heart should transmit them to the lung. In autumn, however, the lung acts as king, and a king does not accept evil. Therefore, the heart wishes to return [the evil qi] to the kidneys, but the kidneys are unwilling to accept them. Hence they stay [in the heart] and conglomerate, causing accumulations. Hence one knows that "hidden beams" are contracted in autumn on a *geng xin* day. (16) Accumulations in the spleen are called "blocked qi." (17) They are located in the stomach duct[1] and are several times the size of a bowl.[2] (18) When they last a long time without being healed, they cause the [afflicted] person to be unable to pull in his four limbs, and they cause jaundice. (19) They prevent the generation of flesh and skin from food and beverages. (20) [Such diseases] are contracted in winter on a *ren gui* day. (21) Why do I say so? When the liver is ill, it will transmit [evil qi] to the spleen, and the spleen should transmit them to the kidneys. In winter, however, the kidneys act as king, and a king does not accept evil. Therefore, the spleen wishes to return [the evil qi] to the liver, but the liver is unwilling to accept them. Hence they stay [in the spleen] and conglomerate, causing accumulations. Hence one knows that "blocked qi" are contracted in winter on a *ren gui* day. (22) Accumulations in the lung are called "rest and run." (23) They are located below the ribs on the right side and are several times the size of a cup. (24) When they last a long time without being healed, they let the [afflicted] person shiver due to [alternating perceptions of] cold and heat, and [they let him] pant and cough and develop blockages in his lung. (25) [Such diseases] are contracted in spring on a *jia yi* day. (26) Why do I say so? When the heart is ill, it will transmit [evil qi] to the lung, and the lung should transmit them to the liver. In spring, however, the liver acts as king, and kings do not accept evil. Therefore, the lung wishes to return [the evil qi] to the heart, but the heart is unwilling to accept them. Hence they stay [in the lung] and conglomerate, causing accumulations. Hence one knows that "rest and run" is contracted in spring on a *jia yi* day. (27) Accumulations related to the kidneys are called "running piglets." (28) They develop in the lower abdomen and extend upward to below the heart. (29) Like a piglet, they move up or down unexpectedly. (30) When they last a long time without ending, they let the [afflicted] person pant due to [qi] moving contrary to

---

1   The entire stomach is understood here as a duct.

2   The wording of this last phrase may not reflect the original sequence of the characters. I suspect that it corresponds to sentence 4 and should be read *ru fu da pan* 如覆大盤 ("they resemble a large bowl turned upside down"). The same applies to sentence 3.

their proper direction. (31) [They cause] the bones to weaken and to have few qi. (32) [Such diseases] are contracted in summer on a *bing ding* day. (33) Why do I say so? When the spleen is sick, it will transmit [evil qi] to the kidneys, and the kidneys should transmit them to the heart. In summer, however, the heart acts as king, and a king does not accept evil. Therefore, the kidneys wish to return [the evil qi] to the spleen, but the spleen is not willing to accept them. Hence they stay [in the kidneys] and conglomerate, causing accumulations. Hence one knows that "running piglets" are contracted in summer on a *bing ding* day. (34) These are the important patterns of the five accumulations.[3]

COMMENTARIES

(2) *Liao Ping:* All these [passages] stick closely to the Five Phases [doctrine]. Modern scholars say that this is not a correct paradigm of medicine. It should be thrown out as soon as possible in order to eliminate this screen of errors.

(4) *Zhang Shixian:* The position of the liver is below the left flank. Hence an accumulation [in the liver] is located at the same place.

   Xu Dachun: "A cup turned upside down" means that its base is large while its top is small.

   Liao Ping: The character *zuo* 左 ("left") should be deleted.

(5) *Hua Shou:* "They have head and foot" means that they are specific in their size, that they have origin and end.

(6) *Hua Shou:* "A cough [with qi] moving contrary to their proper direction" refers to a separate connection [between the lung and] the foot ceasing yin [conduit through which the qi] move from the diaphragm upward and flow into the lung. Hence in the case of a disease in the liver, there is coughing in the chest with [qi] moving contrary to their proper direction. One outbreak occurs every second day; these are *jie* 痎 and *yao/nue* 瘧 [fevers]. In the *Nei jing*, each of the five long-term depots is [associated with a particular] *yao/nue* 瘧 fever].[4] The one in the liver is the "wind *yao/nue*". One could also identify these *yao/nue* [fevers] as diseases of cold and heat. They belong mostly to the minor yang [conduit],

---

3   This difficult issue is another example of the consistent application of the Five Phases doctrine to pathology. Once again, terms and concepts originating from the *Nei jing* are systematically redefined, a fact which irritated later conservative commentators, who considered the contents of the *Nei jing* – heterogeneous and inconsistent as they are – to be binding. Also, in the absence of any tangible evidence, the author(s) of the *Nan jing* again resorted to social symbolism to legitimate their ideas. For some of the disease terms mentioned here, see *Ling shu* treatise 13, "Jing jin" 經筋, and *Su wen* treatise 40, "Fu zhong lun" 腹中論.

4   See *Su wen* treatise 35, "Yao/nue lun 瘧論."

which is related to the liver like outside to inside. Hence [the text] states: "The left flank is the section of the liver."

Zhang Shixian: Those [fevers] breaking out every other day are called *jie* 痎; those breaking out every consecutive day are called *yao/nue* 瘧.

Liao Ping: Later generations have created false [diagnostic] patterns on the basis of these [statements]. To treat diseases by relying on the [Celestial] Stems and [Earth] Branches, on yin and yang [associations], and on the [mutual] generation and destruction [of the Five Phases] – without taking recourse to the four diagnostic [methods] – means to cause great harm. These are all wooden figurines made by this book.[5]

(8) *Li Jiong*: The sixth month in late summer is exactly the month when the soil of the spleen serves as king. [The constellation] *wu ji* 戊己 represents the soil. Hence the qi of the spleen contract this disease on the *wu ji* day.

Zhang Shixian: "Late summer" refers to the sixth month. The soil acts as king during this month; *wu ji* is the day when it is king. Both the entire month and [that specific] day represent the period during which the soil flourishes. Hence the liver is not able to overcome the spleen [during this time], and one contracts an accumulation of fat qi during that month and day.

(3)–(9) *Yang*: *Ji* 積 ("accumulation") stands for *xu* 蓄 ("collection"). That is to say, when the blood vessels are not passable, accumulations occur causing diseases. All accumulations originate in the five long-term depots. If the camp qi proceed continuously [through the body] and do not miss the proper amount of circulation, one speaks of a normal person. A normal person is without disease. If one long-term depot contracts a disease, [the course of] the camp qi is obstructed. Hence the disease will be located in that [depot]. Now, if any of the five long-term depots contracts a disease, it transmits it to the [depot] which it can overcome. When the one [depot] that it can overcome happens to act as king at that moment, it will not be willing to accept the transmission. Because it is not willing to accept [the disease] it will return it, transmitting it to the one [depot] by which it can be overcome. But the [depot] by which it can be overcome will not take it. Therefore, [the qi] stay where they are and conglomerate, forming accumulations. Gradually they grow large. As a consequence, the disease takes shape. As to *fei qi* 肥氣, *fei* 肥 ("fat") stands for *sheng* 盛 ("rich"). That is to say,

---

5   Wooden figurines of men and women were buried with the dead in Chinese antiquity. Confucius believed that this practice gave rise to burying living persons with the dead and condemned it as evil. Liao Ping appears to have resorted to this metaphor because he considered the *Nan jing* to be a source of "false" ideas and practices that killed many patients later on.

fat qi concentrate below the left flank, protruding like a cup turned upside down and resembling fat, rich flesh. Small children have this disease often.

Ding Jin: Yueren's description of the principle behind the formation of accumulations is quite off the point. Obviously, locations suffering from a depletion accept evil [qi], while locations flourishing [with contents] will not take them. In treating accumulations, today's people consider attacking as their duty. That means that they greatly miss the message of the [*Nei*] *jing*. That is truly sad!

(9) *Liao Ping*: This kind of talk is really nothing but child's play! When the spleen does not accept the evil [qi], that should be the end of the disease. How could it return them to the lung?!

(10) *Yang*: "Hidden beams" means that an accumulation extends from above the navel to below the heart. Its size is that of an arm. It resembles the ridgepole of a house.

Hua Shou: [The *fu* 伏 in] *fu liang* 伏梁 ("hidden beams") means "lying hidden without movement," like a wooden beam.

(14) *Li Jiong*: In autumn the vessels [display a] string-like [movement]. These are exactly the months when the metal acts as king. [The constellation] *geng xin* 庚辛 represents the metal. A "hidden beam" is contracted on a *geng xin* day.

(1)–(14) *Xu Dachun*: The treatise "Jing jin" 經筋 of the *Ling* [*shu* states for] the hand minor yin sinew:[6] "Its diseases are internal tensions with hidden beams supported by the heart. In the case of hidden beams accompanied by spitting of blood and pus, death is immanent and no cure is possible." A look at these words shows that they too refer to a disease related to the heart, but the actual appearance of that [disease] is not elucidated clearly. In the [treatise] "Fu zhong lun" 腹中論 of the *Su* [*wen*], it is stated: "[Huang] Di: 'A disease is [as follows]: The lower abdomen [gives the patient a feeling of] abundance. Above, below, to the left and to the right, everywhere are roots. Which disease is that? Can it be treated, or not?' Qi Bo: 'The name of the disease is hidden beams. [The lower abdomen] holds massive pus and blood, located outside of the intestines and the stomach. This must not be treated. If one treats it, each time one presses the [lower abdomen] this brings [the patient] closer to death. When this passes downward, then it is by way of yin [passageways]. It is inevitable that what is passed downward is pus and blood. When this is moved upward, then it presses against the stomach duct where it generates a barrier. [That is:] obstruction illness inside the stomach duct, on both sides. This is a chronic disease; it is dif-

---

6   In correspondence to the concept of the twelve major conduits, the *Ling shu* espouses the idea that the body contains twelve major muscles. They are supposed to run basically parallel to the conduits and are named accordingly. As with the twelve conduits, they may have specific diseases with specific symptoms.

ficult to cure. When it resides above the navel, this is opposition; when it resides below the navel, this is compliance'." The [text] says further: "Someone has his body and limbs, thigh bones, thighs, and shins, all swollen. The region around his navel is painful. Which disease is that?' Qi Bo: 'The disease is named hidden beams. These are wind roots. The [wind] qi has spilled into the large intestine and has attached itself to the *huang*. The plain of the *huang* 肓 is below the navel. Hence, the region around the navel has pain. One cannot move these [qi]. If one moves them, this causes the disease of roughened urination of water'." If one looks at these [passages], hidden beams are not associated with the heart. [Hidden beams are described] there as major swelling, as are intestinal or stomach ulcers. They are called "rooted in wind" because they consist of conglomerations of wind poison. Also, one does not necessarily contract them during a day in autumn. What Yueren has referred to here carries the same name but is an entirely different disease [from the ailment described in the *Ling shu*].

(15) *Liao Ping*: This is what [Zhang] Zhongjing 張仲景 calls: "If it is not transmitted further, the disease will come to an end." ... If neither the lung nor the kidneys accept the evil [qi] why should one fall ill in autumn? ... The apocryphal *Mai jing* 脈經 discusses diseases in terms of days and [Celestial] Stems. Such errors are based on these [statements here].

(18) *Li Jiong*: In the case of *huang dan* 黃疸 ("jaundice"), the body, the arms, the hands, and the feet all turn yellow.

Hua Shou: *Dan* 疸 means that. one develops a yellow [color]; it is caused by moisture and heat.

Xu Dachun: In the case of jaundice one's skin, nails and eyes develop a yellow color.

(16)–(21) *Yang*: *Pi* 痞 stands for *pi* 否 ("clogged"). That is to say, [the passage] is clogged and conglomerations develop forming accumulations. When the spleen qi are depleted, the stomach will be hot, drawing food [to the stomach]. Now, if the spleen has a disease, it cannot send its qi [through the body] and it cannot pass on the bodily liquids. Hence, although food is present in large amounts, one will become emaciated.

(21) *Liao Ping*: To match the ten days [associated with the Ten Celestial Stems] with the five long-term depots is a symbolism of correspondence [used] by the astrologers and diviners .... Each of the earlier [difficult issues] discussed one conduit; the [circumstances of the] remaining [conduits] could be inferred from this [one example]. Here all the five long-term depots are dealt with exhaustively, but the edifice constructed is superficial – it has no basis. To eliminate it would be the right thing to do.

(22) *Li Jiong*: Xi 息 ("to rest") stands for *biao* 表 ("external");[7] *ben* 賁 ("to run") stands for *ge* 鬲 (here, "diaphragm"). That is to say, the lung is located above the diaphragm. When its qi do not proceed, it gradually grows larger, pressing against the diaphragm. Hence accumulations in the lung are called "rest and run."

Hua Shou: Xi ben 息賁 ("rest and run") means "sometimes they rest, sometimes they run." The right flank is the section of the lung. The lung rules the skin [and its] hair. Hence one shivers from [perceptions of] cold and heat. Somewhere else it is said that diseases in the long-term depots are static and do not move. Here, an accumulation in the lung sometimes rests, sometimes runs. Why is that? It is like this. That it either rests or runs does not imply that it does not reside at a permanent location, like the diseases of the short-term repositories. Because it is especially the lung which rules the qi, its qi have certain times when they move or rest. The kidneys also rule qi. Hence the same applies to the "running piglets."

Zhang Shixian: Xi 息 ("to rest") stands for *an jing* 安靜 ("quiet"). *Ben* 賁 ("to run") is identical with *ben* 奔; they both mean *zou dong* 走動 ("to move around"). An accumulation in the lung is sometimes quiet, sometimes it moves around. Hence it is called "rest and run."

(25) *Li Jiong*: The spring months are the time when the wood of the liver acts as king. [The constellation] *jia yi* 甲乙 represents the wood. A "rest and run" is contracted on a *jia yi* day.

(22)–(26) *Yang*: Xi 息 stands for *zhang* 長 ("to grow"); *ben* 賁 stands for *ge* 鬲 (here, "diaphragm"). That is to say, the lung is located above the diaphragm. When its qi do not proceed, it gradually grows larger, pressing against the diaphragm. Hence this is called *xi ben*. Another [explanation] says *ben* stands for *ju* 聚 ("collection"). That is to say, [the accumulation of blocked qi] gradually grows larger, turning into a collection. The lung constitutes the upper cover [of the long-term depots]. Among the long-term depots, it represents the yang. When yang qi are present in abundance, they cause man to develop obstructions in the lung.

(15)–(26) *Xu Dachun*: The treatise "Jing jin" 經筋 of the *Ling* [shu states for] the hand major yin sinew: "Its diseases are at the locations passed by. They include [aching] divergences and torn sinews. In the case of a strong pain, *xi ben* develops. The flanks are tense and [the patient] spits blood." Here, too, *xi ben* is referred to as a disease related to the lung. The [*Ling shu*] states further concerning the hand heart ruler sinew: "Its diseases are at the locations passed by. They include

---

7   *Biao* 表 is probably a mistake for *zhang* 長 ("to grow"). See *Yang's* otherwise identical commentary on sentences 22 through 26.

[aching] divergences and torn sinews in [the patient's] front, as well as chest pain and *xi ben*." Here, then, *xi ben* is a disease related to the [heart] enclosing network. The [treatise] "Yin yang bie lun" 陰陽別論 of the *Su wen* states: "Diseases in the second yang break out in the heart and in the spleen. [As a result] one cannot [use] the hidden bend; females do not have their monthly [period]. Their transmission generates wind wasting. [Further] transmission causes *xi ben*. [Once this stage is reached, the patient] will die; no cure is possible." This [passage] regards *xi ben* as a disease that is transmitted by the heart. It corresponds to the meaning [expressed in the *Nan jing* – namely, that it is a disease] transmitted from the heart to the lung.

(26) *Liao Ping*: Other sections point out that a long-term depot must fall ill during a [season associated with a phase] that it cannot overcome. For instance, [the lung, which is associated with] metal, will fall ill in summer, [which is associated with fire]. Here, [a depot] falls ill during a season [associated with the phase] that it can overcome. That is strange.

(27) *Hua Shou*: "Running piglets" [means that this disease] resembles a piglet that runs around and never settles down. The nature of piglets is [characterized by] quick temper. Hence one has named this [disease accordingly].

(30) *Hua Shou*: "They let the [afflicted] person pant due to [qi] moving contrary to their proper direction" [refers to the fact that] a branch of the foot minor yin [conduit] leaves the lung and ties up with the heart, pouring [qi] into the chest.

(32) *Li Jiong*: The summer months are the time when the fire of the heart acts as king. [The constellation] *bing ding* 丙丁 represents the fire. A "running piglet" is contracted on a *bing ding* day.

(27)–(34) *Yang*: This disease resembles a piglet moving upward against the heart. Also, there are "running piglet" qi.[8] They have nothing to do with this accumulation disease. The names are identical but the diseases are different.

　Xu Dachun: In its treatises on the *tai yang* diseases, the *Shang han lun* 傷寒論 states: "If perturbations occur below the navel after sweating, a tendency exists to develop a running piglet." It states further: "The burning needle[9] lets [the patient] sweat. A cold lump arises at the location where the needle was inserted, and a reddening occurs. Running piglet will inevitably develop." These [statements] seem to refer to a sudden disease. That is different from [what is outlined in the *Nan jing*] here. The *Jin kui yao lüe* 金匱要略 states: "The disease 'running

---

8　See *Ling shu* treatise 4, "Xie qi zang fu bing xing" 邪氣藏府病形.

9　Another name for the *shao zhen* 燒鍼 ("burning needle") treatment technique is *huo zhen* 火鍼 ("fire needle"). A needle with heated tip is quickly inserted into the subcutaneous tissue at a specific location and is then withdrawn again.

piglet' rises from the lower abdomen and pushes upward against the throat. When it develops, one wishes to die, but it may also turn [downward] again and stop. One contracts this [disease] because of fright or fear." This statement comes close to the one here [in the *Nan jing*]. Among the prescriptions recorded, [the *Jin kui yao lüe*] quotes also a passage from the text of the *Shang han lun*. The disease, then, [as it is described] here [in the *Nan jing*, develops over] a long time once it is acquired, and does not come to an end. It develops because of an accumulation in the kidneys, and it is difficult to cure. However, if it is caused by an external affection that – due to a mistaken treatment – has resulted in a collection [of qi], this is not an accumulation in the kidneys, and it is easy to cure. Thus, the appearances of these diseases are similar but their causes are different.

五十七難曰：（一）泄凡有幾？皆有名不？
（二）然：泄凡有五，其名不同。有胃泄，有脾泄，有大腸泄，有小腸泄，
有大瘕泄，名曰後重。（三）胃泄者，飲食不化，色黃。（四）脾泄者，腹脹
滿，泄注，食即嘔吐逆。（五）大腸泄者，食已窘迫，大便色白，腸鳴切
痛。（六）小腸泄者，溲而便膿血，少腹痛。（七）大瘕泄者，裏急後重，數
至圊而不能便，莖中痛。（八）此五泄之法也。

The fifty-seventh difficult issue: (1) How many kinds of diarrhea exist; do they all have names?

(2) It is like this. Altogether, there are five kinds of diarrhea, and all are named differently. They include the "diarrhea of the stomach," the "diarrhea of the spleen," the "diarrhea of the large intestine," the "diarrhea of the small intestine," and the "diarrhea of large conglomeration-illness." [Another] designation [for the latter] is "heavy behind." (3) In the case of a diarrhea of the stomach, food and beverages are not transformed, and the color [of the stools] is yellow. (4) In the case of a diarrhea of the spleen, the abdomen is swollen and full. Liquid diarrhea rushes down; solid food is vomited, proceeding contrary to its proper course. (5) In the case of a diarrhea of the large intestine, one has cramps [in the abdomen] after having consumed food. The stools are white. One hears sounds in the intestines and feels a cutting pain. (6) In the case of a diarrhea of the small intestines, one passes pus and blood with the urine and with the stools, and one feels pain in the lower abdomen. (7) In the case of a diarrhea of large conglomerations, one feels tensions inside [the abdomen] and heaviness at the behind. One goes to the latrine frequently and is still unable to pass any stools. Pain is felt in one's stalk. (8) These are the important patterns of the five kinds of diarrhea.

COMMENTARIES

(1) *Yang: Xie* 泄 ("diarrhea") stands for *li* 利 ("to pass through").

(2) *Katō Bankei*: If any of the five kinds of diarrhea turns very serious, it will cause a "heavy behind." "Heavy behind" stands for *li* 痢 ("dysentery"). Hua commented that a "heavy behind" occurs [only] in the case of a diarrhea of large conglomerations. That is incorrect.

(3) *Yang*: The stomach belongs to the soil; hence its diarrhea is of a yellow color. Food and beverages are not transformed. *Hua* 化 ("transformed") stands for *bian* 變 ("changed") or *xiao* 消 ("digested"). That is to say, all items eaten do leave the body complete and undigested.

Yu Shu: This [condition results] from wind entering the intestines and moving up against the stomach. As a consequence, food is not digested. In the [treatise] "Feng lun" 風論 [of the *Su wen*], it is stated: "If wind enters one's center over an extended period of time, this causes intestinal wind diarrhea." Diarrhea means that food [passes through the body] without being digested.

Zhang Shixian: When evil [qi] reside in the stomach, the lower opening of the stomach does not close firmly. Food and beverages enter the interior [of the stomach] and do not wait there until [they are digested by] the rubbings of the spleen. Instead, they are transmitted directly to the large intestine, from which they leave [the body]. Hence the color of that diarrhea is the color of the stomach. Hence it is yellow.

Ding Jin: When the stomach has received evil [qi], it cannot move and transform food and beverages. Yellow is the color of the soil. The evil [qi] are evil [qi] either of moisture or of cold.

(4) *Yang*: *Zhu* 注 ("to rush") means *wu jie du* 五節度 ("excessive"). That is to say, the diarrhea passes down like rushing waters; it cannot be stopped. When the spleen has a disease, it cannot transform the grains. Hence when one eats one will vomit – that is, [the food] moves contrary to its proper direction.

Yu Shu: The center generates moisture. Moisture generates soil. The soil generates the spleen. The spleen dislikes moisture. If it is overcome by humid qi, the abdomen will be swollen and liquid diarrhea rushes out. The nature of soil is responsible for confidence and for the flavors. Here, the soil has a disease related to the flavors and there is no confidence. Hence as soon as one eats one will vomit – that is, [the food] moves contrary to its proper direction. The [treatise] "Yin yang ying xiang [da] lun" 陰陽應象大論 [of the *Su wen*] states: "If moisture prevails, soft diarrhea results." That is to say, when humid qi enter [the abdomen], attacking spleen and stomach, water and grains will not be separated. Hence liquid diarrhea rushes down.

Zhang Shixian: *Zhu* 注 ("to rush") means that the diarrhea is violent. When the spleen is depleted [of proper qi] and receives evil [qi], it cannot digest the water and the grains [in the stomach] by rubbing [the latter, and it will not] disperse the essence qi of the stomach to the five long-term depots and six short-term repositories. Water and grains remain in the stomach. Hence the abdomen is swollen and full and violent diarrhea occurs. The food is vomited and does not move downward.

Ding Jin: All the six short-term repositories are supplied with qi by the stomach. The five long-term depots are supplied with qi by the spleen. When the spleen and the stomach receive evil [qi], all qi are blocked and no transformations occur. Hence the [abdomen is] swollen and full, and violent rushes [of diarrhea] occur. When the qi are not transformed, they move contrary to their proper course. Hence food is vomited.

(5) *Yang*: *Jiong po* 窘迫 ("cramp") stands for *ji* 急 ("tensions"). As soon as the meal is finished, one has a desire to pass [stools]. Cramps result that cannot be stopped. "White" is the color that comes from the lung. "One hears sounds in the intestines and feels a cutting pain" means that [the intestines and their contents are] cold. "Cutting" means that the pain cuts like a knife. That is [a description of] the condition of the intestines.

Yu Shu: [In this case] qi of the large intestine are depleted. After having finished a meal, one must go to the latrine immediately. Because the [proper qi of the large intestine are] depleted, evil [qi] are transmitted into it. The evil and the [remaining few] correct [qi] clash against each other; hence a cutting pain results.

(6) *Yang*: The small intestine belongs to the heart. The heart rules the blood vessels. Hence the stools carry pus and blood. The small intestine is located in the lower abdomen; hence one feels pain in the lower abdomen.

Li Jiong: The small intestine is the short-term repository to the heart. The heart generates the blood. Hence the stools are bloody.

Xu Dachun: The qi of the small intestine move downward into the urinary bladder. The urinary bladder is located close to the lower abdomen. Hence pain is felt in the lower abdomen.

(7) *Yang*: *Jia* 瘕 ("conglomeration-illness") stands for *jie* 結 ("knottings"). This is a condition in which conglomerations are present in the lower abdomen and one still [attempts to] pass [his stools]. Another name is "heavy behind." That is to say, at the time of [passing] stools, one feels a heavy pain. Again and again one feels a desire to pass [the stools]; he goes to the [latrine] but then does not pass anything. Also, the pain extends into the yin stalk. This is a diarrhea of the kidneys.

Yu Shu: The orifices kept open by the kidneys are the two yin [gates]. When the qi are depleted, one frequently thinks of going to the latrine. The behind [feels] heavy but one cannot relieve [his nature]. Pain is felt in the stalk. When the qi in the kidneys are not sufficient, harm is caused to the throughway vessel. Hence internal tensions result.

Ding Deyong: "Tensions inside" means intestinal pain. "Heaviness at the behind" means [a feeling of] extreme heaviness from the loins downward.

Xu Dachun: The qi of the stools cannot pass. As a result, evil qi move into the urine. Hence pain is felt in one's stalk.

(1)–(8) *Xu Dachun*: The characteristics of these diseases are distinguished in this paragraph quite clearly and properly. The diarrhea of the small intestine as well as [the diarrhea] of large conglomerations are the so-called *li* 痢 ("dysentery") diseases of later times. The first three kinds are *sun xie* 飧泄 ("undigested meal diarrhea").

Katō Bankei: The *Nei jing* mentions numerous kinds of *xie* 泄 and *li* 痢 diarrheas. These include the *sun xie* 飧泄 ("undigested meal diarrhea"), the *dong xie* 洞 泄 ("penetrating diarrhea"), the *ru xie* 濡泄 ("soft diarrhea"), the *wu tang* 鶩溏 ("ducks' slop"), the *jia xie* 瘕泄 ("conglomeration diarrhea"), the *bao zhu* 暴注 ("sudden rushes"), and the *xia po* 下迫 ("downward pressure") [as *xie* 泄 kinds of diarrhea], as well as *chang pi bian xue* 腸澼便血 ("intestinal cleansing with bloody stools"), *xia bai mo* 下白沫 ("white foam passing down"), and *xia nong xue* 下膿血 ("pus and blood passing down") as so-called *li* 痢 kinds of diarrhea. Bian Que has eliminated this excessive abundance [of terms and concepts] and has approached a simple [categorization]. Hence the three kinds of diarrhea associated with spleen, stomach, and large intestine are called *xie* 泄 diarrhea; the two diarrheas associated with the small intestine and with large concentrations are called *li* 痢 diseases. Xian [Yuan] and Qi [Bo] called them *chang pi* 腸澼 ("intestinal cleansing"); [Zhang] Zhongjing 張仲景 called them *zhi xia* 滯下 ("blocked passage downward"). The meaning is always the same. Briefly speaking, there are five kinds of *xie* 泄 diarrhea. As soon as these *xie* diarrheas develop into a "heavy behind," they become *li* 痢 dysentery. Thus, diarrhea and dysentery have the same origin but are two different [phenomena]. The *Su wen* says: "In the lower [part of the body this] causes outflow of [undigested] food (*sun xie* 飧泄). If this lasts for long, it causes intestinal flush." That is correct. *Xie* diarrhea is often associated with cold; *li* dysentery is often associated with heat.

五十八難曰：(一)傷寒有幾？其脈有變不？

(二)然：傷寒有五，有中風，有傷寒，有濕溫，有熱病，有溫病，其所苦各不同。(三)中風之脈，陽浮而滑，陰濡而弱；(四)濕溫之脈，陽濡而弱，陰小而急；(五)傷寒之脈，陰陽俱盛而緊濇；(六)熱病之脈，陰陽俱浮，浮之而滑，沉之散濇；(七)溫病之脈，行在諸經，不知何經之動也，各隨其經所在而取之。

(八)腸寒有汗出而愈，下之而死者；有汗出而死，下之而愈者，何也？

(九)然：陽虛陰盛，汗出而愈，下之即死；(十)陽盛陰虛，汗出而死，下之而愈。

(十一)寒熱之病，候之如何也？

(十二)然：皮寒熱者，皮不可近席，毛髮焦，鼻槀，不得汗；(十三)肌寒熱者，皮膚痛，唇舌槀，無汗；(十四)骨寒熱者，病無所安，汗注不休，齒本槀痛。

The fifty-eighth difficult issue: (1) How many kinds of "harm caused by cold" exist; are they accompanied by any changes in the [movement of the qi in the] vessels?

(2) It is like this. There are five kinds of harm caused by cold. These include to be struck by wind, to have been harmed by cold, moisture and warmth, the heat disease, and the warmth disease. In each case the complaints are different. (3) In case one was struck by wind, the [movement in the] vessels is at the surface and smooth at the yang [section] while it is soft and weak at the yin [section]. (4) [The movement in the] vessels in the case of moisture and warmth is soft and weak at the yang [section] while it is minor and tense at the yin [section]. (5) [The movement that can be felt in the] vessels in the case of harm caused by cold is full, tight, and rough at both the yin and yang [sections]. (6) [The movement that can be felt in the] vessels in the case of a heat disease is at the surface at both the yin and yang [sections. If one touches] the surface, [he perceives a] smooth [movement; if one presses one's fingers to] the depth, [the movement perceived there is] dispersed and rough. (7) [The movement in] the vessels in the case of a warmth disease [is characterized by the fact that this disease] proceeds through all conduits. It is impossible to know to which [specific] conduit a movement is related. In this case one takes [the evil qi] away from the specific conduit where they just happen to be.

(8) In the case of harm caused by cold, one may induce sweating and a cure will be achieved, but if a purging is induced [the patient will] die. There are other cases where sweating causes death while purging would lead to a cure. Why is that?

(9) It is like this. In the case of a depletion of yang [qi] and an abundance of yin [qi], sweating will lead to a cure and purging will lead to death. (10) In the case of an abundance of yang [qi] and a depletion of yin [qi], sweating will lead to death and purging will bring about a cure.

(11) How can the [different] cold-heat diseases be diagnosed?

(12) It is like this. When cold and heat have affected the skin, the skin will not approach the mat, the hair will be scorched, and the nose will be dry. One must not induce sweating. (13) When cold and heat have affected the flesh, pain will be felt in the skin. The lips and the tongue will dry out, and there will be nothing that could be sweated. (14) When cold and heat have affected the bones, one suffers from unrest all over [the body]. Sweat will flow ceaselessly; the roots of the teeth will dry out and be in pain.

COMMENTARIES

(1) *Hua Shou*: Bian 變 ("changes") should be read as *bian* 辨 ("to distinguish"); that is to say, "[is it possible to] distinguish [them on the basis of different movements in the] vessels?"

Ye Lin: This is discussed in great detail in the [treatises] "Feng lun" 風論 ("On Wind") and "Re lun" 熱論 ("On Heat") of the *Su wen*. But why was no separate section entitled "Han lun" 寒論 ("On Cold") included [in the *Nei jing*]? Well, all the [diseases] discussed at the beginning of the [treatise] "Re lun" 熱論, which are heat diseases according to modern understanding, belong to the "harm caused by cold" category. That is to say, if they are categorized as harm caused by cold, [the *Nei jing*] obviously contains a special discussion focussing on harm caused by cold! Unfortunately, the entire seventh chapter [of the *Nei jing*] was lost due to military actions and fire. Yueren knew also that the ancient medical classics used the term "harm caused by cold" as an all-encompassing designation for affections caused by external [qi]. Hence he feared that later generations might not [be able to] distinguish between [diseases due to] cold and heat, and wrote his discourse on the existence of five [kinds of] harm caused by cold in order to distinguish between their [respective movements in the] vessels and [other] symptoms. Mr. Hua has commented that *bian* 變 ("changes") should be read *bian* 辨 ("to distinguish"). That is correct.

Liao Ping: Here the character *mai* 脈 ("[movement in the] vessels") should refer inclusively to the appearance of the color, the voice, the skin, and the network [vessels].

(2) *Yang*: When someone is ill because he was struck by wind chill in the time between [the solar terms] *shuang jiang* 霜降 ("hoar-frost descends") and *chun fen* 春分 ("vernal equinox"), that is called *shang han* 傷寒 ("harm caused by cold"). If someone is ill because he received qi of cold during winter and then, during spring, was struck again by spring winds, that is called *wen bing* 溫病 ("warmth-disease"). *Re bing* 熱病 ("heat diseases") develop frequently during summer; if someone has such a disease and suffers from frequent sweating, this is called *shi wen* 濕溫 ("moisture and warmth"). If someone is harmed by a depletion evil at one of the eight seasonal terms,[1] that is called *zhong feng* 中風 ("to be struck by wind"). According to the words of the [*Nan*] *jing* here, *wen bing* 溫病 ("warmth-disease") refers to an epidemic disease, not to a spring disease. "Epidemics" means that in one year both the old and the young of one entire province or district suffer from one [and the same] disease.

Zhang Shixian: When someone has been struck by wind evil and suffers from a bad wind,[2] that is called *zhong feng* 中風 ("to be struck by wind"). When someone is affected, in the depth of winter, by cold and, after a certain time, develops heat and has a bad cold, that is *shang han* 傷寒 ("harm caused by cold"). If someone has already been harmed by moisture and is then struck by heat, the moisture and the heat will clash against each other, resulting in disease. The entire body will be in pain. That is called *shi wen* 濕溫 ("moisture and warmth"). When someone has been harmed by cold in winter and develops heat only in summer, together with a bad cold, headache, and bodily pain, that is called *re bing* 熱病 ("heat disease"). If during the entire year cold and warmth do not appear at their proper times, and if man is thus affected by inappropriate qi, old and young alike will show the same effects. That is called *wen bing* 溫病 ("warmth disease"). A vernacular expression is *tian xing* 天行 ("epidemics"). These are the five different complaints from which one may suffer [in the case of harm caused by cold] diseases.

---

1   This is a reference to the ancient idea that diseases are caused by winds originating from the cardinal direction opposite to the direction where Tai yi 太一 happens to reside on the eight seasonal terms. See Unschuld, *Medicine in China: A History of Ideas*, 67-73.

2   The term *e feng* 惡風 ("malign wind") can also be read as *wu feng* ("to have an aversion against wind"). Both readings are possible. The same applies to the terms *e han* 惡寒 ("malign cold") and *wu han* ("to have an aversion against cold"). Several commentators of the present difficult issue have used these terms but it is difficult to determine in each case which reading they had in mind. Hence one should remember, when reading these comments, that the concept of "suffering from a bad wind" (possibly referring to paralysis) could also include an "aversion against wind," and that a "bad cold" could be or could include an "aversion against cold."

(3) *Ding Deyong*: The yang vessels proceed above the flesh. If one presses them with a light hand and [the movement in them] appears greatly excessive, that is called "smooth." The yin vessels proceed below the flesh. If one presses them with a heavy hand and [the movement in them] appears insufficient, that is called "weak." This [kind of a condition is revealed through] an insufficient [movement in the vessels that is felt] by pressing [the vessels heavily, and through a] surplus [movement that is felt with slightly] lifted [fingers]. Hence one knows [the patient] was struck by wind.

Yang: If one presses [the vessels] and perceives the presence of a movement, and if one lifts [the fingers slightly] and has a perception as if there were no [movement], that would be called a "weak" [movement]. That is [a movement which is] at the surface and smooth in front of the gate [section] and soft and weak in the foot [section].

(4) *Ding Deyong*: As to "[the movement is] soft and weak at the yang [section]," the yang vessels proceed above the flesh; "soft and weak" indicates that qi of moisture have overcome the fire. The yin vessels proceed below the flesh. "Minor and tense" indicates that the moisture of the soil does not overcome the wood. Hence one perceives a "minor and tense" [movement]. For this reason [the text] states: "[The movement is] soft and weak at the yang [section], and minor and tense at the yin [section]."

Yang: Xiao 小 ("minor") stands for *xi* 細 ("fine"); *ji* 急 ("tense") stands for *ji* 疾 ("urgent").

Yu Shu: In the case of a "moisture and warmth" disease, the patient will sweat profusely on his head. Why do I say so? [The text] says that the yang [movement in the] vessels at the inch opening appears soft and weak. This indicates that the water has seized the [location of the] fire. The original [text in the *Nei*] *jing* states: "The kidneys are responsible for the penetration of liquids into the heart and for the formation of sweat." That is [what is] meant here.

Liao Ping: All these sentences speak of yin or yang repletion, but I do not know to what they refer.

(5) *Ding Deyong*: "[The movement is] full at both the yin and yang [sections]" means that it is extreme. That is to say, [the movement that can be felt in both] the inch [section] and the foot [section] is extremely full and also tight and rough. Such [a condition results from one's] being struck by the cold of fog or dew. When water is subjected to the cold of wind it congeals. Hence one knows that if the kidneys are subjected to cold, this [kind of movement in the] vessels appears.

Yu Shu: If [the vessels] appear as if one touched a rope, that is called "tight"; if [the movement in the vessels] resembles knives cutting bamboo, that is called "rough."

Liao Ping: In distinguishing between [diseases caused by] wind, cold, moisture, and heat, the *Shang han* [*lun* 傷寒論 of Zhang] Zhongjing 張仲景 considers the symptoms as most decisive, while it regards the movement in the vessels [as it is conditioned by the affected] conduits themselves as secondary. It is a false doctrine of the *Nan jing* to determine diseases on the basis of the [movements in the] vessels alone. One must also compare this with the text of the *Shang han* [*lun*] and the mistakes here will become obvious by themselves.

(6) *Ding Deyong*: "[The movement is] at the surface at both the yin and yang [sections]" means that [the movement that can be felt] in both the foot [section] and inch [section] is at the surface. "At the surface it is smooth" means that if one presses [the vessels] with a light hand, [one perceives a] smooth [movement]. That is a [movement in the] vessels [characteristic] of the heart being damaged by heat. "In the depth it is dispersed and rough" means that if one presses [the vessels] with his hand to the depth, [one will perceive] a dispersed and rough [movement]. That is [a sign of] a depletion of bodily liquids.

Yang: To press with a light hand is called "at the surface"; to press with a heavy hand is called "in the depth."

Liao Ping: The *Nei jing* discusses the heat diseases in several treatises. How could one identify them through the [movement in the vessels]! Also, how could anybody [describe heat diseases] exhaustively with just the one word, "surface"?! This is nothing but fool's talk!

(7) *Ding Deyong*: The lung represents the metal; it rules the qi and disperses them through all conduits. One does not know which conduit – following its depletion – has received these particular evil [qi] in the first place before they were transmitted further.[3] Hence one takes the evil [qi causing] the disease away from the location where they just happen to be.

Yang: All demonic or *li* 癘 qi[4] disperse through all the conduits. Hence one cannot know in advance [where they may proceed]. One must diagnose the individual patient. As soon as is known in which conduit [these qi] happen to move, the treatment must be applied there.

Zhang Shixian: "The [movement in the] vessels in the case of a warmth disease" [means the following]. When [seasonally] inappropriate qi disperse through all

---

3   I read the *chuan shou* 傳受 of the text as *shou chuan* 受傳.

4   The term *li* 癘 has been used since ancient times to designate particularly evil qi responsible for epidemic diseases.

conduits, it is difficult to distinguish which conduit has received them [first]. In this case one must examine to which conduit the disease belongs before a treatment can be applied.

Ye Lin: Warmth (*wen* 溫) diseases are epidemic (*wen yi* 瘟疫) diseases. In ancient times the character *wen* 瘟 ("epidemic") did not exist. Hence [the characters] *wen* ("warmth") and *wen* ("epidemic") were used interchangeably [for some time after the latter was created]. *Yi* 疫 ("epidemic") stands for *yi* 役 ("military service"), as in *yao yi* 徭役 ("compulsory service"). [Epidemics] occur often in the aftermath of ravages and burning committed by soldiers, or after such calamities of unbalanced [weather conditions that result] in floods and droughts. Large [epidemics affect] an entire city; small [epidemics affect] a market or a village. [Epidemics] are transmitted to everybody.

(1)–(7) *Katō Bankei:* The *Nei jing* categorizes all heat diseases as *shang han* 傷寒 ("harm caused by cold"). Obviously, then, the meaning of "heat disease" is very broad. In discussing the respective diseases, [the *Nei jing*] talks only about the conduits through which they are transmitted, but it does not differentiate clearly among the five different symptom [clusters] related to affections caused by, for instance, two [different] external agents. Also, it names only two diseases – warmth and heat. Bian Que was the first to discuss the five kinds of harm caused by cold because the *Nei jing*, in its discussion of heat [diseases], did not talk about the appearances of the [movements in the] vessels [associated with the individual heat diseases]. Hence he introduced the names and the [respective movement in the] vessels of the diseases resulting from having been affected by an [external] evil [qi. Disease] names are quite important in human therapeutic efforts. When the naming [of a disease] is not correct, its discussion cannot be to the point. When the discussion [of a disease] is not to the point, the problem cannot be handled successfully. When medical problems cannot be handled successfully, the people have nobody to turn to in the case of a disease. [This difficult issue asks] how many kinds of harm caused by cold exist, and [the answer] differentiates among [the five kinds of harm caused by cold] on the basis of the causation of the respective diseases. These, then, are all the so-called heat diseases of the *Nei jing*. The "harm caused by cold" listed as one of the five diseases [categorized broadly as harm caused by cold] is the true harm caused by cold. The remaining four diseases – namely, [harm caused by] wind, heat, warmth, and moisture – fall in one category with [the true] harm caused by cold. This coincides with the statement [in the *Nei jing*] that they all belong to the category of harm caused by cold. All these diseases have heat as one of their symptoms. That is, the actual complaints are identical in all cases. But when [the

Nan jing] says that [the complaints] are different in each case, it says so because it distinguishes between [manifestations of the diseases in] the yin or yang [section], in the external or internal [section], near the surface or in the depth. The *Nei jing* emphasized the [differences between the respective manifestations of heat diseases on the basis of the] symptoms related to the transmission [of the respective diseases] through the conduits. That, too, was detailed and exhaustive. But it did not talk about the differences among the heat diseases due to the [fact that they are caused by] five [different] evil [qi]. Therefore, Bian Que set aside the question of the complaints; he did not differentiate among them. Instead, he pointed out the appearances of the [movements in the] vessels in order to distinguish the characteristics of the five diseases concerned. Thus he provided proper targets and facilitated treatment. [When writing] the *Shang han lun* 傷寒論, [Zhang] Zhongjing 張仲景 relied on this treatise in all respects, proving [his remarks] by analogy. Hardly anything else [could be said about this issue]. Students should consult his [work].

(8)–(10) *Ding Deyong*: Abundance or depletion of yin and yang [qi] does not refer to [a movement in the] vessels [that can be felt] at the surface or in the depth. It means that diseases due to cold or heat are different; that dryness and moisture are not the same. Man's five long-term depots and six short-term repositories have twelve conduits. They all can be subjected to diseases. The hand major yang and the [hand] minor yin [conduits] belong to the fire; it rules the warmth. The hand yang brilliance and the [hand major yin [conduits] belong to the metal; it rules the dryness. The hand minor yang and the [hand] ceasing yin [conduits] belong to the minister fire; it rules the heat. These are the six conduits of dryness, heat, and warmth; they are penetrated by the qi of heaven. When they have a disease, the body will not [feel] heavy and will not suffer from bad wind;[5] it will be affected by dryness. The *Su wen* states: "Whenever [a movement] at the surface is accompanied by dryness, the disease is in the hand [conduits]." That is correct. If one purges [the disease] with a "supporting the qi" [preparation, the patient] will be cured. If one asks him to consume *gui* 桂 branch [preparations][6] to take away [his disease through] sweating, he will die as soon as sweat leaves [his body]. The foot major yang and the [foot] minor yin [conduits] belong to the water, which rules the cold. The foot yang brilliance and the [foot] major yin [conduits] belong to the soil, which rules the moisture. The foot ceasing yin and the [foot] minor yang [conduits] belong to the wood, which rules the wind. These are the six conduits of wind, cold, and moisture; they are penetrated by the

---

5   See note 2.

6   These are preparations containing cinnamon bark (*gui zhi* 桂枝, *Cortex Cinnamomi*).

qi of the earth. When they have a disease, the body will feel heavy and [suffer from] bad cold. Hence the *Su wen* states: "Whenever [a movement] is at the surface while no dryness is present, the disease is in the foot [conduits]." That is correct. If one takes away [the patient's disease by means of] sweating, using a *gui* 桂 branch [preparation, the patient] will be cured as soon as the sweat leaves [the body]. If one purges him with a "supporting the qi" [preparation], he will die. This is the great pattern of the matching of the five long-term depots and the six short-term repositories with yin and yang. Thus, when the [*Nan*] *jing* states: "In the case of a depletion of yang [qi] and an abundance of yin [qi], sweating will lead to a cure and purging will lead to death. In the case of an abundance of yang [qi] and a depletion of yin [qi], sweating will lead to death and purging will bring about a cure," the meaning [of this statement] is directly opposite [to what would be correct].

Yang: These explanations are contrary [to what is right]. They do not agree with the meaning [expressed in the *Su wen*]. One cannot rely on them in one's practice. If one acted contrary to them, that would be appropriate.

Yu Shu: The meaning expressed in the [classic] scriptures cannot be wrong. The meaning outlined here in the [*Nan*] *jing* must be the result of an error in writing in the course of the transmission [of this text through the ages]. Whenever someone is ill due to harm caused by cold, the [movement in his] vessels is at the surface, strong, and frequent. One can achieve a cure through causing [the patient] to sweat. [In this case] the disease is in the exterior [sections]. When the [movement in the] vessels is in the depth, fine, and frequent, one can achieve a cure through purging. [In this case] the disease is in the interior [sections]. If one acts according to these [standards], he will not miss one case out of ten thousand.

(8) *Liao Ping*: The *Shang han* [*lun*] 傷寒論 ("On Harm Caused by Cold") is a very compact book, designed entirely to outline [the diseases referred to by its title. The *Nan jing*, in contrast,] discusses [these diseases] with but a few sentences. Later people appreciated its simple and easily understandable [contents], and it is for this reason that it reached wider circulation than any other [book]. But is there any other [work] matching [the *Nan jing*] in the confusion of principles?[7] If everything is indeed as simple [as it is portrayed by the *Nan jing*], then [Zhang] Zhongjing 張仲景 and [Wang] Shuhe 王叔和 must have pretended to write about a difficult subject!

---

7   *Luan dao* 亂道 ("confused path") is, of course, a metaphor for the "confused principles" (*luan dao*) borrowed, in the eyes of Liao Ping, by Zhang Zhongjing from the *Nan jing*.

(9) *Li Jiong*: A depletion of yang [qi] indicates external cold; an abundance of yin [qi also] indicates external cold. The cold poison battles among the camp and guard qi; heat must develop and a dislike for cold. [The movement in the vessels to be felt at] both the foot [section] and the inch [section] is near the surface and strong. Internally no annoyance occurs; if [the patient feels] a minor irritation, he will long for warm drinks and food, and he will dislike anything chilled. This is a condition of yang depletion and yin abundance. Sweating the [patient] will bring about a cure; purging him is a mistake and results in death.

Zhang Shixian: A depletion of yang [qi] and an abundance of yin [qi] indicates external disease and internal well-being. In the case of an external disease one should induce sweating. As soon as the sweat leaves [the body], the disease is cured. If, by mistake, one purges, that will result in death.

(10) *Li Jiong*: An abundance of yang [qi] indicates internal heat; a depletion of yin [qi also] indicates internal heat. The cold poison clashes against the camp and guard qi. When the yang is present in abundance, the yin is at its weakest. The yin then changes into yang. [Similarly,] when cold is present in abundance, it generates heat. [As a consequence] the qi of yang heat are abundant and enter the interior [sections of the body]. The heat poison resides in the stomach. Water and other [liquids] dry up. The stool conglomerates. The respective person does not dislike external cold; he cannot avoid steaming. Steaming develops heat and causes extreme desiccation. This, then, results in incoherent talk. Purging will bring about a cure; sweating is a mistake and leads to death.

Zhang Shixian: A depletion of yin [qi] and an abundance of yang [qi] indicates internal disease and external wellbeing. In the case of an internal disease one should purge. Hence, as soon as the disease is purged, it will be cured. If, by mistake, one induces sweating, this will result in death. If someone dies like this, one knows that medicine killed him because a crude practitioner did not know [how to distinguish] external and internal [diseases].

Liao Ping: Whether it is possible to induce sweating or whether it is not possible to induce sweating, whether it is possible to purge or whether it is not possible to purge – all of this cannot be discussed in detail exhaustively in two sentences.

(11)–(12) *Ding Deyong*: The [condition of the] lung can be diagnosed through [the condition of] the body's skin [and its] hair. The large intestine [and the lung] constitute exterior and interior. When the long-term depot [i.e., the lung] has a disease, one feels cold; when the short-term repository [i.e., the large intestine] has a disease, one feels hot. Hence [the text] states: [When] cold and heat have affected the skin." "The skin will not approach the mat" means that the three yin and the three yang [conduits] of the hands reflect heaven; heaven moves. Hence in the case of a disease one does not wish to lie down and approach the mat. "The hair will be scorched; the nose will be dry; one must not induce sweating" means that the fire of the heart below [the hair and the nose causes] dryness and heat, resulting in disease. One must not cause sweating in the [patient]. If one causes him to sweat, he will die. If one purges him, he will be cured. This is so because the lung rules the dryness.

(11) *Zhang Shixian*: "Cold and heat" means that one is cold at night and hot in the morning.

Xu Dachun: "Cold and heat" means that one is suddenly cold or hot.

(12) *Xu Dachun*: If evil qi are present in the skin, one cannot touch anything.

(13) *Ding Deyong*: The [condition] of the spleen can be diagnosed through the [condition of the] flesh. The stomach [and the spleen] constitute exterior and interior. When the long-term depot [i.e., the spleen] has a disease, the body will be cold; when the short-term repository [i.e., the stomach] has a disease, the body will be hot. Hence [the text] states: "[When] cold and heat have affected the flesh." "Pain will be felt in the skin; the lips and the tongue will dry out" [means that] the spleen corresponds to the soil. The soil controls the moisture. Hence the bodily liquids leave through the skin and the body is heavy. When the bodily liquids are drained toward the outside, the lips and the tongue will dry out. This disease is called "dried up moisture." No [liquids are left in the body that could serve as a source for] sweating. If one induces sweating [anyway], the intestines and the stomach will be drained and become impassable. If one purges, a rushing diarrhea will be the result. This disease is caused by qi of moisture. One must provide warmth to the center and harmonize the qi.

(14) *Ding Deyong*: The kidneys rule the bones; the urinary bladder [and the kidneys] constitute exterior and interior. When the disease is in the yang [section, i.e., in the urinary bladder], the body is hot and heavy and one [suffers from] a bad cold.[8] When [the disease] is in the yin [section, i.e., in the kidneys, the body is] cold. "One suffers from total unrest" means that the kidneys rule the water. Sweat rushes out without a break. The roots of the teeth dry out and ache. Sweating causes the cure; purging results in death. When the yin [qi] are abundant while the yang [qi] are depleted, one will die.

(11)–(14) *Xu Dachun*: This paragraph should not be listed together with "harm caused by cold" in one difficult issue. Because cold-heat diseases are manifestations of various diseases which are not transmitted through the conduits, the *Ling shu* has listed cold-heat diseases as the heading of a separate treatise. There it outlines, in detail, the respective needling techniques. From this one can see

8   See note 2.

that [cold-heat diseases] do not belong to the "harm caused by cold" diseases mentioned in the preceding [section of this] text. I do not know whether Yueren considered them to be related and, for this reason, joined them. If he considered the cold and heat [of the cold-heat diseases] as resulting from harm caused by cold, that would be a grave mistake. Furthermore, this is [a quotation of an] original text in the treatise "Han re lun" 寒熱論 of the *Ling* [*shu*].⁹ However, from the paragraph "Cold and Heat of Bones" [of the *Ling shu* treatise], numerous words have been omitted [here in the *Nan jing*]. As a result, the meaning is incomplete. The text of the [*Nei*] *jing* states: "When the bones have alternating sensations of cold and heat, with the patient finding no place where to rest, and sweat flowing without end, if [in such a situation] the teeth have not dried up completely yet, one chooses [for therapy] the network [vessels] of the minor yin [conduit] at the inner side of the thigh. If the teeth have dried up entirely, [the patient] will die. No cure is possible." One can see that, originally, minor and serious symptoms were distinguished here. Now, the [*Nan jing*] states only: "The roots of the teeth will dry out and be in pain." Thus [the *Nan jing* lists], for the case that cold and heat have affected the bones, only symptoms indicating death but no symptoms indicating survival. The [complete quotation] provided an important clue for [an understanding of] the relationships between death and survival. How could one make such omissions?

Ding Jin: *Han re bing* 寒熱病 ("cold-heat diseases") is an all-encompassing term for harm caused by cold and for being struck by wind.

---

9   Cf. *Ling shu* treatise 21, "Han re bing" 寒熱病.

五十九難曰：（一）狂癲之病，何以別之？

（二）然：狂之始發，少臥而不饑，自高賢也，自辨智也，自貴倨也，妄笑好歌樂，妄行不休是也。（三）癲疾始發，意不樂，直視僵仆。（四）其脈三部陰陽俱盛是也。

The fifty-ninth difficult issue: (1) By what [criteria] can the diseases of madness and peak-illness be distinguished?

(2) It is like this. During the initial development of madness, [patients] rest only rarely and do not feel hungry. They will [speak of] themselves as occupying lofty, exemplary positions. They will point out their special wisdom, and they will behave in an arrogant and haughty way. They will laugh – and find joy in singing and making music – without reason, and they will walk around heedlessly without break. (3) During the initial development of peak-illness, one's thoughts are unhappy. [The patient] lies down and stares straight ahead. (4) The yin and the yang [movements in the] vessels are full in all three sections.

COMMENTARIES

(1) *Liao Ping*: This was discussed in the [*Nei*] *jing* in great detail. Why should one ask about this again?

(2) *Ding Deyong*: Diseases of madness [originate as follows]: If one induces, in the case of a disease in any of the three hand yang [conduits], sweating when this is contrary to what would be appropriate, an abundance of yang [qi] results and madness develops. If, in the case of a disease of the three foot yin [conduits], one purges when this is contrary to what would be appropriate, an abundance of yin [qi] results and peak-illness develops.

Yang: To find out whether someone suffers from madness, one observes the respective person at the first outbreak [of his disease]. In case he does not wish to lie down and sleep or is not willing to drink and eat, and if he speaks of himself as an exemplary person and wise man, worthy of being honored and praised, or sings or laughs and runs around without break, all these [phenomena] are caused by an abundance of yang qi. Hence the [*Nan*] *jing* states: "A doubling of the yang [qi results in] madness." That is [what is] meant here. Today's people believe [madness] to be identical with peak-illness. That is an error.

Hua Shou: Madness develops in the yang [vessels]; hence all its manifestations result from a surplus [of yang qi], which are responsible for the [continuous] moving around [of the patients].

(3)*Yang*: *Dian* 癲 ("peak-illness") stands for *dian* 顛 ("to fall"). During an outbreak [of peak-illness] one falls down. Hence one speaks of *dian jue* 顛蹶 ("to fall"). The yin qi are present in great abundance. Hence one cannot walk or stand and falls down. Today's people believe [the peak-illness] to be identical with *xian* 癇 convulsions. That is a mistake.

    Hua Shou: Peak-illness develops in the yin [vessels]. Hence all its manifestations result from an insufficiency [of yang qi, a condition which is] responsible for the quiet [attitude of the patients].

(4) *Ding Deyong*: [Earlier,] the [*Nan*] *jing* stated: "A doubling of the yang [qi results in] madness. A doubling of the yin [qi results in] peak-illness."[1] Here [the text says]: "The yin and yang [movements in the vessels] are full in all three sections." The inch [section] constitutes the yang; the foot [section] constitutes the yin. [In this case, then, the movements that can be felt in the] inch and foot [sections appear] full and in the depth.

    Li Jiong: The inch opening is the yang section; the foot [section] is the yin section. The [movement in the] vessels is full in all three sections.

    Hua Shou: "The yin and yang [movements in the] vessels are full in all three sections" means [the following]: Madness develops in the yang [vessels. In this case, the movement that can be felt in] all the yang vessels is full. Peak-illness develops in the yin [vessels. In this case the movement that can be felt in] all the yin vessels is full.

    Zhang Shixian: The three sections are the inch, the gate, and the foot. In front of the gate [section] is the yang [section]; behind the gate is the yin [section]. In the case of madness, yang [qi] appear in the vessels in both the yin and yang sections. In the case of peak-illness, both [sections are marked by a] yin [movement in the] vessels.

    Liao Ping: The two characters [*san bu* 三部 ("three sections")] must have been added later.

(1)–(4) *Hua Shou*: The four sentences of the twentieth difficult issue [which read,] "a doubling of the yang [qi results in] madness; a doubling of yin [qi results in] peak-illness; when the yang [qi] are gone one sees demons; when the yin [qi] are gone one's eyes turn blind" should be part of the present [paragraph]. *Chong* 重 is to be read like the *Chong* in *zai chong* 再重 ("twice"). If one considers [the statement] "a doubling of yang [qi results in madness]; a doubling of yin [qi results in peak-illness]" on the basis of [*chong* being read as] "twice," the meaning of the [statement] "the yin and the yang [movement in the vessels] are full in all [three sections]" in the text above becomes evident. If one traces such [a

_____

1   See the twentieth difficult issue.

condition] to its extreme – namely to "when the yin [qi] are gone" and "when the yang [qi] are gone" – [it becomes obvious that] the process [of an increase in the unilateral presence of specific qi] does not end with the "doubling of yin [qi]" and with the "doubling of yang [qi]". An extreme abundance of yin [qi] represents [a situation where] the yang [qi] are gone. Demons are beings of the darkness and of yin. Hence they become visible [in such a situation]. An extreme abundance of yang [qi] represents [a situation where] the yin [qi] are gone. One water cannot overcome five fires. Hence the eyes turn blind.

Xu Dachun: In the treatise "Dian kuang" 癲狂 of the *Ling* [*shu*], the symptoms of peak-illness and madness, the needling and cauterization techniques, and the application of a treatment in accordance with the symptoms are outlined both in detail and comprehensively. In this paragraph here, however, only one or two symptoms from the [*Nei*] *jing* are pointed out. These are by no means two different diseases; it is just that the appearance of this disease takes three or four shapes. If one examines the text of the [*Nei*] *jing* carefully, everything will become obvious by itself. This here is [an example of the saying]: "One item recorded, tens of thousands omitted!"

Ding Jin: This [difficult issue] has the same meaning as the twentieth difficult issue. However, the twentieth difficult issue discussed only the [movement in the] vessels; the present [paragraph] talks about the appearances of these diseases. [Together, they] serve to impart the knowledge of how to treat [madness and peak-illness]. "During the initial development of madness, one rests only rarely and does not feel hungry" means that the stomach is replete with evil yang [qi] from the six short-term repositories. When the stomach is marked by such repletion rather than by a balance [of yin and yang qi], one rests only rarely and does not feel hungry. The nature of yang is movement and excitement. Hence one will assume for oneself a lofty and exemplary position, one will point out one's special wisdom, and one will be arrogant and haughty. When the yang fire burns excessively and rushes against the heart, one will laugh and sing without reason, and one will walk around heedlessly without break. For treatment, one must drain the fire of the yang brilliance [short-term repository][2] and harmonize its qi. "During the initial development of peak-illness, one's thoughts are unhappy" means that evil yin [qi] of the seven emotions have accumulated in the heart. The nature of yin is quietness and occlusion. When a fire burns internally and cannot find its way out, one will lie down and stare straight ahead. For treatment, one must drain the fire of the minor yin [long-term depot][3] and har-

---

2   That is, the stomach; it is associated with the foot yang brilliance conduit.

3   That is, the heart; it is associated with the hand minor yin conduit.

monize its blood. "The yin and the yang [movements in the] vessels are full in all three sections" means that in the case of madness, the yang [movement in the vessels] in the inch, gate, and foot [sections] of both hands are full; this disease is associated with the short-term repositories. In case of peak-illness, the yin [movements in the vessels] in the inch, gate, and foot [sections] of both hands are full; this disease is associated with the long-term depots. Yang [movements in the] vessels are at the surface, smooth, and extended; yin [movements in the] vessels are in the depth, rough, and short. "Full" has in both cases the meaning of "frequent and replete."

Katō Bankei: The *Ling shu* refers to peak-illness and madness with many statements .... The present paragraph quotes only one or two points, thus eliminating verbosity and approaching a concise [discussion of these diseases. The *Nan jing*] allows one to understand the respective yin and yang associations [of madness and peak-illness]. On the whole, one may say that the statements and elucidations recorded in the *Nan jing* always present the general meaning. Pang Anchang[4] 龐安常 stated: "[The *Nan jing*] alludes but does not develop." That is correct. Also, if one compares, for instance, the present paragraph with the *Ling shu,* what was [presented] without any order in the latter is [presented] concisely here. Hence one is able to recognize the basic [principles] of all diseases. The development of the diseases may proceed along many lines, but most fundamental is the [dichotomy between] repletions and depletions of yin and yang [qi]. For instance, if in the case of madness or peak-illness one clearly distinguishes whether [the disease is associated with a repletion or depletion of] yin or yang [qi] and then applies the treatment, there will be no grief resulting from treading the wrong path or from sinking into marshy grounds. When Bian Que disregarded here any further ramifications and selected only the yin and yang [manifestations of these diseases] as their two [basic] symptoms, he did so in order to demonstrate to later students nothing but the final principles. That is the intention of the ancients.

---

4 Pang Anshi 龐安時, *Zi* name Anchang (1042-1099), was a famous physician and medical author of the Song dynasty. His works include a commentated *Nan jing* edition (see appendix A) which is no longer extant.

六十難曰：（一）頭心之病，有厥痛，有真痛，何謂也？
（二）然：手三陽之脈，受風寒，伏留而不去者，則名厥頭痛；（三）入連在
腦者，名真頭痛。（四）其五藏氣相干，名厥心痛；（五）其痛甚，但在心，
手足青者，即名真心痛。（六）其真心痛者，旦發夕死，夕發旦死。

The sixtieth difficult issue: (1) Among the diseases of head and heart are "receding
[qi] pain" and "genuine pain." What does that mean?

(2) It is like this. When the three hand yang vessels have received [qi of] wind-
cold – which remain hidden where they are and do not move away – that is called
"headache resulting from receding [qi]." (3) When [these qi] enter and join with the
brain, that is called "genuine headache." (4) When the qi of [any of] the five long-
term depots turn against [the heart], that is called "pain in the heart resulting from
receding [qi]." (5) When the pain is extreme, and when it is limited to the heart,
while the hands and the feet are virid,[1] that is called "genuine pain in the heart." (6)
When the onset of genuine pain in the heart is in the morning, death will occur at
night; when the onset is at night, death will occur in the morning.

COMMENTARIES

(1) *Hua Shou*: For details, see the twenty-fourth treatise of the *Ling shu*, "Jue ni" 厥
逆[2].

Liao Ping: The brain is considered [here] as "heart." "Pain in the heart," then, is
"headache." [The heart alluded to here] is not the heart attached to the lung.

(2) *Ding Deyong*: The three hand yang [conduits] represent the yang-in-yang. Here,
they have received [qi] of wind-cold which remain hidden where they are and
do not move away. As a consequence, the [qi in these] three yang [conduits]
move upward, which is contrary to their proper direction. Hence [the text]
speaks of "headache resulting from receding [qi]."

Yang: *Qu* 去 ("move away") stands for *xing* 行 ("to proceed"). *Jue* 厥 ("receding")
stands for *ni* 逆 ("to move contrary to a proper course"). [The text] says: "When
the three hand yang vessels [have received qi of wind cold which] remain hidden
where they are and do not move away." Because of such a blockade, [the yang

---

1 The character *qing* 青 ("virid") may be a mistake for *qing* 清 ("cool"), as some commentators have assumed, because the corresponding passage in the *Nei jing* (see *Ling shu*
treatise 24, "Jue bing" 厥病) says: "In case of true heartache, hands and feet are cool."
However, one should be cautious in interpreting changes in the *Nan jing* on the basis of
the *Nei jing*. Interestingly enough, Xu Dachun accepted the reading of *Qing* as "virid."

2 This should be "Jue bing" 厥病. *Su wen* treatise 47, "Qi bing" 奇病, speaks of headache as
"Jue ni" 厥逆.

qi] move contrary to their proper course and clash against the head. Hence one speaks of "headache resulting from receding [qi]." When [evil qi in the] three foot yang [vessels] cause a blockade because they remain where they are, this, too, will lead to headache. The [*Nan*] *jing* does not mention this here for reasons of space.

Yu Shu: Qi of wind-cold enter the three yang conduits. Hence headache resulting from receding [qi] results. This kind of pain comes to an end quickly.

Li Jiong: Jue 厥 ("receding") stands for *leng* 冷 ("cold").

Zhang Shixian: Jue 厥 ("receding") stands for *ni* 逆 ("to move contrary to a proper course"). *Zhen* 真 ("genuine") means *wu ta za* 無他雜 ("nothing else involved"). The three yang [conduits] of the hands move from the hands to the head. When wind-cold settles down in the head, an obstruction [of these conduits] results. [The respective qi] move contrary to their proper course and cannot continue their flow through [the entire organism]. Therefore, they cause pain which is called "headache resulting from receding [qi]." There are six kinds of headache resulting from receding [qi]. If one has a headache and a perception as if [his head] were swelling, and if he feels distressed in his heart, that is the first [kind of headache resulting from receding [qi]. If the vessels on the head ache and if the heart is sad, and if one has a tendency to cry, that is the second [kind of headache resulting from receding [qi]. If the head feels really heavy and aches, that is the third [kind of headache resulting from receding [qi]. If the head aches, if the intellect tends to be forgetful, and if one cannot stand it being touched, that is the fourth [kind of headache resulting from receding [qi]. If the head aches first, and if the loins and the back follow, that is the fifth [kind of headache resulting from receding [qi]. If one has [a feeling as if the movement in] the vessels in front and behind the ears was rushing with great vigor, and if he is hot, that is the sixth [kind of headache resulting from receding [qi]. For details, see the *Ling shu*.[3]

Xu Dachun: The three hand yang [conduits] are those of the small intestine, the large intestine, and the Triple Burner. According to the *Su* [*wen*], the three hand yang [conduits] extend from the hands to the head. Hence, if they are blocked by [qi of] wind-cold residing in them, headache results.

(3) *Ding Deyong:* When [these qi] enter and join with the brain, that is called "genuine headache." The brain is the sea of marrow. If [qi of] wind-cold enter here, death will follow.

---

3   This is another reference to *Ling shu* treatise 24, "Jue bing" 厥病.

Yu Shu: "Genuine headache" means that the qi of wind-chill have entered the *ni wan* mansion[4] which constitutes the sea of marrow. When evil [qi] enter there, genuine headache results. Severe pain develops in the brain, and hands and feet turn cold up to the elbows and knees. This is called genuine headache because the qi of cold enter the depth [of the head]. The qi of wind-cold enter the brain by way of the wind palace. Hence [the text] says: "Enter and join with the brain."

Hua Shou: In the case of genuine headache, the pain is severe. The entire brain aches. Hands and feet are cool up to the joints [of elbows and knees]. Death will occur; no treatment [is possible]. The brain, as the sea of marrow, is the place where the true qi are accumulated. It must not receive evil [qi]. If it receives evil [qi], death will occur.

Xu Dachun: When the evil [qi] have entered the brain, they are no longer present in the conduits but reside in the brain. Hence this is called "true [headache]."

Liao Ping: If [the words "enter and join with the brain"] were omitted, and if [the remaining words] were joined to form one statement, that would be correct.

(4) *Yang*: All conduits and network [vessels] are tied to the heart. If one single conduit has a disease, [the contents of] this vessel proceed contrary to their proper course. When they move contrary to their proper course, they will seize the heart. When they have seized the heart, the heart will ache. Hence this is called "pain in the heart resulting from receding [qi]." This is [a condition in which] the qi of [any of] the five long-term depots move contrary to their proper course, clashing [with the heart] and causing pain. It is not a pain [developed] by the heart itself.

Hua Shou: The *Ling shu* lists five kinds of pain in the heart resulting from receding [qi], including "stomach pain in the heart," "kidneys pain in the heart," "spleen pain in the heart," "liver pain in the heart," and "lung pain in the heart." In all [these cases] evil qi from one of the five long-term depots have turned against [the heart].

Zhang Shixian: The heart is the lord-ruler official; it governs the entire body. If any conduit has received evil [qi, its contents] will move contrary to their proper course and turn against [the heart], which results in pain. That is called "pain in the heart resulting from receding [qi]."

Ye Lin: All conduits and network [vessels] are tied to the heart; the heart rules [the movement in] all the vessels. The camp [qi moving in the latter – i.e.,] the blood – originate from the heart and penetrate the twelve conduits and network

---

4   This term appears in reconstructed versions of *Su wen* treatise 73, "Ben bing lun" 本病論. It is identified as referring to the "Upper Field of Cinnabar," a term denoting the head in the terminology of the Daoist Interior Gods hygiene school. See H. Welch, *Taoism: The Parting of the Way*, (Boston 1966), 106-107.

[vessels]. If one conduit is affected by a disease, [the contents of] this vessel will move contrary to their proper course. When they move contrary to their proper course, they will seize the heart. When they seize the heart, the heart will ache. Hence that is called "pain in the heart resulting from receding [qi]." This is [a situation where] the qi of [any of] the five long-term depots clash [against the heart, because they] move contrary to their proper course, with pain being the result. This is not a disease of the heart itself.

Liao Ping: [The term *gan* 干 ("to attack"; here, "to turn against")] is a mistake for *xi* 襲 ("to invade"). It was appropriate during the time of Huai nan [zi] 淮南子.[5] It is an expression [borrowed] from the political doctrine of the Five Phases school.

(5) *Ding Deyong*: The true heart cannot have a disease. When the external conduits[6] are affected by an onslaught of any of the five evil [qi], that is called "pain in the heart resulting from receding [qi]." When the pain is severe, hands and feet are cool and chilled. If the [qi at the] "spirit gate" hole[7] are cut off, death will occur. This disease is called "genuine pain in the heart."

(5)–(6) *Yang*: The heart is the ruler of the five long-term depots and six short-term repositories. According to the law, it should not receive any disease. If it is affected by a disease, its spirit will move away and its qi will vanish. As a consequence, hands and feet will be cool and chilled. If in the case of pain in the heart hands and feet are chilled, it is genuine pain in the heart. If [in the case of pain in the heart], the hands and the feet are warm, that is pain in the heart resulting from receding [qi]. The same applies to headache. From this morning to tomorrow morning is one day. Here [the text] says: "When the onset is in the morning, death will occur at night; when the onset is at night, death will occur in the morning." That is to say, death occurs exactly after one half day.

(5)–(6) *Hua Shou*: The *Ling shu* states: "In the case of genuine headache, hands and feet are cool up to the joints; the pain in the heart is severe," that is genuine pain in the heart. Further, in the seventy-first treatise, it says: "The minor yin [conduit] is the vessel associated with the heart. The heart is the great ruler of the five long-term depots and six short-term repositories. The heart is the lord-ruler; it is the lodging place of the essence spirit. As a long-term depot it is firm and

5 Liu An 劉安 (died 122 BCE), grandson of the founder of the Han dynasty and Prince of Huainan.

6 "External conduits" may refer to the conduits associated with the heart-enclosing network.

7 This sentence is quoted from *Su wen* treatise 74, "Zhi zhen yao da lun" 至真要大論. The "spirit gate" hole is located below the palm at the inner side of the wrist on the hand-minor yin conduit, which is associated with the heart.

enduring; evil [qi] cannot settle down in it. If they settle down in it, they will harm the heart. When the heart is harmed, the spirit will move away; when the spirit has moved away, one dies." In the [phrase] "when the [onset of] genuine pain in the heart," the character *tou* 頭 ("head") appears to be missing below the character *xin* 心 ("heart"). Obviously, the text is corrupt here. The [character] *qing* 青 ("virid") in "hands and feet are virid" should be *qing* 清 ("cool"). It stands for *leng* 冷 ("cold").

(6) *Zhang Shixian:* "In the morning" and "at night" means "early" and "late." That is to say, death occurs quickly. If the time of death lies within such a short period, one cannot apply a treatment. That is evident. Cases of genuine headache will also lead to death and cannot be treated.

(5) *Xu Dachun:* "The hands and the feet are virid" [means that] when evil cold attacks the position of the ruler fire, the color of the blood changes.

(1)–(6) *Xu Dachun:* According to the treatise "Jue bing" 厥病 of the *Ling* [*shu*], the disease of "headache resulting from receding [qi]" has several manifestations. For its treatment, one selects either yang conduits or yin conduits. From this one can see that it is not [a condition where] only the three yang [conduits] are affected by a disease. If [the text] had said that [the evil] was transmitted from the three yang [conduits] to the other conduits, that would have been correct. As to the "genuine headache," the text of the [*Nei*] *jing* states: "Hands and feet are cold up to the joints; death will occur; no treatment can be applied." Hence, there are symptoms also indicating death for headache. This parallels [the statement] that in the case of [true] pain in the heart, hands and feet are virid up to the joints, with death being imminent and no treatment applicable. As to the symptoms of "pain in the heart resulting from receding [qi]," the text of the [*Nei*] *jing* mentions five different kinds of manifestations of [receding] pain in the heart, including kidneys [pain in the heart], stomach [pain in the heart], spleen [pain in the heart], liver [pain in the heart], and lung [pain in the heart]. In each case the appearance of the disease differs. Hence one cannot say "the [qi of any of the] five long-term depots turn against [the heart]," because the stomach is a short-term repository and cannot be called "long-term depot." If [qi from] the heart turn against the heart, this results in "genuine pain in the heart." This should not be listed with pain in the heart resulting from receding [qi. The author] should have written his statements as clearly as the text in the [*Nei*] *jing*. Why did he put down his words so foolishly, causing the text of the [*Nei*] *jing* to become obscured rather than [clarified]?!

Ding Jin: The intention of the present chapter is to make it very clear that diseases in the long-term depots are more serious than diseases in the short-term repositories. When the qi in the long-term depots clash against each other, that is more serious than when wind-cold remains hidden [in some conduit]. Hence [the text] speaks of imminent death in the case of pain in the heart; it does not speak of imminent death in the case of headache. When, for instance, wind-cold remains hidden in [any of] the six short-term repositories, the true qi of the three yang [conduits] move contrary to their proper course. Hence the evil [qi] will be able to proceed straight upward and the head will ache. The brain is the sea of marrow; it is difficult for any evil [qi] to attack it. Only if essence or marrow suffer major harm can evil [qi] attack [the brain]. When they attack it, a cure is difficult to achieve. In case [any of] the qi of the five long-term depots clashes against the heart, the yin qi will move upward – which is contrary to their proper direction – and [cause] severe pain. However, the heart is the lord-ruler; it is difficult for any evil [qi] to attack it. Only if any of the seven emotions has severely harmed its true qi can evil [qi] attack [the heart]. Such an attack is focussed on the heart; pain [will result] and one must die immediately. "Hands and feet are virid" refers to the color associated with the liver. In this case the qi of the mother of the heart are cut off, and the color of the true long-term depot becomes visible. In the development of diseases due to the five evil [qi], only madness and the peak-illness – as well as headache and pain in the heart – have special characteristics. For this reason they were mentioned here first, before the next chapter refers to the development of diseases caused by the five evil [qi] in general.[8]

---

8   Ding Jin listed this difficult issue as the forty-seventh, followed by the tenth difficult issue of the version adopted here as the forty-eighth.

六十一難曰：（一）經言望而知之謂之神，聞而知之謂之聖，問而知之謂之工，切脈而知之謂之巧，何謂也？

（二）然：望而知之者，望見其五色，以知其病。（三）聞而知之者，聞其五音，以別其病。（四）問而知之者，問其所欲五味，以知其病所起所在也。（五）切脈而知之者，診其寸口，視其虛實，以知其病，病在何藏府也。（六）經言以外知之曰聖，以内知之曰神，此之謂也。

The sixty-first difficult issue: (1) The scripture states: Anybody who looks and knows it is to be called a spirit; anybody who listens and knows it is to be called a sage; anybody who asks and knows it is to be called an artisan; anybody who feels the vessels and knows it is to be called a skilled workman. What does that mean?

(2) It is like this. Those who "look and know it" are those who look for the five colors [in a person's complexion] in order to know his disease. (3) Those who "listen and know it" are those who listen to the five tones [in a person's voice] in order to distinguish his disease. (4) Those who "ask and know it" are those who ask [the patient which of] the five flavors he longs for in order to know where his disease has emerged and where it is located now. (5) Those who "feel the vessels and know it" are those who examine the [patient's] inch opening and see whether he is marked by depletion or repletion in order to know in which long-term depot or short-term repository his disease is located.[1] (6) That is [what is] meant when the scripture states: Those who know the [disease] from its external [manifestations] are called sages; those who know the [disease] from its internal [manifestations] are called spirits.

COMMENTARIES

(1) *Zhang Shixian*: A spirit looks at the [patient] and knows [his disease]; he does not have to ask him, listen to him, or feel [his vessels]. A sage looks [at the patient] and listens to him and then knows [his disease]. An artisan looks [at the patient], listens to him and asks him, but he does not have to feel [his vessels]. The skilled workman, finally, feels the vessels and, in addition, must look [at the patient], listen to him, and ask him; only then does he know about his disease.

Xu Dachun: The treatise "Xie qi zang fu bing xing" 邪氣藏府病形 of the *Ling* [*shu*] states: "Someone who looks at the [patient's] complexion and knows his disease, he is called 'enlightened'. Someone who presses the [patient's] vessels and knows his disease, he is called 'divine'. Someone who asks the [patient] about his disease and knows the location of the disease, he is called 'practi-

---

1   Most later editions have omitted one of the two consecutive characters *bing* ("illness") in this sentence. I have retained both in the text, but have disregarded one in my translation.

tioner'." This is different from [the statement] here [in the *Nan jing*]. I do not know on what source Yueren has based [his classification].

Liao Ping: This is yet another uninteresting and dull difficult issue.

(2) *Yang*: To look for the colors means that if, for instance, one sees in the [facial] region [associated with the] liver a virid color, the disease is in the liver itself. If one sees a red color [in the facial region associated with the liver, qi from] the heart have seized the liver and the liver has fallen ill too. Hence, from looking for the five colors [in a person's complexion] one knows which of the five [long-term depots has a] disease.

Hua Shou: The *Su wen* treatise "Wu zang sheng cheng" 五藏生成 states: "Hence, if the complexion appears green-blue like young grasses, death [is imminent]; yellow like hovenia-fruit, death [is imminent]; black like soot, death [is imminent]; red like rotten blood, death [is imminent]; white like withered bones, death [is imminent]. This is how death is visible in the five complexions. [If the complexion appears] green-blue like the feathers of the kingfisher, [the person will] survive; red like a chicken comb, [the person will] survive; yellow like the abdomen of a crab, [the person will] survive; white like the lard of pigs, [the person will] survive; black like the feathers of a crow, [the person will] survive. This is how survival is visible in the five complexions. If [the complexion] is generated by the heart, it resembles vermilion wrapped up in white silk. If [the complexion] is generated by the lung, it resembles red wrapped up in white silk. If [the complexion] is generated by the liver, it resembles virid wrapped up in white silk. If [the complexion] is generated by the spleen, it resembles a *gua-lou* fruit wrapped up in white silk. If [the complexion] is generated by the kidneys, it resembles violet wrapped up in white silk. These are the external splendors generated in the five depots." The *Ling shu* states in its treatise 49: "Greenish and black are associated with pain. Yellow and red are associated with heat. White stands for cold." It states further: "When a red complexion as big as a thumb appears on both cheekbones, a [patient's] disease may have improved and is almost healed, he will die all of a sudden nevertheless. When a black complexion as big as a thumb appears in the courtyard,[2] [a person may] not have had a disease and will die all of a sudden nevertheless."

Zhang Shixian: The five colors are virid, yellow, red, white, and black.

(3) *Yang*: The five notes are *gong* 宮, *shang* 商, *yue* 角, *zhi* 徵, and *yu* 羽; they are matched with the five long-term depots. If the patient tends to cry, he has a disease in the lung; if he loves to sing, he has a disease in the spleen. Hence [the text] says: "They listen to the tones [in a person's voice] and know [his] disease."

---

2 The metaphor ,courtyard' is identified in the *Ling shu* as the forehead.

Hua Shou: Mr. Chen from Siming says: "The five long-term depots [develop specific] sounds and these sounds [reflect specific] tones. The sound [associated with the] liver is shouting; [shouting] corresponds to the tone of *yue*, which should be balanced and straight. If tone and sound correspond to each other, no disease is present. If, however, the tone *yue* appears to be disorderly, a disease is in the liver. The sound [associated with the] heart is laughter. The corresponding tone is *zhi*, it should be harmonious and extended. If tone and sound correspond to each other, no disease is present. If the [tone] *zhi* appears to be disorderly, a disease is present in the heart. The sound [associated with the] spleen is singing. The corresponding tone is *gong*; it should be strong and harmonious. If tone and sound correspond, no disease is present. If the [tone] *gong* appears to be disorderly, a disease is present in the spleen. The sound [associated with the] lung is wailing. The corresponding tone is *shang*; it should be light and unyielding. If tone and sound correspond, no disease is present. If the [tone] *shang* appears to be disorderly, a disease is present in the lung. The sound [associated with the] kidneys is groaning. The corresponding tone is *yu;* it should be deep and heavy. If tone and sound correspond to each other, no disease is present. If the [tone] *yu* appears to be disorderly, a disease is present in the kidneys.

(4) *Yang*: To ask the patient means to inquire, [for instance,] whether he likes [food with] an acrid flavor. [If so.] one knows that he has a disease in the lung. If someone loves chilled food, one knows that he has internal heat. Hence [the text] says: "To know where [his disease] has emerged and where it is located now."

Zhang Shixian: The five flavors are sour, sweet, bitter, acrid, and salty. "Where [a disease] is located now" refers to the conduit where the disease appears [at the moment of the examination]; "where it has emerged" refers to the conduit from which the disease started. For example, if a disease in the heart results from being struck by wind, "the disease is in the heart" refers to its present location, while "being struck by wind" refers to the place where it emerged.[3]

Xu Dachun: "To ask" means to ask the patient where he suffers and what he loves or dislikes, what gives him pleasure and what makes him angry.

(5) *Ding Deyong*: *Shi* 眡 ("to look") should be *chi* 持 ("to grasp") – that is to say, one grasps the [patient's] inch opening with his hand.

Yang: *Qie* 切 ("to press into") stands for *an* 按 ("to press") – that is to say, one presses the vessel at the inch opening. If [the movement felt] is like a string and rapid, the liver is ill. If it is vast and rapid, the heart is ill. If it is at the surface and frequent, the disease is in the short-term repositories; if it is in the depth

---

3   See difficult issue 49, note 2. Wind evil affects the organism by hitting the liver first.

and fine, the disease is in the long-term depots. Hence [the text] says: "[In order to know] in which long-term depot [or short-term repositorythe disease] is located."

(6) *Ding Deyong*: The [movement in the] vessels corresponds to the five colors; the colors correspond to the five flavors; the flavors correspond to the five tones. Hence these patterns of looking, listening, asking, and feeling exist. All these [patterns] have been discussed in the preceding chapters of the [*Nan*] *jing*. Anybody who studies them will know [what is meant] here, he will be a good physician belonging to any of the classes of spirit, sage, artisan, or skilled workman.

Yang: To look for the color, to listen for the sounds, and to feel the vessels are [methods] to recognize internal diseases by checking their external [manifestations].

Hua Shou: To know [about a disease] from its external [manifestation refers to] looking and listening. To know [about a disease] from its internal [manifestation refers to] asking and feeling [the vessels]. "Spirit" implies "subtlety" and "sophistication." "Sage" implies "penetration" and "understanding." Here [those who control these techniques are] summarily called "sages and spirits." This includes the "artisans and skilled workmen."

Zhang Shixian: "External [manifestations]" refers to a situation where symptoms are visible externally and can be examined. "Internal [manifestations]" refers to a situation where a disease is present that is not yet manifest externally. The examination of external [manifestations] makes it easy to know [what disease is present], but the interior is dark and difficult to inspect. Those who know about an internal disease because [they examine] symptoms that appear externally are called sages. Those who recognize an internal disease that has not yet resulted in external [symptoms] that could be examined are called spirits.

Xu Dachun: The initial question called those who [recognize a disease] through looking and listening spirits and sages. Here, the [*Nei*] *jing* is quoted as calling those who look and listen sages, and those who ask and feel [the vessels] spirits. Furthermore, the two categories of artisans and skilled workmen are omitted [here]. The [*Nei*] *jing* contains no passage that could be checked against this quotation. The reason [for these differences] is not clear. Also, the patterns of listening and asking are discussed in both [sections of the *Nei*] *jing*[4] under many aspects. Here the outline is limited to the five sounds and five flavors. The meaning [of these patterns as presented by the *Nan jing*] remains incomplete.

---

4 "Both [sections of the *Nei*] *jing*" may refer to *Su wen* and *Ling shu*.

Ding Jin: This paragraph combines the meaning of the entire text of the three volumes.[5] "External [manifestations]" means that one looks at [a patient's] complexion and listens to his voice. That is to say, one knows the disease before it becomes manifest. "Internal [manifestations]" means that one asks about [the patient's] preferences concerning any of the five flavors and feels his vessels in order to examine his disease, and then knows whether it is a depletion or a repletion. Yueren looked forward to the physicians of later generations who had to attain this level [of proficiency] in order to join the path of Xian [Yuan] and Qi [Bo]. If they did not [attain this level of proficiency], they were bound to remain crude artisans and nothing else!

---

5   The meaning of *san juan* ("three volumes") is not clear. The term could refer to the present and to the preceding two chapters in the *Nan jing* (difficult issues 59 and 60 of Ding Jin's edition correspond to issues 42 and 43 of the present edition). "Three volumes" might also refer to the *Su wen,* the *Ling shu,* and the *Nan jing.*

Chapter Five
Transportation Holes

THE SIXTY-SECOND DIFFICULT ISSUE

六十二難曰：（一）藏井滎有五，府獨有六者，何謂也？

（二）然：府者，陽也。三焦行於諸陽，故置一俞，名曰原。府有六者，亦
與三焦共一氣也。

The sixty-second difficult issue: (1) The [vessels associated with the body's] long-term depots have five [holes each; these are the] "wells," "creeks," [etc]. Only the [vessels associated with the body's] short-term repositories have six [holes each]. What does that mean?

(2) It is like this. The short-term repositories are yang. The Triple Burner passes [its qi] through all the yang [conduits and short-term repositories]. Hence an [additional] transportation [hole] has been established, named "origin." [When it is said] "the short-term repositories have six," this is so because the [three sections of the] Triple Burner have one qi in common, which is added [to those of the remaining five short-term repositories].[1]

---

1   This is the first of a series of seven difficult issues discussing the locations and functions of holes suitable for needling. The *Nei jing* advocates at least two systems of needling: (1) the (older?) system of piercing locations distributed all over the body and located on the conduit-circuit, and (2) the system of extremities' needling, which recognizes only a limited number of holes – holes that are not situated on the conduit-circuit. The *Nan jing* took over extremities' needling only, and appears to have disregarded the system of circuit-needling completely. (see the Prolegomena, section I.B.). The system of extremities' needling is based on a recognition of twelve conduits. The names of these conduits are identical with those of the classical conduits (hand major yin, etc.), but their courses and conceptual basis are entirely different. The twelve conduits of extremities' needling are not part of the conduit-circuit passed by the constantly circulating *qi* 氣, although the holes to be needled on the former also appear in the system of circuit-needling. Invisible to the human eye, the twelve conduits of extremities' needling are conceptualized as streams; the term *ching* 經, which denotes these conduits, is henceforth rendered as "stream." These streams spring forth from the feet or hands, extend to the knees or elbows, respectively, and submerge there again. The six streams associated with the five (plus one) long-term depots have five holes each, while the six streams associated with the six short-term repositories have six holes each. Together, these are the so-called transportation holes. They carry generic names that apply to all twelve streams alike. The

(1) *Li Jiong*: "Wells," "rapids," "creeks,"[2] "streams," and "confluences" are the five [holes on the conduits associated with] the five long-term depots. Now, the [conduits associated with the] six short-term repositories have, in addition to the holes called] "well," "rapids," "creek," "stream," and "confluence," one [hole] where [the qi] cross over, and that is the "lowland [hole]." How is that?

Xu Dachun: For details on these holes, see the treatise "Ben shu" 本輸 of the *Ling* [*shu*].

Liao Ping: The twelve conduits are grounded in the long-term depots and short-term repositories, of which there are six each. This is most evident and does not wait for questions! To omit one long-term depot as not worth counting because heaven [is associated with the number] six and because earth [is associated with the number] five – these are all erroneous doctrines which have been arrived at because [someone] was completely ignorant of the meaning conveyed by the classic.

(2)*Xu Dachun*: Yu 俞 stands for *xue* 穴 ("hole"). The "Ben shu" 本輸 treatise of the *Ling* [*shu*] calls the hole where [the qi of the Triple Burner) cross over *yuan* 原 "lowland." The distance to be passed by the [qi of the] Triple Burner is long.

---

locations where the streams originate are called "wells"; next come the "creeks," "rapids," "streams," and "confluences." On the streams associated with the short-term repositories, a sixth hole – called *yuan* 原 – is identified between the "rapids" and the "streams." Originally, this term *yuan* may have been inserted carrying the meaning of "lowlands." The underlying image resorted to by all these designations is that of a river which comes from the mountains, rushes down the cliffs, crosses the lowlands, and becomes a stream before it flows into the ocean. The *Nan jing* itself and most of the commentators equate *yuan* 原 with *yuan* 元 ("origin"), relating the *yuan* hole to the "original" qi emitted by the Triple Burner. This may be seen as a breaking away from the original metaphor, but it should be recalled that the character used for *yuan* remains identical for both readings and may therefore continue to convey the old image, as hinted at by a statement in the *Ling shu* to the effect that at this point the stream "crosses over" or "passes through" (*guo* 過). More problematic is an adequate rendering of the term *yu* 俞. In accordance with traditional Chinese interpretations, I have translated *yu* here as "rapids" – that is, as the place where the young stream "rushes forth" (*zhu* 注). The etymology of the term suggests meanings such as "boat on water" (Karlgren, *Analytic Dictionary of Chinese and Sino-Japanese*, 1923, 374) or "the making of a boat by hollowing out a tree" (*Shuo wen* 說文). Hence, *yu* has also often been interpreted as being identical with *shu* 輸 ("to transport"), suggesting a translation of *yu* 俞 as "transportation" [hole]. Linking all these meanings might be the idea, in the present context, that transportation on a stream becomes possible only once the latter has passed its rapids. Where the term *yu* 俞 is used to designate holes for needling in general, I have translated it as "transportation [hole]"; in that context, the underlying idea appears to be the possibility of transporting qi in the organism by means of needling. A third meaning of *yu* will appear in difficult issue 67.

2   The sequence should be "creeks," "rapids."

Five holes would not suffice to cover all the locations where these qi flow and accumulate. Hence an additional hole was established, called *yuan* 原, "lowland."

Liao Ping: To add the Triple Burner as the sixth short-term repository is the same as to add the heart ruler[3] as the sixth depot. Here attention focuses on the Triple Burner, and where is the heart ruler to be left?

(3) *Xu* Dachun: *Gong yi qi* 共一氣 ("the qi are identical") means that [the qi of the Triple Burner] also pass through all the yang [conduits]; it does not mean that all the [qi passing through the yang conduits and short-term repositories] originate from the Triple Burner. This is discussed in detail in difficult issue 66.

Ye Lin: The Triple Burner is the source of the yang qi. The six short-term repositories are all yang, and all their qi originate from the Triple Burner. Hence [the text says] *gong yi qi* 共一氣 ("the qi are identical").

(1)–(3) *Ding Deyong*: The Triple Burner serves as messenger-official; its position corresponds to that of the minister fire. As such, it carries out the orders of the ruler fire. [Hence] an [additional] transportation [hole] was established [for it] and it was given the designation "lowland." "The [vessels associated with the] short-term repositories have six [holes each]" because the Triple Burner, [although consisting of three sections, is considered to emit only] one [type of] qi. Hence [the text] states: "The [three sections of the] Triple Burner have one common qi."

Yang: Where the vessels [associated with] the five long-term depots emerge, these locations are always [called] "wells"; where [their contents] flow are the "creeks"; where [their contents] rush are the "rapids"; where their contents pass are the "streams"; where they disappear are the "confluences." These [locations together] are called "five transportation [holes]"; they correspond to metal, wood, water, fire, and soil. The same applies to the [vessels associated with the] six short-term repositories. The locations where they emerge are the "wells"; where [their contents] flow are the "creeks"; where [their contents] rush are the "rapids"; where [their contents] cross over are the "lowlands"; where [their contents] pass are the "streams"; where [their contents] disappear are the "confluences." These transportation [holes of the short-term repositories] also correspond to the Five Phases. The only exception are the "lowland" [holes], which do not correspond to the Five Phases. *Yuan* 原 stands for *yuan* 元 ("origin"). The "original qi" (*yuan qi* 元氣) are the qi of the Triple Burner. These qi are eminent and strong; hence they do not correspond to the Five Phases. The six short-term repositories have six transportation [holes] so that they correspond to the six *he* 合 [i.e., the four cardinal directions, as well as above and below] of the way of heaven. However,

---

3   The "heart ruler" is the heart-enclosing network.

the [vessels associated with the] five long-term depots also have an origin/low-land [hole. Here] the third hole is considered to be the origin/lowland [hole]. A separate hole was not established [on the conduits associated with the five long-term depots] because the five long-term depots reflect the earth. The earth is less important. Hence the qi of the Triple Burner simply cross over it. For this reason no separate hole exists [on the vessels associated with the five long-term depots to account for the qi of the Triple Burner]. The six short-term reposito-ries represent the yang. The Triple Burner represents the yang, too. Hence [the text] states: *gong yi qi* 共一氣 ("all their qi move together").

Yu Shu: Heaven governs what is below it with the six qi; the earth provides what is above it with the Five Phases. Wind, cold, heat, dryness, moisture, and fire are the six qi; metal, wood, water, fire, and soil are the Five Phases. [Altogether, these] eleven qi interact with each other and constitute [all phenomena]. Man corresponds to that. His six short-term repositories reflect the six qi; his five long-term depots reflect the Five Phases. These too are eleven qi which interact with each other and constitute [man]. Heaven gets six. That is to say, heaven be-longs to yang; it is matched with a yin number.[4] The earth gets five. That is to say, the earth belongs to yin; it is matched with a yang number. In this way, [the dual combination of] yin and yang is generated. The same applies to man's short-term repositories and long-term depots. The six short-term repositories match the six qi. That is to say, the gall bladder [corresponds to] wood and is matched with wind. The bladder [corresponds to] water and is matched with cold. The small intestine [corresponds to] fire and is matched with heat. The large intes-tine [corresponds to] metal and is matched with dryness. The stomach [corre-sponds to] soil and is matched with moisture. The Triple Burner [corresponds to] minor yang and is matched with fire. The Triple Burner is responsible for the original qi. It has [a hole of] its own among the [holes on the] yang vessels [associated with the] six short-term repositories. [This hole is called] "origin/lowland." The five long-term depots are matched with the Five Phases. [That is to say,] the liver [is matched with the] wood. The heart [is matched with the] fire. The spleen [is matched with the] soil. The lung [is matched with the] metal. The kidneys [are matched with the] water. The five long-term depots reflect the yin; the [vessels associated with them] have no "origin/lowland" as a separate hole. That is to say, the Five Phases rule the original qi secretly among the holes on the yin vessels. Hence [on these vessels] "origin/lowland" and "rapids" consti-tute one and the same hole. Hence [when the text] states: "The qi of the Triple Burner [and of the remaining five short-term repositories] are identical," the

---

4   Yin numbers are even; yang numbers are odd.

underlying principle has become clear now. If one looks closely at the meaning of [this paragraph of the *Nan] jing*, and at the questions and answers preceding and following it, [it appears] that some [passages have been] omitted from the text here.

Hua Shou: Mr. Yu states: "I suspect that [some passages are] missing from this paragraph; it should be checked against difficult issue 66."

Zhang Shixian: The five [holes on the conduits associated with the long-term depots] are the "wells," "creeks," "rapids," "streams," and "confluences." The six [holes on the conduits associated with the short-term repositories] are the "wells," "creeks," "rapids," "origins/lowland," "streams," and "confluences." The Triple Burner controls all qi, hence the conduits [associated with] the six short-term repositories have one additional transportation [hole], which is called "origin/lowland." [The text states] "the short-term repositories have six" because the qi of the six short-term repositories and the qi of the Triple Burner are all yang [qi].

Katō Bankei: The question in this paragraph [asks the following]. Each of the five conduits associated with the long-term depots has [holes called] "well," "creek," "rapids," "stream," and "confluence." Each of the six conduits associated with the short-term repositories has one additional [hole called] "origin/lowland." [Hence] they have six [holes altogether]. Why is that? The answer states that the "lowland" is the place where the qi of the Triple Burner cross over. Whenever one pierces the holes on the twelve conduits at the limbs [beyond] the four joints of hands and feet, he must add to the transportation [holes] the "lowland" if he wishes to regulate the transformation of qi by the Triple Burner. However, on the yin conduits the rapids [hole] is also the lowland [hole]; only the yang conduits have a separate lowland [hole]. This is so because the Triple Burner is counted among the six short-term repositories. Although it has no physical appearance, how could the [remaining] five short-term repositories manage to move and transform water and grains, if it were not for the qi [of the Triple Burner]? Thus, the functioning of the short-term repositories relies on the utilization of these qi. Hence [the text] states: "The short-term repositories have six because their qi are identical with those of the Triple Burner."

六十三難曰：(一)《十變》言，五藏六府滎合，皆以井為始者，何也？
(二)然：井者，東方春也，萬物之始生。諸蚑行喘息，蜎飛蠕動，當生之
物，莫不以春而生。故歲數始於春，日數始於甲，故以井為始也。

The sixty-third difficult issue: (1) The *Ten Changes* states: The [sequence of holes located on the streams associated with the body's] five long-term depots and six short-term repositories, [including] "creeks," ["rapids," "streams," and] "confluences," is always preceded by a "well." Why is that?

(2) It is like this. The "wells" are [associated with] the Eastern regions and with spring. [That is the season when] all things come to life, when all the *qi* [insects start to] move, when the *zhui*¹ [insects start to] breathe, when the *yuan* [insects start to] fly, and when the *ru* [insects start to] wriggle. All things that must come to life will come to life in spring. (3) Hence the counting of the [seasons of the] year begins with spring, and the counting of the days² begins with *jia*. Hence the "wells" constitute the begin [in the sequence of holes on the streams associated with the five long-term depots and six short-term repositories].

COMMENTARIES

(1) *Ding Jin*: *Shi bian* 十變 ("Ten Changes") is the title of an ancient book.
(2) *Yu Shu*: The [*Nan*]*jing* states: "The 'wells' are [associated with] the eastern regions and with spring." Spring bestows on [all things] its transforming and nourishing [qi], without asking for anything in return. "Spring" stands for "benevolence." Among the five constant [relationships], benevolence reflects water. The water that has benevolence is the water in a well. The water in a well supports the people too without asking for anything in return. Hence the [*Nan*]*jing* states: "The 'wells' are [associated with] the Eastern regions and with spring." The *Yi* [*jing*] 易經 states: "Wells nourish and cannot be exhausted." They reflect, indeed, spring and benevolence. All things come to life because of the transforming and nourishing [qualities] of the qi of spring. Similar benevolence is practiced by the wells. Hence, when the sages selected spring [as the season when all] things are nourished [again], they had the image of a well in mind. That is, when the ash of the reed is flying,³ the hibernating insects begin to be excited. The *qi* insects [start to] move, the *zhui* insects [start to] breathe, the *yuan* insects [start to] fly,

---

1 I interpret *chuan* 喘 here as an error in writing for *zhui* 惴
2 Some editions have *yue* 月 ("months") instead of *ri* 日 ("days").
3 A metaphor for winter.

and the *ru* insects [start to] wriggle. They all come to life because of the qi of spring. *Ru* are insects living in wells.

Xu Dachun: According to the treatise "Ben shu" 本輸 of the *Ling* [*shu*], the wells of all the [streams associated with the] long-term depots belong to [the phase of] wood, while the wells of all the [streams associated with the] short-term repositories belong to [the phase of] metal. That is also clearly outlined in the text of the following [difficult issue]. Here, however, a general classification is given of all the wells of the [streams associated with the] long-term depots and short-term repositories as belonging to [the phase of] wood. That contradicts the text of the [*Nei*] *jing;* it also contradicts the text below. If it had said [here] that only the wells of the [streams associated with the] long-term depots belong to [the phase of] wood, but not those of the [streams associated with the] short-term repositories, [that would have implied that the streams associated with] the short-term repositories start from wells, too, but that [these wells] do not belong to [the phase of] wood. What is the meaning of this? [The author of the *Nan jing*] was extremely careless in writing down his words.

(3) *Yu Shu*: Spring represents wood. The [Celestial Stem] *jia* 甲 – mentioned further below – also [represents] wood. Wells have benevolence. Benevolence also [represents] wood. If, here, the wells are said to precede everything else, that is to say that the principle of benevolence is most important. Hence, in the course of a year, spring comes first. In the course of the days, *jia* comes first. On the conduit vessels, the "wells" come first.

Yang: All [the streams associated with] the long-term depots and short-term repositories have a „spring" as their first [hole]. *Jing* 井 refers to "valley spring"; it does not mean a well dug up [by man]. The places in mountain valleys where spring water appears first are called "spring."„Spring" carries the meaning of "ruling the appearance." After water has come to light in a spring, it stays near [its source]. It winds around and does not yet constitute a major stream. Hence it is called *rong* 榮 ("creek"). A creek appears as a small water. Where it stands without moving, it develops depth and there are places where it rushes and shoots, turning here and there like a line. Hence one speaks here of *yu* 俞 ("rapids"). The rapids are responsible for the accumulation and subsequent moving away [of the water]. Over time, they generate huge tracks. *Jing* 經 ("stream," "conduit") stands for *jing* 徑 ("track"). Another meaning is *jing ying* 經營 ("transaction"). The movement in the streams finally reaches its destination; it meets with the sea. Hence [this place] is called *he* 合 ("confluence"). *He* stands for *hui* 會 ("to meet"). The meaning implied here is that of water flowing and moving on. [The contents of] man's conduit vessels reflect this [image], hence the designations ["well/spring," "creek," etc.] were chosen. The "wells/springs" constitute "beginning" and [they reflect the season of] spring because of their inherent meaning of "generating life." "The counting of the [seasons of the] year begins with spring" means that the first month is the beginning of the year. "The counting of the days begins with *jia*" means that the East is represented by [the dual combination of Celestial Stems] *jia yi* 甲乙. The first month and [the combination] *jia yi* are both associated with spring.

Zhang Shixian: Spring is the first of the four seasons. *Jia yi* represents [the phase of] wood. Both the first month and [the dual combination] *jia yi* are associated with spring. Hence [each of] the twelve months begins with *jia*; it is not so that the [counting of the twelve] months begins with *jia*. Some [texts] say "day" instead of "month." That is wrong.

六十四難曰：（一）《十變》又言，陰井木，陽井金；陰滎火，陽滎水；陰
俞土，陽俞木；陰經金，陽經火；陰合水，陽合土。陰陽皆不同，其意何
也？

（二）然：是剛柔之事也。陰井乙木，陽井庚金。陽井庚，庚者，乙之剛
也；陰井乙，乙者，庚之柔也。乙為木，故言陰井木也；庚為金，故言陽
井金也。餘皆倣此。

The sixty-fourth difficult issue: (1) The *Ten Changes* states further: The yin wells are wood; the yang wells are metal; the yin creeks are fire; the yang creeks are water; the yin rapids are soil; the yang rapids are wood; the yin streams are metal; the yang streams are fire; the yin confluences are water; the yang confluences are soil. In each case, the yin and yang [categories are associated with] different [phases]. What is the meaning of that?

(2) It is like this. This is a case where hardness and softness [are matched with each other]. The yin wells are [associated with the Celestial Stem] *yi* and [with the phase of] wood; the yang wells are [associated with the Celestial Stem] *geng* and [with the phase of] metal. The *geng* of the yang wells' *geng* is the hardness of *yi*. The *yi* of the yin wells' *yi* is the softness of *geng*. [The Celestial Stem] *yi* [represents the phase] wood. Hence [the *Ten Changes*] states: "The yin 'wells' are wood." [The Celestial Stem] *geng* [represents the phase] metal. Hence [the *Ten Changes*] states: "The yang 'wells' are metal." The same applies to all the remaining [holes].[1]

---

1   In this difficult issue, the *Nan jing* perfects the theoretical systematization of the holes on the "streams" in the extremities by linking them to both the yinyang and the Five Phases categories. The "wells," "creeks," and so on are divided into two groups following their location on a stream associated with a long-term depot (i.e., yin) or short-term repository (i.e., yang). Each pair of yin and yang wells, creeks, and so forth is then matched with a pair of two of the Five Phases in such a way that the yang partner always represents a phase which is able, according to the sequence of mutual destruction, to control the phase represented by the yin partner. This control is expressed by reference to the matching of a hard component (i.e., yang) with a soft component (i.e., yin). Later commentators equated this metaphor with the image of husband and wife. In sentence 2, the pattern is further clarified by reference to the system of the Ten Celestial Stems. The usual sequence in which these stems appear is as follows:

The Five Phases	Wood	Fire	Soil	Metal	Water
yang stems	*jia* 甲	*bing* 丙	*wu* 戊	*geng* 庚	*ren* 壬
yin stems	*yi* 乙	*ding* 丁	*ji* 己	*xin* 辛	*gui* 癸

COMMENTARIES

(1) *Yang*: All the five long-term depots are [categorized as] yin. The yin wells represent the [phase of] wood; the [yin] creeks represent the [phase of] fire; the [yin] rapids represent the [phase of] soil; the [yin] streams represent the [phase of] metal; the [yin] confluences represent the [phase of] water. The six short-term repositories are [categorized as] yang. The yang wells represent the [phase of] metal; the [yang] creeks represent the [phase of] water; the [yang] rapids represent the [phase of] wood; the [yang] streams represent the [phase of] fire; the [yang] confluences represent the [phase of] soil. The wood of the yin wells is matched with the metal of the yang wells. The meaning implied here is that yin and yang [match each other like] husband and wife. Hence [the text] states: "*Yi* is the softness of *geng; geng* is the hardness of *yi*." All the other [holes] follow the same pattern.

Hua Shou: The twelve conduits start from the well holes. The yin wells represent the wood. Hence the wood of the yin wells generates the fire of the yin creeks. The fire of the yin creeks generates the soil of the yin rapids. The soil of the yin rapids generates the metal of the yin streams. The metal of the yin streams generates the water of the yin confluences. The yang wells represent the metal. Hence the metal of the yang wells generates the water of the yang creeks. The water of the yang creeks generates the wood of the yang rapids. The wood of the yang rapids generates the fire of the yang streams. The fire of the yang streams generates the soil of the yang confluences.

Xu Dachun: In the treatise "Ben shu" 本輸 of the *Ling* [*shu*], the text states clearly that the wells of the [conduits associated with the] long-term depots belong

To achieve a matching of yin and yang holes on the basis of mutual control between the two phases concerned, the Ten Stems appear in pairs in the present difficult issue, as follows:

The Five Holes	Wells	Creeks	Rapids	Streams	Confluences
The Five Phases (yang)	Metal	Water	Wood	Fire	Soil
The Five Stems (yang)	*geng*	*ren*	*jia*	*bing*	*wu*
The Five Stems (yin)	*yi*	*ling*	*ji*	*xin*	*gui*
The Five Phases (yin)	Wood	Fire	Soil	Metal	Water

Horizontally, the Five Phases appear in the sequence of mutual generation; vertically, the Five Phases appear in the sequence of mutual destruction.

to the [phase of] wood, while the wells of the [conduits associated with the] short-term repositories belong to the [phase of] metal. The [*Ling shu*] text does not elucidate the associations of the remaining creeks, rapids, and so on. I do not know on which book the [categorizations in the] *Nan jing* are based .... Furthermore, the [conduits associated with the] six short-term repositories have an additional hole, the "lowland". The [association of the] lowland hole with one of the Five Phases can be concluded from the associations of the [remaining] five [holes with the Five Phases]. Needling and cauterization experts have henceforth relied on the data provided [here] .... [The lowland holes] are located near the rapids [holes]. They should both be associated with [the phase of] wood. Also, where [the contents] rush down, these are the rapids; where they cross over, these are the "lowlands". The meanings [of these two images] are close to each other, too.

(2) *Hua Shou*: "Hardness" and "softness" refers to the matching of *yi* and *geng*. The Ten Celestial Stems are [counted] here starting with *yi* and *geng* because of the following. All the holes [on the conduits associated with the] long-term depots and short-term repositories start with a "well." The wells on the yin vessels start with [the Celestial Stem] *yi,* and with [the phase of] wood, while the wells on the yang vessels start with *geng* and metal. Hence the matching of hardness and softness is outlined beginning with *yi* and *geng*. The matching of all the remaining Five Phases follows this example.

Xu Dachun: This section outlines the principles of the matching of yin and yang. The meaning [expressed] is both sophisticated and correct.

(1)–(2) *Ding Jin*: This quotation from the ancient scripture *Shi bian* 十變 ("Ten Changes") refers to the matching of the wells, creeks, rapids, streams, and confluences with both the Five Phases and yinyang. But the particular yin and yang [associations selected are those that] control each other. What does that mean? That is to say, in the matching of yin and yang, the image of hardness and softness has been drawn upon. For instance, the yin wells are wood; the yang wells are metal. That is a matching of *yi* 乙 and *geng* 庚. *Yi* represents the yin [aspect of the phase of] wood; it is matched with *geng* – that is, with the yang [aspect of the phase of] metal. Hence [the text] states: "*Geng* is the hardness of *yi*; *yi* is the softness of *geng*." Similarly, the yin creeks are fire, and the yang creeks are water. That is a matching of *ding* 丁 and *ren* 壬. *Ding* represents the yin [aspect of the phase of] fire; *ren* represents the yang [aspect of the phase of] water. The yang rapids are wood, and the yin rapids are soil. That is a matching of *jia* 甲 and *ji* 己. *Jia* represents the yang [aspect of the phase of] wood; *ji* represents the yin [aspect of the phase of] soil. The yin streams are metal; the yang streams are fire.

That is a matching of *bing* 丙 and *xin* 辛. *Xin* represents the yin [aspect of the phase of] metal; *bing* represents the yang [aspect of the phase of] fire. The yin confluences are water, and the yang confluences are soil. That is a matching of *wu* 戊 and *gui* 癸. *Gui* represents the yin [aspect of the phase of] water; *wu* represents the yang [aspect of the phase of] soil. With this kind of matching, hardness and softness support each other. As a consequence, the *qi* and the blood can flow without break. It is obvious, then, that the conduits and the holes, as well as the long-term depots and the short-term repositories of the human body are all matched with [either the yin or yang aspects of] the Five Phases. [Hence] their mutual interaction never comes to an end.

Liao Ping: Mr. Huang [Yuanyu] 黃元禦, *hao* name Kunzai 坤載,[2] has said: The great physicians rank this book together with the *Ling shu*, the *Su wen*, and [the work of Zhang] Zhongjing 張仲景 among the four [scriptures] written by the sages. But by substituting Celestial Stems for the names of the long-term depots and short-term repositories, [the author of the *Nan jing*] has integrated [medicine] into astrology. That was his great mistake.

---

2   An author of numerous medical works of the mid-eighteenth century.

六十五難曰：（一）經言所出為井，所入為合，其法奈何？
（二）然：所出為井，井者，東方春也，萬物之始生，故言所出為井
也。（三）所入為合，合者，北方冬也，陽氣入藏，故言所入為合也。

The sixty-fifth difficult issue: (1) The scripture states: Where [they] appear are the wells; where they disappear are the confluences. What kind of a pattern is that?

(2) It is like this. "Where [they] appear are the wells" [means the following]. The wells are [associated with] the Eastern region and with spring. [During spring] all things come to life. Hence [the scripture] states: "Where [they] appear are the wells." (3) "Where [they] disappear are the confluences" [means the following]. The confluences are [associated with] the Northern region and with winter. [During winter] the yang qi disappear and are stored away. Hence [the scripture] states: "Where [they] disappear are the confluences."

_{COMMENTARIES}

(1)–(3) *Ding Deyong*: Man's yang qi appear and disappear in accordance with the four seasons. Hence, in spring the qi are in the wells, in summer they are in the creeks, in autumn they are in the streams, and in winter they are in the confluences. For piercing, the qi holes are always selected in accordance with the four seasons.

Yang: Spring and summer rule generation and nourishment. Hence the yang qi are present outside. Autumn and winter rule intake and storage. Hence the yang qi are present inside. Man also reflects this pattern.

Li Jiong: The East is the first of the four regions. Spring is the first of the four seasons. A well is the source of any river. Hence wells are [associated with] the Eastern region and with spring. The North is the final of the four regions. Winter is the final of the four seasons. A confluence marks the end of any river. Hence confluences are [associated with] the Northern region and with winter.

Zhang Shixian: Wells are springs where [water] comes out [of the ground. The water] bubbles forth without interruption; there is never "too much" or "not enough." Confluences are places where [waters] come together. For instance, when a water flows toward the sea it starts from a shallow [spring and ends when] it enters the depth [of the ocean]. The Eastern region represents the first of the four regions; spring is the first of the four seasons. The wells are the first [holes on the conduits, preceding] the creeks, rapids, streams, and confluences. Hence [the text] states: "The wells are [associated with] the Eastern region and with spring." Spring is the season when all things come to life. Hence places where the water of the streams comes out [of the ground] first are called wells. The northern region is the final of the four regions; winter is the final of the four seasons. The confluences are the last [holes, following the] wells, creeks, rapids, and streams. Hence [the text] states: "The confluences are [associated with] the Northern region and with winter." In winter the yang qi hide in the depth. Hence places where the water of the streams enters [a larger reservoir] are called "confluences."

Liao Ping: This was outlined quite clearly by the [*Nei*] *jing.* Why should such a question be posed again? *Chu* 出 ("to appear," "to come out") and *ru* 入 ("to disappear," "enter") stand for *nei* 内 ("inside") and *wai* 外 ("outside"). [In the *Nei jing*], these [terms] denote the paths of the [main] conduits and of the network [vessels]. It is impossible to match the four seasons with the Five Phases. Similarly, if one were to associate the Five Phases with the six [holes on each conduit, including the] "origin/lowland", one transportation [hole] would be left over. Whenever someone displays such ignorance, demonstrates such absurd behavior, and is so confused in what he sees and hears, one should no longer communicate with him!

六十六難曰：（一）經言肺之原出于太淵，（二）心之原出于太陵，（三）肝之原出于太衝，（四）脾之原出于太白，（五）腎之原出于太谿，（六）少陰之原出于兌骨，（七）膽之原出于邱墟，（八）胃之原出于衝陽，（九）三焦之原出于陽池，（十）膀胱之原出于京骨，（十一）大腸之原出于合谷，（十二）小腸之原出于腕骨。（十三）十二經皆以俞為原者，何也？

（十四）然：五藏俞者，三焦之所行，氣之所留止也。

（十五）三焦所行之俞為原者，何也？

（十六）然：臍下腎間動氣者，人之生命也，十二經之根本也，故名曰原。（十七）三焦者，原氣之別使也，（十八）主通行三氣，經歷於五藏六府。（十九）原者，三焦之尊號也，故所止輒為原。五藏六府之有病者，取其原也。

The sixty-sixth difficult issue: (1) The original [qi] of the lung appear at the *tai yuan* [hole]. (2) The original [qi] of the heart appear at the *da ling* [hole]. (3) The original [qi] of the liver appear at the *tai chong* [hole]. (4) The original [qi] of the spleen appear at the *tai bai* [hole]. (5) The original [qi] of the kidneys appear at the *tai xi* [hole]. (6) The original [qi] of the minor yin appear at the *dui gu* [hole]. (7) The original [qi] of the gall bladder appear at the *qiu xu* [hole]. (8) The original [qi] of the stomach appear at the *chong yang* [hole]. (9) The original [qi] of the Triple Burner appear at the *yang chi* [hole]. (10) The original [qi] of the urinary bladder appear at the *jing gu* [hole]. (11) The original [qi] of the large intestine appear at the *he gu* [hole]. (12) The original [qi] of the small intestine appear at the *wan gu* [hole].

(13) On all the twelve streams the rapids [holes] constitute the origin [holes]. Why is that?

(14) It is like this. The rapids [holes on the conduits associated with the] five long-term depots are the locations where the qi that are sent out by the Triple Burner stop and rest.

(15) Why are the transportation [holes] where the [qi] sent out by the Triple Burner [stop and rest called] "origin" [holes]?

(16) It is like this. The qi moving below the navel and between the kidneys constitute man's life. They are the source and the basis of the twelve conduits. Hence they are called "original [qi]." (17) The Triple Burner is the special envoy that transmits the original qi.(18) It is responsible for the passage of the three qi through the [body's] five long-term depots and six short-term repositories. (19) "Origin" is an honorable designation for the Triple Burner. (20) Hence [the place] where [its qi] come to a halt is [called] "origin." (21) In case the [body's] five long-term depots and

six short-term repositories suffer from a disease, one always selects their respective [conduits'] origin [holes for piercing].[1]

COMMENTARIES

(1) *Ding Deyong*: Behind the palm of the right hand, below the fish-line, is the great meeting point of the [movement passing through the] vessels.[2] Hence [the text] states: "The original qi of the lung appear at the *tai yuan* [hole]."

(2) *Ding Deyong*: Behind the palm, in the hollow between the two muscles, is the origin [hole of the conduit associated with] the heart enclosing network.

  Yu Shu: Behind the palm between the two bones.

  Liao Ping: "Heart" should be "heart ruler."

(3) *Yu Shu*: It is located two inches behind the basic joint of the big toe. It is also said to be located two inches or one and a half inches behind the basic joint of the big toe.

(4) *Ding Deyong*: At the inner side of the foot below the *he* 核 bone.

(5) *Ding Deyong*: It is located between the inner ankle and the heel bone.

(6) *Ding Deyong*: That is the *shen men* 神門 hole. It is [located on] the vessel of the true heart.

(1)–(6) *Yang*: In each case these [origin holes] are the rapids [holes on the conduits associated with] the five long-term depots because [on the conduits associated with] the five long-term depots the rapids [holes] are always considered as origin [holes]. The minor yin [vessel] is the vessel of the true heart. It too has an origin [hole], located behind the palm in the hollow at the end of the *dui* 兌 bone. Other names [for this hole] are *shen men* 神門 and *zhong du* 中都. Earlier, [the text] had stated: "The original [qi] of the heart appear at the *da ling* 大陵 [hole]." That, however, was a reference to the vessel of the heart enclosing network. Whenever it is stated "the heart has a disease," this refers to the vessel of the heart enclosing network. The true heart itself cannot be ill. Hence it has no rapids [hole associated with it]. Here, an origin [hole] is listed for the [treatment of diseases in the] conduit outside [of the heart], not for a treatment of the inner long-term depot [itself].

---

1 Taken by itself, this difficult issue contains rather unambiguous information. But in comparison with various treatises in the *Nei jing*, a number of incongruities became apparent to those commentators of later centuries who did not perceive the innovative nature of the *Nan jing*. The resulting discussion ranged from syncretistic attempts to harmonize the differing statements of the *Nan jing* and *Nei jing* to outright rejection of the *Nan jing* data as wrong.

2 See the first difficult issue.

Hua Shou: Someone [could] say: "According to the *Ling shu*, the *tai ling* 太陵 [hole] is the origin [hole associated with] the heart. The *Nan jing* writes the same but, in addition, it distinguishes the *dui gu* 兌骨 [hole] as the origin [hole associated with] the minor yin [long-term depot, i.e., the heart]. The authors of all the books on needling and cauterization [from subsequent times] agree that the *tai ling* [hole] is the rapids [hole] on the [conduit associated with the] hand ceasing yin heart ruler, while the *shen men* [hole] behind the palm at the end of the *dui* bone [i.e., the *dui gu* hole] is the rapids [hole] where the [contents of the] conduit [associated with the] heart rush down. There seems to be a discrepancy here [between the contents of the *Ling shu* and those of all the later books on needling and cauterization]. Why is that?" Well, the seventy-first treatise of the *Ling shu* states: "[The Yellow Thearch said:] 'If the minor yin [vessel] is the only one that has no transport [opening], will it never have a disease?' Qi Bo replied: 'The conduits outside of it may have a disease, but the long-term depot itself cannot have a disease. Hence [for a treatment] one chooses only the conduit behind the palm, at the tip of the pointed bone. As for the turns and windings of all the remaining vessels, the slow and swift nature of their movements, all that is identical with the course of the hand minor yin vessels of the heart ruler'." Furthermore, the second treatise [of the *Ling shu*] states: "The heart qi] exit through the *zhong chong* [opening]. They flow to the *lao gong* [opening]. From there they pour into the *da ling* [opening]. They move further on into the *jian shi* [opening]. From there they enter the *qu ze* [opening]. That is the [course of the] hand minor yin [conduit]." Furthermore, in the treatise "Miu ci" 繆刺 of the *Su wen* it is stated: "Then pierce the hand heart ruler [conduit] and the [hand] minor yin [conduit], one wound each at the tip of the *dui* bone [i.e., at the *dui gu* hole; the disease] ends immediately." Also, the treatise "Qi xue" 氣穴 states: "The [conduits associated with the] long-term depots have fifty transportation holes." In his comment, Mr. Wang 王 referred, in his list of transportation [holes associated with] the five long-term depots, only to a „well" transportation hole on the conduit [associated with the] heart enclosing [network], but he did not mention a „well" transportation hole on the conduit [associated with the] heart. Furthermore, the seventy-ninth difficult issue [of the *Nan jing*] states: "In the case of a disease in the heart, drain at the rapids [hole] of the hand heart ruler [conduit] and supplement at the well [hole] of the hand heart ruler [conduit]." A close look at the meaning of all these passages from scriptures [like the *Su wen*, the *Ling shu*, and the *Nan jing*] makes one realize that the treatment applied to the hand minor yin [conduit] is identical to [the treatment applied to] the heart ruler [conduit].

Liao Ping: Earlier, the five long-term depots have been discussed in terms of the Five Phases. Here, the heart ruler is named as an additional depot, which brings about a total of six long-term depots. Really, [right and wrong] are turned upside down here in daydreams beyond imagination!

(7) *Ding Deyong*: [This hole] is located below the external ankle slightly to the front.

(8) *Ding Deyong*: This refers to the vessel movement [that can be felt] between the bones five inches above the instep.

(9) *Ding Deyong*: [This hole] is located in the hollow behind the basic joint of the finger next to the small finger.

(10) *Ding Deyong*: [This hole is located] on the line between the red and white flesh below the large bone at the outside of the foot.

(11) *Ding Deyong*: [This hole] is located in the "tiger-mouth" between the thumb and the next finger.

(12) *Ding Deyong*: [This hole] is located inside of the wrist bone of the small finger. *Yang*: [This hole] is located in the hollow of the wrist of the hand. [Ding Deyong's wording] "wrist of the finger" is a mistake.

(1)–(12) *Yu Shu*: All the twelve conduits mentioned above are matched with the Five Phases. Whenever, in the course of a year, one of the Five Phases reaches a position where it dominates [the others], one should first drain the respective origin [holes] before that [particular phase has assumed its] ruling position. In a year when [any of the Five Phases is represented] insufficiently, one must supplement first at the origin [hole]. The origin [holes] are those referred to here.

Xu Dachun: The *da ling* [hole] is a hole on the hand ceasing yin [conduit which is associated with the] heart ruler. Why is it called here the "origin" [hole of the conduit associated with the] heart? In the treatise "Jiu zhen shi er yuan" 九鍼十二原 of the *Ling* [shu], it is stated: "The major yang in the yang is the heart. Its origin [opening] exits through the *da ling* [opening." The treatise "Xie ke" 邪客 of the *Ling* [shu] states: "[The Yellow Thearch asked:] 'The hand minor yin vessel, it is the only one that has no transport [openings]. Why?' [Qi Bo] responded: 'The minor yin [conduit] is the heart vessel. The heart is the big ruler among the five long-term depots and six short-term repositories. It is the place where the //essence// spirit resides. As long as this long-term depot is firm and stable, evil [qi] will not be accepted there. The fact is: All evil [qi] that are present in the heart, they all are present in the heart enclosure'." For this reason, the *da ling* [hole] is named here as the origin [hole] of the heart. There is also an explanation for the fact that the *shen men* [hole] was selected [as an origin hole]. The treatise "Xie ke" states: "If the minor yin [vessel] is the only one that has no rapids [opening], will it never have a disease? Qi Bo: The conduits outside of it may have a disease, but the long-term depot itself cannot have a disease. Hence [for a treatment] one chooses only the conduit behind the palm, at the tip of the pointed bone." That is [a hole which is] called *dui gu* 兌骨 here [in the *Nan jing*]. However, the present [statement in the *Nan jing* was written to outline] a pattern for the selection of holes in the treatment of diseases but the *dui gu* [hole] is by no means the origin/lowland [hole] of the minor yin [conduit]. Here, the *da ling* [hole] is presented as the origin/lowland [hole] of the heart and, in addition, the *dui gu* [hole] is named as the origin/lowland [hole] of the minor yin [conduit]. The heart, though, is the minor yin [long-term depot]. Consequently, the minor yin [conduit] not only has [one] rapids [hole] but has two rapids [holes]! Why didn't [the author of the *Nan jing*] give [this issue] some deep thought? Furthermore, the treatise "Ben shu" 本輸 of the *Ling* [*shu*] states: "The [conduit associated with the] heart appears at the *zhong chong* 中衝 [hole]; that is the well [hole which represents the phase of] wood. [Its qi] start flowing at the *lao gong* 勞宮 [hole]; that is the creek [hole]. They rush down at the *da ling* 大陵 [hole]; that is the rapids [hole]. They pass at the *jian shi* 間使 [hole]; that is the stream [hole]. They disappear at the *qu ze* 曲澤 [hole]; that is the confluence [hole]." All of these are holes of the hand ceasing yin [conduit, which is associated with the heart enclosing network], but the [*Nei*] *jing* refers to them as locations where the [qi of the] heart appear and disappear. The [*Nei*] *jing* text does not outline any [separate] wells, creeks, and other holes situated on the ceasing yin conduit itself. It is obvious, then, that the rapids [hole] of the hand minor yin [conduit] is the rapids [hole] of the hand ceasing yin [conduit]. The *Jia yi jing* 甲乙經 was the first to consider, for the [hand] minor yin conduit itself, the *shao chong* [hole] as "well," the *shao fu* 少府 [hole] as "creek," the *shen men* 神門 [hole] as "rapids," the *ling dao* 靈道 [hole] as "stream," and the *shao hai* 少海 [hole] as "confluence." With this [innovation, the list of] wells, creeks, [etc.] was completed for all the twelve conduits. That, however, was achieved solely through inductive reasoning. The two scriptures [*Su wen* and *Ling shu*] in fact contained no such data. The reference here [in the *Nan jing*] to the *dui gu* [hole] as the origin [hole] of the minor yin [conduit] provided the basis for the statement in the *Jia yi jing*.

Katō Bankei: The first treatise of the *Ling shu* adds up the five rapids [holes] – *tai yuan, tai ling, tai bai, tai chong,* and *tai xi*[3] – as well as the *jiu wei* 鳩尾 and the *bo yang* 脖胦 [holes], and reaches a total of twelve origin [holes]. The second treatise [of the *Ling shu*] discusses the origin [holes on the conduits associated with] the five long-term depots and six short-term repositories and refers to

---

3   All of these exist twice, on the extremities of the left and right, respectively.

only eleven origin [holes]. The second treatise consistently lists the rapids [hole on the hand-]ceasing yin [conduit] as the origin [hole of the] hand minor yin [conduit] because whenever evil qi are present in the heart, they are, in fact, always situated in the heart enclosing network. Therefore one knows that the treatments applied to these two conduits are identical. Hence one origin [hole] could be omitted. Bian Que, now, started from the text of the second treatise and added a rapids [hole] on the [hand] minor yin [conduit, which is associated with] the true heart. [Consequently,] he reached a total of twelve. In the first treatise of the *Ling shu*, one reaches a sum of twelve if one counts the number of holes [mentioned]; one reaches a number of five if one counts only the rapids [holes] on the [main] conduits. The two holes *jiu wei* and *bo yang* belong to the controller vessel. To add these [two holes] to the origin [holes] is an old pattern, too, but still, they are not origin [holes] on the proper conduits. Hence [the *Nan jing*] has added, in the present difficult issue, the sentence, "the [original qi of the] minor yin appear at the *dui gu* [hole]," in order to point out [all] the origin [holes] of the twelve proper conduits.

(13) *Li Jiong*: Yu 俞 refers here to [the rapids hole in the sequence of] well, creek, rapids, stream, and confluence. It is not used here in reference to all the transportation [holes] (*yu* 俞).

Xu Dachun: This is a double error. According to the treatise "Ben shu" of the *Ling* [*shu*], the [conduits associated with the] five long-term depots have only wells, creeks, rapids, streams, and confluences. The [conduits associated with the] six short-term repositories have, in addition, one origin hole. [On the conduits of] the five long-term depots, the rapids [holes] constitute the origin [holes], while [on the conduits of] the six short-term repositories, the rapids [holes] represent the rapids [holes] and the origin [holes] represent the origin [holes]. Why was the word "all" added here [in the *Nan jing*]? As far as the statement that the rapids [holes] constitute the origin [holes on the conduits associated with the five long-term depots] is concerned, the treatise "Jiu zhen shi er yuan" 九鍼十二原 of the *Ling* [*shu*] originally said: "When any of the five long-term depots has an illness, this must be removed through the twelve origin [openings]. ... The minor yin in the yang, that is the lung. Its origin [opening] exits through the *tai yuan* [opening]. Of the *tai yuan* [openings], there are two. The major yang in the yang is the heart. Its origin [opening] exits through the *da ling* [opening]. Of the *da ling* [openings], there are two. The minor yang in the yin is the liver. Its origin [opening] exits through the *tai chong* [opening]. Of the *tai chong* [openings], there are two. The extreme yin in the yin is the spleen. Its origin [opening] exits through the *tai bai* [opening]. Of the *tai bai* [openings], there are two. The major yin in the yin is the kidney. Its origin [opening] exits through the *tai xi* [opening]. Of the *tai xi* [openings], there are two. The origin [opening] of the fatty membrane exits through the *jiu wei* [opening]. Of the *jiu wei* [openings], there is one. The origin [opening] of the skinny membrane exits through the *bo yang* [opening]. Of the *bo yang* [openings], there is one. All these twelve origin [openings] serve to treat the five long-term depots and six short-term repositories when they have an illness." The names of these twelve origin [holes] refer to [conduits associated with] the short-term repositories. There are altogether twelve [origin] holes, but that does not mean that there are origin [holes located] on all the twelve conduits! The ten holes from the *tai yuan* through the *tai ji* mentioned above are the so-called rapids holes of the treatise "Ben shu" in the *Ling* [*shu*]. Because the [conduits associated with the] five long-term depots have rapids [holes] but do not have origin [holes], the [*Nei jing*] refers to the rapids [holes] as origin [holes]. How was it possible that [the author of the *Nan jing*] included the [conduits associated with the] six short-term repositories [in his statements]? Why didn't he give [this issue] some profound thought?

Liao Ping: [This sentence] should read: "All the twelve conduits have transportation holes (*yu* 俞); on the [conduits associated with the] five long-term depots, the rapids [holes] (*yu* 俞) represent the lowland [holes]. Why is that?"

(14) *Li Jiong*: The Triple Burner sends its qi from this rapids [hole] to penetrate [the entire organism]; also, this rapids [hole] is the place where [the qi of the Triple Burner] stop and rest.[4]

(13)–(14) *Hua Shou*: "On all the twelve conduits the rapids [holes] constitute the lowland [holes]" means the following. The rapids [holes] of all the twelve conduits are tied to the Triple Burner. They are the locations where [the Triple Burner] passes its qi and also where these qi stop and rest.

(14) *Katō Bankei*: The character *yu* 俞 here is not the *yu* 俞 of [all] the twenty-five *yu* 俞 ("transportation holes") of the conduits [associated with] the long-term depots. Rather it is the *yu* 俞 of *yu* 俞 ("rapids") and *yuan* 原 ("lowland"). From this one can see that only on the conduits [associated with] the long-term depots the *yu* 俞 ("rapids") [holes] are the *yuan* 原 ("lowland") [holes].

(16) *Yang*: The qi moving below the navel and between the kidneys are [called] "cinnabar field" (*dan tian*) 丹田. The cinnabar field is man's source and root. It is the long-term depot of the essence and the spirit; it is the origin of the five qi. It is the mansion of the Imperial Prince. In males the essence is stored here; in females [the cinnabar field] regulates the monthly period. It constitutes the gate where yin and yang [qi] unite to create posterity. It is located three inches below

4 I read *liu* 流 ("to flow") here as *liu* 留 ("to rest").

the navel; its circumference measures four inches. It is attached to the vessels of the spine and to the root of the kidneys. It has a yellow color in its center; it is virid on the left, white on the right, red on top and black on its bottom. The three inches reflect the three powers; the four inches reflect the four seasons; the five colors reflect the Five Phases. The [location] between the two kidneys is called "great sea" (*da hai* 大海); another name is "submerged in water" (*ni shui* 溺水). Inside of it is the spirit turtle. It exhales and inhales the original qi. When [the original qi] flow [out of the cinnabar field], they penetrate the four limbs as wind and rain; they reach everywhere. The [two] kidneys are distinguished by [their storing] the essence of the sun and of the moon, [respectively. This essence] consists of immaterial qi; it constitutes man's source and root .... Hence it is obvious that the cinnabar field is the basis of life. When the Daoists contemplate the spiritual, when the Buddhist monks meditate, they all cause the qi of their heart to move below the navel. That corresponds exactly to what is meant here. Hence [the text] states "'origin/lowland' is an honorable designation for the Triple Burner" because the Triple Burner's qi are accumulated in the kidneys.

Li Jiong: For comments, see the eighth difficult issue.

(17) *Li Jiong*: For comments, see the thirty-eighth difficult issue.

(18) *Li Jiong*: Man's Triple Burner reflects the qi of the three primordial [forces] – heaven, earth, [and man]. Therefore [the text states: "It is responsible for] the passage of the three qi." The upper [section of the Triple] Burner encompasses heart and lung. The central [section of the Triple] Burner encompasses spleen and stomach. The lower [section of the Triple] Burner encompasses liver and kidneys. [This explains why] the passage [of the qi of the Triple Burner] affects the entire [organism].

Liao Ping: This book emphasizes the [importance of the] kidneys. Here, in addition, it emphasizes the [importance of the] Triple Burner. Nothing of this appears in the *Nei jing*. These are all doctrines fabricated by [the author of] this book.

Nan jing 1962: "Three qi" [refers to] *zong qi* 宗氣 ("stem qi"), *ying qi* 營氣 ("camp qi"), and *wei qi* 衛氣 ("guard qi"). They constitute the "true qi."

(19) *Li Jiong*: Yuan 原 stands for *yuan* 元 ("origin"). The original qi are the Triple Burner's qi. These qi are honorable and great. Hence [the text states]: "'Origin' is an honorable designation [for the Triple Burner]".

(15)–(19) *Hua Shou*: "The rapids [holes] where the Triple Burner passes [its qi] are the origin [holes]" means the following. The moving qi below the navel and between the kidneys constitute man's life; they are the source of the twelve conduits. Consequently, the Triple Burner is the special envoy [transmitting] the original qi. It is responsible for the passage of the upper, central, and lower qi through the body's five long-term depots and six short-term repositories. "[The Triple Burner is responsible for] the passage of the three qi" means, according. to Mr. Ji, [the following]: The lower [section of the Triple] Burner is endowed with the true primordial qi; these are the original qi. They move upward and reach the central [section of the Triple] Burner. The central [section of the Triple] Burner receives the essential but unrefined qi of water and grains and transforms them into camp and guard [qi]. The camp and guard qi proceed upward together with the true primordial qi and reach the upper [section of the Triple] Burner. "Origin" represents an honorable designation for the Triple Burner, and all the locations where [its qi] stop represent origin [holes] because [the movement of the qi of the Triple Burner] resembles the arrival of the imperial herald, announcing the places where [the Emperor] will pass by and rest. When any of the five long-term depots or six short-term repositories has a disease, it is always appropriate to remove it from these [holes].

(19) *Liao Ping*: Suddenly the Triple Burner is considered to be the master of the twelve origin [holes]; in addition, [the Triple Burner is said] to be tied to the gate of life. The *Nei jing* definitely contains no such doctrine. The *Nan jing* was the first to create such wooden figurines. Later people caused further confusion when they integrated these doctrines into the *Tai su*, thus inventing particularly fabulous stories!

(14)–(21) *Xu Dachun*: The treatise "Ben shu" 本輸 of the *Ling* [*shu*] states that the places where [the contents of the conduits associated with] the five long-term depots rush down are the rapids [holes; at the same time] they constitute the origin [holes. On the conduits associated with] the six short-term repositories, the places where [the qi] cross over are the origin [holes]. There is no reference to the Triple Burner. Now, the places where the qi of all the conduits rest and stay in the depth are the origin [holes]. Hence the treatise "Jiu zhen" 九鍼 states: "The exits of the twelve origin [openings] are in the four key joints." These holes are all located where the muscles and the bones move and join each other. Hence diseases also often stay there. When [the text] says, "the Triple Burner is responsible for the [passage of the three] qi," the wells, creeks, and so on should also all be provided with qi by the Triple Burner. Why is only the place where [the qi] rush down called "lowland"? Also, the Triple Burner has its own conduit as a passageway [of its qi]. Why does it have to be tied [to any other conduit]?

六十七難曰：（一）五藏募皆左陰，而俞在陽者，何謂也？
（二）然：陰病行陽，陽病行陰，（三）故令募在陰，俞在陽。

The sixty-seventh difficult issue: (1) All the levy [holes associated with] five long-term depots are located at the yin [side of the body; all] the transportation [holes] are located at the yang [side]. What does that mean?

(2) It is like this. Yin diseases [may] move to the yang [section of the body]; yang diseases [may] move to the yin [section of the body]. (3) It is for this reason that the levy [holes] are located at the yin [side of the body], while the transportation [holes] are located at the yang [side of the body].[1]

(1)–(3) *Ding Deyong*: Man's back is yang; his abdomen is yin. When [the text] here states: "All the transportation [holes associated with the] five long-term depots are located on the yang [side]," this refers to the transportation [holes] on the back. Hence the two transportation holes [associated with the] lung are located on both sides below the third vertebra at a mutual distance of one and a half individually standardized inches. The two transportation holes [associated with the] heart are located on both sides below the fifth vertebra at a mutual distance of one and a half individually standardized inches. The two transportation holes [associated with the] liver are located on both sides below the ninth vertebra at a mutual distance of one and a half individually standardized inches. The two transportation holes [associated with the] spleen are located on both sides below the eleventh vertebra at a mutual distance of one and a half individually standardized inches. The two transportation holes [associated with the] kidneys are located on both sides below the fourteenth vertebra at a mutual distance of one and a half individually standardized inches. The levy [holes associated with the]

---

1 Sentence 1 may be based on a statement in *Su wen* treatise 39, "Ju tong lun" 舉痛論, where a *mu* location is associated with the stomach while a *yu* location is associated with the back. Another, even less informative reference to the *mu* and *yu* locations appears in Su wen treatise 47, "Qi bing lun" 奇病論, where it is stated: "For treatment use the *mu* and *yu* of the gall bladder." In his commentary, Wang Bing added: "Chest and abdomen are called *mu*; the back and the spine are called *yu*." Subsequently, he outlined the exact positions of the *mu* and *yu* locations associated with the gall bladder on the abdomen and on the back, respectively. The origin of this concept is not clear. It must have been of interest to the author of the *Nan jing* because it permitted an application of the yinyang theory to a therapeutic needling of the trunk without resorting to circuit-needling. As may be recalled, difficult issue 45 introduced another alternative to circuit-needling of the trunk by proposing the "eight gathering points."

lung are the two *zhong fu* 中府 holes; they are located one inch below the *yun men* 雲門 and three ribs above the breast nipples. The levy [hole associated with the] heart is the one *ju que* 巨闕 hole; it is located one inch below the *jiu wei* 鳩尾.² The levy [holes associated with the] spleen are the two *zhang men* 章門 holes; they are located directly [on one level with the] navel below the youngest ribs. The levy [holes associated with the] liver are the two *qi men* 期門 holes. They are located in a distance of one and a half inches on both sides of the *bu rong* 不容 [hole]. The levy [holes associated with the] kidneys are the two *jing men* 京門 holes. They are located in the hips at the basis of the youngest ribs.

Yang: The abdomen is yin. The levy [holes] of the five long-term depots are all located on the abdominal [side of the body]. Hence [the text] states: "All the levy [holes] are located on the yin [side]." The back is yang. The transportation [holes] of the five long-term depots are all located on the back. Hence [the text] states: "All the transportation [holes] are located on the yang [side]." When the long-term depots inside [of the body] have a disease, [its qi] move out toward the yang [side]. The yang transportation [holes] are on the back. When the external sections of the body have a disease, [its qi] move inward to the yin [section]. The yin levy [holes] are on the abdominal [side of the body]. Therefore the patterns of needling demand: "From the yang pull the yin; from the yin pull the yang."³ That is [what is] meant here.

Hua Shou: *Mu* 募 ("levy") and *yu* 俞 ("transportation") are general designations for the holes [associated with the] five long-term depots. On the abdominal [side of the body], which represents the yin, these [holes] are called *mu*; on the back, which represents the yang, these [holes] are called *yu*. *Mu* is the *mu* of *mu jie* 募結 ("to levy"). That is to say, the qi of the conduits are levied here. In the Bian Que biography [of the *Shi ji*], the *yu* are called *shu* as in *wei shu* 委輸 ("to transport"). That is to say, the qi of the conduits are transported from these locations elsewhere. As to [the statement] "*yin diseases move to the yang [section]; yang diseases move to the yin [section]*," that refers to the fact that] the qi of the yin and yang conduits and network [vessels] are mutually interconnected and that the qi of the back and of the abdominal side, of the long-term depots and of the short-term repositories mutually penetrate and correspond to each other.

---

2 *Jiu wei* 鳩尾 ("pigeon-tail") is a designation of a hole and of the sternum.

3 A reference to *Su wen* treatise 5, "Yin yang ying xiang da lun" 陰陽應象大論. The Chinese wording *cong yang yin yin cong yin yin yang* 從陽引陰從陰引陽 has been interpreted differently by various authors. In *Tai su* treatise 3, "Yin yang" 陰陽, Yang Shangshan 楊上善 reads *cong* ("from") as *xie* 瀉 ("to drain") and *yin* 引 ("to draw") as *bu* 補 ("to supplement"), assigning the following meaning to the phrase: "[In case of yang repletion and yin depletion], drain the yang in order to supplement the yin, [and vice versa]."

For this reason, yin diseases sometimes move into yang [regions] and yang diseases sometimes move into yin [regions].

Zhang Shixian: "Yin diseases move to the yang [section" refers to] the evil [qi] of wind and cold that come from outside and enter through man's back. "Yang diseases move to the yin [section" means that] when the cold or the heat of water and grains affect a person, they will harm his six short-term repositories, from which they will be transported to his five long-term depots. Hence all the levy holes are located on the abdominal [side], while all the transportation holes are located on the back. Since yin diseases move to the yang [side], yin [diseases] must be drawn away from the yang [side]. Their treatment is applied at the transportation [holes]. Since yang diseases move to the yin [side], yang [diseases] must be drawn away from the yin [side]. Their treatment is applied at the levy [holes]."

(1) *Xu Dachun*: The levy [holes associated with the] short-term repositories are located on the yin [side of the body] too, and the transportation [holes associated with the short-term repositories] are also located on the yang [side of the body]. It is not so that only the [levy and the transportation holes associated with the] five long-term depots [are located on the yin and yang sides, respectively]. Also, the next chapter discusses yin and yang together [too]. I suspect that below [the words] "five long-term depots" should be the two characters "six short-term repositories."

(2)–(3) *Xu Dachun*: The [*Nei*] *jing* contains no complete outline of all the levy and transportation [holes]. I do not know on what source [the present difficult issue] is based. In the *Su* [*wen* treatise] "Tong ping xu shi lun" 通評虛實論, [it is stated]: "When suddenly the abdomen is full and when pressure is unable [to push the abdominal wall] down, [in such a situation] one selects the hand major yang conduit and network [vessels]. These are levy [holes associated with the] stomach." It is not made clear exactly which holes are meant here.

(1)–(3) *Ding Jin*: The concentration and transportation holes are places where the qi and the blood may leave their normal course of circulation through the yin and yang [sections of the body]. Similarly, the evil [qi] of diseases appear only through these [holes]. For instance, if someone has a disease in his yin section, [that disease] can move into the yang [section] because of the transportation [holes]. If a disease is in the yang section, it can move into the yin [section] because of the levy [holes]. If this [possibility] did not exist, [the yin and yang sections of the body] would be separated from each other and no mutual penetration could occur. For this reason, the levy [holes] are located on the yin [side] while the transportation [holes] are located on the yang [side]. The meaning of this [pattern] can be best elucidated by the example of *nüe* 瘧 [fevers].⁴ All *nüe* diseases result from being affected by evil [qi] of external heat and moisture. These [evil qi] harm the vital cold qi inside [the body]. The evil [qi] gradually accumulate at the levy holes.⁵ When the evil qi move into the yang [section], they will cause heat. When they move into the yin [section], they will cause cold. When the evil enters [the organism] only superficially, its way is short. Hence there are daily outbreaks. When the evil enters the depth [of the organism], its way is long. Hence outbreaks occur only every second day. The deeper [the evil] penetrates, the longer [the distance it has to travel]. Hence its outbreaks may occur only every third or fourth day. Is this not clear evidence of [the statement]: "Yin diseases move to the yang and yang diseases move to the yin [sections of the body]"?

(2)–(3) *Ye Lin*: "Yin diseases proceed to the yang [section]; yang diseases proceed to the yin [section" means the following]: The back is yang; the abdomen is yin. The transportation [holes] are located on the back. "Transportation [holes]" refers to locations where the yin qi of the long-term depots are transported. Therefore [the text states]: "Yin diseases move to the yang [section of the body]." The levy [holes] are located on the abdomen. "Levy [holes]" refers to locations where the yang qi of the long-term depots accumulate. Therefore [the text states]: "Yang diseases move to the yin [section of the body]." [All this is said] in order to demonstrate that the yin and yang conduits and network [vessels] are mutually interconnected and that the qi of the back and of the abdominal side, of the long-term depots and of the short-term repositories mutually penetrate and correspond to each other. Hence all the locations where disease qi accumulate or move around are interconnected. When the [*Nei*] *jing* states, "from the yang pull the yin; from the yin pull the yang," that is [what is] meant here.

(1)–(3) *Katō Bankei*: Because the previous chapter⁶ discussed all the wells, creeks, rapids, streams, and confluences, the present [difficult issue is concerned with] the meaning of the levy and transportation holes located on the abdomen and on the back. *Mu* 募 stands for *jie* 結 ("accumulation"); it is a designation for the yin holes, which are located on the abdomen. *Yu* 俞 stands for *shu* 輸 ("trans-

---

4 *Nüe* fevers may have included malaria. See Miyashita Saburō 宮下三郎, "Malaria (*yao*) in Chinese Medicine during the Jin and Yuan Periods," *Acta Asiatica* 36 (1979): 90-112.

5 The text has *mu yuan* 募原. That may be a mistake for *mu xue* 募穴 ("levy hole"). The term *mu yuan* is identical with *mo yuan* 膜原, which appears in the *Su wen* treatise "Ju tong lun" 舉痛論. Its meaning is not entirely clear. Tamba Genkan 丹波元簡 (alias Taki Mototane) interpreted it as "the origin of the diaphragm at the seventh vertebra of the spine."

6 Katō Bankei's *Nan jing* edition places the present difficult issue between issues 73 and 74.

portation"); it is a designation for the yang holes, which are located on the back. The levy and transportation [holes] of the conduits are places where the qi of the long-term depots stop and rest. But there is a difference between levy and transportation [holes]. The transportation [holes] belong to the section of the back. The blood and the qi of the major yang conduit are collected there to be transported somewhere else. The levy [holes] are located in the chest and in the abdominal section; some of them belong to a basic conduit, some belong to other conduits. Blood and qi rest at these places, which reach into the depth and provide a link to the long-term depots. Hence in the case of a disease, yang diseases move to the yin [section] and yin diseases move to the yang [section]. All these [holes] are selected [as places to apply treatment] for this reason. That is meant when the needling experts [say]: "From the yang pull the yin; from the yin pull the yang." ... A general designation of the qi holes all over the body is *yu* 俞 ("transportation hole"). The *yu* 俞 referred to here are only the transportation [holes associated with the] five long-term depots on the back. Readers should not confuse [the two meanings of this term].

Nan jing 1962: The levy and the transportation [holes] are holes of central importance in the circulation of qi and blood. Therefore, evil [qi causing] diseases frequently enter and leave [the body] through these [holes] as well. Obviously, if "yang diseases move to the yin [section, and if] yin diseases move to the yang [section]," for treating the diseases in the five long-term depots by means of needling, one should employ the principal pattern "from the yang pull the yin; from the yin pull the yang." The yang and yin diseases discussed in the present difficult issue include, in fact, [those caused by] evil qi belonging to the yin and yang [categories], as well as symptoms such as cold or heat, depletion or repletion. In the case of yin diseases, one can pierce the transportation [holes] on the back in order to harmonize the qi in the conduits and draw out the evil [qi]. That is [what is meant by] "from the yang pull the yin." In the case of yang diseases, one can needle the levy [holes] on the abdomen in order to harmonize the qi in the conduits and draw out the evil. That is [what is meant by] "from the yin pull the yang."

六十八難曰：（一）五藏六府，各有井滎俞經合，皆何所主？
（二）然：經言所出為井，所流為滎，所注為俞，所行為經，所入為
合。（三）井主心下滿，（四）滎主身熱，（五）俞主體重節痛，（六）經主喘咳
寒熱，（七)合主逆氣而泄。（八)此五藏六府其井滎俞經合所主病也。

The sixty-eighth difficult issue: (1) Each of the [conduits associated with the body's] five long-term depots and six short-term repositories has a "well," "creek," "rapids," "stream," and "confluence." What [diseases can] be controlled through them respectively?

(2) It is like this. The scripture states: Where they appear are the "wells"; where they flow[1] are the "creeks"; where they rush down are the "rapids"; where they proceed are the "streams"; where they disappear are the "confluences." (3) [Through] the wells [one can] control fullness below the heart. (4) [Through] the creeks [one can] control body heat. (5) [Through] the rapids [one can] control a heavy body and pain in the joints. (6) [Through] the streams [one can] control panting and coughing as well as [alternating spells of] cold and heat. (7) [Through] the confluences [one can] control qi proceeding contrary to their proper course, as well as diarrhea. (8) These are the diseases [that can be] controlled [through] the wells, creeks, rapids, streams, and confluences of the [conduits associated with the body's] five long-term depots and six short-term repositories.[2]

COMMENTARIES

(1) *Li Jiong*: [On the conduit associated with] the liver, the *da dui* 大敦 [hole] is the well; the *xing jian* 行間 [hole] is the creek; the *da chong* 大衝 [hole] is the rapids; the *zhong feng* 中封 [hole] is the stream; and the *qu quan* 曲泉 [hole] is the confluence. [On the conduit associated with] the lung, the *shao shang* 少商 [hole] is the well; the *yu ji* 魚際 [hole] is the creek; the *da yuan* 大淵 [hole] is the rapids; the *jing qu* 經渠 [hole] is the stream; and the *chi ze* 尺澤 [hole] is the confluence. [On the conduit associated with] the heart, the *shao chong* 少衝 [hole] is the well; the *shao fu* 少府 [hole] is the creek; the *shen men* 神門 [hole] is the rapids; the *ling dao* 靈道 [hole] is the stream; and the *shao hai* 少海 [hole] is the confluence. [On the conduit associated with] the kidneys, the *yong quan* 湧泉 [hole] is the well; the *li gu* 麗谷 [hole] is the creek; the *da xi* 大谿 [hole] is

---

1   The corresponding passage in *Ling shu* treatise 1, "Jiu zhen shi er yuan," has *liu* 溜 ("to stream") instead of *liu* 流 ("to flow").

2   Sentences 3 through 8 were added by the *Nan jing* author; they are not part of the *Nei jing* quotation referred to by sentence 2.

the rapids; the *fu liu* 復溜 [hole] is the stream; and the *liu gu* 溜谷 [hole] is the confluence. [On the conduit associated with] the spleen, the *yin bai* 隱白 [hole] is the well; the *da du* 大都 [hole] is the creek; the *da bai* 大白 [hole] is the rapids; the *shang qiu* 商丘 [hole] is the stream; and the *yin ling quan* 陰陵泉 [hole] is the confluence. [On the conduit associated with] the heart enclosing network, the *zhong chong* 中衝 [hole] is the well; the *lao gong* 勞宮 [hole] is the creek; the *da ling* 大陵 [hole] is the rapids; the *jian shi* 間使 [hole] is the stream; and the *qu ze* 曲澤 [hole] is the confluence. These are the wells, creeks, rapids, streams, and confluences of the [conduits associated with the] five long-term depots. [On the conduit associated with] the gall bladder, the *qiao yin* 竅陰 [hole] is the well; the *xia xi* 俠谿 [hole] is the creek; the *lin qi* 臨泣 [hole] is the rapids; the *yang fu* 陽輔 [hole] is the stream; the *yang ling quan* 陽陵泉 [hole] is the confluence; and the *qiu xu* 丘虛 [hole] is the lowland. [On the conduit associated with] the large intestine, the *shang yang* 商陽 [hole] is the well; the *san jian* 三間 [hole] is the creek; the *yang xi* 陽谿 [hole] is the stream; the *qu chi* 曲池 [hole] is the confluence; and the *he gu* 合谷 [hole] is the lowland. [On the conduit associated with] the small intestine, the *shao ze* 少澤 [hole] is the well; the *qian gu* 前谷 [hole] is the creek; the *hou xi* 後谿 [hole] is the rapids; the *yang gu* 陽谷 [hole] is the stream; the *shao hai* 少海 [hole] is the confluence; and the *wan gu* 腕骨 [hole] is the lowland. [On the conduit associated with] the stomach, the *li dui* 厲兌 [hole] is the well; the *nei ting* 內庭 [hole] is the creek; the *yin gu* 隱谷 [hole] is the rapids; the *jie xi* 解谿 [hole] is the stream; the *san li* 三里 [hole] is the confluence; and the *chong yang* 衝陽 [hole] is the lowland. [On the conduit associated with] the urinary bladder, the *zhi yin* 至陰 [hole] is the well; the *tong rong* 通容 [hole] is the creek; the *shu gu* 束骨 [hole] is the rapids; the *kun lun* 崑崙 [hole] is the stream; the *wei zhong* 委中 [hole] is the confluence; and the *jing gu* 京骨 [hole] is the lowland. [On the conduit associated with] the Triple Burner, the *guan chong* 關衝 [hole] is the well; the *ye men* 液門 [hole] is the creek; the *zhong du* 中都 [hole] is the rapids; the *zhi man* 支滿 [hole] is the stream; the *tian jing* 天井 [hole] is the confluence; and the *yang chi* 陽池 [hole] is the lowland. These are the wells, creeks, rapids, streams, and confluences, as well as – in addition – the lowland [holes] of the [conduits associated with the] six short-term repositories, respectively.

Hua Shou: Zhu 主 stands for *zhi* 治 ("to rule") .... Yu 俞 stands for *shu* 輸 ("transportation") and *zhu* 注 ("to rush down"). Where a creek develops into rushing water, that [point] represents a *yu* 俞.

Xu Dachun: That is to say, what diseases can be controlled by piercing all these holes.

(2) *Ye Lin*: "The scripture states" refers to the text of the treatise "Jiu zhen shi er yuan" 九鍼十二原 of the *Ling shu*.

(3) *Lü Guang*: The "wells" are [associated with the phase of] wood. The wood is [associated with] the liver. The liver is responsible for fullness.

  Yu Shu: The "wells" reflect the wood; they correspond to liver and spleen. The position [of liver and spleen] is below the heart. Here, evil [qi] are present in the liver. These [evil qi of the] liver seize the spleen. Hence there is "fullness below the heart." The treatment must be applied at the wells; one must not allow the wood to seize the soil.

(4) *Lü Guang*: The "creeks" are [associated with the phase of] fire. The fire is [associated with] the heart. The heart is responsible for body heat.

  Yu Shu: The "creeks" constitute the [phase of] fire; they reflect the heart. The lung belongs to the [phase of] metal; externally it rules the skin [and its] hair. Here the fire of the heart burns the metal of the lung. Hence body heat results. That is to say, evil [qi] are present in the heart. Hence the treatment must be applied at the creeks; one must not allow the fire to seize the metal. In this way, body heat will be cured.

(5) *Lü Guang*: The "rapids" are [associated with the phase of] soil. The soil rules the spleen. The spleen is responsible for a heavy body.

  Yu Shu: The "rapids" reflect the soil; they correspond to the spleen. Here, evil [qi] are present in the [long-term depot associated with the] soil. The soil must punish the water. The water [represents] the kidneys. The kidneys rule the bones. Hence in the case of a disease [in the kidneys] one has pain in his joints. If the evil [qi] are present in the [long-term depot associated with the] soil, the soil has the disease itself and a heavy body results. The treatment should be applied at the rapids holes.

(6) *Lü Guang*: The "streams" are [associated with the phase of] metal. The metal rules the lung. The lung is responsible for [alternating spells of] cold and heat.

  Yu Shu: The "streams" reflect [the phase of] metal; they correspond to the lung. Here, evil qi are present in the [long-term depot associated with the phase of] metal.[3] Hence the lung is ill. If it is affected by cold, coughing results; if it is affected by heat, panting results. Here, evil [qi] are present in the [long-term depot associated with the phase of] metal. The metal must punish the wood. The wood [is associated with] the liver. The mental condition associated with the liver is anger. If one is angry, his qi will proceed contrary to their proper direction and seize the lung. Hence panting results. Why is that so? The meaning is

---

3 The text has *jing* 經 ("conduit," "stream"). This sentence appears again after the next sentence, with jin 金 ("metal") instead of *jing*. The passage may be somewhat corrupt.

that the various branches of the liver start from the liver – where a ramification occurs – and are tied to [the area above] the diaphragm where [their contents] rush into the lung. The [treatise] "Mai yao jing wei lun" 脈要精微論 states: "Blood that is below the flanks lets a person pant because of a movement contrary to its proper course." That is [what is] meant here. The treatment must be applied at the streams lest the metal punish the wood.

(7) *Lü Guang*: The "confluences" are [associated with the phase of] water. The [phase of] water rules the kidneys. The kidneys are responsible for diarrhea.

Yu Shu: The "confluences" reflect the [phase of] water; they correspond to the kidneys. If the qi of the kidneys are insufficient, the throughway vessel will be harmed. As a consequence, the qi will proceed contrary to their proper direction and internal cramps result. The kidneys are responsible for the opening of the two yin orifices. If the qi of the kidneys do not prohibit it, diarrhea and the rushing out [of liquids from the body] will result. When evil [qi] are present in the [long-term depot associated with the phase of] water, the water must seize the fire. The fire [corresponds to] the heart; it must not receive a disease. The wood of the liver represents the mother of the fire of the heart; it is the child of the water of the kidneys. As a first [result of] sadness, the mother will receive evil [qi from her child]; as a second [result of continuing] sadness, the child will be punished. The mental condition associated with the liver is anger. Sadness will result in anger. Anger is the reason for a movement of qi contrary to their proper direction. These are [examples] of the way in which the Five Phases mutually seize and overpower each other. Hence there are differences and parallels among the diseases. Here, the treatment is to be applied at the streams lest one allow the water to seize the fire. As a result, the wood of the liver will not be affected by sadness and the qi will stop moving contrary to their proper course. If no evil [qi] are present in the kidneys, there will be no rushing and no diarrhea. The wells, creeks, rapids, streams, and confluences referred to above reflect the Five Phases and correspond to the five long-term depots. When evil [qi] accumulate in [these long-term depots, one can] control them as is described here. Those who are experts in diagnosis will examine [the patient] and recognize [the disease]. They will know whether a disease has emerged in the long-term depot [where it is located now] itself, or whether it resulted from [the fact that evil qi from another depot] have seized [the long-term depot which is ill now]. In the case of a depletion one must supplement; in the case of a repletion one must drain.

(3)–(8) *Xu Dachun*: According to the associations [of the wells, creeks, etc.] with the Five Phases, as listed in the sixty-fourth difficult issue, a fullness below the heart is a disease of the liver, [which is associated with] the wood. Body heat is a disease of the heart, [which is associated with] the fire, [etc. See Lü Guang's and Yu Shu's comments on sentences 3 through 7]. However, this is but a reference to one single principle. The categorization of diseases and the selection of holes [for treatment] in the two [books of the *Nei*] *jing* follow a pattern that differs substantially from the one outlined here. One should not rely on only a single doctrine, and one must be familiar with possible modifications.

Chapter Six
Needling Patterns

THE SIXTY-NINTH DIFFICULT ISSUE

六十九難曰：（一）經言虛者補之，（二）實者瀉之，（三）不實不虛，以經取之，何謂也？

（四）然：虛者補其母，（五）實者瀉其子，（六）當先補之，然後瀉之。（七）不實不虛，以經取之者，是正經自生病，不中他邪也，（八）當自取其經，故言以經取之。

The sixty-ninth difficult issue: (1) The scripture states: In the case of depletion, supplement it. (2) In the case of repletion, drain it. (3) When neither a repletion nor a depletion are present, remove the [disease] from the conduits. What does that mean?

(4) It is like this. In the case of depletion, supplement the respective [conduit's] mother. (5) In the case of repletion, drain the respective [conduit's] child. (6) One must supplement first and drain afterwards. (7) The removal of [a disease] from the conduits [themselves] because neither a repletion nor a depletion is present is [appropriate] if a regular conduit has fallen ill by itself rather than as a result of having been struck by evil [qi transmitted from] another [conduit]. (8) In this case one must select [for treatment] just this one conduit. Hence the scripture states: Remove it from the conduit.[1]

---

1 With this difficult issue, the final section of the *Nan jing* is introduced – that is, the section devoted to actual therapy. The *Nan jing* advocates only one therapeutic approach – namely, the needling of the so-called transportation holes on the short conduits running in the four limbs from hands and feet to elbow and knees, respectively. The sixty-ninth difficult issue introduces a therapeutic approach that directly follows the pathological patterns outlined in difficult issues 49 and 50. Sentence 1 alludes to *Ling shu* treatise 10, "Jing mai" 經脈, where all the conduits are listed with their various diseases. The three approaches discussed here are mentioned among the five general therapeutic approaches listed there. However, when the *Ling shu* speaks of "depletion" or "repletion," it does so in a very concrete sense: A conduit may be overly full or empty. Hence it may have to be drained or supplemented. When the *Ling shu* states, "if neither a repletion nor a depletion is present, remove the [illness] from the conduits," it appears to refer to rather tangible illness-causing qi (like humidity) that have entered the conduit and have to be removed from it. Some later commentators interpreted the contents of the present

(1) *Liao Ping*: The pattern of the Five Phases as outlined in this book implies that everybody's brain is nothing but a battlefield with grace and hatred, generation and destruction, troublemaking and alliances, as well as rival doctrines. That is a very great mistake. It reminds one of vulgar expressions like "the heart is fire, the lung is metal; the metal is on top, the fire is below." How could [the body] stand a fire that actually burns something down? We will recall: It should not be that some members of a family are hot like fire while others are cold like water.

Ye Lin: "The scripture states" refers to the treatise "Jing mai" 經脈 of the *Ling shu*.

(1)–(8) *Ding Deyong*: First the [*Nan*] *jing* has introduced the wells, creeks, rapids, streams, and confluences and has matched them with the Five Phases. Then it has outlined how each of the twelve conduits has a child and a mother [conduit], mutually generating and nourishing each other. Now [the *Nan jing*] discusses the pattern of how to employ the needles in order to supplement or drain. For example, in the case of a depletion in the network [vessel] of the foot ceasing yin [conduit associated with] the liver, one supplements at the confluence of this foot ceasing yin conduit; it is the mother. In the case of repletion, one drains at the creek of the foot ceasing yin conduit; it is the child. If no evil [qi] from other [conduits] are present, one must select [for treatment holes on] just this one conduit [which is ill]. Hence [the text] states: "Remove it from the conduit."

Yang: If in spring one feels a [movement in the] vessels that is [associated with] the kidneys, this represents a depletion evil. In such a situation the kidneys are depleted and cannot transmit any qi to the liver. Hence one supplements the

difficult issue on the basis of these concepts. However, the meaning expressed here is rather different from that of the *Nei jing* – as already noted by Xu Dachun and Liao Ping. Here the *Nan jing* continues its tendency to systematize the contents of the *Nei jing* – and whatever other "scripture" it may have had as its starting point – strictly on the basis of the paradigm of systematic correspondence. In accordance with difficult issues 49 and 50, a "repletion" is not simply a state of the affected conduit being overly full; it is a disease transmitted to the affected conduit by its child-conduit. Similarly, a "depletion" is a disease transmitted by the mother-conduit. "Mother" and "child" refer to the mutual generation order of the Five Phases. A disease in a conduit which is "neither a depletion nor a repletion" does not mean, as some commentators have written, that this is the only case where external pathological qi have affected the body; rather, it simply refers to the fact that the affected conduit has been hit directly from outside. In case of "repletion" or "depletion," other conduits have been affected by outside qi first and have transmitted these evil qi to the sick conduit in question. The therapeutic principle emphasized here underscores the necessity not only of treating the functional unit in the organism that happens to be affected by a disease at the time of diagnosis but also of searching for and treating the unit that was weak enough in the first place to be affected by primarily external, illness-causing qi.

kidneys. If the kidneys have a disease, they will transmit it to the liver. The liver is the child of the kidneys. Hence [the text] states: "Supplement the mother." If in spring one feels a [movement in the] vessels that is [associated with] the heart, this represents a repletion evil. In such a situation the heart is replete with abundant qi. These [qi] move contrary to their proper direction and come to seize the liver. Hence one drains the heart. When the heart is in a normal condition, nothing impedes the movement of the qi of the liver. The liver represents the mother of the heart. Hence [the text] states: "Drain the child." If neither repletion nor depletion are present, no [qi from] one of the long-term depots have seized any other [depot]. If in spring one feels a string-like and rapid or simply a string-like [movement in the vessels], these are indications that the liver long-term depot itself has fallen ill. Consequently one must supplement or drain at the foot ceasing yin or [foot] minor yang [conduits].[2] Since [each] conduit has [holes associated with one of the Five Phases of] metal, wood, water, fire, and soil [respectively], one must remove the disease [from a hole associated with the phase characterizing] the current season.

Hua Shou: The tenth treatise of the *Ling shu* notes for all the twelve conduits: "If the [evil] qi abound, they are to be drained. If the [proper qi] are depleted, they are to be supplemented. When [the qi] neither abound nor are depleted, then [the disease] is to be removed from the [respective] conduit." In the case of a depletion, one supplements the respective mother; in the case of repletion, one drains the respective child. A child may cause repletion in its mother; a mother may cause depletion in her child. For example, in case the liver suffers from a depletion, one supplements at the confluence of the ceasing yin [conduit] – that is, the *qu quan* 曲泉 [hole]. In case [the liver suffers from] repletion, one drains at the creek of the ceasing yin [conduit] – that is, the *xing jian* 行間 [hole]. "One must supplement first and drain afterwards" means something that is elucidated in a later discourse – namely, if there are not enough yang qi and if there is a surplus of yin qi, one must first supplement the yang and afterwards drain the yin [qi]. However, this meaning appears to be out of place here; something may be missing or [the presence of this sentence here] is a mistake. The passage is superfluous. "In case neither a repletion nor a depletion is present, remove the [disease] from the respective conduit" refers to the meaning expressed in the forty-ninth difficult issue – namely, sadness and pondering harm the heart; if the body is cold and if drinks are chilled, that harms the lung, and so on. These are situations where the respective conduit has fallen ill by itself.

---

2   The former is associated with the liver itself; the latter is associated with the liver's short-term repository–that is, with the gall bladder.

Xu Dachun: According to the patterns of supplementing and draining [as listed in] the *Nei jing*, one either selects the [sick] conduit itself [for treatment] or one selects several other conduits; one [may have to] drain first and supplement afterwards, or one [may have to] supplement first and drain afterwards; or one just supplements and does not drain, or one just drains but does not supplement. In some cases one single conduit is selected, in other cases three or four conduits are selected [for treatment]. All these teachings are equally important; it is impossible to pick one of them as the dominant one. The pattern of supplementing the mother and draining the child represents but one principle among [all those listed in the *Nei jing*]. If one takes only the principle of supplementing and draining into consideration as it is outlined here [in the *Nan jing*], that is inadequate.

Nan jing: The therapeutic method of "supplementing the mother in the case of depletion and of draining the child in the case of repletion" can be applied in two ways in the practice of needling – first, by differentiating between well, creek, rapids, stream, and confluence holes on the [affected] conduit itself and by selecting [one of these holes] for treatment, and, second, by utilizing the relationships among the twelve conduits as a whole. (1) The method of supplementing and draining at the wells, creeks, rapids, streams, and confluences of the [affected] conduit itself: If, for instance, the conduit [associated with the] lung suffers from a depletion of qi, one selects the rapids hole of the conduit [associated with the] lung – that is, the *tai yuan* [hole]. The *tai yuan* 太淵 hole belongs to the [phase of] soil. The soil can generate metal. That is an [example of] "in the case of depletion supplement the mother." If, for instance, the conduit [associated with the] lung suffers from a repletion of qi, one must employ the method of "in the case of repletion, drain the child." One selects for treatment the confluence hole of the conduit [associated with the lung] – that is, the *chi ze* 尺澤 hole, which is associated with water. (2) The method of supplementing and draining through the five transportation holes on the twelve conduits: here man is seen as a whole and the twelve conduits are considered as the basis [of treatment]. For example, in the case of a depletion of qi in the conduit [associated with the] liver, one must select [for treatment] the transportation holes of the foot major yin conduit of the spleen in accordance with the method of "in the case of depletion supplement the mother." The lung belongs to the [phase of] metal; the soil is the mother of the metal. At the same time one may select the *tai bai* 太白 hole of this particular conduit for treatment – it belongs to the soil. In contrast, if the lung conduit is marked by a repletion of qi, one may select the transportation holes of the kidney conduit – [in accordance with the method of] "in the case

of repletion drain the child" – or one could select [only] the confluence hole of
this particular conduit – that is, the *yin gu* 隱谷 [hole] – in order to apply the
treatment. The children of the lung are the kidneys; the kidneys belong to [the
phase of] water. The *yin gu* [hole] belongs to [the phase of] water. If one drains
the child, one cures the repletion of the mother. This is the principle that a child
can cause depletion in its mother.

(4)–(5) *Liao Ping*: In the [*Nei*] *jing*, supplementing and draining are applied mostly to the [sick] conduit itself. This book pastes [these approaches] to the Five
Phases and establishes a special theory of "child" and "mother" that was not
pointed out by the [*Nei*] *jing* itself.

(6) *Li Jiong*: A mother may cause repletion in her child. Accordingly, [a treatment]
to supplement the mother must be [applied at the conduit of the long-term
depot] preceding [the sick long-term depot in the order of mutual generation].
A child may cause depletion in its mother. [A treatment] to drain the child must
be [applied at the conduit of the long-term depot] following [the sick long-term
depot in the order of mutual generation].

   Ding Jin: "One must supplement first and drain afterwards" means that if one
wishes to drain the respective [conduit's] child, one should first supplement its
mother. Obviously, the ancient people greatly emphasized the strengthening of
the basis.

(8) *Xu Dachun*: "Select [for treatment] just this one conduit" means that one must
pierce the holes of the [sick] conduit itself; one must not supplement the mother
or drain the child.

七十難曰：（一）經言春夏刺淺，秋冬刺深者，何謂也？

（二）然：春夏者，陽氣在上，人氣亦在上，故當淺取之；（三）秋冬者，陽氣在下，人氣亦在下，故當深取之。

（四）春夏各致一陰，秋冬各致一陽者，何謂也？

（五）然：春夏溫，必致一陰者，初下針，沉之至腎肝之部，（六）得氣，引持之陰也；（七）秋冬寒，必致一陽者，初內針，淺而浮之至心肺之部，（八）得氣，推內之陽也。（九）是謂春夏必致一陰，秋冬必致一陽。

The seventieth difficult issue: (1) The scripture states:[1] In spring and summer piercing is shallow; in autumn and winter piercing is deep. What does that mean?

(2) It is like this. In spring and summer the yang qi are in the upper [regions], and man's qi are also in the upper [regions]. Hence one must [insert the needle] superficially in order to remove them. (3) In autumn and winter the yang qi are in the lower [regions], and man's qi are also in the lower [regions]. Hence one must [insert the needle] deeply in order to remove them.

(4) In spring and summer reach all yin; in autumn and winter reach all yang. What does that mean?

(5) It is like this. Spring and summer are warm; one must reach all the yin [qi. That is to say,] upon the initial insertion of the needle, one must penetrate deeply into the regions of the kidneys and of the liver. (6) The qi one gets hold of there are to be pulled out; they constitute the yin [qi alluded to above]. (7) Autumn and winter are cold; one must reach all the yang [qi. That is to say,] the initial insertion of the needle must be shallow; it must reach to the regions of heart and lung near the surface. (8) The qi one gets hold of there are to be pushed into the interior; they constitute the yang [qi alluded to above]. (9) That is [what is] meant by "in spring and summer reach all the yin; in autumn and winter reach all the yang."[2]

COMMENTARIES

(2)–(3) *Ding Deyong*: As for "in spring and summer piercing is shallow; in autumn and winter piercing is deep," the [*Nei*] *jing* states: "In spring and summer pierce

---

1 The two characters *jing yan* 經言 ("the scripture states") are omitted in several editions (including, among others, those by Hua Shou, Xu Dachun, Liao Ping, and Katō Bankei, but not those by Wang Jiu'en and Li Jiong).

2 The preceding difficult issue introduced a therapeutic approach of needling based entirely on the Five Phases doctrine. The present difficult issue introduces an innovative approach based exclusively on the yinyang doctrine.

the wells and the creeks because these are locations where the flesh is shallow and thin. In autumn and winter pierce the streams and the confluences because these are locations where the flesh is deep and thick."³ That means that the locations where piercing is applied should be [selected] in accordance with the seasons.

Yang: The scripture states: "In spring the qi are in the fine hair; in summer the qi are in the skin; in autumn the qi are in the flesh [close to the bones]; in winter the qi are in the muscles and in the bones." These are the [different locations of the] qi in the course of the four seasons. If, in the course of the four seasons, one is affected by a disease, the location of this [disease] will be shallow or deep following the [position of the] proper qi [of the current season]. Hence, in applying needles for the treatment of diseases, one must remove [the disease-causing qi] in accordance with the deep or shallow position of the qi of the four seasons.

Hua Shou: In spring and summer the yang qi are near the surface and move upward. Man's qi do the same. Hence, in piercing them one must [remain in] shallow [regions]. The aim is not to have greatly excessive [yang qi]. In autumn and winter the yang qi are in the depth and move downward. Man's qi do the same. Hence, in piercing them one must [reach into] deep [regions]. The aim is not to have insufficient [yang qi].

Xu Dachun: "Yang qi" refers to the qi of heaven and earth; "man's qi" refers to the camp and guard qi. "Upper" refers to the upper [regions] of skin and flesh. "Lower" refers to the central [regions] of muscles and bones. "Remove them through superficial [insertion]" and "remove them through deep [insertion" is to say that] one must [use the needle to] hit the location where the disease is situated. [With such an approach, the disease] will be cured easily.

Zhang Shixian: That is to say, there are differences in the insertion of needles in the course of the four seasons. The main goal in needling is to get hold of qi [in order to remove or transmit them]. When the qi are in the upper [regions] one inserts the needle only superficially; when the qi are in the lower [regions] one inserts the needle deeply.

(4) *Xu Dachun*: *Zhi* 致 stands for *qu* 取 ("to remove"). That is to say, one uses the needles to remove the qi.

(5)–(6) *Yu Shu*: The [*Nei*]*jing* states: "In spring and summer nourish the yang." That is to say, remove all the qi from the yin [region] to nourish the yang. One must be concerned about a [possible] isolation of the yang [qi]. *Zhi* stands for *du*

---

3   *Ling shu* treatise 2, "Ben shu" 本輸, states that one should pierce the "creeks" in spring, the "origins" in summer, the "confluences" in autumn, and the "wells" in winter. The same pattern is also recommended in *Ling shu* treatise 44, "Shun qi yi ri fen wei si shi" 順氣一日分爲四時. See also difficult issue 74.

("abundant," "refined"); it means *ji* ("to arrive at," "extreme"). That is to say, one reaches to the [regions of the] kidneys and of the liver and leads all the yin qi away from there. Liver and kidneys are yin.

Hua Shou: "In spring and summer the qi are warm; one must reach all the yin [qi]" means that in spring and summer one nourishes the yang [with yin qi]. At first one lowers the needle deeply until it reaches the regions of the kidneys and of the liver. As soon as one gets hold of qi there, one pulls the needle up and lifts these [qi] all the way up to the section of the heart and of the lung. That is the so-called "reaching of all the yin [qi]".

Xu Dachun: "Warm" refers to seasonal warmth. When yang [qi] are present in abundance, not enough yin [qi] are available [to support the yang qi]. Hence one removes yin qi [from deeper sections] in order to nourish the yang [qi at the surface]. "Penetrate deeply" means to insert the needle deeply into the section of muscles and bones – that is, of kidneys and liver. "Pull out" means to pull the qi out into the yang section.

Liao Ping: The meaning of this text lies just at the borderline of what can be understood and what cannot be understood. The people of later times have considered this book as a guideline because it is so simple. They did not know that medicine is not something that can be comprehended easily.

(7)–(8) *Yu Shu*: The [*Nei*] *jing* states: "In autumn and winter nourish the yin." That is to say, the extreme yin is in command. No yang qi are present to nourish the yin. Hence one removes all the qi from the yang [regions] in order to provide nourishment to the yin [qi]. One must avoid an isolation of the yin [qi]. Heart and lung are yang. Hence [the text] states: "Reach to the regions of heart and lung."

Yang: If one enters the skin three *fen* 分 [deep, one reaches] the region of heart and lung. That is where the yang qi move. If one enters the skin five *fen* [deep, one reaches] the region of kidneys and liver. That is where the yin qi move. The yang [qi] are the guard [qi]; the yin [qi] are the camp [qi]. In spring and summer diseases proceed through the yang [region]. Hence one draws yin [qi] there in order to restore harmony in the yang [region]. In autumn and winter diseases proceed through the yin [region]. Hence one sends yang [qi] to the interior in order to restore harmony to the yin [region].

Hua Shou: "In autumn and winter the qi are cold; one must reach all the yang [qi]" means that in autumn and winter one nourishes the yin [with yang qi]. At first one inserts the needle only superficially and brings it to below the surface. That is exactly the region of heart and lung. As soon as one gets hold of qi there, one pushes the needle and brings it to the interior until it reaches the section of the kidneys and of the lung. That is the so-called "reaching of all the yang [qi]".

Xu Dachun: "Cold" refers to seasonal cold. When yin [qi] are present in abundance, not enough yang [qi] are available [to support the yin qi]. Hence one removes yang qi [from the regions at the surface] in order to nourish the yin [qi in the depth]. "Shallow insertion" means to insert the needle only superficially into the section of skin and blood – that is, of heart and lung. "Push" means to push these qi into the yin section. That is the meaning of the statement in the [*Nei*] *jing*: "From the yin pull the yang; from the yang pull the yin."[4]

(9) *Hua Shou*: The doctrine of the "transmission of yin and transmission of yang" [outlined in] this difficult issue is a concept created by Bian Que himself. The underlying principle is indeed [applicable in certain situations]. However, whenever one employs the needles one should supplement or drain according to the requirements [of the individual patient). One must not rely primarily on the [approach introduced here].

Zhang Shixian: Zhi 致 stands for *bei* 備 ("to complete").

Xu Dachun: The doctrine of the "transmission of yin and transmission of yang" is not outlined in the [*Nei*] *jing*. [Here it is stated first:] "In spring and summer piercing is shallow." [Then the text says] that one should first [insert the needle] into the regions of kidneys and liver. That means that one still has to pierce deeply. This is difficult to reconcile with the meaning of the [initial statement of the text. I do not know on what [source] this is based.

Katō Bankei: The *Su wen* states in treatise 64: "In spring the qi are in the conduit vessels; in summer the qi are in the tertiary network [vessels]; in late summer the qi are in the muscles and the flesh; in autumn the qi are in the skin; in winter the qi are in the bones and in the marrow." Furthermore, in treatise 9, the *Ling shu* states: "The qi of spring are in the fine body hairs. The qi of summer are in the skin. The qi of autumn are in the partings of the flesh. The qi of winter are in the sinews and bones. ... The fact is: When piercing a fat person, this must be in agreement with autumn and winter. When piercing an emaciated person, this must be in agreement with spring and summer." The present paragraph starts from these statements to discuss the patterns of deep and shallow piercing. Its message is quite subtle. Of course, spring and summer themselves are differentiated by shallow and deep [piercing]; and the same applies to autumn and winter. Hence one knows that the seasonal [qi] of heaven are tied together with the qi of man like the two halves of a tally in their movement up and down and in their being located at the surface or in the depth. Also, one should realise from this that for [needling] a thin person, one must apply the pattern of spring and summer even in autumn and winter, and that for [needling] a fat person, one must

---

4   See also difficult issue 67.

apply the pattern of autumn and winter even in spring and summer. In each case one must proceed according to the individual requirements. The subtle meaning expressed here [is reflected in the sayings] "change your approach according to the situation you encounter" and "always stick to the golden mean." One must observe [these guidelines]!

七十一難曰：（一）經言刺榮無傷衛，刺衛無傷榮，何謂也？
（二）然：鍼陽者，臥鍼而刺之；（三）刺陰者，先以左手攝按所鍼榮俞之
處，氣散乃內針。（四）是謂刺榮無傷衛，刺衛無傷榮也。

The seventy-first difficult issue: (1) The scripture states: When piercing the camp
[qi] do not harm the guard [qi]; when piercing the guard [qi] do not harm the camp
[qi]. What does that mean?

(2) It is like this. When needling the yang [qi], one performs the piercing with a
lying needle. (3) When piercing the yin [qi], one first presses, with one's left hand,
the location of the transportation [hole] where the camp [qi] are to be needled. As
soon as the [guard] qi are dispersed, one inserts the needle. (4) That is [what is]
meant by "when piercing the camp [qi] do not harm the guard [qi]; when piercing
the guard [qi] do not harm the camp [qi]."

COMMENTARIES

(1)–(4) *Ding Deyong*: Man's camp [qi] are yin; his guard [qi] are yang. The two constitute outside and inside. One removes [guard qi] with a lying needle because
otherwise one might harm the camp [qi]. When piercing the camp [qi] one
first presses, with the left hand, the hole to be pierced, causing the yang [qi] to
disperse, and only then inserts the needle lest one harm the guard [qi].

Yang: Three *fen* 分 deep in the skin are the guard qi. If a disease is situated in the
[region of the] guard qi, one inserts the needle only superficially. Hence [the text
states]: "One performs the piercing with a lying needle." The reason is that one
might harm the camp qi if one inserts [the needle] deeply. Five *fen* 分 deep in
the skin are the camp qi. Hence one first presses the hole where the needle is to
be applied. As soon as the [guard] qi are dispersed, one inserts the needle. The
reason is that otherwise one might harm the guard qi.

Yu Shu: The three yin and the three yang [conduits] are all responsible for [the
passage of] qi and blood. It is just that the amounts [of these two compo-
nents contained in the individual conduits] are different. Hence, when the sages
outlined the principles of applying the needles, they saw to it that neither the
camp nor the guard [qi] received any harm. The treatise "Xue qi xing zhi" 血氣
星志[1] states: "The major yang [conduits] regulary [contain] much blood, few
qi; the minor yang [conduits] regulary [contain] a little blood and much qi;
the yang brilliance [conduits] regulary [contain] much qi and much blood; the

---

[1]   *Su wen* treatise 24.

ceasing yin [conduits] regulary [contain] much blood and little qi; the minor yin [conduits] regulary [contain] much qi and a little blood; the major yin [conduits] regulary [contain] much qi and little blood." Qixuan zi 啓玄子² noted in his commentary: "The amounts of blood and qi reflect the regular numerical conditions of heaven. Hence the principles of needling generally require the draining of what is present in large amounts."

(1) *Xu Dachun*: The guard [qi] are responsible for the blood; they [are located] in the interior [sections of the organism]. The guard [qi] generate the qi that proceed through the exterior [sections of the organism]. If a disease is present in the [region of the] camp qi or the guard qi, one should always hit its exact location; one must not reach beyond [the proper target]. The meaning expressed here is that of the [treatise] "Ci qi lun" 刺齊論 of the *Su* [*wen*]: "When piercing the bones do not harm the sinews; when piercing the sinews do not harm the flesh; when piercing the flesh do not harm the vessels; when piercing the vessels do not harm the skin; when piercing the skin do not harm the flesh; when piercing the flesh do not harm the sinews; when piercing the sinews do not harm the bones."

(3) *Xu Dachun*: The yin [qi] are the camp [qi]. The camp [qi proceed] in the depth. When inserting a needle, one must cross through the [region of the] guard [qi] to reach the camp [qi]. However, the guard [qi] belong to the qi. One can cause them to disperse. Hence one presses the [respective hole to be needled with one's finger], causing the guard qi gradually to leave this place. Then, if one inserts the needle straight down to the camp [qi], he will not harm the guard [qi].

(1)–(4) *Xu Dachun*: The method of applying a lying needle corresponds to the method of superficial piercing mentioned in the treatise "Guan zhen" 官鍼 of the *Ling* [*shu*]. To disperse the qi through pressure corresponds to the method of "squeeze and disperse, push and press" outlined in the *Su* [*wen* treatise] "Li he zhen xie lun" 離合眞邪論. However, the meaning implied in the [*Nei*] *jing* is different in both cases [from the meaning expressed in the *Nan jing*]. Here, these [methods] are employed as principles for the piercing of yin and yang [qi], respectively. This meaning is simple but appropriate and can serve as a guideline.

(1) *Liao Ping*: The [*Nei*] *jing* has no such statement. In the [*Nei*] *jing*, the camp [qi] rule the vessels while the guard [qi] rule the network. The network is the section of the flesh. The [*Nei*] *jing* employs the method of fivefold diagnosis;³ here the five terms – skin, flesh, vessels, muscles, and bones – are transformed into but the

---

2   *Hao* name of Wang Bing 王冰.

3   The term *wu zhen* 五診 ("fivefold diagnosis") appears in *Su wen* treatise 80, "Fang sheng shuai lun" 方盛衰論. It is not clear, though, whether Liao Ping had in mind the meaning implied there when he used the term here.

two words "camp [qi]" and "guard [qi]." That is a great mistake! The [*Nei*] *jing* offers a clear account; Xu [Dachun's argument] is muddled.

(4) *Liao Ping*: The [*Nei*] *jing* has no such words. How can [the *Nan jing*] say: "That is [what is] meant."

(1)–(4) *Katō Bankei*: The *Ling shu* states: "There are three different [approaches employed in] needling. These include the piercing of the camp [qi; the piercing] of the guard [qi, and the piercing] of cold *pi* 痹 which has settled down in the conduits." The [text] states: "The piercing of the camp [qi] causes an outflow of blood; the piercing of the guard [qi] causes an outflow of qi."[4] Also, the *Su wen* states: „When piercing the skin do not harm the flesh; when piercing the flesh do not harm the sinews; when piercing the sinews do not harm the bones. When piercing the bones do not harm the sinews; when piercing the sinews do not harm the flesh; when piercing the flesh do not harm the vessels; when piercing the vessels do not harm the skin." From these texts one may conclude that "no harm" refers to the outflow of blood when the camp [qi are pierced], and to the outflow of qi when the guard [qi are pierced]. "Harm" means that qi flow out when the camp [qi are pierced] and that blood flows out when the guard [qi are pierced]. When piercing the camp [qi], one aims at the blood. Hence one presses, with the left hand, the transportation [hole] to be needled and lets the guard qi disperse before he inserts the needle. In this way, the qi moving at the surface will not be disturbed. That is a piercing of camp [qi] without harming the guard [qi]. When piercing the guard [qi], one aims at the qi. Hence one brings the needle into an oblique position before inserting it. In this way, one avoids too deep a penetration. That is a piercing of guard [qi] without harming the camp [qi]. The *Ling shu* refers to these [approaches] solely on the basis of the fact that the qi and the blood move near the surface and in the depth, respectively. The present paragraph offers a straightforward outline of the patterns of needling [involved here]. In fact, both [texts] serve to explain each other.

---

4   See *Ling shu* treatise 6, "Shou yao gang rou" 壽夭剛柔..

七十二難曰：（一）經言能知迎隨之氣，可令調之；調氣之方，必在陰陽，何謂也？

（二）然：所謂迎隨者，知榮衛之流行，經脈之往來也。（三）隨其逆順而取之，故曰迎隨。（四）調氣之方，必在陰陽者，知其內外表裏，隨其陰陽而調之，故曰調氣之方，必在陰陽。

The seventy-second difficult issue: (1) The scripture states: If one is able to recognize whether the qi move against or follow [their proper course], he will be in a position to restore their harmony. The pattern of restoring harmony among the qi must be tied to yin and yang. What does that mean?

(2) It is like this. When [the scripture] speaks of "moving against or following," [that implies] an understanding of the course the camp and guard [qi] have taken, and of the coming and going [of the qi] in the conduit vessels. (3) The [qi] have to be removed following their moving contrary to or in accordance with [their proper course]. Hence [the scripture] speaks of "moving against or following." (4) As for [the statement] "the pattern of restoring harmony among the qi must be tied to yin and yang," [that implies] that harmony among the [qi] is to be restored only after one has understood whether [a disease] is located in the inner or outer, or in the interior or exterior [regions of the body] – that is, whether [it is located] in a yin or yang [region].[1]

COMMENTARIES

(1)–(4) *Ding Deyong*: The camp and the guard [qi] penetrate [the entire body] by flowing through all the twelve conduits. This [flow] has start and end. Starting

---

1 The question in sentence 1 quotes a passage from *Ling shu* treatise 9, "Zhong shi" 終始. However, the first half of the version given here differs from the original in the *Ling shu* both in its wording and – I assume – in its meaning. The *Ling shu* statement reads *zhi ying zhi sui qi ke ling he* 知迎知隨氣可令和, ("if one knows about moving against and following, one will be able to cause harmony among the qi"). In a statement immediately preceding this one, the *Ling shu* mentions the two needling techniques that have to be applied if one intends to drain or supplement qi: "To drain [qi] one moves [the needle] against them; to supplement [qi] one follows them." The *Nan jing* redefines the terms *ying* ("to move against") and *sui* ("to follow") by equating them with the terms *ni* ("to move contrary to a proper course") and *shun* ("to move in accordance with a proper course"). That is to say, in the *Nei jing*, "moving against" and "following" refer to the movement of the needle (for details, see the commentaries by Ding Deyong and Zhang Shixian), while in the *Nan jing*, these terms refer to the movement of the qi. As is typical of the *Nan jing*, it does not state openly that it reinterprets the old terms; rather, it presents them in a new conceptual context, which it claims to be that of the "scripture" (i.e., the *Nei jing*).

from the Central Burner, [the qi] flow into the hand major yin conduit and network [vessel]. Then they flow into the hand yang brilliance conduit and network [vessel]. There are twenty-four such conduits and network [vessels] and each day has twenty-four hours. They are all matched with each other. If one removes the qi with a needle as long as they are still in the starting period of their arrival [in a specific conduit], that is called "to withdraw [qi] by moving against them."[2] If one inserts the needle while the qi end their flow [through a specific conduit], then pulls [the needle] out and [closes] the hole by laying a finger on it, that is called "to add [qi] by following them." Furthermore, to supplement a [particular conduit's] mother is also called "to supplement [qi] by following them," and to drain a [particular conduit's child] is also called "to withdraw [qi] by moving against them." Furthermore, if one withdraws or inserts the needle in accordance with [the patient's] exhalation and inhalation, this too is called "moving against" or "following." These are the patterns of restoring harmony among yin and yang. Hence [the text] says: "They must be tied to yin and yang."

Yang: The camp qi proceed along their regular course without ever coming to a stop. The guard qi proceed through the body during the daytime; they proceed through the long-term depots and short-term repositories during the nighttime. *Ying* 迎 ("to move against") stands for *ni* 逆 ("to move contrary to a proper course"); *sui* 隨 ("to follow") stands for *shun* 順 ("to move in accordance with a proper course"). That is to say, the guard qi move contrary to the proper course; the camp qi move in accordance with the proper course. When a disease is located in the yang [section], one must observe [the moment] when the camp qi and the guard qi arrive in the yang section and then pierce it. When a disease is located in the yin [section], one must observe [the moment] when the camp qi and the guard qi arrive in the yin section and then pierce it. That is the meaning of "moving against" and "following." Furthermore, *ying* ("to move against") stands for *xie* 瀉 ("to drain"); *sui* ("to follow") stands for *bu* 補 ("to supplement"). Hence the scripture states: "In withdrawing [qi] by moving against them, how can one avoid creating a depletion."[3] This means that draining leads to depletion. [And it states further:] "In adding [qi] by following them, how can one avoid creating a repletion?" This means that supplementing leads to repletion. [The statement] "the pattern to restore harmony among the qi must be tied to yin and yang" [means the following]. In the case of a yin depletion and a yang repletion, supplement the yin and drain the yang. In the case of a yang depletion and a yin repletion, supplement the yang and drain the yin. There may be cases where

---

2   See difficult issue 79.

3   See difficult issue 79.

the yang [qi] have joined the yin [qi], or where the yin [qi] have joined the yang [qi]. Or both yin and yang [qi] may be depleted, or both may be replete. In all cases one must restore harmony among the yin and the yang [qi] in accordance with the course the disease takes. In this way, no disease will remain uncured.

(4) *Yu Shu*: "The pattern of restoring harmony among the qi must be tied to yin and yang" means that from the external [condition, one seeks to] understand the internal [condition]; from the internal [condition, one seeks to] understand the external [condition].[4] This means that at the time of crescent moon, do not drain; at the time of full moon, do not supplement. [When needling] determine the [respective] person's [rhythm of] inhalation and exhalation, and take into consideration whether the day is cold or warm. From the yang pull the yin; from the yin pull the yang.[5] In spring and summer reach all yin; in autumn and winter reach all yang.[6] Hence [the text] states: "The pattern of restoring harmony among the qi must be tied to yin and yang." "To understand whether [a disease] is located in the inner or outer, or in the interior or exterior [regions of the body]" means that one must examine whether the [movement in the] vessels is at the surface or in the depth, and one must recognize whether a disease consists of a depletion or of a repletion. From the external [condition], one must understand the internal [condition]; one looks at the exterior [appearance] and compares it with the interior [condition]. Hence [the text] states: "[After] one has understood whether a [disease] is located in the inner or outer, or in the interior or exterior [regions of the body]." "Harmony is to be restored [only after one has understood] whether [a disease is located] in a yin or yang [region]" means that the harmonizing treatment must be applied in accordance with the yin or yang [categorization of the] vessels in which the disease is located.

Li Jiong: *Ying* ("to move against") stands for *ni* ("to move contrary to a proper course") and for *qu* 取 ("to remove"). *Sui* ("to follow") stands for *shun* ("to move in accordance with a proper course") and for *bu* 補 ("to supplement").

(4) *Hua Shou*: "Inner" is yin; "outer" is yang; "exterior" is yang; "interior" is yin. [That is to say] one examines whether the disease is in a yin or in a yang [section] and harmonizes accordingly. Mr. Xie has stated: "Males are 'outer'; females are 'inner'; 'exterior' is yang; 'interior' is yin."

(1)–(4) *Zhang Shixian*: The three yang [conduits] of the hands and feet proceed from the hands to the head and from the head to the feet, respectively. The three yin [conduits] of the hands and feet proceed from the feet to the chest and from the

---

4   I read *yin* 引 here as *yin* 因, and *zhi* 至 as *zhi* 知.
5   See difficult issue 67.
6   See difficult issue 70.

chest to the hands. These are the fixed patterns of the coming and going of the
conduit vessels. Whenever one wishes to drain, the point of the needle should
face the location from which the conduit vessel comes; [upon insertion of the
needle] one moves against the direction from which the qi [come]. As soon as
the qi come - but before they are present in abundance – one moves the needle
contrary to their flow in order to withdraw them. That is called *ying* ("to move
against"). Whenever one wishes to supplement, the point of the needle should
face the direction in which the conduit vessels are leaving; [upon inserting the
needle] one follows the direction the qi will take. When the qi move away – but
before there is a depletion – one moves the needle in accordance with their flow
in order to add [qi] to them. That is called *sui* ("to follow"). Whether one applies
a [draining treatment by] "moving against" or a [supplementing treatment by]
"following" should depend on the kind of harmonization of qi intended. The
restoration of harmony among the qi must be based on an awareness of whether
the disease is located in a yin or in a yang [region]. One applies the [approaches
of] "moving against" or "following" – that is, the [treatments of] supplementing
or draining – in accordance with the prevailing conditions of depletion or repletion in a yin or yang [region]. In this way, one can restore harmony among the
qi. The inner and the interior [sections] are yin; the outer and the exterior are
yang. The inner has an exterior and an interior; the outer, too, has an exterior and
an interior. The ancient people had a saying: "The exterior of the exterior; the
interior of the interior."[7] That is exactly the meaning implied here. In the case
of a depletion of yang and a repletion of yin [qi], drain the yin and supplement
the yang; in the case of a repletion of yang and a depletion of yin, drain the yang
and supplement the yin. That is [what is meant by] "harmony is to be restored
[only after one has understood] whether [a disease is located in] a yin or yang
[region]."

(1) *Xu Dachun*: The treatise "Zhong shi" 終始 of the *Ling* [*shu*] states: "The yang
[conduits] receive their qi from the four limbs; the yin [conduits] receive their qi
from the five long-term depots. Hence one drains them by moving against, one
supplements them by following [their respective courses]. If one knows about
moving against and following, one will be able to cause harmony among the qi.
The pattern of harmonizing the qi must be based on an understanding of [the
patterns of] yin and yang." This passage of the [*Nei*] *jing* was quoted here [in
the *Nan jing*] as the basis [of the present difficult issue]. Now, the yang conduits

7   Possibly a reference to *Su wen* treatise 4, "Jin kui zhen yan lun" 金匱眞言論, which explains the fourfold subcategorization of yin and yang into yang-in-yin and yin-in-yin
and yin-in-yang and yang-in-yin.

rule the outer [sections of the body]; hence they originate from the four limbs. The yin conduits rule the inner [sections of the body]; hence they originate from the five long-term depots. "To move against" means that [during insertion] the point of the needle moves against this place [of origin of the qi in the conduits]; in this way, one withdraws [qi]. Hence this is called "draining." "To follow" means that [during insertion] the point of the needle follows the [qi in the direction they take to] move away; in this way, one adds [qi]. Hence this is called "supplementing." "An understanding of [whether a disease is located in a] yin or yang [region]" means that one must examine whether the yin or the yang [conduits] suffer from depletion or repletion; one must not make any mistakes in applying [a treatment of] supplementing or draining. For details, see difficult issue 79.

(2) *Katō Bankei*: "To move against" and "to follow" are the techniques of supplementing and draining. However, they do not consist of only one pattern. "The course of the camp and guard [qi], and the coming and going [of the qi] in the conduit vessels" [refers to the following]. The camp [qi] proceed inside the vessels; they complete fifty passages during day and night;[8] their flow is determined by the passage of time and by the frequency of breathing. The guard [qi] proceed through all the yang [regions] during the daytime; they proceed through all the yin [regions] during the nighttime. That is "the course of the camp and guard [qi]." The three hand yang [conduits proceed] from the hands to the head; the three foot yang [conduits proceed] from the head to the feet; the three hand yin [conduits proceed] from the chest to the hands; the three foot yin [conduits proceed] from the feet to the abdomen. That is the "coming and going of the [qi in the] conduit vessels." Hua [Shou] commented that these two expressions [i.e., the course of the camp and guard qi, and the coming and going of the qi in the conduit vessels] have one meaning. That was an unsophisticated [opinion].

---

8   See difficult issue 1.

七十三難曰：（一）諸井者，肌肉淺薄，氣少，不足使也，刺之奈何？
（二）然：諸井者，木也；滎者，火也。火者，木之子，當刺井者，以滎瀉
之。（三）故經言補者不可以為瀉，瀉者不可以為補，此之謂也。

The seventy-third difficult issue: (1) All wells [are located where] the flesh is shallow
and thin, and where the qi are too few to be employed [for any treatment]. How
does one proceed if one has to pierce them?

(2) It is like this. All wells are [associated with] wood. All creeks are [associated
with] fire. Fire is the child of wood. Thus, when one has to pierce the wells, one
should drain them through the creeks. (3) Hence the scripture states: [The loca-
tions] where one supplements [the conduits with qi] cannot be used to drain [qi],
and [the locations] where one drains [qi] cannot be used to supplement [the con-
duits]. That is [what is] meant here.[1]

COMMENTARIES

(1)–(3) *Ding Deyong*: All wells are located at the tips of fingers and toes. Hence [the
text] states: "The flesh is shallow and thin." The wells are [associated with] wood,
which is the mother of fire. The creeks are [associated with] fire, which is the
child of wood. Hence in the case of a repletion of [qi of the phase of] wood in
the liver, one drains the respective creek; in the case of a depletion of the qi of
the [phase of] wood in the liver, one supplements at the respective confluence.
Where one has drained one cannot supplement again. Hence [the text] states:
"[The locations where one drains qi] cannot be used to supplement [the con-
duits]."

---

1   By referring in sentence 3 to a statement that has no counterpart in the *Nei jing*, this
    difficult issue continues the argument of the preceding issue – namely, the rejection
    of the idea that one can drain or supplement at the same hole. The idea of draining or
    supplementing a conduit at one and the same hole by merely pointing the needle in
    different directions is based on a mechanical understanding both of the flow of qi in the
    vessels and of the nature of repletion and depletion. With his emphasis on the doctrines
    of systematic correspondence, the author of the *Nan jing* could not accept such obviously
    archaic mechanical thinking. As several commentators have noted, the present difficult
    issue introduces a new consequence of the doctrine of the Five Phases. Since each hole
    on the conduits corresponds to one of the Five Phases, treatments of draining and sup-
    plementing at the individual holes on a single conduit must have effects that can be
    explained within the conceptual framework of systematic correspondence. The example
    offered here refers to the mutual generation sequence of the Five Phases.

Yang: In winter pierce the wells.² If a disease is present in the long-term depots, one should remove it from the wells. In such a situation, where one should pierce the wells, one [in fact] drains through the respective creek in order to eliminate the disease. Hence the scripture states: "In winter the [movement of the] yin qi is tight, and the [movement of the] yang qi is subdued. Hence one selects a 'well' in order to suppress the yin qi moving contrary to their proper course, and one selects a 'creek' in order to let the yang qi pass."³

(2) *Li Jiong*: [Consider a situation where] the wood of the liver is replete. In the case of repletion one drains the respective child. Creeks are [associated with] fire, [and fire] is the child of wood. Hence one should drain at the [creeks]. In spring one pierces at the creeks if the fire has stolen the rule from the wood, although the [period of] rule by the wood had not yet come to an end. According to the pattern, this is a repletion evil. Hence one drains the creeks. In case the liver suffers from a disease of repletion that has arisen in itself, one selects the fire [hole on the conduit associated with the] liver in order to drain there. In the case of a depletion one selects the wood [hole on the conduit associated with the] liver in order to supplement there.

(1)–(3) *Zhang Shixian*: The wells represent the wood, [and the wood] is the mother of the fire. The creeks represent the fire, which is the child of wood. Consider a repletion in the kidneys. In this case one should drain the wood of the wells. But the wood of the wells is located at the tips of fingers and toes where the flesh is shallow and thin and where there are so little blood and so few qi that they do not suffice for the application of a treatment. Thus, one drains the fire in order to effect a change. If one drains the child, a depletion will result in the mother. Also, even though one does not drain qi [from the wood directly], there will still be a depletion [in the liver]. If one spares the creek and pierces the rapids, a depletion of the soil will result so that the water is no longer under control; the evil [qi] in the kidneys will increase further. If one pierces the stream, the metal will generate water and, contrary [to the intention of the treatment], the kidneys will be [even more] replete. Hence one does not pierce there either. The wells

---

2　See difficult issues 70 and 74. The wells are associated with spring; spring is the child of winter. Hence, in case of an illness, one should drain not the confluence itself (which is associated with winter) but its child (i.e., the well). However, because of the lack of sufficient qi there, one must move one step further and drain the creek instead.

3　*Su wen* treatise 61, "Shui re xue lun" 水熱穴論, has a statement worded such that it roughly corresponds to the statement quoted here: "In winter, the yang qi are weak and few, while the yin qi are tight and abundant. The major yang conduit is subdued and deep, the yang [movement in the] vessels is gone. Hence one selects a well in order to suppress the yin qi moving contrary to their proper course, and one selects a creek in order to replenish the yang qi."

can only be drained through the creeks. Hence the [*Nan*] *jing* states: "[The lo-
cations] where one supplements [the conduits with qi] cannot be used to drain
[qi], and [the locations] where one drains [qi] cannot be used to supplement
[the conduits]." That is exactly what is meant here.

(2) *Xu Dachun*: This is the pattern of draining a child. [Accordingly,] a supplementing [treatment] should be applied at the respective confluence. However, these
[instructions] apply only to the well holes because the qi there are too few; they
are insufficient to carry out a supplementing or a draining. If one drains the
child or supplements the mother, the qi [at the well] will respond automatically.
The sixty-ninth difficult issue distinguishes among separate conduits as child
and mother. The present [difficult issue] distinguishes [among different holes
on] a single conduit as child and mother. The meaning is different but the principle is quite subtle.

(3) *Xu Dachun*: Above the word "hence," some text appears to be missing which
must have discussed the pattern of supplementing the mother. With these two
sentences, [both the pattern of draining the child and the pattern of supplementing the mother] could have been summarized [adequately] here. Otherwise, the structure of the text remains incomplete. A further comment: These
statements cannot be checked against any doctrine in the scriptures [because
neither the *Su wen* nor the *Ling shu* contain any corresponding passage].

(1) *Liao Ping*: The [*Nei*] *jing* takes [a patient's] symptoms [as its guideline] and distinguishes among [separate] conduits where [treatments of] supplementing or
draining are to be applied. Only rarely does it [recommend] the piercing of the
fingertips. The present [difficult issue] follows the [doctrine of the] Five Phases.
Hence it includes the wells among the gates to be pierced.

(2) *Liao Ping*: It is quite possible to discuss such [associations] with regard to the
four seasons. But it is impossible to divide the flow of the qi within a single
vessel into five separate entities! These are instructions [that have been created
by the author of the *Nan jing*] at will; they do not differ from the false patterns
employed in geomancy. How can one say that the long-term depots and the
short-term repositories correspond to [treatments such as advocated here]?! A
single vessel has turned here into a complicated affair! [The *Nan jing*] has established numerous false doctrines which cannot but cause everyone to laugh
who knows [the truth]; the [claim that one can] diagnose the [condition of the]
twelve conduits, the long-term depots, and the short-term repositories at [a
location of only] two inches [is one of these false doctrines].

(1)–(3) *Katō Bankei*: The [treatise] "Ci yao lun" 刺瘧論 states: "[Pierce also] the well
holes of all the yin [conduits]. Do not cause blood to leave." For this reason, the

present paragraph warns against the piercing of the wells. All the so-called wells are located at the edges of the fingernails and toenails. These places are quite void of any liquid. Similarly, the flow in the vessels [there] bubbles weakly and only a few [qi] are sent down [the stream of the conduits from there]. Hence, if one plans to supplement there, no objection exists at all. But if one plans to drain there, this is definitely prohibited. Hence [the text] states: "The qi are too few to be employed [for any draining]." Hua [Shou] states, in his comment, that they are too few to be employed for any supplementing or draining. However, the discussion in this [paragraph] focuses on the piercing of the wells; it prohibits only the draining but not the supplementing [of the wells]. Hence the original text states quite clearly that if one has to pierce the wells for draining, one uses the creeks. All it elucidates is the method of substituting the creeks for the wells when the latter have to be drained. As far as supplementing is concerned, why should that be prohibited?

七十四難曰：（一）經言春刺井，夏刺滎，季夏刺俞，秋刺經，冬刺合者，何謂也？

（二）然：春刺井者，邪在肝；夏刺滎者，邪在心；季夏刺俞者，邪在脾；秋刺經者，邪在肺；冬刺合者，邪在腎。

（三）其肝、心、脾、肺、腎而繫於春、夏、秋、冬者，何也？

（四）然：五藏一病，輒有五也。假令肝病，色青者肝也，臊臭者肝也，喜酸者肝也，喜呼者肝也，喜泣者肝也。（五）其病眾多，不可盡言也。（六）四時有數，而並繫於春夏秋冬者也。（七）鍼之要妙，在於秋毫者。

The seventy-fourth difficult issue: (1) The scripture states: In spring pierce the wells; in summer pierce the creeks; in late summer pierce the rapids; in autumn pierce the streams; in winter pierce the confluences. What does that mean?

(2) It is like this. In spring one pierces the wells [only if] evil [qi] reside in the liver. In summer one pierces the creeks [only if] evil [qi] reside in the heart. In late summer one pierces the rapids [only if] evil [qi] reside in the spleen. In autumn one pierces the streams [only if] evil [qi] reside in the lung. In winter one pierces the confluences [only if] evil [qi] reside in the kidneys.

(3) How is it that the liver, the heart, the spleen, the lung, and the kidneys are attached to spring, summer, autumn, and winter?

(4) It is like this. Each single disease in any of the five long-term depots may, [in turn, be the result of] five [diseases]. Take for example a disease in the liver. A virid complexion [indicates that the disease originated in the liver and is still located in] the liver. A fetid odor [indicates that the disease originated in the heart and is now located in] the liver. A preference for sour flavor [indicates that the disease originated in the spleen and is now located in] the liver. A tendency to shout [indicates that the disease originated in the lung and is now located in] the liver. A tendency to weep [indicates that the disease originated in the kidneys and is now located in] the liver.

(5) [If one takes origin and transmission in the organism into account,] there are very many diseases; they cannot be outlined exhaustively here. (6) [However,] the four seasons have a [fixed] number and all [the diseases] are attached [through their associations with the Five Phases] to the four seasons [and to the respective holes

on the conduits]. (7) The principles of needling are quite sophisticated; they are [as fine as] autumn down.[1]

(1)–(2) *Ding Deyong*: When [the scripture] states: "In spring pierce the wells," this means that if [during that period] evil [qi] are present in the liver, one should not allow these evil [qi] of the wood of the liver to cause harm to the soil of the spleen. Hence one pierces them at the wells. "In summer pierce the creeks" means that if [during that period] evil [qi] are present in the heart, one should not allow these evil [qi] of the fire of the heart to cause harm to the metal of the lung. Hence one pierces them at the creeks. "In late summer pierce the rapids" means that if [during that period] evil [qi] are present in the spleen, one should not allow these evil [qi] of the soil of the spleen to cause harm to the water of the kidneys. Hence one pierces them at the rapids. "In autumn pierce the streams" means that if [during that period] evil [qi] are present in the lung, one should not allow these evil [qi] of the metal of the lung to harm the wood of the liver. Hence one pierces them at the streams. "In winter pierce the confluences" means that if [during that period] evil [qi] are present in the kidneys, one should not allow these evil [qi] of the water of the kidneys to harm the fire of the heart. Hence one pierces them at the confluences. That is the pattern of how to cut off the sources of the five evil [qi].

Yang: The application of the needles [in therapy] is extremely complicated; [it is governed by] innumerable patterns. If one does not fully understand how to modify and adapt [these patterns to the individual circumstances of a disease], it will be difficult to save a patient. The present [difficult issue] conveys the idea of adaptation through modification. The [*Nei*] *jing* states: "In winter pierce the

---

1 Some Chinese commentators of past centuries have claimed that the text of the present difficult issue is corrupt; others have regarded it as highly esoteric. My attitude is that of Hua Shou, who stated that we have to interpret what we have in hand. Sentence 2 appears to relativize the rather mechanistic pattern outlined in the question. Therefore I have added the "only if." My interpretation of sentence 3 follows the concepts outlined in difficult issues 49 and 50. One might speculate that, originally, the text was worded differently – namely, *jia ling gan bing se qing zhe gan ye sao chou zhe xin ye xi suan zhe pi ye xi hu zhe fei ye xi qi zhe shen ye* 假令肝病色青者肝也臊臭者心也喜酸者脾也喜呼者肺也喜泣者腎也. This translates as "Take for example a disease in the liver. A virid complexion [indicates that the disease originated in] the liver. A fetid odor [indicates that the disease originated in] the heart. A tendency for sour [flavor indicates that the disease originated in] the spleen, [and so forth]." In sentence 6, one might wonder whether the character *bing* 並 ("all") is not a mistake for *bing* 病 ("illness"). In the latter case, the meaning would remain virtually the same as in my rendering, but the structure of the Chinese sentence would be more elegant, and in the translation one bracket would be unnecessary.

wells, in spring pierce the creeks." Here it is stated: "In spring pierce the wells, in summer pierce the creeks." The underlying principles are highly refined and noteworthy. One should pay special attention to [all of] them. One must not stick to just one pattern as if it included all [there is to needling].

(1) *Xu Dachun*: [No passage corresponding to] these five statements can be found in the text of the [*Nei*] *jing*.

(2) *Xu Dachun*: This is yet another discussion of the associations of the five long-term depots. The wells and spring are both associated with wood. The creeks and summer are both associated with fire. The rapids and autumn are both associated with metal. The confluences and winter are both associated with water. Hence if one has a disease, the qi in the long-term depots will act in accordance with the [currently prevailing season of the] four seasons. Hence the pattern of needling must correspond to the [course of the] seasons too .... The treatise "Shun qi yi ri fen wei si shi" 順氣一日分爲四時 of the *Ling* [*shu*] states: "The long-term depots are controlled by winter. In winter one pierces the well [openings]. The colors are controlled by spring. In spring one pierces the creek [openings]. The time periods [of severity and weakness of diseases] are controlled by summer. In summer one pierces the transport [openings]. The [musical] tones/voices are controlled by late summer. In late summer one pierces the stream [openings]. The flavors are controlled by autumn. In autumn one pierces the confluence [openings]." In comparison with what is said here [in the *Nan jing*, the associations of the seasons with the holes on the conduits as listed in the *Nei jing* are] shifted by one hole. The treatise "Ben shu" 本輸 [of the *Ling shu*] states: "In spring select the network vessels and the creeks; they are situated between the major conduits and the flesh. In summer select the rapids and the secondary network [vessels]; they are located on the skin. In autumn select the confluences. In winter select the wells and the rapids." In the treatise "Si shi [qi]" 四時氣 [also of the *Ling shu*], it is stated:[2] "In spring [diseases] are removed from the conduits, the blood vessels and the partings in the flesh. In summer one chooses [for therapy] those conduits, tertiary vessels and network [vessels] that abound [with qi]. One chooses the partings and opens the skin. In autumn one chooses [for therapy] the conduit transport [openings]. When the evil [qi] are in the short-term repositories, they are to be removed from the [conduit] confluence [openings]. In winter one chooses [for therapy] the well and creek [openings]. It is essential to pierce into the depth, and to let [the needle] remain inserted for

---

2   Here I have followed the original text of the *Ling shu*; the version of this "Si shi qi" 四時
氣 quotation given in the *Xu Dachun* edition at my disposal appears to be quite corrupt.

a while." All these [passages] differ from [what is said] here. I do not know on what source Yueren has based his remarks.

(3)–(7) *Ding Deyong*: Man's five long-term depots are attached to the four seasons. Each single disease in any of the five long-term depots may be [reflected by any of the] five [different indicators]. That is to say, by the five sounds [displayed by the patient's voice], by the five colors [displayed in his face], by the five flavors [the patient longs for], by the five liquids [his body emits], and by the five odors [his body produces]. One can cut off the [course of the] five evil [qi through the organism] by hitting the source of the disease with a needle. Hence one knows that the principles of needling are quite sophisticated; they are [as fine as] autumn down. One must fully comprehend them [if one intends to apply this kind of therapy].

Yang: Any disease in the five long-term depots or six short-term repositories has its physical manifestation. Here the one long-term depot of the liver has been chosen as an example to elucidate the [entire] pattern. [The text] states: "In spring pierce the wells; in summer pierce the creeks." But if a specific long-term depot has a disease, the [necessary treatment at its] vessel must change in accordance [with the character of that particular disease]. One should examine [the situation] and then select [the appropriate hole for treatment]. Take for example a disease [that has arisen] in the liver itself. In case it is a repletion, one selects the [hole associated with] fire on the [conduit associated with the] liver and drains there. If it is a depletion, one selects the [hole associated with] wood on the [conduit associated with the] liver and supplements there. All remaining [possibilities] can be inferred from this. "Extremely fine like autumn down" means that the [pattern underlying the] use of needles is extremely fine, like autumn down.

Hua Shou: The diseases of the five long-term depots are not limited to five. The diseases of the [long-term depots] are very many. Although they are very many, they are [still classified according to] the number of the four seasons. Hence the diseases are attached to spring, summer, autumn, and winter, [and through this association] links are established with the wells, creeks, rapids, streams, and confluences. Whenever one [intends to] apply the needles, he must carefully examine [these correspondences]. A close look at the meaning of the text of this paragraph shows that something must have been mistakenly omitted. Nevertheless, an interpretation must be based on what is left until we know [more about the original extent of this text].

Zhang Shixian: The wells are [associated with the phase of] wood. Spring rules the wood of the liver; it corresponds to the wells. When the wood of the liver is affected by evil [qi], one may control them through the wells. In spring one pierces the wells in order to eliminate evil [qi] from the liver, lest the wood overpower the soil. The creeks are [associated with the phase of] fire. Summer rules the fire of the heart; it corresponds to the creeks. When the fire of the heart is affected by evil [qi], one may control them through the creeks. In summer one pierces the creeks in order to eliminate evil [qi] from the heart, lest the fire overpower the metal. The rapids are [associated with the phase of] soil. Late summer rules the soil of the spleen; it corresponds to the rapids. When the soil of the spleen is affected by evil [qi], one may control them through the rapids. In late summer one pierces the rapids in order to eliminate evil [qi] from the spleen, lest the soil overpower the water. The streams are [associated with the phase of] metal. Autumn rules the metal of the lung; it corresponds to the streams. When the metal of the lung is affected by evil [qi], one may control them through the streams. In autumn one pierces the streams in order to eliminate evil [qi] from the lung, lest the metal overpower the wood. The confluences are [associated with the phase of] water. Winter rules the water of the kidneys; it corresponds to the confluences. When the water of the kidneys is affected by evil [qi], one may control them through the confluences. In winter one pierces the confluences in order to eliminate evil [qi] from the kidneys, lest the water overpower the fire. The five long-term depots are attached to the four seasons. When a long-term depot has a disease, that will become apparent through the five [indicators], as are the sounds, the colors, the odors, the flavor [preferences], and the liquids. "There are very many diseases" means that one cannot enumerate them all. The four seasons have a fixed number, and the well, creek, rapids, stream, and confluence holes are all attached to spring, summer, autumn, and winter. Hence, in spring one does not only pierce the wells; in summer one does not only pierce the creeks; in late summer one does not only pierce the rapids; in autumn one does not only pierce the streams; and in winter one does not only pierce the confluences.

(6) *Xu Dachun*: That is to say, although the diseases may appear in ten thousand variations, there is, nevertheless, a fixed number of treatment patterns corresponding to the four seasons. The entirety [of all diseases] remains within this [frame]. The underlying principle is simple and concise and easily applicable.

(3)–(7) *Xu Dachun*: The question asks how the diseases of the five long-term depots correspond to the four seasons. The explanation should focus on the principles of mutual correspondences [between diseases and seasons]. The answer, however, merely outlines disease symptoms. It does not respond to the question at all. It is really meaningless.

(1)–(7) *Ding Jin*: When this chapter states that in spring, summer, autumn, and win-ter one pierces the wells, creeks, rapids, streams, and confluences [respectively], that does not mean that one must pierce the wells in spring [etc.]. If the evil is in the liver, one pierces the well [of its conduit]. The wells are associated with wood and spring. Hence [the text] states: "In spring pierce the wells." The same applies to the remaining long-term depots. Then there is the question why liver, heart, lung, and kidneys are attached to spring, summer, autumn, and winter. [Here the *Nan jing*] once more refers to the virid [complexion], the fetid [odor], the [preference for] sour [flavor], the [tendency to] shout, and the [tendency to] weep in order to point out that there may be very many diseases in the five long-term depots and six short-term repositories, and that all of them alike are associated with [the Five Phases, i.e., with] metal, wood, water, fire, and soil. Just as the four seasons have their [fixed] number, all [diseases] are attached to either spring, summer, autumn, or winter.

(3)–(7) *Ye Lin*: This [section] once again raises the question of why the liver, heart, spleen, lung, and kidneys are attached to spring, summer, autumn, and winter. Now, any disease in the five long-term depots may be caused by one of five evil [qi]. That must not be overlooked! Take, for instance, a disease in the liver. A virid color [indicates that] the liver [has been affected directly from outside], because the liver is responsible for the colors. A fetid odor [also indicates that] the liver [has been affected, but in this case the patient has been] hit [primarily] by a disease in the heart, because the heart is responsible for the odors. [If odor qi emitted by the heart] enter the liver, they become fetid. If someone prefers sour [flavor, that indicates that] the liver [has been affected, but in this case the patient has been] hit [primarily] by a disease in the spleen, because the spleen is responsible for the flavors. [If flavor qi emitted by the spleen] enter the liver, they become sour. A tendency to shout [indicates that] the liver [has been af-fected, but the patient has been] hit [primarily] by a disease in the lung, because the lung is responsible for the sounds. [If sound qi from the lung] enter the liver, they become shouts. A tendency to weep [indicates that] the liver [has been affected, but the patient has been] hit [primarily] by a disease in the kidneys, be-cause the kidneys are responsible for the liquids. [If liquid qi from the kidneys] enter the liver, they become tears. The liver long-term depot was chosen here as only one example; the [conditions of all the] others can be inferred from it.

Huang Weisan: This difficult issue elucidates the *Nei jing* concept of piercing the five transportation [holes] in accordance with the four seasons; it points out that one should take advantage of the therapeutic pattern of the five transportation [holes]. Now, through the five transportation [holes] one may regulate the diseases as they manifest themselves in the systems of the five long-term depots. That has been stated earlier. However, the [disease] manifestations that belong to the systems of the five long-term depots are very many; they cannot be enumerated easily. Hence, by referring to the concept of diseases that have arisen in the conduit itself where they just happen to be, [the *Nan jing* recalls] the five classification categories – namely, the sounds, colors, flavor [preferences], odors, and liquids. Here the main intention of the *Nan jing* is to link all kinds of [disease] manifestations that are related to the systems of the five long-term depots to the five [transportation] holes, as they are matched with the mutual relationships among the Five Phases – with the four seasons and the Five Phases representing the basis [of this linkage]. For example, all disease manifestations that belong to the system of the liver long-term depot can be said to be [caused by] "evil [qi] in the liver." According to the pattern outlined in the first section of this paragraph, one must select the well hole as the main hole for treating [such an affliction]. That is the approach of "investigating the symptoms, discussing the treatment, and selecting the hole." Furthermore, [for treating] all disease manifestations that belong to the [category of] diseases that have arisen in the conduit itself where they just happen to be, one selects the [appropriate hole for treatment from the] five transportation [holes] of that particular conduit. If the disease manifestations indicate a relation [of the disease concerned] with other conduits, one must select [for treatment], from the five transportation [holes, those holes] of these other conduits that belong to the same category as the original conduit under concern.

七十五難曰：（一）經言東方實，西方虛，瀉南方，補北方，何謂也？
（二）然：金木水火土，當更相平。（三）東方木也，西方金也。（四）木欲
實，金當平之；火欲實，水當平之；土欲實，木當平之；金欲實，火當
平之；水欲實，土當平之。（五）東方肝也，則知肝實；西方肺也，則知肺
虛。（六）瀉南方火，補北方水。南方火，火者，木之子也；北方水，水
者，木之母也。（七）水勝火，子能令母實，母能令子虛，故瀉火補水，欲
令金不能平木也。（八）經曰：不能治其虛，何問其餘。此之謂也。

The seventy-fifth difficult issue: (1) The scripture states: In the case of repletion in
the eastern regions and depletion in the western regions, drain the southern regions
and supplement the northern regions. What does that mean?

(2) It is like this. Metal, wood, water, fire, and soil should level[1] each other. (3) The
eastern regions are [associated with the phase of] wood; the western regions are [as-
sociated with] metal. (4) If the wood is on the point of repletion, the metal should
level it. If the fire is on the point of repletion, the water should level it. If the soil
is on the point of repletion, the wood should level it. If the metal is on the point
of repletion, the fire should level it. If the water is on the point of repletion, the soil
should level it. (5) The Eastern regions are [associated with] the liver. One knows,
therefore, [that if the wood of the Eastern regions is replete,] the liver is replete. The
Western regions are [associated with] the lung. One knows, therefore, [that if the
metal of the Western regions is depleted,] the lung is depleted. (6) In the case of a
repletion in the liver,] one drains the fire of the Southern regions and supplements
the water of the Northern regions. [One drains] the fire of the southern regions
because fire is the child of wood. [One supplements] the water of the Northern
regions because water is the mother of wood. (7) Water keeps fire in check. A child
can cause repletion in its mother; a mother can cause depletion in her child. Hence
one drains the fire and supplements the water if one wishes the metal to be in a
position where it does not have to level the wood. (8) The scripture states: If one is
unable to cure a depletion, how could one take care of all the other [diseases]? That
is [what is] meant here.[2]

---

1   The term *ping* 平 ("to level") does not appear in this context in the *Nei jing*. It seems to
     have been introduced by the *Nan jing* to denote the relationship of mutual domination
     among the Five Phases, which was alluded to by other authors with the terms *ke* 克 ("to
     overpower," "to destroy"), *sheng* 勝 ("to overcome"), *qi* 齊 ("to array"), and *fu* 伏 ("to sub-
     due").

2   This difficult issue provides a concrete example for the rather abstract therapeutic pattern
     outlined in difficult issue 69. Although its message appears to be rather straightforward,
     the "indirect" approach recommended here prompted rather controversial comments and

(1) *Xu Dachun*: This is the pattern of draining the child [which was referred to] in difficult issue 69.

   Liao Ping: The [*Nei*] *jing* has no such statement; the doctrine [presented here] is fabricated and false. One of the greatest errors among the apocryphal doctrines of needling is the [concept of] child and mother. Hence it appears frequently in such texts. It is always tied to the Five Phases [doctrine]. The Five Phases [doctrine] is not an orthodox pattern of medicine. As a general paradigm, it may be all right. But as presented here, it is highly reminiscent of astrological speculations with their special study of the Celestial Stems and Earth Branches. All of these [doctrines] obstruct the truth.

(2) *Zhang Shixian*: Ping 平 ("to level") means "to eliminate a surplus." Metal, wood, water, fire, and soil should level each other. Otherwise depletions and repletions will appear.

   Liao Ping: [The concept of the Five Phases' leveling each other] is a mistake within a mistake.

(1)–(8) *Ding Deyong*: The four cardinal regions constitute the proper positions of the Five Phases. Their [periods of] domination correspond to the four seasons. Hence spring corresponds to the Eastern regions, [which are associated with

---

interpretations in subsequent centuries. The following graph once more repeats the correspondences and the mutual relationships of generation and destruction among the Five Phases, the long-term depots, and the cardinal directions, as far as they are referred to in this discussion:

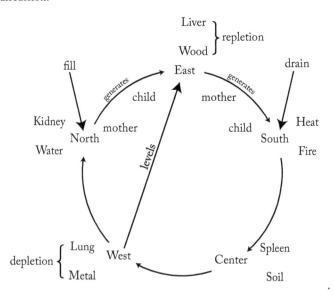

the phase of] wood; summer corresponds to the Southern regions, [which are associated with] fire; autumn corresponds to the Western regions, [which are associated with] metal; winter corresponds to the Northern regions, [which are associated with] water. Late summer corresponds to the center, [which is associated with the] soil. If the fire of the southern regions is replete, it will keep the metal of the Western regions in check. In this case the water of the Northern regions arrives to check, in turn, [the fire]. When fire and water are engaged in a struggle, that will nevertheless cause damage to the lung. Here one should first drain the fire of the Southern regions. That will cause the water of the Northern regions to become replete again. [As a result,] the metal of the lung will be in a position to level [the wood of the Eastern regions]. To "level" is a pattern of restoring harmony among the four cardinal regions in [situations of] depletion and repletion.

Yang: The attitude of the Five Phases towards each other is to keep each other in check. Hence wood keeps soil in check; metal keeps wood in check. Wood is the liver; metal is the lung. When the qi of the lung are depleted or weak, and when, [at the same time,] the qi of the liver are strong and replete, the wood, in contrast [to the normal course], will attack the metal. The metal people do not capitulate; they intend to come to level the wood. When metal and wood are thus engaged in a battle, both long-term depots will be harmed. Hence, when employing the needles [to treat such a situation], one must examine it and comprehend its symptoms. [In the case presented here] it is necessary to drain [qi from] the heart. When the qi of the heart circulate through [the organism], the qi of the liver will recover. Furthermore, one must supplement the kidneys. When the kidneys receive qi, they will transmit them further and nourish the liver. When the qi of the liver are settled, the lung does not show up again to level the liver. Afterwards, one supplements the qi of the spleen. The spleen is the mother of the lung; a mother transmits its qi to her child. The child will then be pacified and settled. Hence [the scripture] states: "If one is unable to cure a depletion, how could one take care of all the other [diseases]? That is [what is] meant here."

Yu Shu: The five long-term depots and the Five Phases level and subdue each other. One must rely on draining and supplementing in order to restore harmony among them and regulate their [relationships]. The *Su wen* states: "When evil qi are present in abundance, that is repletion; when the true qi have been lost, that is depletion." All further situations of depletion and repletion should be approached [according to] this [statement]. The [*Nan jing*] recommends to drain the fire and supplement the water when the wood is replete while the metal is depleted. Now, when the wood is replete, that is to say that the wood has a surplus. As a consequence, the soil fears it. When the soil is in fear of the [wood], the metal has nothing that nourishes it. This, in turn, causes a depletion of metal. If [in such a situation] one does not drain the fire, the fire will flourish and melt the metal. The metal will then become subject to the hostility of wood. [Consequently,] metal and wood [attempt to] keep each other in check, which leads to damage for both of them. Hence one drains the fire. Fire is the child of wood. A child shares qi with its mother. As long as there is no repletion of wood, the fire will not be [able to] level [the metal]. Metal and soil have nothing to fear [from each other]; hence [the latter] will send qi to nourish the metal. When the metal is depleted, one supplements the water and controls the fire. By supplementing the water [one] nourishes the wood. By controlling the fire [one ensures that] the fire does not level the metal. When the wood is provided with nourishment, it will be pacified and can recover. Hence [the text] states: "A child can cause repletion in its mother." When the wood has a surplus, the soil fears the wood. As a result, the soil cannot transmit qi to the metal. The metal will then be depleted. Hence [the text] states: "A mother can cause depletion in her child."

(7) *Hua Shou*: The word "not" in "one wishes the metal to be in a position where it does not have to level the wood" is superfluous .... The basic idea expressed here by Yueren is [as follows. In a situation where] the [qi of the] East exceed repletion and where the qi of the Western regions are insufficient, one drains the fire in order to curb the wood, and one supplements the water in order to support the metal. As a result, metal and wood will enter a stalemate. Hence [the text] states: "If one wishes the metal to be in a position where it can level the wood."

Xu Dachun: Difficult issue 69 states: "In the case of a depletion supplement the mother; in the case of repletion drain the child." Here, in the case of a repletion, [the text recommends] draining the child and supplementing the mother; conversely, in the case of a depletion, [it recommends] supplementing the child. The reason is always plausible but the respective patterns contradict each other. I am not sure why that is so. The child of wood – namely, the fire – is overpowered by the mother of wood – that is, by water. Hence fire is capable of augmenting the qi of water. Hence [the text] states: "A child can cause repletion in its mother." Water overpowers fire; it is able to remove the qi of fire. Hence [the text] states: "A mother can cause depletion in her child." "A child can cause repletion in its mother" [means that] if one drains the child, the strength of the fire is gradually weakened and the water is brought into a situation where it can throw off any restraints considering an attack. "A mother can cause depletion in her child" [means that] if one supplements the mother, the strength of the water will increase and the fire will not dare to retain its surplus. In this way, the fire will not overpower the metal; rather, it will consume the qi of the wood and cause the qi of the metal to expand, while the qi of the wood are weakened every day. As a result, the metal itself is able to level the wood. The word "not" is considered to be superfluous by all authors.

Katō Bankei: When the liver [is replete with qi] to an extreme, the reason is a surplus of fire in the heart. If a child has a surplus, it does not consume the qi of the mother. Therefore the wood of the liver is plentiful and replete. A weakness of [qi in] the kidneys results from an insufficiency of the metal of the lung. If the mother does not have enough qi, it has nothing to assist her child. Hence if the metal of the lung suffers from extreme depletion, one must regulate this [condition] on the basis of the laws of mutual control of the Five Phases. One must supplement the lung and drain the liver and thus level [what is too much and what is too small]. Now when [such a treatment of] East and West is ignored and North and South are treated instead, that is not the usual pattern. It may be compared to the non-classical [doctrines] of the Confucians and to the unconventional [strategies] of the militarists. The sentence "a child can cause repletion in its mother" refers to the pattern of treatment. The mother is the kidneys; the child is the liver. Someone asked whether this could really be so. "If," [he said,] "the heart has a surplus, it causes a repletion in the liver. Now the liver is replete and it should, in turn, cause a repletion in the kidneys. How, then, can the kidneys be depleted?" [I] said: When the heart causes a repletion in the liver, the qi of the [liver] move contrary to their proper course and become evil. When wood generates fire, that is the proper path [of the qi]. Here the heart has a surplus and does not consume the qi of the mother. Hence the qi of the mother do not reach [their destination] and return. They move contrary to the stream and become evil. The kidneys are depleted because they lack the qi of their mother. Now, water generates wood; that is the normal path [of the qi]. However, if its qi are insufficient, it has nothing that it could send out elsewhere. And what could flow back to it? Furthermore, the qi transmitted from the heart to the liver are evil; the qi transmitted from the kidneys to the liver are proper. This may be compared to the flow of water. If its final outlet is obstructed and impassable, the [water] will flow back. When water flows back, there will be strong turbulences. Turbulences create muddy water and the spring [of the stream] will bubble with unrest. Is that [in accordance with] the nature of water? That is the reason for the repletion in the liver. When the spring is rather weak, the flow [of the water emerging from it] will not reach far. Even if one takes all necessary precautions to ensure that it will flow downward, its strength is weak [from the very beginning]. It will be exhausted before it has reached half its way. Nothing remains but mud and sand. What could flow back? That is the reason of the depletion of the kidneys.

Liao Ping: In this book, [the individual units] in the body are seen as hating each other like water and fire; liver and gall bladder are considered to be as distant as [the states of] Hu and Yue. Consequently, [the situation] in the body is reminiscent of the Warring States: there is not one moment of peace and tranquility. [Those who propose such concepts] do not know the basic nature of the Five Phases [doctrine]. Originally, it referred to the inhabitants of the five cardinal regions. It did not say that the interior of the body is to be divided into this and that, and into [individual parts with a] natural disposition to love or hate, to be close with or kill [each other]. [Zhuangzi's idea of the] fighting [kingdoms on each] horn of the snail; Mengzi's [idea of] the ruler who considers his officials as his hands and feet, while the officials consider their ruler as abdomen and heart; or [the idea] of the Emperor representing all mankind under the skies – these are all examples of doctrines considering the individual parts as one whole organism nourishing the ten thousand things. In contrast, the medical people have divided the body into units endowed with kindness and hostility, hating and killing each other, and they believe this to be the principle of nature. By linking [this concept] to the sayings of the Five Phases school, they have made everything even worse, causing the five long-term depots to resemble the evil spirits and malicious demons of the fortune-tellers who are engaged in battle with each other. [The one concept] can be considered to be as unbelievable as [the other].

(1)–(8) *Ye Lin*: Of the authors who have commented on this paragraph, not a single one has sufficiently understood Yueren's advice. Only Mr. Xu [Dachun] in his [*Nan jing*] *jing shi* has come close to it. Now I shall elucidate its meaning. "Repletion in the Eastern regions and depletion in the Western regions" [means the following]. The Eastern regions stand for wood and for the liver. The Western regions stand for metal and for the lung. Man's five long-term depots correspond to the Five Phases. They all must be leveled and subdued; they should not dominate individually. However, if one long-term depot alone dominates, disease develops. One must rely on supplementing and draining in order to restore harmony. It is with regard to the patterns of restoring harmony that the text states "drain the Southern regions and supplement the Northern regions." [That is to say,] the fire of the Southern regions is the child of wood. The water of the Northern regions is the mother of wood. If one discusses this along the principle of the original nature of the Five Phases, a repletion of wood should be leveled by metal; a repletion of fire should be leveled by water; a repletion of soil should be leveled by wood; a repletion of metal should be leveled by fire; a repletion of water should be leveled by soil. That is the principle of nature. Here, a repletion in the liver, [which is associated with the] Eastern regions, [is accompanied by] a depletion in the lung, [which is associated with] the Western regions. If the metal is depleted, how can it level the wood? If we discuss treatment, one must curb what is excessive and one must support what is insufficient. Hence [the text] states: "Drain the fire of the Southern regions, and supplement the water of the Northern regions." This is the case of a repletion where one drains the respective child. Now, fire is the child of wood; water is the mother of wood. If one drains the fire, the fire weakens and removes qi from its mother. As the strength of the fire decreases, it becomes unable to attack the metal. If one supplements the water, the qi of the fire are weakened even further and it snatches even more qi from the wood. Therefore it is stated [in the text]: "Water keeps fire in check." Furthermore, as the qi of wood leak away, the metal is no longer the subject of attacks. As a result, its depletion recovers by itself. Through this recovery, it can once again fulfill its function of leveling the wood. When the water overpowers the fire, the strength [of the metal] increases even further. Therefore, water, the mother of wood, keeps the fire – that is, the child of wood – in check. When [the text] states, "a child can cause repletion in the mother; a mother can cause depletion in the child," [that means the following]. If the child of wood – namely, fire – is overpowered by the mother of wood – namely, water – the fire is, in fact, able to augment the qi of water. Hence [the text] states: "A child [of a particular long-term depot] can cause repletion in the mother [of that depot]." But the water may also overpower the fire and remove the qi of fire. Hence [the text] states: "A mother [of a particular depot] can cause depletion in the child [of that depot]." Looking at the text above and below [these statements, it becomes obvious that] the two words "child" and "mother" refer to the wood of the liver. [If one intends to] suppress the wood, that is achieved by supporting the metal. Still, Yueren feared that the reader might misunderstand this. Therefore, he once again elucidated the meaning [of this passage] and stated: "Hence one drains the fire [i.e., the child of wood] and supplements the water [i.e., the mother of wood] if one wishes the metal to be in a position where it can level the wood." Hence, if one does not know the pattern of treating the depletion of metal and applies supplementing and draining solely on a single conduit, one will not be able to treat all the other diseases. The word "not" following [the word] metal was considered to be superfluous by Mr. Hua [Shou, who said] it should be eliminated. He was quite correct.

(7) *Tamba Genkan*: Not a single commentary [by earlier authors] on this passage has been correct. Xu [Dachun's] explanations were relatively clear and complete. This [paragraph] states that, originally, the nature of metal overpowers wood. When the wood is on the point of repletion, [the metal] must level it. Here the metal cannot execute its orders; instead it is oppressed by the wood itself. Hence, if one supplements the water – which is the mother of wood – the strength of the water will increase; it will suffice to aid the metal. If one drains the fire – which is the child of the wood – the strength of the fire will decrease; it will turn to the wood for help. When the wood helps [the fire], the strength of its excessive repletion will decrease too; it will no longer be in a position to oppress the metal. When the metal is no longer subject to oppression, it will recover from its depletion. When it has recovered, it will once again be in a position to level the repletion of the wood. When the water overpowers the fire, its strength will be increasingly replete. That is to say, the mother of the wood keeps the child of the wood in check. Therefore [the text] states: "The child causes repletion in the mother; the mother causes depletion in the child."

(1)–(8) *Huang Weisan*: This difficult issue discusses a situation where two conduits have a disease at the same time, and it outlines a therapeutic pattern of treating them simultaneously. The pattern does not consist of selecting holes on the two conduits affected by the disease themselves, and it does not recommend selecting holes on the respective mother or child conduits. Rather, it select the holes on two other conduits to achieve the effect of "one treatment, two successes." This [pattern] belongs, in fact, to the therapeutic [approaches focusing on conduits] that are separated [from the sick conduits] by one or two positions. That is the most sophisticated therapeutic pattern in traditional Chinese medicine.

七十六難曰：（一）何謂補瀉？當補之時，何所取氣？當瀉之時，何所置氣？（二）然：當補之時，從衛取氣；當瀉之時，從榮置氣。（三）其陽氣不足，陰氣有餘，當先補其陽，而後瀉其陰；（四）陰氣不足，陽氣有餘，當先補其陰，而後瀉其陽。（五）榮衛通行，此其要也。

The seventy-sixth difficult issue: (1) What is meant by „supplementing" and "draining"? When it is advisable to supplement, whence shall one remove the qi? When it is advisable to drain, whence shall one release the qi?

(2) It is like this. When a supplementation is required, qi are to be removed from the guard [qi]; when a drainage is required, qi are to be released from the camp [qi]. (3) When there are not enough yang qi while there is a surplus of yin qi, one must supplement the yang [qi] first and then drain the yin [qi]. (4) When there are not enough yin qi while there is a surplus of yang qi, one must supplement the yin [qi] first and drain the yang [qi] afterwards. (5) The flow of the camp and guard [qi through the organism] is the major [goal] of the [therapeutic interventions of supplementing and draining].

(1) *Liao Ping:* There is no need to pose such a question. The [*Nei*] *jing* provides detailed and clear [information] on all the patterns of supplementing and draining by means of needling and cauterization. One must not refer to a "removal" or "release" [of qi]. It is a great error to state that supplementing is the removal of guard [qi] while draining is the removal of camp [qi]. Supplementing and draining are applied in accordance with an abundance or weakness [of qi] in the individual conduits. There is no such doctrine that one distinguishes between guard and camp [qi].

(2) *Yu Shu:* The lung moves the five qi; it pours them into the five long-term depots. [The qi] penetrate the six conduits and find their way into the one hundred vessels. Whenever one removes qi [from one location to supplement a depletion elsewhere], they are to be removed them from the guard qi. As soon as [one feels that guard] qi have accumulated [around the needle], the needle is to be inserted further [into the depth] to push [the qi] into the conduit vessel that is depleted. [To exercise this technique,] one must distinguish between sections that are near the surface and others that are in the depth. This is the way to supplement. Hence [the text] states: "When one has to supplement, he removes qi from the guard [qi]." That is [what is] meant here. When evil [qi] are present in the section of the camp [qi], the needle is inserted into the conduit affected

by repletion. As soon as one feels that qi have accumulated [around the needle], the needle is pulled [out of the depth] to drain [the repletion]. Hence [the text] states: "When one has to drain, he releases qi from the camp [qi]." *Zhi* 置 ("to release") stands for *qu* 取 ("to remove") and for *ying* 迎 ("to move against").

Katō Bankei: "The removal of qi from the guard [qi" means the following]. After inserting the needle only slightly, one lets it remain for a while. As soon as qi have accumulated around it, one pushes [the needle] into the depth. In this way, one causes qi that were dispersed below the surface to be accepted by the vessels. That is the supplementing of the [camp qi in the vessels]. "One releases qi from the camp [qi" means the following]. One inserts [the needle] deeply and lets it remain for a while. As soon as qi have accumulated around it, one pulls [the needle out of the vessel] and causes the qi that were in the vessel to disperse in the [section of the] guard [qi] outside [of the vessels]. That is the draining of the [vessels].

(3) *Yu Shu*: If, for instance, the gall bladder does not have enough [qi] while the liver has a surplus, one supplements the foot minor yang [conduit] first and drains the foot ceasing yin [conduit] afterwards.

(4) *Yu Shu*: This pattern is the opposite of the one mentioned above.

(5) *Yang*: This [refers to] changes resulting from the yin and yang [units'] inflicting of depletion and repletion upon each other.

(1)–(5) *Hua Shou*: The fifty-second treatise of the *Ling shu* states: "Those qi that proceed outside of the conduits below the surface are the guard qi; those essence qi that move within the conduits are the camp qi." Hence, for supplementing, one removes those qi that move outside of the vessels below the surface in order to supplement a place that is depleted. For draining, one releases camp qi so that they have no further use. *Zhi* 置 ("to release") is used here like the *zhi* in *qi zhi* 棄置 ("to discard"). However, man's diseases may appear in many variations of depletion and repletion. Hence the principles of supplementing and draining are multifaceted, too. Thus, if the yang qi are not enough while there is a surplus of yin qi, one supplements the yang first and drains the yin afterwards in order to harmonize [their balance]. When the yin qi are not enough while there is a surplus of yang qi, one supplements the yin first and drains the yang afterwards in order to harmonize [their balance]. If one applies such [a treatment], the camp and the guard [qi] will proceed through [the body] by themselves. For patterns of how to supplement or drain, see a later paragraph.[1]

Xu Dachun: This [paragraph] is a continuation of the text of the preceding [difficult issue]; it discusses the pattern of supplementing and draining and empha-

---

1   See difficult issue 78.

sizes that one must investigate whether the yin or the yang [section] is affected by a depletion or repletion. The guard [qi] are yang; the camp [qi] are yin. In the case the guard [qi] are depleted while the camp [qi] are replete, one supplements the yang and drains the yin. In the case the camp [qi] are depleted while the guard [qi] are replete, one supplements the yin and drains the yang. The pattern of supplementing and draining is further differentiated by [considerations] of which [of these interventions is to be carried out] first and which is second. In the treatise "Zhong shi" 終始 of the *Ling* [*shu*], it is stated: "When the yin [qi] abound while the yang [qi] are in a state of depletion, the yang [qi] are to be supplemented first. Only then the yin [qi] are to be drained to achieve harmony. When the yin [qi] are in a state of depletion while the yang [qi] abound, the yin [qi] are to be supplemented first. Only then the yang [qi] are to be drained to achieve harmony." That is the basis of what is said here [in the *Nan jing*].

Liao Ping: The [condition of the] long-term depots counts here and nothing else; one does not distinguish between camp and guard [qi in the context of draining and supplementing]. In the case of an abundance, the camp and the guard [qi] are both present in abundance. In the case of a depletion, the camp and the guard [qi] are both depleted. If one were depleted and the other were replete, they would balance each other and one could not speak of „supplementing" and "draining." To neglect the long-term depots and short-term repositories and to distinguish among camp and guard [qi] for separate supplementing and draining is a great mistake.

七十七難曰：（一）經言上工治未病，中工治已病者，何謂也？
（二）然：所謂治未病者，見肝之病，則知肝當傳之與脾，（三）故先實其脾
氣，無令得受肝之邪，故曰治未病焉。（四）中工治已病者，見肝之病，不
曉相傳，但一心治肝，故曰治已病也。

The seventy-seventh difficult issue: (1) The scripture states: The superior practitioner initiates a cure where there is no disease yet; the mediocre practitioner treats where there is a disease already. What does that mean?

(2) It is like this. The so-called treatment of where there is no disease yet [implies the following]. When one sees a disease in the liver, one should know that the liver will transmit it to the spleen. (3) Hence one prevents this [transmission] by supplementing the qi of the spleen, with the effect that it will not accept the evil [qi] from the liver. Hence [the scripture] speaks of "treating what is not yet ill." (4) When a mediocre practitioner sees a disease in the liver, he does not know about mutual transmission, and he will focus all his efforts on treating the liver. Hence [the scripture] speaks of his "treating where there is a disease already."[1]

---

1 Various commentators, including Hua Shou and Ye Lin, have pointed to the close relationship between the present difficult issue and a statement found in *Ling shu* treatise 55, "Ni shun" 逆順. Yet the phrasing of the question in sentence 1 should also remind one of *Su wen* treatise 2, "Si qi tiao shen da lun" 四氣調神大論, with the famous statement: "As for the DAO, the sages practice it; the stupid wear it [for decoration only]. If one follows yin and yang, then life results. If one opposes them, then death results. If one follows them, then order results. If one opposes them, then disorder results. To act contrary to what is appropriate, this is opposition. This is called inner obstruction. Hence, 'the sages did not treat those already ill, but treated those not yet ill.' (*gu sheng ren bu zhi yi bing zhi wei bing* 故聖人不治已病治未病). They did not put in order what was already in disorder, but put in order what was not yet in disorder." This passage appears to be a general advice to value prevention more highly than curative efforts. The last line of the corresponding passage in *Ling shu* treatise 55 repeats the *Su wen* literally, except for a replacement of *sheng ren* 聖人 ("sages") by *shang gong* 上工 ("superior practitioner"). Although the Chinese wording *bu zhi yi bing zhi wei bing* is identical, the meaning in the *Ling shu* is different; it points out that in treating an individual patient, one must focus on those parts of the organism that have not yet been affected by a disease in order to prevent a further transmission of evil qi within the organism. The general preventative effort recommended in the *Su wen* statement for keeping an individual person from falling ill was narrowed down in the *Ling shu* to preventative efforts aimed at the protection of healthy functional units in the individual organism when other units have fallen ill already. The *Nan jing* elucidated the *Ling shu* statement by providing a concrete example based on the Five Phases paradigm.

(1) *Li Jiong*: A superior practitioner is a medical practitioner who takes up ten thousand [cases] and cures ten thousand [cases]. In all [cases] he treats diseases that are not yet manifest [as diseases]. A mediocre practitioner cannot yet fully understand and resolve [the dynamics of a disease]. Hence he will simply take care of one long-term depot and that is it.

Liao Ping: The text of the [*Nei*] *jing* was extremely clear. To ask such a mistaken question creates nothing but barriers.

(2) *Liao Ping*: "To treat what is not yet ill" [corresponds to] the so-called ordering of the state before a revolt has arisen, and to the protection of the country before it is in danger. To extend this to [a statement that only the mediocre practitioner treats] what is ill already does not agree at all with the idea expressed in the [*Nei*] *jing*.

(4) *Li Jiong*: He realizes that the liver has a disease but does not know the principle that the liver will transmit [the disease] to the spleen. He will focus all his attention on treating the conduit of the liver.

(1)–(4) *Ding Deyong*: The *Su wen* states: "Spring keeps late summer in check; late summer keeps winter in check; winter keeps summer in check; summer keeps autumn in check; autumn keeps spring in check." That is the principle of the four seasons and Five Phases keeping each other in check. With man's five long-term depots, [it is as follows]. Those that have a surplus [of qi] move forward to keep [another depot] in check. Those that do not have enough [qi] receive evil [qi]. The superior practitioner supplements first where there is not enough; thus he prevents evil [qi] from being received. Only afterwards does he drain where there is a surplus. That is [what is meant by] "treating what is not yet ill." The mediocre practitioner takes the needle and simply drains where there is a surplus. Hence [the text] speaks of "treating what is ill already."

Yang: When [one of] the five long-term depots gets a disease, it will always transmit it to [the long-term depot] that it keeps in check. For instance, a disease in the liver is transmitted to the spleen. If the [latter] happens to be in its flourishing period, it will not accept what is transmitted. Hence it is not necessary to move [proper qi] into this direction. For example, a disease in the liver should be transmitted to the spleen. The spleen rules in late summer. If [the transmission] occurs exactly during that ruling period, [the spleen] will not accept the evil. Hence it is not necessary to cause a preventive repletion of [proper] qi in the spleen. If the time is not late summer, [the spleen] will accept the evil [qi] from the liver. Hence one must simply cause a preventive repletion of qi in the spleen, lest it accept the evil [qi] from the liver. Anybody who acts like this is called a superior practitioner. *Gong* 工 ("practitioner") is used here like *miao* 妙 ("excellent"). That is to say, these are [practitioners] who comprehend the origin of a disease in an excellent manner. A mediocre practitioner cannot resolve the entire [dynamics of a disease]. Hence he will simply take care of one long-term depot and that is it.

Hua Shou: If one realizes that the liver has a disease, he will first cause a repletion in the spleen so that the evil [qi transmitted from the liver] have no place to enter. That is "treating what is not yet ill." A man who acts like this is a superior practitioner. If one realizes that the liver has a disease and focuses all his attention on treating the liver, that is "treating what is ill already." A mediocre practitioner acts like this. The fifty-fifth treatise of the *Ling shu* states: "The superior practitioner pierces [diseases] that have not emerged yet. Next he pierces those that are not fully developed yet. Next he pierces those that have begun to weaken again. The inferior practitioner pierces [diseases] that have just launched an attack. They address [their therapy] to those whose physical appearance appears rich [of proper qi, while in fact these are evil qi]. They address [their therapy to situations] where the disease and the [movement in] the vessels contradict each other. Hence it is said: 'When [the evil qi] are just abounding, one must not dare to risk a causing of harm. When piercing [a disease] that has weakened, the action will have significant success.' Hence, when it is said: 'The superior practitioner initiates a cure where there is no disease yet, he does not cure where there is a disease already,' then that is meant here."

Ye Lin: The treatise "Ni shun" 逆順 of the *Ling shu* states: "The superior practitioner pierces where [a disease] has not yet developed ... [see above, Hua Shou's quotation from *Ling shu* treatise 55] ... he does not treat what is ill already." That is to say, the superior practitioner pierces where a disease has not yet developed. Then he pierces where [the evil qi] have just arrived but are not yet present in abundance. Then, afterwards, he pierces where [the evil qi] have already weakened. That resembles the military technique of avoiding the sharp [point of the enemy's] weapon and of attacking [the enemy] when he is careless and retreats. Hence Bo Gao states: "Do not confront those qi that come with a peng-peng [drum roll]. Do not attack battle troops approaching with loud drum rolls. In [the text] *Rules of Piercing* it says: Do not pierce a baking heat. Do not pierce a dripping sweat. Do not pierce vessels with chaotic flow, and do not pierce when the disease and the [movement in the] vessels contradict each other."[2] That is right. The inferior practitioner does not know about these principles. He pierces at that moment when the evil [qi] carry their attack into the conduit vessels.

---

2   See also *Ling shu* treatise 55, "Ni shun."

Or he pierces just at that moment when [the evil qi] abound in the pores of the skin. Or he pierces when the evil and the proper [qi] are battling each other. He cannot look forward to a success [of his treatment]; all [his activities] are appropriate only to spoil the affair. The present [paragraph] discusses the necessity of reaching [into long-term depots] where the disease has not yet developed or where it is just on the point of retreating, and of applying the needle only there. However, against all diseases it is advisable to prepare strategies early. One must not wait until the disease has matured and then begin the treatment; this would only lead to late remorse. If the treatment starts early, the efforts one needs are few but the successes one earns are many. The merit of bending the chimney and removing the fuel is certainly higher than that of being severely burned in assisting to extinguish a fire. In treating diseases, one must definitely act like this; actually, the administration of all affairs in the world should be like this. Why should these [principles] apply only to the techniques of needling?! When the qi in any of the five long-term depots abound, they will [be sent out to] assist the [long-term depot which is] generated [by the long-term depot where the qi abound]. The liver generates the heart; the heart generates the spleen; the spleen generates the lung; the lung generates the kidneys; the kidneys generate the liver. If the transmission [of qi] follows [this course], that is a good sign. In the case of a disease, however, [the affected depot] will annoy the [depot] it can overpower. The liver [can] overpower the spleen; the spleen [can] overpower the kidneys; the kidneys [can] overpower the heart; the heart [can] overpower the lung; the lung [can] overpower the liver. That is a transmission [of qi] contrary [to the proper course]; it is a bad sign. "The superior practitioner treats what is not yet ill" means that he treats the long-term depot to which the disease has not yet been transmitted. Hence, when he realizes that the liver has a disease, he knows that the liver transmits it to the spleen. Therefore, he must first cause a repletion in the spleen. In this way, he ensures that the disease of the liver can not be transmitted and will be cured. Hence the [text] states: "Treats what is not yet ill." The mediocre practitioner is unaware of this. He realizes that the liver has a disease and treats nothing but the liver. Then, before the disease in the liver has come to an end, a disease in the spleen will emerge in turn. Hence [the text] states: "Treats what is ill already."

七十八難曰：（一）針有補瀉，何謂也？

（二）然：補瀉之法，非必呼吸出內針也。（三）然：知為鍼者，信其左；不知為針者，信其右。（四）當刺之時，必先以左手厭按所鍼滎俞之處，彈而努之，爪而下之，其氣之來，如動脈之狀，順鍼而刺之。（五）得氣因推而內之，是謂補；（六）動而伸之，是謂瀉。（七）不得氣，乃與男外女內；（八）不得氣，是謂十死不治也。

The seventy-eighth difficult issue: (1) With needles one may supplement or drain. What does that mean?

(2) It is like this. The patterns of supplementing and draining do not imply that one must withdraw or insert the needle [in accordance with the patient's] exhalation and inhalation. (3) Instead, those who know how to apply the needle, they rely on their left [hand]; those who do not know how to apply the needle, they rely on their right [hand]. (4) When one is about to pierce, he first presses with his left hand the transportation [hole] where he [intends to] needle the camp [qi]. The pressure is to be exerted with full vigor through his fingernail. As soon as the arrival of the qi [felt below the left hand] resembles the [pulsation of the qi at the usual locations] where the movement [in the] vessels [can be felt below the skin], one inserts the needle. (5) When the qi have accumulated [around the needle], one pushes them toward the interior. That is called "to supplement." (6) To move [the needle] and withdraw it [from the section of the camp qi into the section of the guard qi] is called "to drain." (7) If no qi accumulate [around the needle, one must seek them] in males in the external and in females in the internal [sections of the organism]. (8) If [even then] no qi accumulate [around the needle], that is a so-called [situation in which, of ten such patients,] ten will die without any [successful] treatment being possible.[1]

---

1   This difficult issue modifies the techniques of "supplementing" and "draining" as outlined in the *Nei jing*. A comparison of the corresponding passage in *Su wen* treatise 27, "Li he zhen xie lun," 離合眞邪論 with the version given here in the *Nan jing* shows where the latter disagrees with the former. The *Nei jing* version has the following wording: "When [the patient] inhales, one inserts the needle in order to avoid the qi clashing against [the needle]. One lets the needle remain quiet for a while to avoid the evil [qi] dispersing. When the patient inhales [again], one revolves the needle until qi have accumulated [around the needle]. One waits until [the patient] exhales [again] and pulls the needle out. With the completion of the exhalation, [the needle must be] withdrawn. A large amount of qi will have left [the body]. Hence that is called 'draining.' The Thearch said: 'If [the qi] are not enough, how does one supplement them?' Qi Bo replied: 'One must first lay one's hand [on the location to be pierceed] and seek [the depleted section]. Then one presses it down and disperses [the guard qi]. Then one pushes [one's hand into the flesh] and holds it tight. One squeezes [the respective location] and causes [qi to arrive in] great excitement. Then one scratches [the respective location] and lowers the [needle into the

(2) *Yang*: "Supplementing" means that one withdraws the needle while [the patient] exhales. "Draining" means that one inserts the needle while [the patient] inhales. Hence [the text] states: "Withdraw or insert the needle [in accordance with the patient's] exhalation and inhalation."

Xu Dachun: The [treatise] "Li he zhen xie lun" 離合眞邪論 of the *Su* [*wen*] states: "When [the patient] inhales, insert the needle; do not let the [proper] qi revolt. Wait until [the patient] exhales to pull the needle out. When the exhalation is completed, [the needle] is removed. Large [quantities] of qi leave. Hence, this is called 'draining'. When an exhalation is completed, insert the needle. [Hold the needle] calmly and let it remain [inserted] for long to have the qi arrive. Wait for an inhalation and pull the needle. The qi must not leave. At each place [where the needle was inserted], push [the hole] and close the door and thereby let the spirit qi be preserved. Large [quantities of] qi stay where they are. Hence this is called 'supplementation'." That is the pattern of withdrawing or inserting [the needle in accordance with the patient's] exhalation and inhalation. Yueren thought that the principle [of supplementing and draining] was not outlined in sufficient comprehensiveness by these [words. Hence he felt it to be] appropriate to write the text that follows.

---

flesh]. Then one lets [the qi] pass [again] and removes the needle by pulling it toward outside through the gate [opened by the needle. Immediately afterwards, one closes the hole with one's finger] to keep the spirit [qi] from leaving. One inserts the needle at the point of complete exhalation and lets it remain quiet for a while until the qi have arrived. That is just as if one were to wait for someone dear to come – one would be unaware of whether it is morning or already evening. When the qi have arrived, one treats them appropriately and keeps them carefully. If, then, one pulls the needle out at the same time as [the patient] inhales, no qi can leave [the body] – they will remain where they are. One closes the gate [opened by the needle with one's finger] and thus causes [the proper] spirit - qi to be retained and a large amount of qi [from elsewhere comes to] remain [at the location that was pierced]. Hence this is called 'supplementing'." Obviously, the *Nei jing* approach to supplementing and draining is based on the assumption that an artificial hole opened by a needle serves, in addition to mouth and nose, as a further gate where qi may enter or leave the body corresponding to exhalation and inhalation. The *Nan jing*, with its concept of an internal exchange of qi between the sections of the guard and camp qi, states, of course, that it is not necessary to link supplementing and draining to inhalation and exhalation. For the concept of supplementing and draining through internal exchange, see difficult issues 70, 71, 72, and 76. The passage *tan er nu zhi zhua er xia zhi* 彈而努之爪而下之 may be a corrupt version of the *Nei jing* passage quoted above (*tan er nu zhi zhua er xia zhi* 彈而怒之抓而下之). My rendering of sentence 3 however, follows the alternative assumption that the characters *nu* 怒 ("excitement") and *zhua* 抓 ("to scratch") were changed deliberately to *nu* 努 ("vigorous") and *zhua* 爪 ("fingernail"). Thus in the *Nan jing* version *xia zhi* 下之 should not refer to the insertion of the needle but to the lowering of one's fingers or hand into the flesh.

Liao Ping: Xu [Dachun] commented: "The [treatise] 'Li he zhen xie lun' 離合
眞邪論 [see Xu's comment above] ... the text that follows." Later people were
wrong when they took these words as an indication that Yueren supplemented
what was incomplete in the [*Nei*] *jing*. That is a great mistake!

(3)–(8) *Yang*: The pattern of inserting a needle is [as follows]. First, one must know
the location of the hole. This is then pressed with the left hand. Then one
squeezes this location, pressed down as it already is, with the right hand. The
movement [in the] vessel will be felt below the left hand. [The location of the
hole] is then pressed with the fingers of the left hand. Next one seeks [the hole]
with the needle and pierces it. One waits until the qi react below the needle and
then pushes them into the [section of the] camp [qi]. That is the "supplementing." When the qi have accumulated [around the needle], one simply revolves
[the needle] and then withdraws it. That is [the technique of] "draining." If one
lets the needle remain [in the section of the camp qi] over an extended period
of time and waits in vain for the qi to arrive, he then lets the needle remain in
the [section of the] guard qi for a while and waits for qi [to accumulate around
the needle] there. If no [qi] accumulate [there] even after an extended period of
time, one inserts the needle once again into the [section of the] camp qi. If at
all these three locations[2] the qi do not react to the needle, that means that yin
and yang are equally exhausted and cannot be subjected to needling again. Of
ten persons [with such symptoms], ten will die. Hence [the text] states: "Ten
will die without any [successful] treatment being possible." The guard [qi] are
yang; the yang is external. Hence [the text] states: "[Seek them] in males in the
external [section]." The camp [qi] are yin; the yin is internal. Hence [the text]
states: "[Seek them] in females in the internal [section]."

Ding Deyong: "Those who know how to apply the needle rely on their left [hand]"
means [the following]. The left hand first presses the location to be pierced. As
soon as one perceives with his hand an arrival of qi resembling the [pulsation of
the qi at the usual locations] where the movement [in the] vessels [can be felt],
he inserts the needle. That is another [variation of the pattern of] "withdrawal
by moving against." The effect is draining. When the qi have passed and one
pierces by following them with the needle, that is [identical with the pattern
of] "support by following."[3] In males yang qi move in the external [sections of
the organism]; in females yin qi move in the internal [sections of the organism.
Treating] males, one presses the respective hole [to be pierced] with a light hand;

---

2   In his almost identical commentary, Zhang Shixian speaks of two instead of three loca-
     tions.

3   See difficult issues 79 and 72.

[treating] females, one presses the respective hole with a heavy hand. If after some time has passed no qi have arrived – that is, if no [qi] react to the [pressure exerted by the] left hand – one must not pierce. If one pierces, there will be no effect. That indicates that the [flow of the] qi has been cut off. Hence [of ten persons afflicted with such symptoms,] ten will die and no [successful] treatment is possible. Why should one wait for the qi by letting the needle remain [inserted]?

Yu Shu: If one accumulates qi of the guard [section] and pushes them into a depleted section – [that is,] if one opens a hole [between the guard section and the depleted section] and then withdraws the needle – that is called "supplementing." If one removes qi from the guard [section] by pulling the needle out – that is,] if one opens a hole [between the guard section and the external environment] and then withdraws the needle – that is called "draining." If one waits for an inhalation to insert the needle and then, at the point of complete exhalation, withdraws the needle, that is called "supplementing first and draining afterwards." If one acts contrary to this, that is called "draining first and supplementing afterwards." The *Xuan zhu mi yu* 玄珠密語 speaks about the patterns of supplementing and draining as follows: "One presses the [location to be pierced] until qi have accumulated [there. Then one] inserts [the needle] into the section of the heaven. As soon as the qi have accumulated [around the needle] in the section of the heaven, one pushes them into the section of the earth. When the qi of heaven and earth interact, one withdraws the needle. That is called 'draining'. If one proceeds the opposite way, that is called 'supplementing'." This concept [and the present passage of the *Nan jing*] contradict each other.

Zhang Shixian: Those who are experts in needling press the place to be needled with their left hand to inform themselves of whether the flesh of the patient under their fingers is thick or thin, whether muscles and bones are closely attached to each other, and whether the [location selected as a] hole [for needling] is genuine or false. Only then do they insert the needle with the right hand. They always rely on the pressure exerted by their left hand and do not wait until after they have inserted the needle to realize [whether the flesh is thin or thick, etc.]. Those who do not know how to needle do not [first] apply pressure with their left hand. In a senseless manner they insert the needle and only after the needle has reached the interior do they know whether they have hit the hole or not.

(3) *Liao Ping*: That is a false statement! Since when does whether someone knows or does not know depend on a distinction between left and right?!

(4) *Xu Dachun*: *Tan* 彈 ("to press down") stands for *ji* 擊 ("to strike"). *Nu* 弩 ("crossbow") stands for *rou* 揉 ("to bend," "to crush," "to rub"). "[By his] fingernails" means that one sinks his fingernails into the flesh.

Liao Ping: The [*Nei*] *jing* says *zhua er xia zhi* 抓而下之 ("scratch [the respective location] and lower the needle").

(7) *Liao Ping*: To distinguish [in this context] between males and females is an error within an error.

七十九難曰：（一）經言迎而奪之，安得無虛？（二）隨而濟之，安得無實？（三）虛之與實，若得若失；實之與虛，若有若無，何謂也？
（四）然：迎而奪之者，瀉其子也；（五）隨而濟之者，補其母也。（六）假令心病，瀉手心主俞，是謂迎而奪之者也。（七）補手心主井，是謂隨而濟之者也。（八）所謂實之與虛者，牢濡之意也。（九）氣來實者為得，濡虛者為失，故曰若得若失也。

The seventy-ninth difficult issue: (1) The scripture states: To confront [those who come] and [attempt] to remove them [without sufficient strength], how could it be that this will not result in a depletion [of proper qi]?

(2) [The scripture states further:] To pursue [those who go away] and [invariably] assist them, how could it be that this will not result in a repletion [of evil qi]?

(3) [The treatments of] depletion and repletion resemble [attempts to achieve] a gain or [to create] a loss. Repletion and depletion resemble having and not having. What does that mean?

(4) It is like this. [If one intends] to withdraw [qi] moving contrary [to the direction of their regular flow, one should] drain the respective child. (5) [If one intends] to provide support [to qi] following [their proper course, one should] supplement the respective mother. (6) Take for example a disease in the heart. To drain at the rapids [hole] of the hand heart ruler [conduit] would be called "to withdraw [qi] moving against [the direction of their flow]." (7) To supplement at the well [hole] of the hand heart ruler [conduit] would be called "to provide support [to the qi] following [their proper course]." (8) The [concepts of] so-called depletion and repletion convey the meaning of firmness and softness. (9) If the qi arrive firm and replete, that is [comparable to] a "gain"; if they [arrive] soft and depleted, that is [comparable to] a "loss." Hence [the scripture] states: "Resemble a gain or a loss."[1]

---

1   This difficult issue provides another example of a reinterpretation of terms quoted from the *Nei jing*. Three different concepts are combined here. First, there is the concept, outlined in difficult issue 50, that a child who sends its qi backward in the sequence of mutual generation causes a repletion in its mother, while a mother who sends evil qi to her child is responsible for the latter's depletion. Hence one must drain the child in case of a repletion so that it can no longer send a repletion evil to its mother; in case of a depletion evil, one supplements the mother with proper qi so that she will no longer have to transmit evil qi to her child. Second, the concepts of "moving against" and "following" continue the point elaborated in difficult issue 72. The Chinese phrases *ying er duo zhi* 迎而奪之 and *sui er ji zhi* 隨而濟之 are identical here in sentences 1 and 2 (quoting the *Nei jing*) and in sentences 4 and 5, where they offer the understanding of the *Nan jing*. But the meanings are different, so they must be rendered differently into English. As in difficult issue 72, the *Nei jing* concepts of *ying* 迎 ("to move against") and of *sui* 隨 ("to follow") refer to the

COMMENTARIES

(1) *Liao Ping*: When [the *Nan jing*] quotes a passage from the [*Nei*] *jing* in order to pose a question, the following [text] differs in many cases from the [*Nei*] *jing*. [The questions and answers of the *Nan jing*] were not intended to quote the [*Nei*] *jing* but to change and contradict its [contents].

(1)–(3) *Hua Shou*: This [passage] is based on the first treatise of the *Ling shu*. *De* 得 ("gain") means *qiu er huo* 求而獲 ("to ask for something and get it"). *Shi* 适 ("loss") stands for *zong* 縱 ("to let go") and for *yi* 遺 ("to release"). The second paragraph states: "Repletion and depletion resemble having and not having." That is to say, in the case of a repletion qi are present; in the case of a depletion, qi are absent. When [the *Nan jing*] states: "the [treatments of] depletion and repletion resemble a gain or a loss [respectively]," that is to say, supplementing must lead to significant gains; draining must lead to significant loss.

(3) *Zhang Shixian*: For *xu zhi yu shi* 虛之與實, the *Ling shu* says *wei xu wei shi* 為虛為實. For *shi zhi yu xu* 失之與虛, the *Ling shu* says *yan shi yu xu* 言實與虛. The wording here is different from the *Ling shu* but the meaning is the same.

---

mechanics of inserting the needle. In contrast, the *Nan jing* concepts of *ying* and *sui* refer to the movement of the qi arriving at a certain hole, either "moving against their proper course" or "following their proper course." If, for instance, qi move contrary to their proper course in the sequence of mutual generation of the Five Phases, they are responsible for a repletion. A depletion is caused by a mother in her child – that is, by qi following their proper course. However, if we follow difficult issue 69, the disease in the heart described in the present issue appears to be a case in which the respective conduit has fallen ill by itself, because the *Nan jing* suggests (in difficult issue 69) that such diseases be treated on the respective conduit itself. This, then, is the third concept to be taken into account here. The level of theoretical abstraction is noteworthy because the mother-child concept – which was introduced to explain (in an abstract manner) the origins of repletion and depletion – is employed here to guide the selection of holes (through their association with the Five Phases) on a single conduit (that has fallen ill by itself) in order to treat its repletion or depletion. For comparison, I add here the original version of the *Nei jing* passage (*Ling shu* treatise 1) quoted in sentences 1 through 3: "The general [principles of] needling [are as follows]. In case of a depletion, one must replenish the [depleted section]; in case of a repletion, one must drain the [replete section]; in case something remains [in the organism] for too long, one must eliminate it; in case evil [qi] gain dominance, one must clear them out. The *Da yao* 大要 says: 'Through slow [insertion] and quick [withdrawal of the needle] one achieves repletion; through quick [insertion] and slow [withdrawal of the needle] one achieves depletion.' That is to say, depletion and repletion resemble having and not having. One must investigate what are secondary [symptoms] and what were the original [causes of an illness], and whether [the proper qi] are still present or whether they have been lost already. The treatment of a depletion resembles [attempts to achieve] a gain; the treatment of a repletion resembles [attempts to create] a loss." (*Da yao* is the title of an unknown text quoted by the *Nei jing* several times).

Liao Ping: The [concept of] supplementing and draining through child and mother is a false doctrine of this book which does not appear in the [*Nei*] *jing*.

(1)–(3) *Xu Dachun:* For *ying* 迎 ("to move against") and *sui* 隨 ("to follow"), see difficult issue 72; for the [original] wording of the [quotation from the *Nei*] *jing*, see the *Ling* [*shu*] treatise] "Jiu zhen shi er yuan" 九鍼十二原.

(4) *Hua Shou:* *Ying* 迎 ("to move against") means to proceed toward what is ahead. *Sui* 隨 ("to follow") means to follow toward what is behind.

(4)–(5) *Xu Dachun:* The words "child" and "mother" used here refer to the [sequences of mutual] generation and destruction of the Five Phases as applied to the well and rapids [holes] on a particular conduit. They do not, as in the discussion of difficult issue 75, refer to "child" and "mother" among the five long-term depots. In the text of the [*Nei*] *jing*, *ying* 迎 ("to move against") and *sui* 隨 ("to follow") refer to the application of a needle contrary to or in accordance with the flow of the qi in the conduits. The withdrawal and the insertion of the needle in accordance with exhalation and inhalation of qi, and also the direction into which the needle is pointed, determine whether one supplements or drains. The patterns outlined in both [the *Su wen* and the *Ling shu* books of the *Nei*] *jing* are truly complete. Here, needling at the hole at which the qi arrive is called "to move against" and "to drain," while needling at the hole from which the qi departed is called "to follow" and "to supplement." Hence, where the text of the [*Nei*] *jing* considers the [needling] contrary to or in accordance with [the flow of the qi] as "moving against" or "following," here [in the present difficult issue, the needling of] the holes in front or behind the basic hole [associated with the disease] is considered as "moving against" and "following." The underlying concepts are certainly very close but the patterns are different in each case.

(6) *Yu Shu:* In the case of a disease in the heart, one drains at the rapids [hole] of the hand heart ruler [conduit] because it is a rule that the heart receives no disease. That which receives a disease is the heart enclosing network. The hand heart ruler [conduit] is the hand ceasing yin[conduit associated with] the heart enclosing network. The rapids [hole] on the [conduit associated with the heart] enclosing network is [associated with the] soil. The heart is [associated with] fire. The soil is the child of fire. Therefore, draining this rapids [hole] means draining the child. *Ying* 迎 ("to move against") means *qu qi* 取氣 ("to remove qi"). *Duo* 奪 ("to withdraw") means *xie qi* 瀉氣 ("to drain qi").

(7) *Yu Shu:* The heart is fire; the well [hole] is wood. When, in the present case, one supplements at the well [hole] of the [hand] heart ruler, that means that one supplements the mother. Wood is the mother of fire. *Sui* 隨 ("to follow") means

"to remove qi from the [section of the] guard [qi]." *Ji* 濟 ("to provide support") means "to supplement a conduit that does not have enough [qi]".

(8) *Yu Shu*: "Firmness" and "softness" refer to depletion and repletion.

(1)–(9) *Ding Deyong*: If [one of] the five long-term depots is depleted, supplement its mother. That is meant by "providing support [to qi] following [their proper course]." In the case of repletion, drain the respective child. That is meant by "withdrawing [qi] moving against [their proper course]." Thus, if one wishes to perform a supplementing or a draining, he must first diagnose the vessels of the five long-term depots. If the qi at the hole to be pierced arrive firmly and replete, they can be drained. If they come depleted and softly, they can be supplemented. If someone takes a needle and does not know about firmness and softness, [how could he perform a treatment resulting in] gain or loss?

(8)–(9) *Xu Dachun*: The [treatise] "Xiao zhen jie" 小針解 of the *Ling* [*shu*] states: "It is said: 'Repletion and depletion resemble having and not having.' That is to say, In the case of repletion, qi are present; in the case of depletion, qi are absent. [It is said further: 'The treatments of] depletion and repletion resemble a gain or a loss [respectively].' That is to say, supplementing must lead to significant gains; draining must lead to extreme loss." The sentence with [the words] *you* 有 ("to have") and *wu* 無 ("not to have") refers, first of all, to the [presence or absence of] qi. The sentence with [the words] *de* 得 ("gain") and *shi* 失 ("loss") refers to the application of needles. [The presence or absence of qi and the application of needles] are, in fact, two different concepts. Here [in the *Nan jing*,] the text of the [*Nei*] *jing* is quoted and explained but the text of the [*Nei*] *jing* has been altered. The words are reiterated but their meaning is difficult to comprehend. That is the reason why they have never been well interpreted.

八十難曰：（一）經言有見如入，有見如出者，何謂也？
（二）然：所謂有見如入者，謂左手見氣來至，乃內針；（三）針入見氣盡，
乃出針。是謂有見如入，有見如出也。

The eightieth difficult issue: (1) The scripture states: When it is apparent, then insert; when it is apparent, then withdraw. What does that mean?

(2) It is like this. The statement "when it is apparent, then insert" means that as soon as one [notices] with his left hand that the qi appear, he inserts the needle. (3) When the needle is inserted and when it is apparent that the qi have left completely, then he withdraws the needle. That is [what is] meant by "when it is apparent, then insert; when it is apparent, then withdraw."[1]

COMMENTARIES

(1) *Xu Dachun*: The text of the [*Nei*] *jing* contains no [corresponding passage] that could be analysed [in comparison with] these two sentences.

Liao Ping: The present difficult issue [outlines] the pattern that one must wait for the qi [to come if one intends] to apply needling or cauterization. Why would [the *Nan jing*] employ [in this context] terms like "coming," "leaving," "arrival," and "stopping" that were used earlier [in this book in the context of] investigating the vessels at the inch opening?

(1)–(3) *Ding Deyong*: If one wishes to pierce a person, he first waits with his left hand for the qi in the respective hole. As soon as the qi arrive, he inserts the needle. He waits until the qi have [passed the hole] completely and withdraws the needle again. The hole [pierced here] is not [a child or mother hole] at which one drains or supplements [in cases of qi] moving against or following [their proper course]. The present pattern is to be applied [in situations] which are – [as the *Nan jing* has] stated [earlier][2] – neither a depletion nor a repletion but [cases where a disease] is to be removed from the respective conduit itself.

(2) *Hua Shou*: Below the statement *yu xian ru ru* 有見如入 ("when it is apparent, then insert"), the four characters *yu xian ru chu* 有見如出 ("when it is apparent, then withdraw") must be missing. *Ru* 如 should be read here like *er* 而 ("then"). Mengzi wrote: "Watch the road as if (*er* 而) you had never seen it before." Here the word *er* is to be read like *ru*. The two were used with identical [meanings].

---

1 In Katō Bankei's edition, the text of the present difficult issue is combined with that of the seventy-fourth issue to form difficult issue 78.

2 See difficult issue 69.

(1)–(3) *Zhang Shixian*: Skillful needling requires that the application[3] [of the nee-
dle] follows the [movement of the] qi. Whenever one wishes to insert the needle he must first press with his left hand the location to be needled. Then he
must squeeze it with the fingernail [of his right hand] until it swells. In this way,
he causes qi to arrive at the place to be needled, [and the feeling he has below his
fingers] is the same as [that at one of the usual locations where] the movement
[in the] vessels [can be perceived]. Then he begins to insert the needle. He waits
until the qi have [left again] entirely and withdraws the needle afterwards. [The
statement] "until the qi have [left again] entirely" corresponds to the point made
in the *Ling shu* that [it is harmful] to replenish if one has already supplemented
and to deplete if one has already drained.[4] The character *ru* stands for *er*.

(3) *Xu Dachun*: *Qi jin* 氣盡 ("the qi have left completely") means that the qi have
come and then have dispersed again.

(1)–(3) *Ye Lin*: This [paragraph] states that for withdrawing or inserting the needle
one must observe whether the qi have already arrived and whether they have
already left. Only then may one withdraw or insert [the needle].

(2) *Liao Ping*: When the qi arrive, one cannot withdraw the needle; when the qi
have left, one must quickly withdraw the needle and should not let it remain
[in the hole].

---

3   The text has *san* 散 ("to disperse"), but the legend to the graph added to the text in Zhang
    Shixian's edition has *shi* 施 ("to apply").

4   See difficult issue 81.

八十一難曰：（一）經言無實實虛虛，損不足而益有餘，（二）是寸口脈耶？（三）將病自有虛實耶？（四）其損益奈何？

（五）然：是病，非謂寸口脈也。（六）謂病自有實虛也。（七）假令肝實而肺虛，肝者木也，肺者金也，金木當更相平，當知金平木。（八）假令肺實而肝虛，微少氣，用針不瀉其肝，而反重實其肺，故曰實實虛虛，損不足而益有餘，（九）此者中工之要害也。

The eighty-first difficult issue: (1) The scripture states: Do not replenish a repletion or deplete a depletion – [that is, do not] weaken what is insufficient [already, and do not] add to any existing surfeit. (2) Does that concern [a misinterpretation of the movement that is felt at] the inch opening [section of the] vessels? (3) Or [does that refer to] diseases resulting from [an incorrect treatment of] depletions and repletions? (4) "To weaken" and "to add," what does that mean?

(5) It is like this. [The statement quoted] refers to diseases [resulting from malpractice]; it does not refer to [a misinterpretation of the movement that is felt at] the inch opening [section of the] vessels. (6) The diseases referred to are those resulting from [an incorrect treatment of cases of] depletion or repletion. (7) Take for example a repletion in the liver and a depletion in the lung. The liver is [associated with] wood; the lung is [associated with] metal. Metal and wood should level each other, and one should know how to level the [repletion in the liver, which is associated with the] wood, by [employing the functions of the lung, which is associated with the] metal. (8) Take, as another example, a repletion in the lung and a depletion in the liver. [The latter has] very few qi. [If, in this case, a practitioner] employs the needle not to supplement the liver but to even further increase the repletion of the lung, one could, consequently, speak of a "replenishing of a repletion" and of a "depleting a depletion," or of a "weakening of what is [already] insufficient" and of an "adding to an existing surfeit." (9) Mediocre practitioners committing such [mistakes] cause serious damage.[1]

---

1 Various authors have combined this difficult issue with the text of issue 12 to form one paragraph. Huang Weisan explained this as follows: "The former paragraph [i.e., difficult issue 12] discusses [a situation] where the physician does not understand whether the appearance of the [movement in the] vessels indicates a depletion or a repletion. [Hence] he commits mistakes when he applies the methods of supplementing or draining. The latter paragraph [i.e., difficult issue 81] discusses [a situation] where the physician does not investigate whether a disease manifests itself as a depletion or as a repletion. [Hence] he commits mistakes when he applies the methods of supplementing or draining. As a result, he will cause minor afflictions to turn serious and serious afflictions to end in death." (See Huang Weisan, 1969, 122.) The passage *sun bu zu er yi you yu* 損不足而益有餘 in sentence 1 is quoted from *Ling shu* treatise 1 "Jiu zhen shi er yuan 九針十二原."

(1) *Xu Dachun*: That is to say, one supplements in the case of a repletion where a draining is required, or one drains in the case of a depletion where a supplementation is required – that is, one weakens what is already insufficient, or one adds to an existing surfeit. All of these [approaches] represent malpractice. For the [corresponding] text in the [*Nei*] *jing*, see the *Ling* [*shu*] treatise "Jiu zhen shi er yuan" 九針十二原.

　Liao Ping: The text of the [*Nei*] *jing* was originally very clear. As soon as it was incorporated into the present book, it became confusing and misleading.

(2)–(3) *Xu Dachun*: That is to say, [the person] posing these questions did not know whether "depletion" and "repletion" refer, in this context, to the [movement in the] vessels or to diseases.

(2) *Liao Ping*: This entire book was written with the single purpose of developing this one sentence. Hence the inch opening is the most important [concept] from the beginning to the end [of the *Nan jing*].

(2)–(3) *Liao Ping*: The meaning of these two sentences is incomprehensible.

(5) *Hua Shou*: The two characters *shi bing* 是病 ("refers to diseases") are a mistake; they have been added [by people in later times. In a situation where] the liver is replete while the lung is depleted, the metal should level the wood. That [pattern] parallels what was said in the discussion of the seventy-fifth difficult issue. If the lung has a repletion while the liver is depleted, one must curb the metal and support the wood. If, however, by applying the needles one does not supplement the liver but, on the contrary, adds further repletion to the lung, that is "replenishing of a repletion and depleting of a depletion." This kind of weakening of what is [already] insufficient and this kind of adding to an existing surfeit will inevitably kill the patient. *Zhong gong* 中工 ("mediocre practitioner") refers to *zhong chang zhi gong* 中常之工 ("ordinary practitioner"); one could also say *cu gong* 粗工 ("unskilled practitioner").

(7) *Xu Dachun*: For details, see difficult issue 75.

　Liao Ping: The *Nei jing* says the same thing in different words. It was not necessary to tie these [ideas] to the Five Phases.

(9) *Ding Deyong*: *Zhong* 中 ("mediocre," also "to strike") stands for *shang* 傷 ("to injure"). That is to say, a practitioner with inadequate training does not know about hardness and softness of the five long-term depots.[2] His application of needles or drugs is marked by mistakes. Therefore he contributes to even greater damage.

2　See difficult issue 10.

Yang: A superior practitioner treats what is not yet ill; he knows the sources of depletion and repletion. Hence, when he supplements or drains, he applies what is appropriate. The mediocre practitioner has not yet penetrated to the foundations of the transmission of diseases. When he treats he will add even further damage.

Xu Dachun: "Damage" means not only that he is unable to cure these diseases but also that he, contrary [to what is expected from him], causes damage to the people [treated by him].

(5) *Liao Ping*: This sentence, too, is incomprehensible. How can diseases be compared with the inch opening?

APPENDICES

Appendix A

Survey of Commentated *Nan jing* Editions by Chinese Authors from the Third through Twentieth Century

Title	Alternative title(s)	Author(s) / editor(s)	Date of compilation/ publication	Number of *juan*	Text lost (0) or extant (+)
Huang Di zhong nan jing 黃帝眾難經	Nan jing zhu jie 難經注解 Zhu zhong nan jing 註眾難經	Lü Guang(-wang) 呂廣王 Lü Bowang 呂博望	3rd century	1 (2)	+
Nan jing zhu shi 難經注釋	Ji zhu nan jing 集註難經 Nan jing zhu jie 難經注解 Huang Di ba shi yi nan jing zhu 黃帝八十一難經註 Huang Di ba shi yi nan jing 黃帝八十一難經	Yang Xuancao 楊玄操	7th/8th century	13 (5, 1)	+
Ba shi yi nan yin yi 八十一難音義		Yang Xuancao 楊玄操	7th/8th century	?	0

Title	Alternative title(s)	Author(s) / editor(s)	Date of compilation/ publication	Number of *juan*	Text lost (0) or extant (+)
Tian sheng jiao ding Nan jing 天聖校定難經		Chao Zongque 晁宗愨 Wang Juzheng 王舉正 Wang Weiyi (?) 王惟一	1026-1031	?	0
Nan jing bu zhu 難經補注	Bu zhu Nan jing 補注難經	Ding Deyong 丁德用	1062	2 (5)	+
Nan jing zhu 難經注	Yu Shu zhu Nan jing 虞庶注難經	Yu Shu 虞庶	1067	5	+
Zhu jie Nan jing 註解難經		Yang Kanghou 楊康侯	1098	?	+
(Nan jing) yin shi 難經音釋		Shi Youliang 石友諒	Song	?	+
Nan jing bian zheng shi yi 難經辨正釋疑	Bian Que ba shi yi nan jing bian zheng tiao li 扁鵲八十一難經辨正條例條例	Zhou Yuquan 周與權	Song	1	+
Liu shi Nan jing jie 劉氏難經解		Liu 劉	Song	?	0
Nan jing shu 難經疏		Gao Chengde 高承德	Song	?	0

Title	Alternative title(s)	Author(s) / editor(s)	Date of compilation/ publication	Number of *juan*	Text lost (0) or extant (+)
Nan jing shu 難經疏		Hou Ziran 侯自然	Song	13	0
Nan jing shu 難經疏		??	Song	1	+
Nan jing shu yi 難經疏義		Wang Zongzheng 王宗正	12th century	2	0
Nan jing jie yi 難經解義	Nan jing bian 難經辨 / Nan jing jie 難經解	Pang Anshi 龐安時	11th century		0
Ji zhu Nan jing 集註難經		Ji Tianxi 紀天錫	12th century	3 (5)	+
Yao zhu Nan jing 藥註難經	Zhang Jie gu zhu Nan jing 張潔古註難經	Zhang Yuansu 張元素	12th century	?	0
Wang Hanlin ji zhu Huang Di ba shi yi Nan jing 王翰林集註黃帝八十一難經	Ji zhu ba shi yi Nan jing 集註八十一難經 / Nan jing ji zhu 難經集註	Li Yuanli 李元立	12th/13th century	13 (5)	+

Title	Alternative title(s)	Author(s) / editor(s)	Date of compilation/ publication	Number of juan	Text lost (0) or extant (+)
Huang Di ba shi yi Nan jing zuan tu ju jie 黃帝八十一難經纂圖句解	Nan jing ju jie 難經句解 Tu zhu Nan jing 圖註難經 Nan jing tu jie 難經圖解	Li Jiong 李駧	1269	1 (4, 7, 8)	+
Nan jing zhu 難經註		Feng Jie 馮玠	Song	?	0
Huang Di ba shi yi Nan jing zhu shi 黃帝八十一難經注釋		Song Tingchen 宋庭臣	Song	1	0
Nan jing zhu 難經注		Xie Fugu 謝復古	Song	?	0
Nan jing ben yi 難經本義	Bian Que Nan jing 扁鵲難經	Hua Shou 滑壽	1361	2	+
Nan jing bian yi 難經辯疑		Chen Ruisun 陳瑞隆 Chen Zhaizhi 陳宅之	Yuan	?	0
Nan jing ben zhi 難經本旨		Yuan Kunhou 袁坤厚	Yuan	?	0

Title	Alternative title(s)	Author(s) / editor(s)	Date of compilation/ publication	Number of juan	Text lost (0) or extant (+)
Nan jing shuo 難經說		Xie Jinsun 謝縉孫	14th century	?	+
Ba shi yi Nan jing jing luo jie 八十一難經經絡解		Xiong Zongli 熊宗立	ca. 1446	?	+
Wu ting zi su jie ba shi yi Nan jing 勿聽子俗解八十一難經		Xiong Zongli 熊宗立	1446	6	+
Tu zhu ba shi yi Nan jing 圖註八十一難經	Tu zhu ba shi yi Nan jing bian zhen 圖註八十一難經辨真	Zhang Shixian 張世賢	1510	8 (4)	+
Qie Wang shi mi chuan tu zhu ba shi yi Nan jing ping lin jie jing tong zong 鍥王氏秘傳圖註八十一難經評林捷徑統宗	Tu zhu ba shi yi Nan jing ping lin jie jing tong zong 圖註八十一難經評林捷徑統宗	Wang Wenjie 王文潔	ca. 1510	6	+
Ba shi yi Nan jing tu jie 八十一難經圖解		Nie Shangheng 聶尚恒	ca. 1612	2	+
Nan jing fu shuo 難經附說		Lü Fu 呂復	Ming	?	0
Nan jing zheng yi 難經正義		Ma Shi 馬蒔	Ming	?	?

Title	Alternative title(s)	Author(s) / editor(s)	Date of compilation/ publication	Number of juan	Text lost (0) or extant (+)
Nan jing jian shi 難經箋釋		Huang Yuan 黃淵	Ming	?	?
Nan jing kao wu 難經考誤		Yao Jun 姚濬	Ming	?	?
Nan jing bu zhu 難經補註		Xu Shu 徐述	Ming	?	?
Nan jing zhi jie 難經直解		Mo Xi 莫熺	1669	2	+
Bian Que Nan jing 扁鵲難經		??	1723	2	+
Nan jing jing shi 難經經釋		Xu Dachun 徐大椿	1727	2	+
Nan jing ben yi zhai zhu 難經本義摘註		Guo Daming 享大銘	1734	2	+
Gu ben Nan jing chan zhu 古本難經闡註		Ding Jin 丁錦	1736	2	+
Yue ren Nan jing zhen ben shuo yue 越人難經真本說約		Shen Dezu 沈德祖	1739	2	+
Nan jing xuan jie 難經選解		Huang Yuanyu 黃元御	1756	2	+

Title	Alternative title(s)	Author(s) / editor(s)	Date of compilation/ publication	Number of *juan*	Text lost (0) or extant (+)
Bian Que mai shu nan jing 扁鵲脈書難經		Xiong Qinghu 熊慶笏	1817	6	+
Nan jing jie 難經解		Zou Hanhuang 鄒漢璜	1840	?	+
Nan jing zhai chao 難經摘抄		Wang Tingjun 王廷俊	1867	?	+
Nan jing xi jie 難經晰解		Yuan Chongyi 袁崇毅	ca. 1875	2	+
Nan jing qi meng 難經啓蒙		Gong Naijiang 龔迺疆	Qing	2	+
Nan jing zheng yi 難經正義		Ye Lin 棐霖	1895	6	+
Nan jing bi ji 難經筆記		Ren Xigeng 任錫庚	ca. 1910	2	+
Zhu Nan jing 註難經		Dai Zhen 戴震	Qing		?
Chun qiu ben Nan jing shu 春秋本難經疏		Tang Ganqing 唐干頃	Qing		?
Nei Nan yao yu 內難要語		Tang Bingjun 唐秉鈞	Qing		?
Nan jing jing shi bu zheng 難經經釋補証		Liao Ping 廖平	1913	1	+

Title	Alternative title(s)	Author(s) / editor(s)	Date of compilation/ publication	Number of juan	Text lost (0) or extant (+)
Nan jing bian zheng 難經編正		Si Shuping 司樹屏			+
Nan jing hui zhu jian zheng 難經匯註箋正		Zhang Shouyi 張壽頤	1923	4	+
Nan jing zhang ju 難經章句		Sun Dingyi 孫鼎宜	1932	3 + 1	+
Nan jing ji yi 難經集義		Wu Baoshen 吳保神			+
Nan jing zhu lun 難經註論		Wu Qinchai 吳琴儕			+
Nan jing du ben 難經讀本		Wang Yiren 王一仁	I 1936		+
Nan jing 難經		Cai Luxian 蔡陸仙	1936	2	+
Nan jing cong kao 難經叢考		Zhang Ji 張驥	1938		+
Nan jing mi jie jiang yi 難經秘解講義		Meng Shichen 孟世忱	ca. 1948		+
Nan jing hui tong 難經會通		Huang Weihan 黄維翰	1948	1	+

Title	Alternative title(s)	Author(s) / editor(s)	Date of compilation/ publication	Number of *juan*	Text lost (0) or extant (+)
Nan jing yi shi 难经译释		Nan jing zhong yi xue yuan 南京中医学院	1962	6	+
Nan jing zhi yao 難經知要		Huang Weisan 黄稚三	1967	6	+
Nan jing jin shi 难经今释		Tang Xiangqing 唐湘清	1968	6	+
Nei Nan jing xuan shi 内难经选释		Yen Hongchen 闾洪臣 Gao Guangzhen 高光振	1979	6	+
Nan jing benyi 难经本义		Chen Sanbao 陈三宝	1979	6	+
Nan jing ben yi jie shuo 难经本义解说		Yang Guofan 杨国藩	1981	6	+
Nan jing ben yi 难经本义		Zhang Gaoming 张高铭	1982	1	+
Nan jing ben yi 难经本义		Li Yude 李育德	1982		+
Nan jing ben yi xin bian xin yi 难经本义新编新译		Huang Sanyuan 黄三元	1983	2	+

Title	Alternative title(s)	Author(s) / editor(s)	Date of compilation/ publication	Number of *juan*	Text lost (0) or extant (+)
Nan jing editions of unclear date					
Nan jing guang shuo 難經廣說		Wu Sanzhong 五三重			+
Nan jing bian shi 難經辨釋		??			
Nan jing zhong xuan 難經重玄		Wang Shaoqing 王少卿			0
Qin Yue ren Nan jing jian jin 秦越人難經剪錦		Shi Lin 施麟			+
Nan jing zhi jie 難經直解		Zhang Jinggao 張景皋			?

Appendix B

Chinese Twentieth-Century Essays on the Nan jing

Qin Bowei 秦伯未
"*Nan jing* zhi yan jiu" 難經之研究
Zhong guo yi xue yuan yuan kan 6 (1928) 中國醫學院院刊

Yang Yehe 楊野鶴
"*Nan jing yin Neijing wen you Nei jing suo bu zai kao*" 難經引內經文有內經所
不載考
Yi lin yi ngo 9 *(1931)* 醫林一諤

Wei Yuan 衛原
"*Nan jing* zhi zhen wei" 難經之真僞
Zhong yi xin sheng ming 10 (1935) 中醫新生命

Wei Juxian 衛聚賢
"Bian Que de yi shu lai zi Yin du" 扁鵲的醫書來自
印度
Xin zhong yi kan 5 (1939) 新中醫刊

Lu Juefei 盧覺非
"Bian Que yi shu lai zi Yin du zhi yi" 扁鵲的醫書來自印度質疑
Hua xi yi yao za zhi 8 (1947) 華西醫藥雜誌

Yi Siqiu 易斯秋
"*Nan jing* zhang ju yu yi" 難經章句語譯
Xin zhong yi yao 7/8/11/12 (1956) 新中医药

Zong Fen 宗分
"Bian Que yu *Nan jing*" 扁鵲与难经
Jian kang bao 12 (1957) 健康报

Fan Xingzhun 范行准
"*Huang di zhong Nan jing zhu, Yu kui zhen jing* zuo zhe Lü Guang de nian dai
wen ti" 黄帝众难经注玉匮针经作者吕广的年代问题
Shang hai zhong yi yao za zhi 10 (1957) : 32- 35 上海中医药杂志

He Aihua 何爱华
  "Wo dui *Nan jing* zhu zuo nian dai wen ti de shang que" 我对难经著作年代问题的商榷
  Shang hai zhong yi yao za zhi 4 (1958): 41-42 上海中医药杂志

Zhao Shanshan 赵善山
  "Dui *Nan jing* mu shi jin xu bu huo bu shui fa wen ti de tan tao" 对难经木实金虚补火补水法问题的探讨
  Guang dong zhong yi 2 (1960) 广东中医

He Aihua 何爱华
  "Guan yu *Nan jing* de ji ge wen ti" 关于难经的几个问题
  Ren min bao jian 2 (1960): 67-170 人民保健

He Aihua 何爱华
  "Guan yu *Nan jing* de bian ci wen ti" 关于难经的篇次问题
  Ha er bin zhong yi 8 (1965): 41-43 哈尔滨中医

Xiao Gong 肖珙
  "*Nei jing, Nan jing* zhong shi er jing mai yu shi yi jing mai xue shuo de bing cun" 内经难经中十二经脉于十一经脉学说的并存
  Shan dong zhong yi xue yuan xue bao 3 (1980) 山东中医学院学报

Shi Bingsheng 史冰生
  "*Nan jing* si fang zang qi xu shi bu xie fa chu tan" 难经四方脏器虚实补泻法初探
  Zhe jiang zhong yi za zhi 9 (1980) 浙江中医杂志

Gao Hesheng 高和声
  "*Nan jing* 'qi xing chuan xi' ju kao" 难经蚑行喘息句考
  Zhe jiang zhong yi xue yuan xue bao 4 (1981) 浙江中医学院学报

Jiang Wenzhao 蒋文照
  "*Nan jing* xuan shi" 难经选释
  Zhe jiang zhong yi xue yuan xue bao 4 (1981) 浙江中医学院学报

Song Zhixing 宋知行
  "*Nan jing* 'sheng qi zhi yuan' tan yuan qi yu qi jing guan xi" 难经生气之原谈元气与奇经关系
  Zhe jiang zhong yi xue yuan xue bao 4 (1981) 浙江中医学院学报

Feng Heming et al. 冯鹤鸣
  "*Nan jing* xuan shi" 难经选释
  Zhe jiang zhong yi xue yuan xue bao 6 (1981) 浙江中医学院学报

Ye Deming 叶德铭
  "*Nan jing* xuan shi" 难经选释
  Zhe jiang zhong yi xue yuan xue bao 6 (1981) 浙江中医学院学报

Fang Yaozhong 方药中
"Lüe tan dui *Nan jing* yin yang mai de li jie he yun yong" 略谈对难经阴阳脉的理解和运用
Zhe jiang zhong yi za zhi 16 (1981):488 浙江中医雜誌

Sun Runzhai et al. 孙润斋
"Bian Que yu *Nan jing* (Chong du *Nan jing* you gan)"
扁鹊与难经。重读难经有感
Xing tai zhong yi jing yan xuan bian 1 (1982) 邢台中医经验选编

Cheng Hongru 程鸿儒
"Man tan Qin Yue ren yu *Nan jing*" 漫谈秦越人与难经
Zhong hua yi shi za zhi 12 (1982): 147-149 中华医史杂志

Jiang Chunhua 姜春华
"Lüe lun *Nan jing*" 略论难经
Xin zhong yi 12 (1982) 新中医

Liu Guanjun 刘冠军
"Lüe lun *Nan jing* dui zhen jiu xue di gong xian" 略论难经对针灸学的贡献
Zhong yi za zhi 4 (1983) 中医杂志

Liu Guanjun 刘冠军
"*Nan jing* wu shu ci" 难经五输刺
Xing lin zhong yi yao 3 (1984) 杏林中医药

N.N.
"*Nan jing, Nan jing ben yi, Lei jing* jie shao" 难经难经本义类经介绍
Zhong yi za zhi 6 (1984) 中医杂志

N.N.
"*Nan jing* wu ji bing ji qian tan" 难经五积病機浅谈
Hei long jiang yi yao 3 (1984) 黑龙江医药

N.N.
"*Nei, Nan* shi ti da an" 内难试题答案
Jiang su zhong yi 3 (1984) 江苏中医

Appendix C

Commented *Nan jing* Editions by Japanese Authors in the Takeda and Fujikawa Libraries, as well as Lost Titles of Past Centuries

1. Dated manuscripts and publications

Title	Author	Date of Manuscript	Date of Publication	Text lost (o) or extant (+)
Nan-gyō-un-an-snō 難經雲庵抄	Sō Ippaku (Un'an) 僧一柏雲庵	1559		+
Nan-gyō-hō-an-shō 難經蓬庵抄	Sō Dōki 僧道器	1560		+
Nan-gyō-non-gi-shō 難經本義抄.	Jutokuan Gen'yū 壽德庵玄由		1629	+
Nan-gyō-shō-kei 難經捷徑	Jutokuan Gen'yū 壽德庵玄由		1637	+
Nan-gyō-hon-gi-seki-i (alt. title: Nan-gyō-seki-i) 難經本義摭遺 難經摭遺	Teichikusō Gensetsu 貞竹叟玄節		1659	+
Nan-gyō-chū-so 難經註疏	Nagoya Gen'i 名古屋玄医		1684	+

Title	Author	Date of Manuscript	Date of Publication	Text lost (o) or extant (+)
Nan-gyō-hon-gi-shō (alt. title: Nan-gyō-hon-gi-tai-shō) 難經本義鈔 難經本義大鈔	Morimoto Genkan 森本玄閑		1695	+
Nan-gyō-hon-gi-gen-kai 難經本義諺解	Okamoto Ichiku 岡本爲竹		1706	+
Nan-gyō-waku-mon 難經惑問	Furubayashi Kengi 古林見宜	1711	1715	+
Nan-gyō-shichi-jū-go-na-no-kai 難經七十五難之解	Kazuki Gozan 香月牛山	1712		+
Nan-gyō-hon-gi-bi-kō 難經本義備考	Kazuki Gozan 香月牛山	1714		+
Nan-gyō-kei-setsu-ki 難經螢雪解	Keikosai Ikkoho 鷄口齋一壺父	1719		+
Nan-gyō-mon-ku 難經文句	Katō Hiroaki 加藤啓明	1735		o
Nan-gyō-ku-mon-ku-den-shō 難經口問口伝鈔	Nanri-sensei 南里先生	1738		+
Nan-gyō-tatsu-gen 難經達言	Takamiya Tei 高宮貞		1749	+
Nan-gyō-tetsu-kagami 難經鐵鑑	Hirooka Sosen 廣岡蘇仙		1750	+
Nan-gyō-chi-shin-ron 難經知新論	Aoki Zen'an 菁木善庵	1761		o

Title	Author	Date of Manuscript	Date of Publication	Text lost (o) or extant (+)
Nan-gyō-hi 難經祕		1762		+
Nan-gyō-hatsu-bi-shō-gen 難經發微小言	Banri 万里	1766		+
Nan-gyō-ko-gi 難經古義	Katō Bankei 加藤萬卿		1773	+
Nan-gyō-hak-ki 難經發揮	Sugai Kuratsune 菅井倉常		1778	+
Nan-gyō 難經	Matsui Zaian 松井村庵		1781	+
Nan-gyō-so-sho 難經疏證	Tamba Genkan 丹波元胤 (alias Taki Mototane 多紀元胤)		1819	+
Nan-gyō-ki-bun 難經記聞	Tachibana Koshō 橘虎口肅	1827		+
Nan-gyō-in-go-zu-kai 難經韵語圖解	Okada Seian 岡田靜安		1834	+
Nan-gyō-mon-ji-kō 難經文字攷	Ito Kaoru 伊藤馨	1857		+
Nan-gyō-wa-yaku 難經和譯	Kishihara Kotarō 岸原鴻太郎		1939	+

2. Undated manuscripts and prints

Title	Author	Date of Manuscript	Date of Publication	Text lost (o) or extant (+)
Nan-gyō-kai-dai 難經解題	Taki Motohiro 多紀元簡			+
Nan-gyō-chū-kai 難經注解				+
Nan-gyō-kai-i 難經開委	Izumo Hirosada 出雲広貞			o
Nan-gyō-shō-kai 難經小解				+
Nan-gyō-gen-kō 難經原好	Kanda Gensen 神田玄仙			o
Nan-gyō-ko 難經考	Yūi-sensei 由頤先生			+
Nan-gyō-katsu-gi-ho-sei 難經滑義補正	Sugimoto Ryō 杉本良			+
Nan-gyō-kan-ki-sei-gi 難經管窺精義				+
Nan-gyō-gai-den 難經外伝	Ebi Koreyoshi 蝦惟義			o
Nan-gyō-ben-chū 難經辨注	Miura Ranhan 三浦蘭阪			o

Title	Author	Date of Manuscript	Date of Publication	Text lost (o) or extant (+)
Nan-gyō-hon-gi-shu-sho 難經本義首書	Nagoya Gen'i 名古屋玄医			o
Nan-gyō-shin-chu 難經新註	Tezuka Gentsū 手塚玄通			o
Nan-gyō-hon-gi-zu-kai 難經本義図解				+
Nan-gyō-zu-setsu 難經図説				+
Nan-gyō-zu-yō 難經図要				+
Nan-gyō-sei-mon 難經正文	Miura Ranhan 三浦蘭阪			o
Nan-gyō-so-heki 難經蒼璧				+
Nan-gyō-shō 難經抄	Matsushita Kenrin 松下見林			+
Nan-gyō-hon-gi-wa-kai-shaku 難經本義和解釋	Asada Kazue 淺田賈壽衛			+
Nan-gyō-ji-kai 難經自解	Mori Dokuyū 守獨有			+
Nan-gyō-hon-gi-jo-kō-roku 難經本義序講錄	Miura Dōsai 三浦道齋			+

Title	Author	Date of Manuscript	Date of Publication	Text lost (o) or extant (+)
Nan-gyō-son-gi-kō-hon (alt. title: Nan-gyō-hon-gi) 難經存疑稿本 難經本義	Dodo Tō 百夕鯛			+
Nan-gyō-chū-so 難經註疏	Yoshida Sōjun 吉田宗恂			o
Nan-gyō-hon-gi-ki-bun 難經本義記聞	Asai Shūhaku 淺井周伯			+
Hachi-jū-ichi-nan-gyō-sei-gi 八十一難經精義	Ebi Koreyoshi 蝦惟義			o
Ko-tei-hachi-ju-ichi-nan-gyō-gu-toku 黃帝八十一難經愚得	Hattori Ryō 服部良			+
Ko-tei-hachi-ju-ichi-nan-gyō-shu-shaku-bi-kō 黃帝八十一難經輯釋備考	Kiyokawa Gai 清川豈			+

Appendix D

Zhang Zhixian's Graphs
Depicting the Eighty-One Difficult Issues (1510)

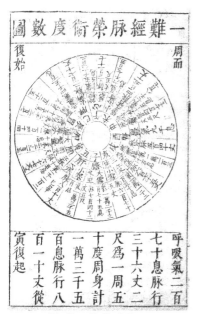

The First Difficult Issue

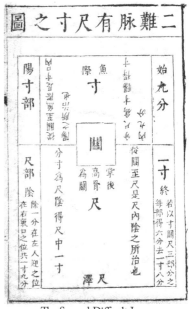

The Second Difficult Issue

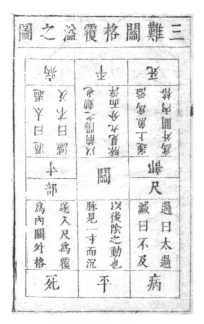

The Third Difficult Issue

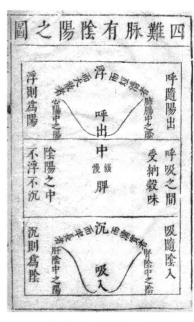

The Fourth Difficult Issue

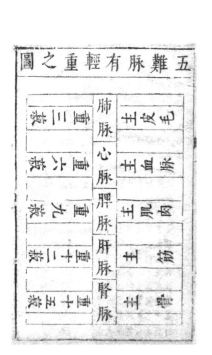

The Fifth Difficult Issue

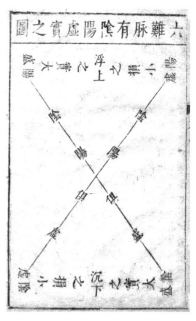

The Sixth Difficult Issue

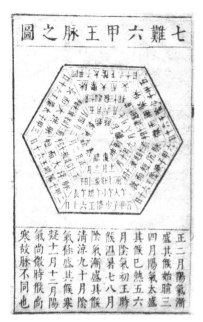

The Seventh Difficult Issue

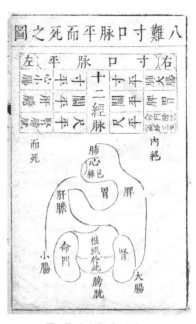

The Eighth Difficult Issue

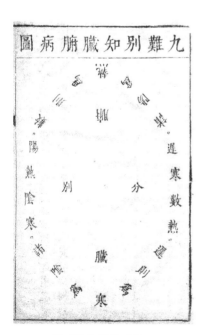

The Ninth Difficult Issue

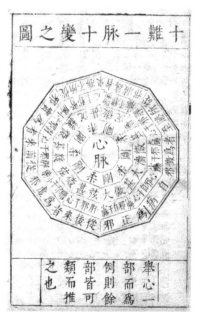

The Tenth Difficult Issue

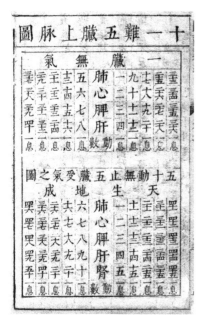

The Eleventh Difficult Issue

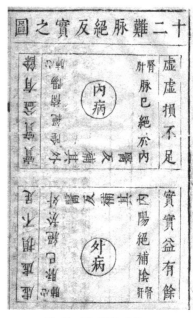

The Twelfth Difficult Issue

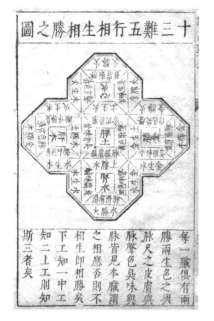

The Thirteenth Difficult Issue

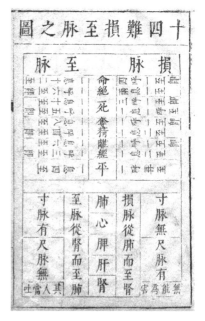

The Fourteenth Difficult Issue

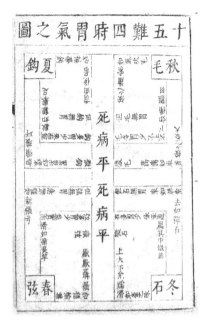

The Fifteenth Difficult Issue

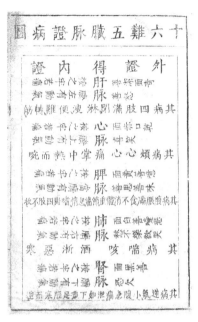

The Sixteenth Difficult Issue

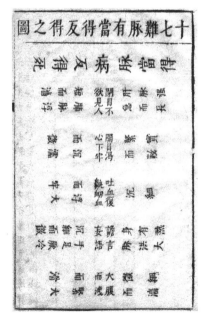

The Seventeenth Difficult Issue

The Eighteenth Difficult Issue

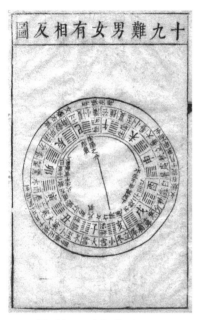

The Ninteenth Difficult Issue

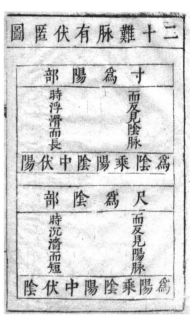

The Twentieth Difficult Issue

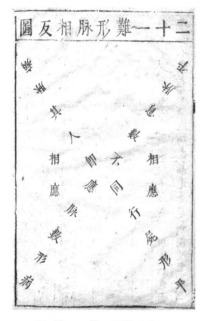

The Twenty-First Difficult Issue

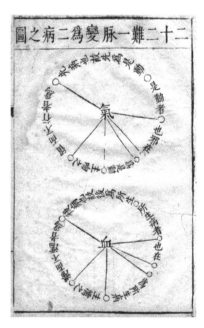

The Twenty-Second Difficult Issue

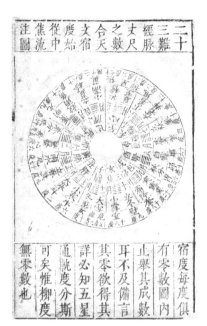

The Twenty-Third Difficult Issue

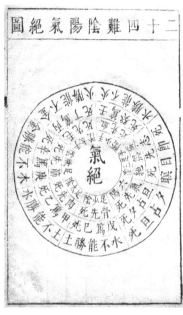

The Twenty-Fourth Difficult Issue

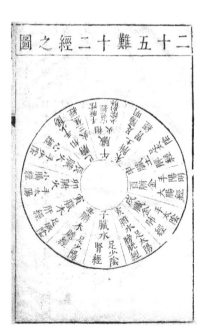

The Twenty-Fifth Difficult Issue

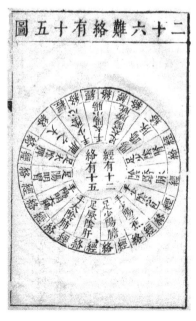

The Twenty-Sixth Difficult Issue

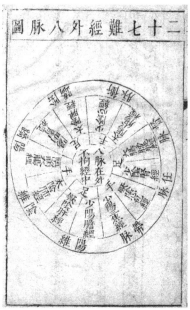

The Twenty-Seventh Difficult Issue

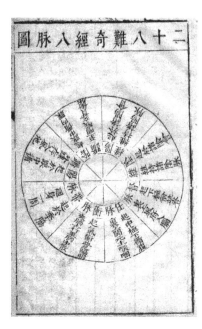

The Twenty-Eighth Difficult Issue

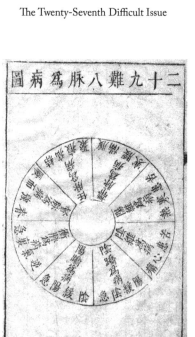

The Twenty-Ninth Difficult Issue

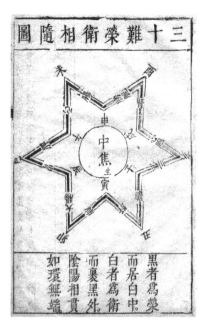

The Thirtieth Difficult Issue

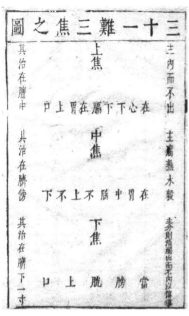

The Thirty-First Difficult Issue

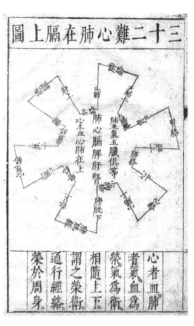

The Thirty-Second Difficult Issue

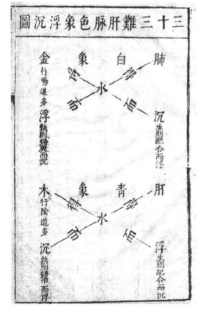

The Thirty-Third Difficult Issue

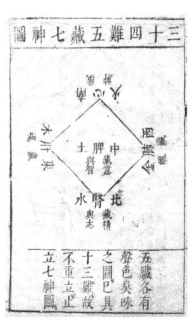

The Thirty-Fourth Difficult Issue

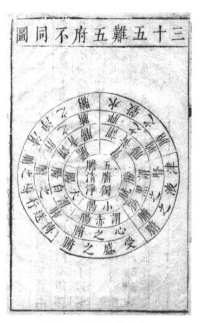

The Thirty-Fifth Difficult Issue

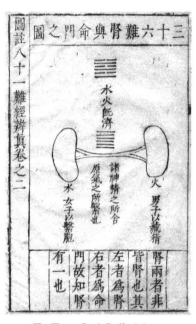

The Thirty-Sixth Difficult Issue

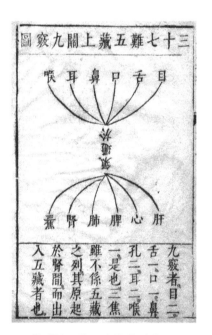

The Thirty-Seventh Difficult Issue

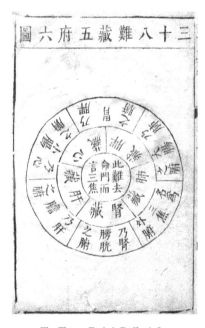

The Thirty-Eighth Difficult Issue

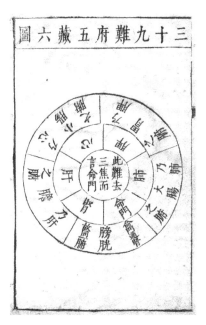

The Thirty-Ninth Difficult Issue

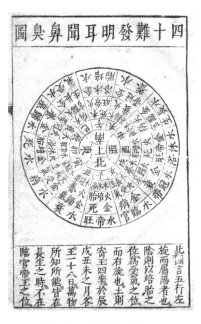

The Fortieth Difficult Issue

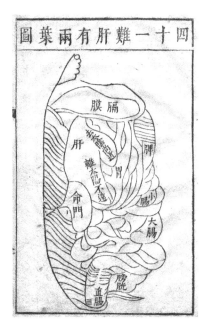

The Forty-First Difficult Issue

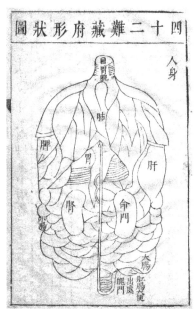

The Forty-Second Difficult Issue

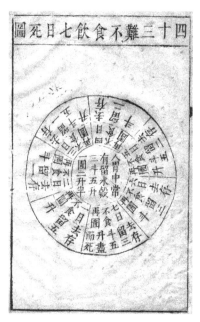

The Forty-Third Difficult Issue

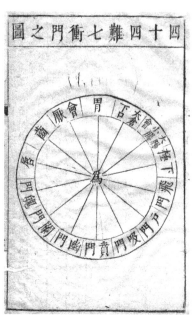

The Forty-Fourth Difficult Issue

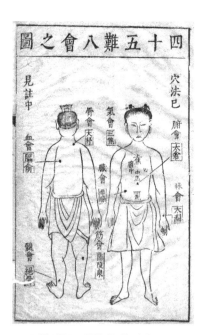

The Forty-Fifth Difficult Issue

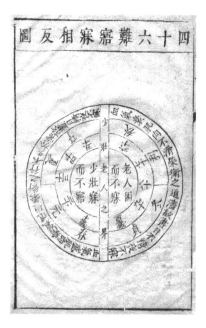

The Forty-Sixth Difficult Issue

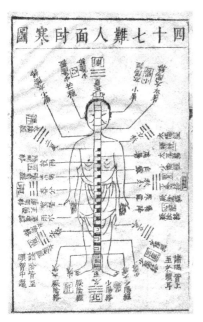

The Forty-Seventh Difficult Issue

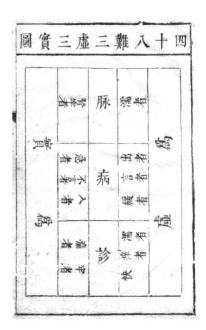

The Forty-Eighth Difficult Issue

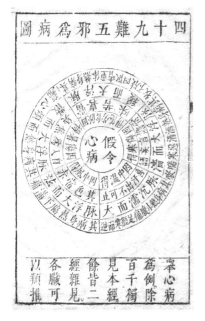

The Forty-Ninth Difficult Issue

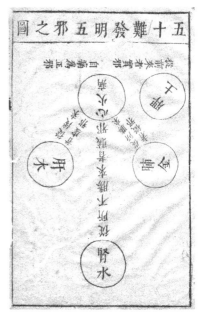

The Fiftieth Difficult Issue

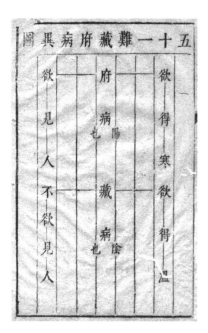

The Fifty-First Difficult Issue

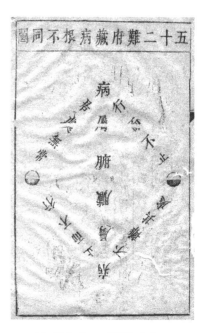

The Fifty-Second Difficult Issue

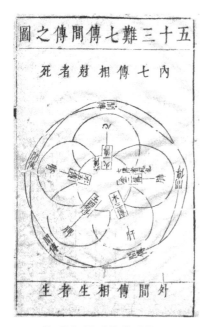

The Fifty-Third Difficult Issue

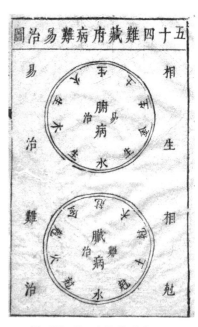

The Fifty-Fourth Difficult Issue

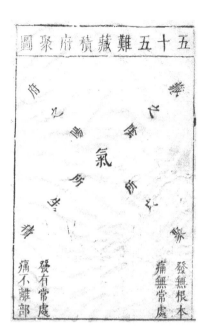

The Fifty-Fifth Difficult Issue

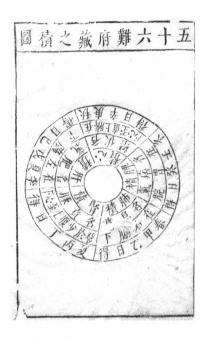

The Fifthy-Sixth Difficult Issue

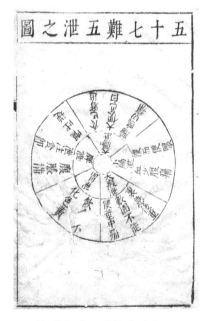

The Fifty-Seventh Difficult Issue

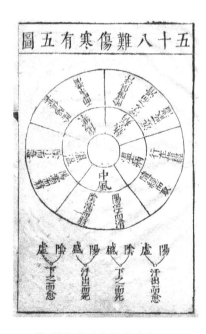

The Fifty-Eighth Difficult Issue

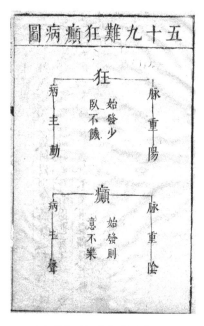

The Fifty-Ninth Difficult Issue

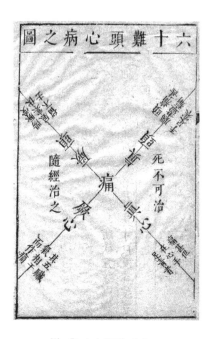

The Sixtieth Difficult Issue

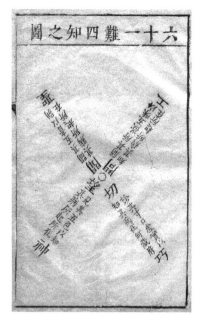

The Sixty-First Difficult Issue

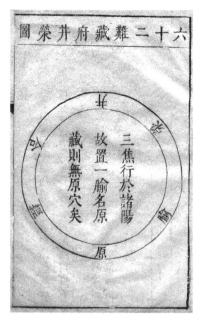

The Sixty-Second Difficult Issue

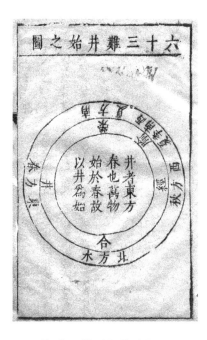

The Sixty-Third Difficult Issue

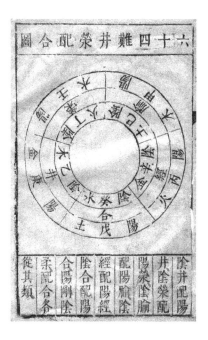

The Sixty-Fourth Difficult Issue

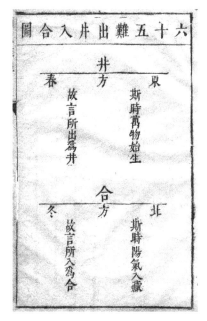

The Sixty-Fifth Difficult Issue

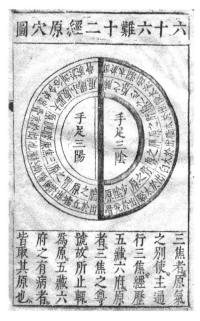

The Sixty-Sixth Difficult Issue

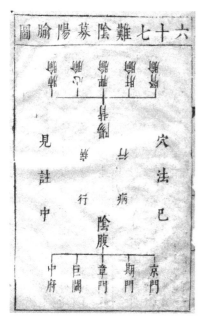

The Sixty-Seventh Difficult Issue

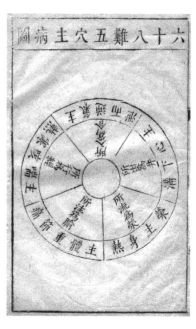

The Sixty-Eighth Difficult Issue

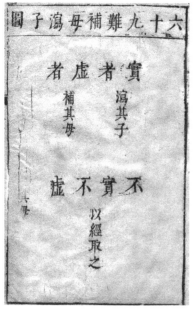

The Sixty-Ninth Difficult Issue

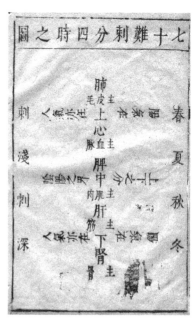

The Seventieth Difficult Issue

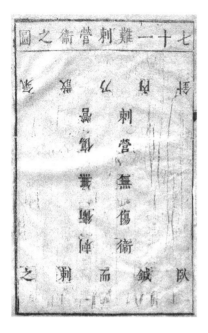

The Seventy-First Difficult Issue

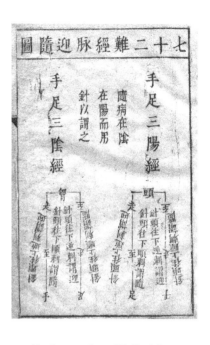

The Seventy-Second Difficult Issue

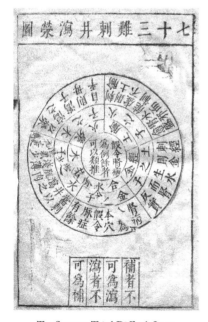

The Seventy-Third Difficult Issue

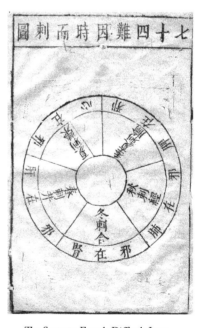

The Seventy-Fourth Difficult Issue

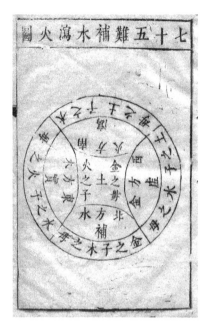

The Seventy-Fifth Difficult Issue

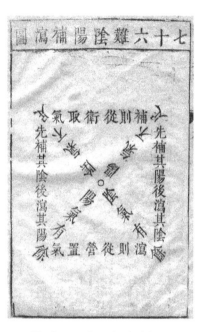

The Seventy-Sixth Difficult Issue

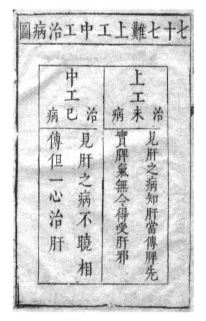

The Seventy-Seventh Difficult Issue

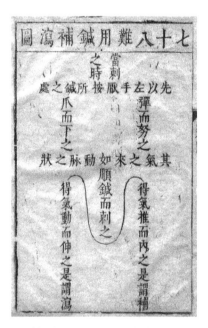

The Seventy-Eighth Difficult Issue

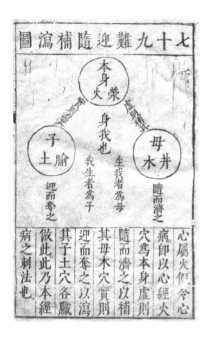

The Seventy-Ninth Difficult Issue

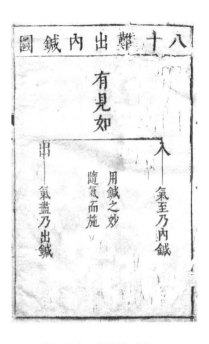

The Eightieth Difficult Issue

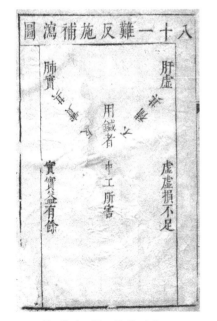

The Eighty-First Difficult Issue

Glossary of Technical Terms in the *Nan Jing*

Radicals with One Stroke

Radical 一
七　七疝　the seven elevation-illnesses: 29[1]
　　七神　the seven spirits: 34
　　七衝門　the seven through-gates: 44
　　七傳　the seven transmissions: 53, 54
上　上焦　the upper [section of the Triple] Burner: 31
　　上關　the upper gates: 37
下　to purge: 58
　　下焦　the lower [section of the Triple] Burner: 31, 55
　　下極　the lower end: 44
三　三焦　the Triple Burner: 8, 25, 31, 38, 39, 45, 62, 66
　　三部　the three sections: 16, 18, 59
　　三虛　the three [kinds of] depletion: 48
　　三實　the three [kinds of] repletion: 48
不　不及　insufficiency: 3, 15
　　不足　not enough: 12, 14, 19, 73, 76, 81

Radical 丨
中　center: 4, 13, 14, 15, 18, 23
　　to be struck: 14, 69
　　中焦　central [section of the Triple] Burner: 23, 31
　　中風　to be struck by wind: 49, 50, 58
　　中濕　to be struck by humidity: 49, 50
　　中工　mediocre practitioner/craftsman: 13, 77, 81
　　中極　the *zhong ji* [hole]: 28

Radical 丿
乘 to seize: 20
　　陰陽相乘　mutual takeover by yin and yang: 3

1　Numbers refer to the difficult issues in which each technical term appears.

Radical 乙

九   九候 the nine indicator[-levels]: 16, 18

       九竅 the nine orifices: 37

乳   the breasts: 31, 45

乾   to dry: 16

Radicals with Two Strokes

Radical 二

五   五藏 the five long-term depots: 1, 8, 10, 12, 13, 14, 25, 30, 32, 34, 35, 37, 39, 42, 55, 56, 60, 63, 66, 67, 68, 74

       五邪 the five evils: 10, 49

       五色 the five complexions: 13, 61

       五味 the five flavors: 37, 61

       五行 the five phases: 18

       五泄 the five diarrheas: 57

       五音 the five notes: 37, 61

       五十度 fifty passages: 1, 30

       五十動 fifty [arrival] movements: 11

井   well [hole]: 62, 63, 64, 65, 68, 73, 74, 79

Radical 亠

交   to intersect: 28

京   京骨 the *jing gu* [hole]: 66

Radical 人

人   人迎 the *ren ying* [location]: 23

伏   1. hidden: 18, 20, 24, 55, 60

       伏梁 2. hidden beams: 56

任   任脈 the controller [conduit-] vessel: 23, 27, 28, 29

便   stools: 16, 57

俞   1. transportation [hole]: 28, 62, 66, 67, 71, 78

       2. rapids [hole]: 64, 66, 68, 74, 79

候   1. to indicate, indicator: 24, 40

       九候 2. the nine indicator [-levels]: 16, 18

倦   exhaustion: 49, 50

倉   太倉 the great granary: 44, 45

傳   transmission, to transmit: 53, 54, 56, 77

傷   1. harm

傷暑 2. to be harmed by heat: 49, 50
傷寒 3. to be harmed by cold: 49, 50, 58

Radical 儿

元　元氣 primordial qi: 14
兌　1. sharp: 15
　　兌骨 2. the *dui gu* [hole]: 66

Radical 入

內　1. internal: 15, 16, 19, 29, 37, 45, 61, 72
　　2. intake: 31
　　內格 3. internal barrier: 3
　　內關 4. internal closure: 3
全　to cure: 13

Radical 八

八　奇經八脈 the eight single-conduit vessels: 27, 28, 29
　　八會 the eight gathering-points: 45
六　六府 the six short-term repositories: 1, 8, 14, 25, 30, 37, 39, 55, 63, 66, 68
　　六十首 the sixty informants: 16

Radical 冫

冬　1. winter: 15, 24, 65, 74
　　冬至 2. winter solstice: 7, 70

Radical 凵

凶　evil auspices: 1, 24
出　to discharge: 31

Radical 刀

切　切脈 to feel [the movement in] the vessels: 17, 18, 61
刺　to apply the needles, to pierce: 18, 70, 71, 73, 74, 78
剛　tough, hardness: 10, 64

Radical 力

動　1. to move
　　動脈 2. [sections where the] movement [in the] vessels [can be felt]: 1, 78
　　動氣 3. moving qi: 8, 16, 66
　　是動 4. excited: 22
勞　weariness: 49, 50

勝 1. to overcome: 52, 53, 54, 75
　　相勝 2. mutual destruction: 13

Radical 匕
北　North: 15, 40, 65, 75

Radical 匚
匿　concealed: 20

Radical 十
十　十變 the ten variations: 10, 34, 63, 64
南　South: 15, 40, 75

Radical 卩
卵　the testicles: 24

Radical 厂
及　不及 insufficiency, insufficient: 3, 15
原　1. origin: 8
　　2. origin [hole]: 62, 66
　　原氣 3. original qi: 36, 38, 66
厥　1. [bent] backward: 29
　　厥陰 2. ceasing yin: 7
　　厥逆 3. to move reversely: 17
　　厥痛 4. receding pain: 60
厭　1. serene: 15
　　會厭 2. epiglottis: 42, 44

Radicals with Three Strokes

Radical 口
口　1. mouth: 16, 24, 37, 42
　　2. opening: 31, 44
　　寸口 3. the inch-opening: 1, 4, 8, 13, 23, 81
吉　good auspices: 1, 24
吐　to vomit, to spit: 14, 17, 57
吸　1. to inhale: 1, 4, 8, 11, 14, 78
　　2. to absorb: 33
　　吸門 3. the inhalation gate: 44
合　1. confluence [hole]: 63, 64, 65

合谷 2. the *he gu* [hole]: 66

味　1. flavor, [-qi]: 4, 37, 49

　　2. flavor (preference): 13, 34, 40, 61

　　3. flvor: 16

　　穀味 4. the grains: 37

呻　groaning: 34, 49

呼　1. to exhale: 1, 4, 8, 11, 14, 78

　　2. to shout: 34, 49, 74

呴　warm flow: 22

命　1. life-span, fate: 14, 37

　　命門 2. the gate of life: 36, 39

　　生命 3. life: 66

周　1. to circulate, to circle: 1, 28, 30, 32

　　2. cycle: 1

咽　咽喉 1. the throat: 28

　　因門 2. the throat-gate: 42

咳　to cough: 49, 56, 68

哭　to cry, to wail: 16, 34, 49

唾　spittle: 34, 49 p

啘　dry vomiting: 16

喘　1. to pant: 16, 68

　　喘咳 2. to pant and cough: 49, 56

喉　咽喉 1. the throat: 28

　　咽囉 2. the windpipe: 42

嘔　to vomit: 57

器　陰器 sexual organ: 24

噫　to belch: 16

嚏　to sneeze: 16

Radical 囗

四　四時 1. the four seasons: 15, 16, 74

　　四肢 2. the four limbs: 16, 19, 49, 56

　　四經 3. the four conduits: 18

困 critical

Radical 土

土　the phase of soil: 18, 64, 75

墮　weary: 16

壅　obstructed, blockage: 22, 56

Radical 士
壯   vigorous: 46

Radical 夂
夏   summer: 15, 70, 74

Radical 夕
外   1. external, outer: 15, 16, 18, 32, 37, 61, 72
      外府 2. external long-term repository: 38
      外關 3, external closure: 3
      外格 4. external barrier: 3
夜   night: 14, 46

Radical 大
大   1. strong: 4, 6, 7, 10, 13, 14, 15, 17, 49
      2. large, great: 17, 26
      大過 3. great excess: 3; see also 太過
      大腸 4. large intestine: 10, 35, 42, 44, 66
      大抒 5. the *da shu* [hole]: 45
      大便 6. stools: 57
      大陵 7. the *da ling* [hole]: 65
      大腸泄 8. diarrhea of the large intestine: 57
      大瘕泄 9. diarrhea of large conglomeration-illnesses: 57
太   太過 1. greatly excessive: 15, 19; see also 大過
      太倉 2. the great granary: 44
      太淵 3. the *tai yuan* [hole]: 45, 65
      太倉 4. the *tai cang* [hole]: 45
      太衝 5. the *tai chong* [hole]:66
      太白 6. the *tai bai* [hole]: 66
      太谿 7. the *tai ji* [hole]: 66
奇   奇經八脈 the eight single-conduit vessels: 27, 28, 29
奪   1. to withdraw: 79
      奪精 2. loss of essence: 14

Radical 女
女   females: 29, 36, 39, 78
妄   妄語 1. to utter nonsense: 17, 49
      妄笑 2. to laugh without reason: 59
      妄行 3. to walk around heedlessly: 59

Radical 子
子   child [long-term depot]: 53, 54, 69, 73, 75, 79
孔   hole: 42
季   季脇 1. the smallest rib: 28
      季夏 2. late summer: 74
      季脇 3. the *ji xie* [hole]: 45

Radical 宀
守   守邪之神 the spirit guarding against the evil: 8
      定 1. to determine: 23
      定息 2. breathing [period]: 1
      害 harm: 14
      寐 to sleep: 46
      寒 cold: 9, 14, 16, 29, 47, 49, 50, 56, 58, 60, 68, 70
      實 1. replete: 4, 6, 12, 15, 17, 49, 79
      2. repletion: 48, 50, 61, 69, 75, 79, 81
      3. to fill, to replenish: 12, 77, 81

Radical 寸
寸   1. inch [-section of the vessels]: 2, 18
      寸口 2. inch-opening: 1, 4, 8, 13, 23, 61, 81
      寸内 3. inch-interior [section of the vessels]: 2
射   砭射 to hit with a sharp stone: 28

Radical 小
小   1. minor: 6, 7, 13, 14, 58
      小腸 2. small intestine: 10, 35, 42, 44, 66
      小腹 3. lower abdomen: 49; see also 少腹
      小腸泄 4. diarrhea of the small intestine: 57
少   少腹 lower abdomen: 16, 56, 57; see also 小腹

Radical 尸
尸   corpse: 14
尺   1. foot [-section of the vessels]: 1, 13, 18, 19
      2. foot [-marsh hole]: 2
      尺内 3. foot-interior [section of the vessels]: 2, 13

Radical 工
工   artisan, practitioner: 13, 61, 77, 81
巧   skilled workman: 61

Radical 巾
帶   the belt [vessel]: 27, 28, 29

Radical 干
干   to attack: 10
      平 1. to level: 75, 81
      平脈 2. normal [movements in the] vessels: 7, 8, 14, 15
      平人 3. healthy person: 42

Radical 幺
幽   幽門 the dark gate: 44

Radical 广
府   1. to collect: 31
      2. short-term repository: 1, 8, 9, 14, 25, 30, 35, 37, 38, 39, 45, 51, 52, 54, 55, 61, 62,
      63, 66, 68
      風府 3. the wind palace: 28
度   五十度 1. fifty passages: 1
      二十五度 2. twenty-five passages: 1
      脈之度數 3. measurements of the vessels: 23
廣   廣腸 the wide intestine: 42

Radical 弓
弦   string-like: 13, 15, 49
弱   weak: 15, 19, 58
強   1. vigorous: 15, 17
      2. stiff: 29

Radical 彡
形   1. physical appearance: 25, 38
      人形 2. a person's physical appearance; body: 21, 23, 49

Radical 彳
後   後重 heavy behind: 57
微   1. feeble: 7, 33
      微邪 2. the weakness evil: 50

Radicals with Four Strokes

Radical 心

心 1. the heart: 4, 5, 10, 12, 14, 15, 16, 17, 29, 31, 32, 34, 35, 37, 40, 41, 42, 49, 50, 53, 56, 60, 66, 68, 70, 74, 79
心主 2. heart-ruler: 18, 23, 25, 79

志 the mind: 24, 29, 34, 42

思 1. to ponder: 16
2. thoughts: 49

急 1, tense: 10, 13, 15, 17, 29, 48
2. tensions: 16, 57

怒 angry, anger: 16, 49

怠 tired: 16

恚 to hate: 49

恐 to be fearful: 16

息 1. breathing: 1, 21
2. break: 30, 37
息賁 3. rest and run: 56

悢 to feel uncomfortable: 29

悲 悲愁 grief: 16

愁 1. anxiety: 16, 49
悲愁 2. grief: 16

愈 to cure, to heal: 17, 56, 58

意 sentiments, thoughts: 33, 34, 41, 42, 59

憂 grief: 49

慮 considerations: 49

應 1. to correspond: 18, 21, 40
相應 2. mutual correspondence: 13

Radical 戶

戶 戶門 the door-gate: 44

所 所生病 illnesses that are generated: 22

Radical 手

手 1. hand: 17, 18, 23, 60
手太陰 2, the hand major yin [conduit]: 1, 18, 23, 24
手陽明 3. the hand yang brilliance [conduit]: 18, 23
手太陽 4. the hand major yang [conduit]: 18, 23
手少陰 5. the hand minor yin [conduit]: 18, 23, 24
手心主 6. the hand heart master: 18, 23, 25, 79

手少陽 7. the hand minor yang [conduit]: 18, 23, 38

手三陽之脈 8. the three hand yang vessels: 60

持　1. to govern: 38

持脈 2. to touch the vessel: 5

收持 3. to support one's stature: 14, 29

引持 4. to pull out [qi]: 70

按　to press the finger [on the vessels in order to feel the movement in them]: 4, 5, 15, 16

掌　the palm: 16

損　1. to diminish: 12, 81

2. diminished: 6

3. injured, injury: 14

Radical 夊

收　1. to contract: 49

收持 2. to support one's stature: 14, 29

數　1. frequent: 9, 13, 15, 17

脈之度數 2. measurements of the vessels: 23

散　1. dispersed: 4, 13, 49, 58

2. to dissipate, to disperse: 28, 71

散膏 3. dispersed fat: 42

敦　generous: 7

Radical 日

日　day: 7, 43, 46, 56, 63

春　spring: 15, 41, 63, 70, 74

是　是動 excited: 22

晝　daytime: 14, 46

暑　heat: 49

Radical 曰

會　八會 1. the eight gathering-points: 45

會厭 2. epiglottis: 42, 44

脈之大會 3. the great meeting-point of [all the] vessels: 1, 2

Radical 月

望　to look: 61

Radical 木

木　[the phase of] wood: 15, 18, 19, 33, 41, 64, 73, 75, 81

本　foundation, basis: 8, 15, 24, 55, 58, 66

東　East: 15, 41, 63, 65, 75
柔　soft, softness: 10, 64
格　barrier: 3, 37
根　root, source: 8, 14, 55, 66
極　下極 the lower end: 44
榮　1. camp [qi]: 1, 14, 30, 32, 35, 46, 71, 72, 76, 78
　　2. to circulate: 14, 32
　　3. to nourish, to supply, 23, 24
　　4. creek [hole]: 62, 63, 64, 68, 73, 74
樂　1. joy: 16, 33
　　2. happy: 59
稟　to dry out: 58

Radical 欠

欠欮 to yawn: 16
欮　to cough: 16
歌　singing: 34, 49

Radical 止

正　正經 1. the regular conduits: 49, 69
　　正邪 2. the regular evil: 50
歲　year: 7, 56, 63

Radical 歹

死　death: 1, 3, 8, 12, 13, 14, 15, 17, 18, 21, 23₅ 24, 37, 43, 53, 58, 60

Radical 殳

殺　to kill: 12

Radical 毋

母　mother [long-term depot]: 69, 75, 79

Radical 毛

毛　1. hair: 5, 14, 24, 42, 58
　　2. hair-like: 15
　　毛際 3. [pubic] hairline: 28

Radical 气

氣　1. qi: 7, 8, 11, 12, 14, 15, 16, 18, 22, 23, 24, 27, 28, 29, 30, 31, 32, 34, 35, 36, 37, 38, 39,
　　45, 46, 49, 55, 56, 60, 62, 65, 66, 68, 70, 71, 72, 73, 76, 77, 78, 79, 80, 81
　　氣衝 2. the *qi chong* [hole]: 28

氣街 3. the street of qi: 31

氣道 4. the passageways for the qi: 3, 46

Radical 水

水　　1. [the phase of] water: 15, 18, 29, 31, 33, 35, 37, 40, 42, 43, 64, 75

水道 2. the passageways for water: 27, 31

汗　　sweat: 24, 34, 49, 58

沈　　1. in the depth: 3, 4, 6, 7, 10, 13, 14, 15, 17, 18, 20, 49, 55, 58, 70

2. to sink: 33

法　　1. pattern: 1, 3, 4, 18, 21, 49, 54, 56, 57, 65, 78

2. method: 14, 16

泄　　1. diarrhea: 16, 57, 68

2. to be drained: 24

注　　to flow: 23

泣　　tears: 34, 49, 74

治　　to rule: 2

to cure: 14, 54, 75

to treat: 17, 77

to regulate: 31

洪　　vast: 7, 14, 17

洒　　to shiver: 16, 49, 56

洩　　diarrhea: 17

涎　　saliva: 34

津　　津液 liquids: 24, 34, 35, 40, 43

水穀之海 the sea of water and grains: 15

消　　1. to digest: 16

消瘦 2. to grow lean: 14

浮　　1. near or at the surface: 3, 4, 6, 7, 13, 14, 15, 17, 18, 20, 49, 55, 58, 70

2. to float: 33

涕　　snivel: 34, 49

清　　clear, clarity: 30, 31, 35

淅　　to shiver: 16, 56

渠　　reservoirs: 27, 28

淺　　shallow: 70, 73

淨　　purity: 35

液　　1. saliva: 49, 63

津液 2. liquids: 24, 34, 35, 40, 43

渴　　thirsty: 17

滑　　smooth: 13, 14, 15, 17, 20, 24, 46, 58

溉　　灌溉 to pour, drainage: 23, 28

溝　ditches: 27, 28
溫　warm, warmth: 14, 24, 51, 58, 70
　　to provide warmth: 37, 42
溢　overflow: 3, 28, 37
　　filled: 27, 28
溶　to be bloated: 29
溺　urine: 42
溲　to urinate: 16, 57
澁　rough: 4, 10, 13, 14, 17, 20, 46, 49, 58
滿　full, swollen, fullness: 14, 16, 24, 27, 28, 29, 49, 57, 68
滯　stagnant: 18
漏　漏水 [the clepsydra's] dripping water: 1, 15
潔　tidy: 16
潤　潤澤 glossy: 24
濁　turbid: 30, 31
濡　1. soft: 4, 15, 17, 24, 48, 49, 58
　　2. moisture: 22
　　3. to moisten: 37
　　4. softness: 79
濕　humidity, moisture: 49, 50, 58
濟　to support: 79
瀉　drainage: 35
　　to drain: 69, 73, 75, 76, 78, 79, 81
漑　灌溉 to pour, drainage: 23, 28

Radical 火
火　[the phase of] fire: 15, 18, 33, 40, 64, 73, 75
無　無魂 absence of *hun*: 14
焦　1. burner: 8, 23, 25, 31, 35, 38, 39, 45, 62, 66
　　2. burned: 24, 34, 49, 58
煩　1. uneasiness: 14
　　2. to feel uneasy: 49
　　煩心 3. uneasiness in the heart: 16, 56
熱　heat: 9, 14, 16, 17, 28, 29, 45, 49, 56, 58, 68
熟　1. to process: 31
　　2. mature: 33
營　to circulate: 37; see also 榮

Radical 牛

牛   1. firm: 4, 16, 17, 48
     2. firmness: 79

Radical 犬

狂   madness: 20, 59

Radicals with Five Strokes

Radical 玉   .

王   1. to govern: 7, 56
     王脈 2. governing [qi moving through the] vessels: 7, 15
玉   玉堂 the *yu tang* [hole] 31
環   1. ring: 23, 30, 37, 53
     環流 2. to circulate: 28

Radical 甘

甘   sweet: 34, 49

Radical 生

生   1. life: 1, 15, 17, 21, 23, 53, 66
     2. to come to life, to be born, to emerge: 18, 40, 41, 55, 63, 65
     3. to generate: 31, 53, 54, 69
     生氣 4. vital influences: 8
     相生 5. mutual generation: 13, 18

Radical 田

男   males: 19, 29, 36, 39, 78
留   to stagnate, to stop: 22, 37, 56, 60
畜   to stagnate: 28

Radical 疒

疝   elevation-illness: 29
病   illness: 3, 4, 7, 9, 13, 14, 15, 16, 17, 18, 19, 21, 22, 23, 29, 45, 48, 49, 50, 51, 52, 53, 54,
     55, 58, 60, 61, 66, 67, 69, 74, 77, 79, 81
疸   jaundice: 56
疾   1. swift: 5, 15
     2. illness: 18
痞   痞氣 blocked qi: 56
痛   pain: 14, 16, 29, 48, 49, 55, 57, 58, 60, 68
痼   痼疾 chronic illnesses: 18

痿　powerless: 14
　　to weaken: 56
瘄　*jie* [fevers]: 56
瘧　*yao* [fevers]: 56
瘦　lean: 14
瘕　瘕聚 1. conglomeration illnesses: 29
　　大瘕泄 2. diarrhea of large conglomeration-illnesses: 57
癰　protuberance-illness: 16
癢　itching: 48
癱　obstruction-illness: 37
癲　peak-illness: 20, 59

Radical 白
白　white: 13, 16, 33, 34, 35, 37, 49, 57

Radical 皮
皮　the skin: 5, 13, 14, 24, 58

Radical 皿
益　1. to add: 12, 14, 81
　　2. increasingly: 15
盛　1. abundance: 6, 35, 58
　　2. full, overfilled, plenty: 19, 28, 37, 46, 58, 59
　　3. peak: 15
盡　1. depleted: 11
　　2. exhausted, exhaustion: 43, 80

Radical 目
目　1. the eyes: 17, 20, 23, 37
　　目眩 2. dizziness: 14, 24
　　目瞑 3. closed eyes: 24
盲　blind: 20
眩　目眩 dizziness: 14, 24
眞　眞藏 true long-term depots: 3
　　眞痛 true pain: 60
督　督脈 the supervisor [conduit] vessel: 23, 27, 28, 29
瞑　目瞑 closed eyes: 24

Radical 矢
短　short: 4, 7, 13, 14, 17, 20

Radical 石
石   stone-like: 15
砭   sharp stone: 28

Radical 示
神   spirit: 8, 34, 36, 39, 42, 61

Radical 禾
秋   autumn: 15, 70, 74
穀   grains: 4, 15, 30, 31, 35, 37, 42, 43
積   accumulations: 18, 55, 56

Radical 穴
穴   hole: 45
窘   窘迫 cramps: 57
竅   九竅 the nine orifices: 37

Radicals with Six Strokes

Radical 竹
笑   to laugh: 16, 59
筋   the muscles: 5, 14, 16, 18, 24, 45
節   1: joints: 16, 24, 68
      2. sections: 42

Radical 米
精   1. essence: 14, 34, 36, 39, 42
      2. alert: 46

Radical 系
累   tied: 15
細   fine: 7, 14, 17
結   1. knotted: 18
      2. knots: 29
      3. to accumulate, to conglomerate: 37, 56
絡   絡脈 network-vessels: 23, 26, 27, 32
絕   命絕 1. severance of fate: 14
      絕骨 2. the *jue gu* [hole]: 45
經   1. conduit: 1, 4, 8, 18, 23, 25, 26, 27, 28, 29, 32, 38, 49, 58, 66, 69, 72
      2. scripture: 7, 11, 12, 13, 15, 17, 19, 20, 21, 22, 23, 30, 35, 37, 39, 40, 44, 46, 49, 53, 61, 65, 68, 69, 70, 71, 72, 73, 74, 75, 77, 79, 80, 81

3. stream [hole]: 64, 68, 74

離經 4. departure from the regular: 14

緊　tight: 7, 17, 48, 58

維　the tie [vessel]: 27, 28, 29

緩　relaxed: 10, 13, 29, 48, 49

縮　to shrink: 24

Radical 老

老　老人 old people: 46

Radical 耳

耳　the ears: 37, 40, 42 聚 1. to contract: 14
　　2. to assemble at: 24
　　3. collections: 55
　　瘕聚 4. conglomeration illnesses: 29

聲　pitch, sound: 13, 34, 40, 49
　　voices: 51

聶　whispering: 15

Radical 肉

肉　flesh: 5, 14, 48, 24, 46, 73

肌　肌肉 flesh: 5, 14, 24, 46, 56, 58, 73

肝　the liver: 4, 5, 10, 11, 12, 14, 15, 16, 17, 24, 33, 34, 35, 37, 39, 40, 41, 42, 49, 53, 56, 66, 70, 74, 75, 77, 81

肛　肛門 the rectum: 42

肺　the lung: 4, 5, 10, 12, 14, 15, 16, 17, 18, 24, 32, 33, 34, 35, 37, 40, 42, 49, 53, 56, 66, 70, 74, 75, 81

肢　the limbs: 16, 19, 49, 56

肥　肥氣 fat qi: 56

胃　1. the stomach: 10, 15, 30, 31, 35, 42, 43, 44, 56, 66
　　胃泄 2. stomach diarrhea: 57

胞　the womb: 36, 39

胱　膀胱 the bladder: 10, 31, 35, 42, 66

脈　1. vessel: 1, 2, 3, 4, 5, 8, 23, 24, 27, 28, 30, 37, 45, 47, 48, 60, 61, 72
　　2. [contents of the] vessels: 1
　　3. [movement in the] vessels: 3, 4, 5, 6, 7, 8, 9, 10, 11, 12, 13, 14, 15, 16, 17, 18, 19, 20, 21, 22, 23, 49, 58, 59, 78, 81

胸　the chest: 14, 18, 23, 28, 47

脅　1. the ribs: 49, 56
　　右脅 2. the right side of the body: 18

季脇 3. the smallest ribs: 28

脊   the backbone, the back: 28, 29

脣   the lips: 24, 43, 44, 58

脛   the shinbone: 16, 49

腙   duct: 31, 56

腎   the kidneys: 4, 5, 8, 10, 11, 12, 14, 15, 16, 34, 35, 36, 37, 39, 40, 42, 49, 53, 56, 66, 70, 74

脹   swollen: 16, 57

脾   1. the spleen: 4, 5, 10, 14, 15, 16, 26, 34, 35, 37, 40, 42, 49, 53, 56, 66, 74, 76

     脾泄 2. spleen diarrhea: 57

腕   腕骨 the *wan gu* [hole]: 66

腠   腠理 the pores: 24, 37

腰   the loins: 29

腸   intestine: 10, 35, 42, 56, 66

腥   frowzy: 34, 49

腫   swelling: 28

腹   the abdomen: 14, 16, 17, 28, 29, 49, 56, 57

腦   the brain: 28, 60

膀   膀胱 the bladder: 10, 31, 35, 42, 66

膈   the diaphragm: 18, 31, 32

腐   1. foul: 34, 49
     2. to spoil: 31

膚   皮膚 the skin: 13, 56, 58

膿   pus: 57

臊   fetid: 34, 39, 74

膽   the gall bladder: 10, 35, 42, 66

膻   膻中 the *dan zhong* [hole]: 31

臍   the navel: 66; see also: 齊

Radical 臣

臥   臥緘 the lying needle: 71

Radical 自

臭   1. odor: 13, 34, 40, 49, 74
     2. stench: 37, 40

Radical 至

至   arrival, arriving: 7, 14

Radical 舌

舌 the tongue: 24, 37, 42, 58

Radical 色

色 complexion: 13, 24, 34, 40, 49, 57, 61, 74

Radical 艸

苦 1. bitter: 34, 49
2. complaints: 58

莖 stalk: 8, 57

葉 leaves: 8, 14, 15, 41, 42

菽 beans: 5

募 levy [hole]: 67

藏 1. long-term depot: 1, 8, 9, 11, 12, 13, 14, 20, 25, 30, 32, 34, 35, 36, 37, 38, 39, 45, 51, 52, 53, 54, 55, 56, 60, 61, 62, 63, 66, 67, 68
2. to store: 15, 34, 39, 42, 65, 66, 74

Radical 虍

虛 1. depletion, depleted: 6, 12, 14, 15, 48, 49, 50, 58, 61, 69, 75, 79, 81
2. to deplete: 12, 81

Radical 血

血 1. blood: 14, 17, 22, 23, 24, 32, 37, 42, 45, 46, 57
血脈 2. blood vessels: 5, 14

衄 nosebleed: 17

Radical 行

行 行尸 1. walking corpse: 14
五行 2. the five phases: 18

街 氣街 street of qi: 31

衝 1. the through-way [vessel]: 27, 28, 29, 31
衝門 2. through-gates: 44
衝陽 3. the *chong yang* [hole]: 66

衛 guard [qi]: 1, 14, 30, 32, 35, 46, 71, 72₃ 76

Radical 衣

衰 1. exhaustion: 15
2. to diminish: 46

補 to fill: 12, 69, 73, 75, 76, 78

Radical 西

西 West: 15, 40, 75

覆 turnover: 3, 37

Radicals with Seven Strokes

Radical 言

言 to talk: 34, 49

診 to examine: 17, 18, 48, 61

調 to balance, to restore harmony: 14, 72

證 evidence: 16

譫 譫言 to speak incoherently: 17, 49

變 variation, change: 10, 15, 16, 22, 58, 63, 64

Radical 豕

象 to reflect: 33

Radical 貝

賁 賁門 1. the strong gate: 44

息賁 2. rest and run: 56

賁豚 3, running piglet: 56

賊 賊邪 the robber evil: 50

Radical 赤

赤 red: 13, 16, 34, 35, 49

Radical 足

足 1. the foot: 17, 18, 23, 49, 56, 60

不足 2. not enough: 12, 14, 16, 19, 73, 76, 81

足少陰 3. the foot minor yin [conduit]: 18, 23, 24

足厥陰 4. the foot ceasing yin [conduit]: 18, 23, 24

足太陽 5. the foot major yang [conduit]: 18, 23

足少陽 6. the foot minor yang [conduit]: 18, 23, 24

足太陰 7. the foot major yin [conduit]: 18, 23

足陽明 8. the foot yang brilliance [conduit]: 18, 23, 28

跟 the heel: 28

踝 the ankle: 28

蹻 the walker-vessel: 23, 26, 27, 28, 29

Radical 身
身   the body: 1, 23, 28, 49, 68

Radical 車
輕   light: 5, 15, 16
轉   轉筋 twisted muscles: 16

Radical 辛
辛   acrid: 34, 49

Radical 走
迎   to move against [a proper course]: 72, 79
迫   窘迫 cramps: 57
迴   迴腸 the returning intestine: 42
逆   to proceed contrary to [the proper course]: 4, 16, 17, 19, 29, 49, 56, 57, 68
逢   相逢 mutual interference: 10
過   太[大]過 great excess: 3, 15
遲   slow: 9, 15

Radical 邑
邪   evil: 8, 10, 22, 28, 37, 49, 50, 56, 69, 74, 77
邱   邱墟 the *qiu xu* [hole]: 66

Radical 酉
酸   sour: 34, 49, 74
醫   physician: 12

Radical 里
重   1. heavy: 5, 16
       2. doubling: 20
       後重 3. heavy behind: 57

Radicals with Eight Strokes

Radical 金
金   [the phase of] metal: 15, 18, 19, 33, 40, 64, 75, 81
針   needle: 70, 71, 78
鉤   hook-like: 15
鍼   needle, to needle: 12, 71, 74, 78, 80, 81

Radical 長

長   extended: 4, 7, 15, 17, 20

Radical 門

門   咽門 1. the throat-gate: 42

     肛門 2. the rectum: 42

     衝門 3. the through-gates: 44

     飛門 4. the flying gate: 44

     戶門 5. the door-gate: 44

     吸門 6. the inhalation-gate: 44

     賁門 7. the strong gate: 44

     幽門 8. the dark gate: 44

     蘭門 9. the screen-gate: 44

     魄門 10. the *po*-gate: 44

閉   1. closure: 16

     2. to close: 17

問   to ask: 61

間   間藏 to skip a depot: 53, 54

聞   to listen: 61

關   1. gate [line], gate-section: 2, 18, 19, 37

     2. closure: 3, 37

     關元 3. the *guan yuan* [hole]: 28

     上關 4. the upper gates: 37

Radical 阜

陰   陰器 sexual organ: 24

陷   fold: 31

陽   陽池 1. the *yang chi* [hole]: 66

     陽陵泉 2. the *yang ling quan* [hole]: 45

隨   to follow [a proper course]: 72, 79

Radical 佳

離   離經 departure from the regular: 14

Radical 雨

霧   mist: 14

露   dew: 14

Radical 青

青   virid: 13, 16, 33, 34, 35, 49, 60, 74

Radicals with Nine Strokes

Radical 面
面　the face: 13, 16, 24, 47

Radical 音
音　五音 the five musical notes: 37, 61

Radical 頁 ,
順　to proceed in accordance with [the proper course]: 4, 19, 72
頭　the head: 14, 18, 23, 47, 56, 60
頸　the neck: 47

Radical 風
風　1. the wind: 60
　　風府 2. wind palace: 28
　　中風 3. to be struck by wind: 49, 58

Radical 飛
飛　飛門 the flying gate: 44

Radical 食
食　food: 14, 16, 43, 49, 50, 56, 57
飲　to drink; beverage: 14, 43, 49, 50, 56, 57

Radical 首
首　informant: 16

Radical 香
香　1. aromatic: 34, 49
　　2. aroma: 37, 40

Radicals with Ten Strokes

Radical 骨
骨　1. the bones: 5, 14, 24, 45, 56, 58
　　絕骨 2. the *jue gu* [hole]: 45
髓　the marrow: 24, 45
體　the body: 16, 68

Radical 彭
髮　the hair: 24, 58

Radical 鬲
鬲   鬲俞 the *ge-shu* [hole]: 45

Radical 鬼
鬼   demons: 20
魂   1. *hun* [spirit]: 34, 42
      無魂 2. absence of *hun*: 14
魄   1. *po* [spirit]: 34, 42
      魄門 2. *po*-gate: 44

Radicals with Eleven Strokes

Radical 魚
魚   魚際 fish-line: 2

Radical 齒
鹹   salty: 34, 49

Radicals with Twelve Strokes

Radical 黃
黃   1. yellow: 13, 16, 34, 35, 49, 57
      黃疸 2. jaundice: 56

Radical 黑
黑   black: 13, 16, 24, 34, 35, 37, 49

Radicals with Fourteen Strokes

Radical 鼻
鼻   the nose: 37, 40, 58

Radical 齊
齊   the navel: 16, 18, 28, 31, 42, 56 (see also 臍)

Radicals with Fifteen Strokes

Radical 齒
齒   the teeth: 24, 42, 44, 58

Index to Prolegomena, Commentaries, and Notes

Abbreviations:
LS = treatise in the *Huang di nei jing ling shu*
P = index refers to Prolegomena only
SHL = treatise in the *Shang han lun*
SW = treatise in the *Huang di nei jing su wen*
TS = treatise in the *Huang di nei jing tai su*

acupuncture,　2, 8, 10

赤掘昭　Akahori Akira,　5

ancestral concepts of illness,　6

八正神明論　"Ba zheng shen ming lun" (SW),　402

百病始生　"Bai bing shi sheng" (LS),　419

百會　*bai hui* hole,　277

暴注　*bao zhu* diarrhea,　432

備急千金要方　*Bei ji qian jin yao fang.* See *Qian jin fang*,　215

本病論　"Ben bing lun" (SW),　392, 450

本草　*Ben cao*,　148, 163

本草綱目　*Ben cao gang mu*,　187

本草經　*Ben cao jing*,　163

本經　*Ben jing*,　163, 164

本神　"Ben shen" (LS),　312

本輸　"Ben shu" (LS),　265, 333, 460, 465, 468, 477, 478, 491, 481, 498, 516

賁豚　*ben tun* ("running piglet"),　197, 427,

本藏　"Ben zang" (LS), 124, 265

痺論　"Bi lun" (SW), 333

扁鵲　Bian Que (P), 24-26, 31, 42, 43, 48 *See also* Qin Yueren,

扁鵲內經　*Bian Que nei jing*, 26

扁鵲外經　*Bian Que wai jing*, 26

標本病傳　"Biao ben bing chuan" (SW), 412

病傳　"Bing chuan" (LS), 412, 415

胕胅　*bo yang* hole, 477, 479

Buddhist prayers, 61

不容　*bu rong* hole, 160, 483

參同契　*Can tong qi*, 134

倉公　Cang gong, 41

曹襃　Cao Bao, 341

長短　*chang duan* hole, 278

腸澼　*chang pi* diarrhea, 432

長強　*chang qiang* hole, 277, 278

長桑君　Changsang jun, 25

腸胃　"Chang wei" (LS), 351, 355, 356

巢元方　Chao Yuanfang, 284

陳四明　Chen from Siming, 304, 308, 328, 342, 343, 347, 365, 366, 367, 415, 456

赤烏神鍼經　*Chi wu shen zhen jing*, 29

尺澤　*chi ze* hole, 52, 65, 487, 495

衝門　*chong men* hole, 55

衝陽　*chong yang* hole, 51, 55, 473, 488

淳于意　Chunyu Yi, 24, 27, 284

刺齊論　"Ci qi lun" (SW), 503

刺瘧論　"Ci yao lun" (SW),　512

刺腰痛論　"Ci yao tong lun" (SW),　273

circulatory movement in the organism,　8

Corpus Hippocraticum,　6

大白　*da bai* hole,　488

大衝　*da chong* hole,　487

大椎　*da chui* hole,　277

大都　*da du* hole,　488

大敦　*da dui* hole,　487

大海　*da hai* ("great sea"),　480

大惑論　"Da huo lun" (LS),　321

大陵　*da ling* hole,　473-478, 488

大抒　*da shu* hole,　363, 366, 367

大唐六典　*Da Tang liu dian*,　29

大谿　*da xi* hole,　487

大迎　*da ying* hole,　51, 55

大淵　*da yuan* hole,　52, 54, 162, 485

戴聖　Dai Sheng,　341

丹田　*dan tian* ("cinnabar field"),　113, 479

膻中　*dan zhong*,　292, 293

膻中　*dan zhong* hole,　248, 291-294, 297, 331, 367, 368

黨永年　Dang Yongnian,　28

Daoism,　29

demonological, demonology, demons,　2-4, 6-8, 33, 44, 226, 228, 229, 400, 445

地倉　*di cang* hole,　51

帝王世紀　*Di wang shi ji*,　25, 27

癲狂　"Dian kuang" (LS), 446

丁德用　Ding Deyong, 34, 35

divinatory doctrines, 45

drugs, 2, 6, 148, 149

洞泄　*dong xie* diarrhea, 432

兌骨　*dui gu* hole, 473, 475, 477, 478

董仲舒　Dong Zhongshu, 21, 228

energy, 4

epidemics, 435, 438

范樞密　Fan Shumi, 28, 30

范行准　Fan Xingzhun, 21, 22, 28-30

方脈舉要　*Fang mai ju yao*, 175

方盛衰論　"Fang sheng shuai lun" (SW), 123, 234, 503

風府　*feng fu* hole, 247, 277

風論　"Feng lun" (SW), 431, 434

Five Phases doctrine, 2, 3, 8 et passim

Franke, Herbert, 32

復溜　*fu liu* hole, 164, 488

婦人瘕　*fu ren jia*, 284

腹中論　"Fu zhong lun" (SW), 422, 424

Fuchs, Walter, 32

肛門　*gang men* ("rectum-gate"), 352

高光振　Gao Guangzhen, 13, 42, 44

膈膜　*ge mo* ("diaphragm"), 366

鬲俞 *ge shu* hole, 365, 366

根結 "Gen jie" (LS), 130, 132, 133, 321, 323

Greco-Latin terminology, 4

賈得道 Gu Dedao, 44, 46

骨空論 "Gu kong lun" (SW), 247, 273, 284, 255, 296

賈維誠 Gu Weicheng, 11

關衝 *guan chong* hole, 488

關元 *guan yuan* hole, 113, 243, 276, 278, 283, 284, 321

官鍼 "Guan zhen" (LS), 504

国語 guo yu, 214

海論 "Hai lun" (LS), 322, 367, 368

韓非子 Han fei zi, 12, 25, 289

寒熱病 "Han re bing" (LS), 65, 443

寒熱論 "Han re lun" (LS), 443

Harper, Donald, 7

何愛華 He Aihua, 13, 22-25

合谷 *he gu* hole, 55, 473, 488

禾窌 *he jiao* hole, 55

何 He, physician, 6

洪範 "Hong fan", 309

後谿 *hou xi* hole, 488

華佗 Hua Tuo, 35, 39, 68

淮南子 *Huai nan zi*, 221, 222, 344, 451

黃疸 *huang dan* ("jaundice"), 425

黃帝 Huang di (P), 25, 26, 31, 68

黃帝內經 *Huang di nei jing* (P), 1, 8, 9, 25, 27, 31

黃帝內經靈樞集注   *Huang di nei jing ling shu ji zhu,*   236

黃帝鍼灸   *Huang di zhen jiu,*   149

黃坤載   Huang Kunzai   373   *See* Huang Yuanyu

黃庭經   *Huang ting jing,*   308, 321

黃元御   Huang Yuanyu,   374

皇甫謐   Huangfu Mi,   23, 25, 27

回骨   *hui gu* hole,   51

會陰   *hui yin* hole,   277, 278, 279

火鍼   *huo zhen* ("fire needle"),   427

醫心方   *Ishinpo,*   22

伊籐馨   Itō Kaoru,   12

Jahn, Karl,   32

Japanese (version of the *Nan jing*),   32

箕門   *ji men* hole,   52, 55

極泉   *ji quan* hole,   52, 55

紀天錫   Ji Tianxi,   48, 67, 216, 404

瘕泄   *jia xie* diarrhea,   432

甲乙經   *Jia yi jing,*   23, 27, 56, 352, 477

間使   *jian shi* hole,   475, 477, 488

竅陰   *qiao yin* hole,   488

解谿   *jie xi* hole,   488

金匱要略   *Jin kui yao lue,*   64, 427

金匱真言論   "Jin kui zhen yan lun" (SW),   195, 346

金門   *jin men,*   280

金韜玉鑑   *Jin tao yu jian,*   29

京骨　*jing gu* hole,　473, 488

經脈別論　"Jing mai bie lun" (SW),　51, 298, 389

京門　*jing men* hole,　483

晴明　*jing ming* hole,　323

經渠　*jing qu* hole,　56

景岳全書　*Jing yue quan shu*,　140

經筋　"Jing jin" (LS),　422, 424, 426

經脈　"Jing mai" (LS),　51, 97, 236, 239-241, 255, 257, 258, 268-270, 332, 366, 368, 592, 493

九宮八風　"Jiu gong ba feng" (LS),　402

九卷　*Jiu juan*,　22

鳩尾　*jiu wei* hole,　364, 477 , 483

九鍼論　"Jiu zhen lun" (LS),　263, 264

九鍼十二原　"Jiu zhen shi er yuan" (LS),　135, 136, 139, 476, 478, 489

巨闕　*ju que* hole,　483

舉痛論　"Ju tong lun" (SW),　8, 321, 482, 485

厥病　"Jue bing" (LS),　448, 449, 452

厥逆　"Jue ni" (LS),　448

決氣　"Jue qi" (LS),　265

Karlgren, B.,　460

客主人　*ke zhu ren* hole,　51

口問　"Kou wen" (LS),　194

崑崙　*kun lun* hole,　488

勞宮　*lao gong* hole,　52, 55, 193, 475, 477, 488

李瀕湖　Li Binhu　187 *See* Li Shizhen

厲兌　*li dui* hole,　488

李東垣　Li Dongyuan,　111

麗谷　*li gu* hole,　487

離合眞邪論　"Li he zhen xie lun" (SW),　503, 536-538

禮記　*Li ji*,　341

李駉　Li Jiong (P),　11, 35, 36 et passim

李時珍　Li Shizhen,　187, 213

奉元立　Li Yuanli,　34-36

廖平　Liao Ping (P),　21, 26, 30, 41 et passim

淋巴管　*lin ba guan* ("lymphatic vessel"),　283

林衡　Lin Heng,　35

臨泣　*lin qi* hole,　488

靈道　*ling dao* hole,　52, 477, 487

靈蘭秘典論　"Ling lan mi dian lun" (SW),　248, 292, 297, 298, 316

靈樞　*Ling shu* (P),　1, 2, 6, 7, 10, 11, 22, 24, 32, 39 et passim

劉安　Liu An,　221, 451

溜谷　*liu gu* hole,　488

六紀正論　"Liu ji zheng lun" (SW),　102

六節藏象論　"Liu jie zang xiang lun" (SW),　57, 72, 78, 86, 104

劉開　Liu Kai,　175,

六元正紀大論　"Liu yuan zheng ji da lun" (SW),　344

呂博望　Lü Bowang,　27, 28

呂復　Lü Fu,　28, 37

呂廣望　Lü Guang(-wang) (P),　21, 28-30, 34, 36, 43 et passim

絡脈　*luo mai* ("network-vessels"),　9

絡卻　*luo que* hole,　366

馬繼興　Ma Jixing,　5, 34, 35

馬堪溫　Ma Kanwen,　4

magic,　7

脈度　"Mai du" (LS),　73, 240, 241, 246, 269, 326, 327, 343

脈法　*Mai fa*,　235, 378

脈經　*Mai jing*,　22, 23, 27, 64, 65, 96, 155, 160, 165, 187, 211, 214, 216, 277, 320, 321, 382, 425

脈訣　*Mai jue*,　32, 155, 187

脈學輯要評　*Mai xue ji yao ping*,　172, 173

脈要精微論　"Mai yao jing wei lun" (SW),　51, 56, 67, 92, 97, 201, 490

馬王堆　Mawangdui texts,　8, 9, 33, 378

medicine of systematic correspondence,　1, 2, 5, 6-8, 31, 34, 154, 186, 235

繆刺　"Miu ci" (SW),　475

明堂鍼灸圖　*Ming tang zhen jiu tu*,　56

宮下三郎　Miyashita Saburō,　485

Mongolian (version of the *Nan-jing*),　32

moxa-cauterization,　41

鶩溏　*wu tang* diarrhea,　433

腦戶　*nao hu* hole,　367

Needham, J.,　8, 304

內經　*Nei jing* (P),　1, 2, 10, 23-25, 27, 32-35, 37-42, 44

內庭　*nei ting* hole,　489

溺水　*ni shui* ("submerged in water"),　480

逆順肥瘦論　"Ni shun fei shou lun" (LS),　322, 323, 376

逆順　"Ni shun" (LS),　219, 532, 534

岡西爲人　Okanishi Tameto,　11, 12, 25, 26, 32, 34

龐安常   Pang Anchang. *See* Pang Anshi,   447

龐安時   Pang Anshi,   447, 561

Persian (version of the *Nan jing*),   32

pharmaceutical knowledge, *See also* drugs,   7

pharmacology of systematic correspondence,   2

脾胃論   *Pi wei lun*,   111

平脈法   "Ping mai fa" (SHL),   94, 155

平人絕穀   "Ping ren jue gu" (LS),   351, 352, 355, 358

平人氣象論   "Ping ren qi xiang lun" (SW),   92, 101, 102, 133, 171, 172, 175, 177, 179,
180, 182, 183, 201

奇病論   "Qi bing lun" (SW),   482

氣衝   *qi chong* hole,   55, 276, 279, 296

氣海   *qi hai* ("sea of qi"),   248, 293, 368

氣海   *qi hai* hole,   368

氣街   *qi jie* hole,   248, 293

七錄   *Qi lu*,   27

期門   *qi men*,   368, 369, 483

氣穴   "Qi xue" (SW),   475

前谷   *qian gu* hole,   475

錢熙祚   Qian Xizuo,   475

千金方   *Qian jin fang*,   155

千金翼方   *Qian jin yi fang*,   27, 155

秦越人   Qin Yueren (P),   25, 26, 31, 34, 35, 37, 43

氣   *qi*-vapors, concept of,   8

啓玄子   Qixuan zi,   395, 503

丘虚   *qiu xu* hole,   475

曲池   *qu chi* hole,   488

曲骨　*qu gu* hole,　278

曲泉　*qu quan* hole,　164, 487, 494

曲澤　*qu ze* hole,　475, 477, 488

Rall, Jutta,　32

熱病　*re bing* ("heat illness"),　435

熱論　"Re lun" (SW),　434

religious healing,　2

人迎　*ren ying* hole, location,　51, 55, 56, 246, 249, 327

榮衛生會　"Rong wei sheng hui". *See* "Ying wei sheng hui" (LS),　51, 55, 56, 65, 69, 73, 82, 97, 115, 178, 240, 246, 248, 252, 327

儒門事親　*ru men shi qin*,　284

濡泄　*ru xie* diarrhea,　432

阮孝緒　Ruan Xiaoxu,　27

阮元　Ruan Yuan,　35

三百种醫籍錄　*San bai zhong yi ji lu*,　11

三部九候論　"San bu jiu hou lun" (SW),　155, 207, 214

三才　san cai,　337

三間　*san jian* hole,　489

三里　*san li* hole,　488

三虛三實　"San xu san shi"（TS),　378

删繁方　*Shan fan fang*,　25

山海經　*Shan hai jing*,　284

上古天眞論　"Shang gu tian zhen lun" (SW),　278

傷寒論　*Shang han lun*,　22, 23, 25-27, 64, 94, 155, 232, 379, 427, 428, 439

傷寒雜病論　*Shang han za bing lun*,　43

傷寒直格　*Shang han zhi ge*,　175

商丘　*shang qiu* hole,　488

商陽　*shang yang* hole,　488

少衝　*shao chong* hole,　163, 477, 487

少府　*shao fu* hole,　473, 487

少澤　*shao ze* hole,　488

燒針　*shao zhen* ("burning needle"),　427

少海　*shao hai* hole,　52, 477, 487, 488

少商　*shao shang* hole,　487

神門　*shen men* ("spirit gate"),　69, 321

神門　*shen men* hole,　474, 477, 487

神秘名醫錄　*Shen mi ming yi lu*,　28

神農本經　*Shen nong ben jing*,　149

生氣同天論　"Sheng qi tong tian lun" (SVC),　389

十變　*shi bian*,　307, 308, 464, 467, 469

十度　*shi duo* ("ten estimates"),　123

史記正義　*Shi ji zheng yi*,　30, 353

史記　*Shi ji*,　9, 12, 24, 25, 27, 30, 43, 284, 353, 483

十四經發揮　*Shi si jing fa hui*,　110, 274

濕溫　*shi wen* ("moisture and warmth"),　435

實邪　*shi xie* ("repletion evil"),　121, 123

十一脈灸經　*Shi yi mai jiu jing*,　9

石友諒　Shi Youliang,　34, 36

壽夭剛柔　"Shou yao gang rou" (LS),　504

束骨　*shu gu* hole,　488

書經　*Shu jing*,　309

水溝　*shui gou* hole,　278

水熱穴論　"Shui re xue lun" (SW),　511

水脹 "Shui zhang" (LS), 284

順氣一日分爲四時 "Shun qi yi ri fen wei si shi" (LS), 498, 516

說文解字 *Shuo wen jie zi*, 289

四部叢刊書錄 *Si bu cong kan shu lu*, 35

四方異診 "Si fang yi zhen", 172

四氣調神大論 "Si qi tiao shen da lun" (SW), 532

四時氣 "Si shi qi" (LS), 516

司馬遷 Sima Qian, 25

蘇東坡 Su Dongpo, 36

素女脈訣 *Su nü mai jue*, 149

素問識 *Su wen shi*, 104

素問 *Su wen* (P), 1, 2, 6, 7, 8, 11, 22, 24, 32, 34, 39

歲露論 "Sui lu lun" (LS), 378, 402

孫脈 *sun mai* ("tertiary vessels"), 9

孫思邈 Sun Simiao, 27, 66, 67, 155

飧泄 *sun xie* diarrhea, 432

surgical knowledge, 7

systematic correspondence, paradigm of, 3, 4, 33, 341, 408, 493

太白 *tai bai* hole, 473, 477, 478, 495

太倉 *tai cang* hole, 363, 364

太衝 *tai chong*, 55, 473, 477, 478

胎化 *tai hua* ("fetal transformation"), 344

太陵 *tai ling* hole, 475, 477

太平御覽 *Tai ping yu lan*, 26, 28, 30

太谿/太溪 *tai xi* hole, 52, 55, 56, 473, 477, 479

太乙 Tai yi, 403

太淵   *tai yuan* hole,   59, 248, 363, 364, 367, 473, 474, 477-479, 495

多紀(丹波)元簡   Taki (Tamba) Motohiro,   22, 188

多紀(丹波)元胤   Taki Mototane (Tamba Genkan),   12, 21, 22, 24-26, 30, 35, 36, 48, 188, 485

terminology, medical,   6

天窗   *tian chuang* hole,   55

天府   *tian fu* hole,   52, 55

天井   *tian jing* hole,   488

天樞   *tian shu* hole,   294, 295, 297

天突   *tian tu* hole,   278

天行   *tian xing*   ("epidemics"),   435

調經論   "Tiao jing lun" (SW),   312

聽會   *ting hui* hole,   51, 55

通評虛實論   "Tong ping xu shi lun" (SW),   197, 485

銅人腧穴鍼灸圖經   *Tong ren shu xue zhen jiu tu jing*,   34

通容   *tong rong* hole,   489

瞳子窌   *tong zi jiao* hole,   51

外臺秘要   *Wai tai mi yao* hole,   26, 215

腕骨   *wan gu* hole,   473, 488

王冰   Wang Bing,   2, 32, 56, 57, 67, 190, 482

王勃   Wang Bo,   26

王誠叔   Wang Chengshu, *See* Wang Zongzheng,   213

王燾   Wang Dao,   25

王鼎象   Wang Dingxiang,   35

王九思   Wang Jiusi,   34, 35

王莽   Wang Mang,   351

王清任   Wang Qingren,   351

王拳正　Wang Quanzheng,　34

王叔和　Wang Shuhe,　23, 32, 68, 213, 249

王惟一　Wang Weiyi,　34, 35

王熙　Wang Xi. *See* Wang Shuhe,　64, 68, 155

王應麟　Wang Yinglin,　34

王皙象　Wang Zhixiang,　34, 35

王宗正　Wang Zongzheng,　213

Watson, Burton,　289

魏伯陽　Wei Boyang,　134

痿論　"Wei lun" (SW),　111

衛氣行　"Wei qi xing" (LS),　51

微邪　*wei xie* ("weakness evil"),　121, 123

委中　*wei zhong* hole,　55, 488

Welch, H.,　450

瘟　*wen* ("epidemic"),　438

溫病　*wen bing* ("warmth illness"),　435

瘟疫　*wen yi* ("epidemic illness"),　437

wind, concept of,　8

wind divination,　27

吳澄　Wu Cheng,　12, 13

五里　*wu li* hole,　55

五癃津液別論　"Wu long jin ye bie lun" (LS),　265

五色　"Wu se" (LS),　145

五十二病方　*Wu shi er bing fang*,　235

五十營　"Wu shi ying" (LS),　51, 289

五行大義　*Wu xing da yi*,　303, 347

五音五味　"Wu yin wu wei" (LS),　111, 272

烏運六氣   *wu yun liu qi* ("doctrine of five periods and six qi"),   100, 304

五藏生成   "Wu zang sheng cheng" (SW),   455

五診   *wu zhen* ("Fivefold diagnosis"),   503

俠白   *xia bai* hole,   52, 55

下白沫   *xia bai mo* diarrhea,   432

下關   *xia guan* hole,   51, 55

下膿血   *xia nong xue* diarrhea,   432

下迫   *xia po* diarrhea,   432

俠谿   *xia xi*,   488

癇   *xian* convulsions,   445

蕭吉   Xiao Ji,   303

孝學   *Xiao xue*,   149

小針解   "Xiao zhen jie" (LS),   136, 544

謝縉孫   Xie Jinsun,   220, 250, 279, 368

邪客   "Xie ke" (LS),   266, 476

邪氣藏府病形論   "Xie qi zang fu bing xing lun" (LS),   144, 375

謝士泰   Xie Shitai,   25

行間   *xing jian* hole,   487, 494

徐大椿   Xu Dachun (P),   11, 26, 28, 38, 39, 41

許慎   Xu Shen,   222

虛邪   *xu xie* ("depletion evil"),   121, 123

宣明五氣論   "Xuan ming wu qi lun" (SW),   138, 310, 311

懸鍾   *xuan zhong* hole,   366

玄珠密語   *Xuan zhu mi yu*,   539

血氣形志   "Xue qi xing zhi" (SW),   502

山田慶兒 Yamada Keiji, 353

閻洪臣 Yan Hongchen, 13, 42

陽池 *yang chi* hole, 473, 488

陽輔 *yang fu* hole, 365, 488

陽谷 *yang gu* hole, 488

楊康侯 Yang Kanghou, 34, 35, 48

陽陵泉 *yang ling quan* hole, 363, 365, 488

陽明脈解論 "Yang ming mai jie lun" (SW), 404

楊上善 Yang Shangshan, 71, 82, 378, 483

陽谿 *yang xi* hole, 51, 55, 488

楊玄操 Yang Xuancao (P), 12, 25, 28, 30, 31, 34, 35

姚振宗 Yao Zhenzong, 29

瘧 *yao* fevers, 389, 422, 423, 485

瘧論 "Yao lun" (SW), 422

液門 *ye men* hole, 488

佚存叢書 *Yi cun cong shu*, 35

易經 *Yi jing*, 105, 110, 223, 309, 322, 464

醫林改錯 *Yi lin gai cuo*, 351

隱白 *yin bai* hole, 488

隱谷 *yin gu* hole, 55, 488, 496

陰交 *yin jiao* hole, 294, 295, 298

陰廉 *yin lian* hole, 55

陰癃泉 *yin ling quan*, 488

瘖門 *yin men* hole, 277

陰陽別論 "Yin yang bie lun" (SW), 51, 427

陰陽二十五人 "Yin yang er shi wu ren" (LS), 124

陰陽離合論 "Yin yang li he lun" (SW), 321, 323

陰陽十一脈灸經　*Yin yang shi yi mai jiu jing*,　235, 236, 241

陰陽應象大論　"Yin yang ying xiang da lun" (SW),　67, 310, 392, 430, 483

陰陽　"Yin yang" (TS),　484

營氣　"Ying qi" (LS),　242, 248, 288

營衛生會　"Ying wei sheng hui" (LS),　51, 58, 265, 286, 288, 289, 296, 314, 319, 371, 372

營衛運行　"Ying wei yun xing" (LS),　58

yinyang doctrine,　3, 498

涌泉/湧泉　*yong quan* hole,　389, 487

憂恚無言　"You wei wu yan" (LS),　361

玉海　*Yu hai*,　35

魚際　*yu ji* hole,　487

玉機眞藏論　"Yu ji zhen zang lun" (SW)　51, 78, 171, 172, 175, 183, 412

玉匱鍼經　*Yu kui zhen jing*,　28, 29

虞庶　"Yu Shu",　34, 36, 48 et passim

玉堂　*yu tang* hole,　291, 297

玉堂　*yu tang*,　367

玉枕　*yu zhen* hole,　366

元氣　*yuan qi* ("original qi"),　21, 461

淵液/淵腋　*yuan ye*,　269

雲門　*yun men* hole,　55, 483

運輸　"Yun shu" (LS),　51, 56, 367

賊風　"Zei feng" (LS),　402

賊邪　*zei xie* ("robber evil"),　121, 123

張機　Zhang Ji,　22, 23, 27, 155

張介賓　Zhang Jiebin,　140

張潔古　Zhang Jiegu. *See* Zhang Yuansu,　325

張景岳　Zhang Jingyue. *See* Zhang Jiebin,　140

脹論　"Zhang lun" (LS),　292

章門　*zhang men* hole,　364, 365, 483

張守節　Zhang Shoujie,　30, 353

張隱庵　Zhang Yin'an,　236

張元素　Zhang Yuansu,　335

張志聰　Zhang Zhicong,　22

張仲景　Zhang Zhongjing　35, 64, 187, 358, 368, 425, 432, 437, 439, 440, 470

張子存　Zhang Zicun,　29

張子和　Zhang Zihe,　284

瘴　*zhang*-illness,　390

趙繼宗　Zhao Jizong,　213

晁宗愨　Zhao Zongque,　34

枕骨　*zhen gu* bone,　365, 366

鍼經　*Zhen jing*,　278, 279, 296

診要經終論　"Zhen yao jing zhong lun" (SW),　251, 260

徵四失論　"Zheng si shi lun" (SW),　61

正邪　*zheng xie* ("regular evil"),　121, 123

鄭玄　Zheng Xuan,　222

脂腸　*zhi chang* ("greasy intestine"),　352

支滿　*zhi man* hole,　488

志室　*zhi shi* hole,　110, 322

至陰　*zhi yin* hole,　321, 323, 488

至眞要大論　"Zhi zhen yao da lun" (SW),　100, 101, 103, 451

中衝　*zhong chong* hole,　475, 477, 488

中都　*zhong du* hole,　474, 488

中風　*zhong feng* ("to be struck by wind"),　435

中封 *zhong feng* hole, 487

中府 *zhong fu* hole, 55, 484

中國醫籍考 *Zhong guo yi ji kao*, 12, 21

中極 *zhong ji* hole, 243, 276, 278, 284,

中脘 *zhong wan* hole, 364, 368

中院 *zhong wan* location, 368,

終始 "Zhong shi" (LS), 78, 251, 328, 505, 508, 531

周禮 *Zhou li*, 150

築賓 *zhu bin* hole, 280

諸病源候論 *Zhu bing yuan hou lun*, 34, 284

朱丹溪 Zhu Danxi, 3

朱熹 Zhu Xi, 149

宗氣 *zong qi* ("stem qi"), 110, 283, 480

足臂十一脈灸癌 *Zu bi shi yi mai jiu jing*, 241

佐傳 *Zuo zhuan*, 6

Comparative Studies of Health Systems and Medical Care

John M. Janzen, *The Quest for Therapy in Lower Zaire*

Paul U. Unschuld,
> *Medical Ethics in Imperial China: A Study in Historical Anthropology*

Margaret M. Lock,
> *East Asian Medicine in Urban Japan: Varieties of Medical Experience*

Jeanie Schmit Kayser-Jones,
> *Old, Alone, and Neglected: Care of the Aged in Scotland and in the United States*

Arthur Kleinman,
> *Patients and Healers in the Context of Culture: An Exploration of the Borderland between Anthropologyy Medicine, and Psychiatry* Stephen J. Kunitz, *Disease Change and the Role of Medicine: The Navajo Experience*

Carol Laderman,
> *Wives and Midwives: Childbirth and Nutrition in Rural Malaysia*

Victor G. Rodwin,
> *The Health Planning Predicament: France9 Quebec, England, and the United States*

Michael W. Dols and Adil S. Gamal,
> *Medieval Islamic Medicine: Ibn Ridwān's Treatise "On the Prevention of Bodily Ills in Egypt"*

Leith Mullings,
> *Therapy, Ideology, and Social Change: Mental Healing in Urban Ghana*

Jean de Kervasdoue, John R. Kimberly, and Victor G, Rodwin,
> *The End of an Illusion: The Future of Health Policy in Western Industrialized Nations* Arthur J. Rubel, Carl W. O. Nell, and Rolando Collado-Ardón, *Susto, a Folk Illness*

Paul U. Unschuld,
> *Medicine in China: A History of Ideas* Paul U. Unschuld, *Medicine in China: A History of Pharmaceutics* Glenn Gritzer and Arnold Arluke3 *The Making of Rehabilitation: A Political Economy of Medical Specialization91890-1980* Arthur Kleinman and Byron Good, editors, *Culture and Depression: Studies in the Anthropology and Cross-Cultural Psychiatry of Affect and Disorder* Judith Justice, *Policies, Plans, and People: Culture and Health Development in Nepal*

Paul U. Unschuld,
> *Nan-jing—The Classic of Difficult Issues*

www.ingramcontent.com/pod-product-compliance
Ingram Content Group UK Ltd.
Pitfield, Milton Keynes, MK11 3LW, UK
UKHW032204150325
456284UK00005B/19/J